AF679351

Skin Cancer: An Issue of Oncology Clinics

Skin Cancer: An Issue of Oncology Clinics

Editor: Rose Parson

FOSTER ACADEMICS

www.fosteracademics.com

www.fosteracademics.com

FOSTER ACADEMICS

Cataloging-in-Publication Data

Skin cancer : an issue of oncology clinics / edited by Rose Parson.
p. cm.
Includes bibliographical references and index.
ISBN 978-1-63242-901-8
1. Skin--Cancer. 2. Skin--Diseases. 3. Oncology. 4. Cancer--Hospitals. I. Parson, Rose.
RC280.S5 S55 2020
616.994 77--dc23

© Foster Academics, 2020

Foster Academics,
118-35 Queens Blvd., Suite 400,
Forest Hills, NY 11375, USA

ISBN 978-1-63242-901-8 (Hardback)

This book contains information obtained from authentic and highly regarded sources. Copyright for all individual chapters remain with the respective authors as indicated. All chapters are published with permission under the Creative Commons Attribution License or equivalent. A wide variety of references are listed. Permission and sources are indicated; for detailed attributions, please refer to the permissions page and list of contributors. Reasonable efforts have been made to publish reliable data and information, but the authors, editors and publisher cannot assume any responsibility for the validity of all materials or the consequences of their use.

Trademark Notice: Registered trademark of products or corporate names are used only for explanation and identification without intent to infringe.

Contents

Preface

This book was inspired by the evolution of our times; to answer the curiosity of inquisitive minds. Many developments have occurred across the globe in the recent past which has transformed the progress in the field.

The cancer that arises from the skin is termed as skin cancer. It occurs due to the development of abnormal cells which can invade or spread to other parts of the body. Melanoma, basal-cell skin cancer and squamous-cell skin cancer are the primary types of skin cancers. Basal-cell carcinomas are those that appear on the sun-exposed areas of the skin, particularly the face. They rarely metastasize and are easily treated with radiation or surgery. Squamous-cell skin cancer metastasizes. Melanomas are the rarest of all skin cancers but frequently metastasize. They can potentially cause death once they spread. Ulcering of the skin, changes in existing moles, patch on skin, enlargement of mole, etc. are some of the signs of skin cancer. It can be diagnosed through a biopsy, histopathological examination, dermoscopy, sonography, etc. The treatment of skin cancer is determined by an assessment of the location of the tumor, specific type of cancer, age and whether it is a primary cancer or a recurrence. Melanomas usually respond poorly to radiation or chemotherapy. Radiation therapy, topical chemotherapy, cryotherapy, electrodesiccation and curettage, photodynamic therapy, Mohs surgery, etc. are some of the strategies in the treatment of skin cancer. This book includes some of the vital pieces of work being conducted across the world, on various topics related to skin cancer. It brings forth some of the most innovative concepts and elucidates the unexplored aspects of oncology. It aims to equip students and experts with the advanced topics and upcoming concepts in this domain.

This book was developed from a mere concept to drafts to chapters and finally compiled together as a complete text to benefit the readers across all nations. To ensure the quality of the content we instilled two significant steps in our procedure. The first was to appoint an editorial team that would verify the data and statistics provided in the book and also select the most appropriate and valuable contributions from the plentiful contributions we received from authors worldwide. The next step was to appoint an expert of the topic as the Editor-in-Chief, who would head the project and finally make the necessary amendments and modifications to make the text reader-friendly. I was then commissioned to examine all the material to present the topics in the most comprehensible and productive format.

I would like to take this opportunity to thank all the contributing authors who were supportive enough to contribute their time and knowledge to this project. I also wish to convey my regards to my family who have been extremely supportive during the entire project.

Editor

1

Evaluation of the Definitions of "High-Risk" Cutaneous Squamous Cell Carcinoma Using the American Joint Committee on Cancer Staging Criteria and National Comprehensive Cancer Network Guidelines

Melinda B. Chu,[1] Jordan B. Slutsky,[2] Maulik M. Dhandha,[1] Brandon T. Beal,[3] Eric S. Armbrecht,[4] Ronald J. Walker,[5] Mark A. Varvares,[5] and Scott W. Fosko[1]

[1] *Department of Dermatology, Saint Louis University, 1402 S. Grand Boulevard, 4th Floor, St. Louis, MO 63104, USA*
[2] *Stony Brook School of Medicine, Department of Dermatology, 181 N. Belle Mead Road, Suite 5, East Setauket, NY 11733, USA*
[3] *School of Medicine, Saint Louis University, 1402 S. Grand Boulevard, St. Louis, MO 63104, USA*
[4] *Center for Outcomes Research, Saint Louis University, 3545 Lafayette Avenue, 4th Floor, St. Louis, MO 63110, USA*
[5] *Department of Otolaryngology-Head and Neck Surgery, Saint Louis University, 3635 Vista Avenue, St. Louis, MO 63110, USA*

Correspondence should be addressed to Melinda B. Chu; chumb@slu.edu

Academic Editor: Günther Hofbauer

Recent guidelines from the American Joint Committee on Cancer (AJCC) and National Comprehensive Cancer Network (NCCN) have been proposed for the assessment of "high-risk" cutaneous squamous cell carcinomas (cSCCs). Though different in perspective, both guidelines share the common goals of trying to identify "high-risk" cSCCs and improving patient outcomes. Thus, in theory, both definitions should identify a similar proportion of "high-risk" tumors. We sought to evaluate the AJCC and NCCN definitions of "high-risk" cSCCs and to assess their concordance. *Methods*. A retrospective review of head and neck cSCCs seen by an academic dermatology department from July 2010 to November 2011 was performed. *Results*. By AJCC criteria, most tumors ($n = 211, 82.1\%$) were of Stage 1; 46 tumors (13.9%) were of Stage 2. Almost all were of Stage 2 due to size alone (≥2 cm); one tumor was "upstaged" due to "high-risk features." Using the NCCN taxonomy, 231 (87%) of tumors were "high-risk." *Discussion*. This analysis demonstrates discordance between AJCC and NCCN definitions of "high-risk" cSCC. Few cSCCs are of Stage 2 by AJCC criteria, while most are "high-risk" by the NCCN guidelines. While the current guidelines represent significant progress, further studies are needed to generate a unified definition of "high-risk" cSCC to optimize management.

1. Introduction

Though it is a rare occurrence, it is well known that prognosis is grim once a cutaneous squamous cell carcinoma (cSCC) has metastasized beyond the skin [1–3]. It would be desirable to be able to identify this small cohort of tumors that are increased risk for metastasis earlier in their presentation to alter treatment approaches and potentially improve outcomes. Recent guidelines from the American Joint Committee on Cancer (AJCC) and National Comprehensive Cancer Network (NCCN) have been proposed to help in the assessment and classification of these "high-risk" cSCCs [4, 5]. Though different in perspective, both guidelines share the common goals of trying to distinguish "high-risk" cSCCs from the bulk of tumors (which are low risk) and trying to optimize patient care. Thus, in theory, both definitions should identify a similar proportion of "high-risk" tumors. In clinical practice, we observed some incongruities between the two definitions. We sought to evaluate the AJCC and NCCN definitions of "high-risk" cSCCs and to assess their concordance.

TABLE 1: AJCC tumor- (T-) staging and "high-risk" features.

Designation	Description
TX	Primary tumor cannot be assessed
T0	No evidence of primary tumor
Tis	Carcinoma in situ
T1	Tumor 2 cm or less in greatest dimension with fewer than 2 high-risk features
T2	Tumor >2 cm in greatest dimension or tumor of any size with two or more high-risk features
T3	Tumor with invasion of maxilla, mandible, orbit, or temporal bone
T4	Tumor with invasion of skeleton (axial or appendicular) or perineural invasion of skull base
	High-risk features
Depth/invasion	>2 mm, Clark level ≥ IV, or perineural invasion
Anatomic location	Primary site ear Primary site hair-bearing lip
Differentiation	Poorly differentiated or undifferentiated

TABLE 2: Abbreviated list of NCCN "high-risk" factors.

NCCN "high-risk" factors[‡]
Area M ≥ 10 mm
Area H ≥ 6 mm
Poorly defined
Recurrence
Immunosuppression
Site of prior RT or chronic inflammatory process
Rapidly growing tumor
Neurologic symptoms
Pathology
Moderately or poorly differentiated histology
Acantholytic, adenosquamous, or desmoplastic subtypes
Depth: ≥2 mm or Clark levels IV, V
Perineural or vascular involvement

Tumor is "high-risk" if ≥1 of 12 risk factors.
M = "medium" risk: forehead, scalp, cheek, neck.
H = "high" risk: "mask areas of the face" central face, ears, periauricular, eyelids, periorbital, nose, temple, and lips.
[‡]Note: The study cohort in this analysis was based on cSCCs from the head and neck only. Risk factors and specifics regarding tumors on Area L ("low" risk anatomic site: trunk and extremities), hands/feet, genitalia are not listed.

TABLE 3: AJCC tumor, node, metastasis (TNM) 2010 cSCC criteria.

Stage	Designation		
	Primary tumor	Regional lymph node	Distant metastasis
0	Tis	N0	M0
I	T1	N0	M0
II	T2	N0	M0
III	T3	N0	M0
	T1	N1	M0
	T2	N1	M0
	T3	N1	M0
IV	T1	N2	M0
	T2	N2	M0
	T3	N2	M0
	T any	N3	M0
	T4	N any	M0
	T any	N any	M1

2. Methods

A retrospective chart review of all cSCCs on the head and neck that were initially seen in the Dermatology Department at Saint Louis University Medical Center in July 2010–November 2011 was performed. Data including patient demographics, tumor anatomic location and size, and histologic subtype was documented for all tumors. In addition, the occurrence of any AJCC "high-risk" tumor features detailed in Table 1 (i.e., Breslow depth >2 mm, Clark level >IV, perineural invasion, location on the ear or hair-bearing lip, and poorly differentiated or undifferentiated histology) and the presence of any of the 12 NCCN "high-risk" factors listed in Table 2 (i.e., size by anatomic location, poorly defined borders, recurrence, immunosuppression, site of prior radiation therapy or chronic inflammatory process, rapidly growing tumor, neurological symptoms, moderately or poorly differentiated histology, acantholytic, adenosquamous, or desmoplastic subtypes, depth: ≥2 mm or Clark levels IV, V, and perineural or vascular involvement) were recorded. Data was recorded as documented in the existing medical record. Additional dermatopathologic review of tumor specimens to collect any missing data was not performed.

In the first part of the analysis, tumors were classified according to the AJCC tumor, node, metastasis (TNM) 2010 criteria for cSCC (Table 3) using tumor size and presence of 2 or more "high-risk features" (Table 1). In the second part, the 2012 NCCN guidelines were applied to all cSCC and tumors with 1 of 12 "high-risk" factors were categorized as "high-risk." Lastly, the proportion of Stage 2 tumors according to AJCC criteria was compared to the proportion of "high-risk" tumors by NCCN guidelines.

3. Results

Clinical information was available for 269 cases of the 296 cases identified. The AJCC analysis was based on 257 cases; eyelid tumors were excluded as there is a separate AJCC staging system for eyelid carcinomas (regardless of histologic subtype). The NCCN analysis (classifying "high-risk" versus "low-risk" cSCCs) was based on 265 cases. In 4 tumors, lymph node involvement was uncovered prior to surgery which excluded them from this analysis as tumors with known lymph node involvement are considered in a separate NCCN algorithm rather than the one examined here.

3.1. AJCC Analysis. Using the AJCC's tumor (T), node (N), metastasis (M) (TNM) criteria, assignments of Stage 1 and

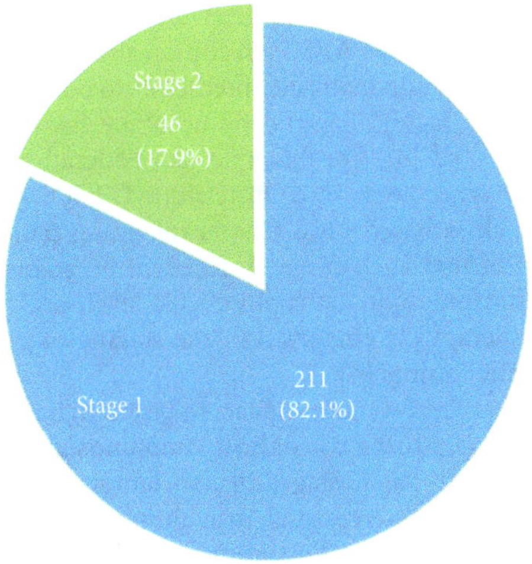

Figure 1: Proportions of Stage 1 versus Stage 2 tumors by AJCC criteria.

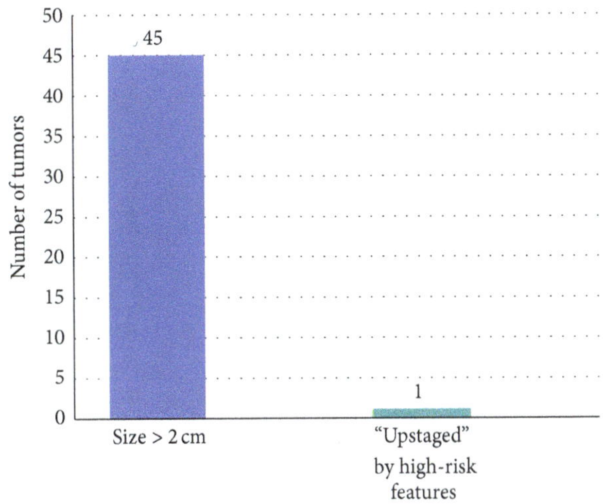

Figure 2: Factor(s) leading to Stage 2 designation by AJCC criteria.

Stage 2 are based on tumor characteristics only (Table 1). Any tumor with a size >2 cm is T2 and thus Stage 2. A tumor that is T1 by size (<2 cm) can be "upstaged" to T2 (and Stage 2) if it possesses ≥2 of the "high-risk" features: depth/invasion >2 mm, Clark level ≥4 mm, perineural invasion, anatomic site on the ear or hair-bearing lip, and poorly differentiated histology. A tumor with an associated positive lymph node is Stage 3 or higher.

In the AJCC analysis, 257 tumors were included. The majority of cSCCs, 211 (82.1%), were Stage 1; 46 tumors (13.9%) were Stage 2 (Figure 1). Almost all (n = 45, 45/46, 98%) were Stage 2 due to size ≥2 cm; only 1 tumor was "upstaged" due to "high-risk features" (Figure 2). This tumor was 1.5 cm in diameter, located on the ear with poorly differentiated histology.

"High-risk" features were not prevalent in our cohort (i.e., perineural invasion (n = 12), hair-bearing lip (n = 12), ear (n = 38)) or almost never recorded. Only 2 tumors had Breslow depth (BD) recorded and Clark level (CL) was never recorded. Of the 2 tumors with BD recorded, only 1 tumor had BD of >2 mm; this tumor met criteria for Stage 2 by size. Histologic subtype was recorded for all 257 tumors; only one tumor had poorly differentiated histology.

3.2. NCCN Analysis. The NCCN guidelines are evidence-based algorithms that are intended to guide a clinician through the management of a tumor step-by-step. Unlike the AJCC staging system, within the NCCN guidelines, eyelid carcinomas are grouped together with cSCCs on any anatomic site; thus, eyelid tumors were included in this investigation aimed at classifying tumors as "high-risk" or "low-risk" by NCCN. However, as noted previously tumors with lymph node involvement detected prior to surgery (either by physical exam or by imaging) are considered on a separate different algorithm rather than the one evaluated here and were excluded from this analysis. Taking this into consideration, 265 of 269 tumors were included in the NCCN analysis.

Only 1 of 12 risk factors (Table 2) is required for "high-risk" tumor classification by the NCCN guidelines. Tumors that do not possess any one of these risk factors are considered "low-risk."

Using NCCN nomenclature, 231 (87%) of tumors were classified as "high-risk," and 43.2% of tumors had 2 or more NCCN risk factors (Figure 3). Size (≥6 mm on "mask areas of the face" and ≥10 mm on forehead, scalp, cheeks, and neck) was most common risk factor listed. Twenty-seven tumors did not meet "high-risk" by size criteria and were "upstaged" by other clinical risk factors. In this group, the majority of tumors exhibited one "high-risk" factor that led to "upstaging" tumors to "high-risk." Histologic features were most frequent (moderately/poorly differentiated (n = 6) and acantholytic, adenosquamous, or desmoplastic subtypes (n = 6)). Clinical designations such as "rapidly growing" (n = 4) and "poorly defined borders" (n = 6) were also frequently observed.

4. Discussion

Our preliminary analysis shows that there is discordance between the AJCC and NCCN definitions of "high-risk" cSCC. Few cSCCs are Stage 2 (14%) by AJCC staging criteria, while most (87%) are "high-risk" by the NCCN guidelines (Figure 4). The AJCC definition of "high-risk" cSCC is narrow, while the NCCN definition is broad.

The purpose of the AJCC staging system is distinct from that of the NCCN treatment guidelines [4, 5]. The goal of the AJCC staging system is to stratify patients with similar outcomes into groups to offer accurate prognostic estimates. AJCC staging is almost entirely based on the "anatomic" characteristics of a primary tumor, using the tumor (T), node (N), and metastases (M) classification [4]. This approach has been criticized as simplistic and in the introduction the authors concede that the restrictive nature of the tumor-based approach has led clinicians to develop other prognostic systems and even led some to conclude that TNM is "obsolete" and "anachronistic" [4]. In fact, most lymphomas and

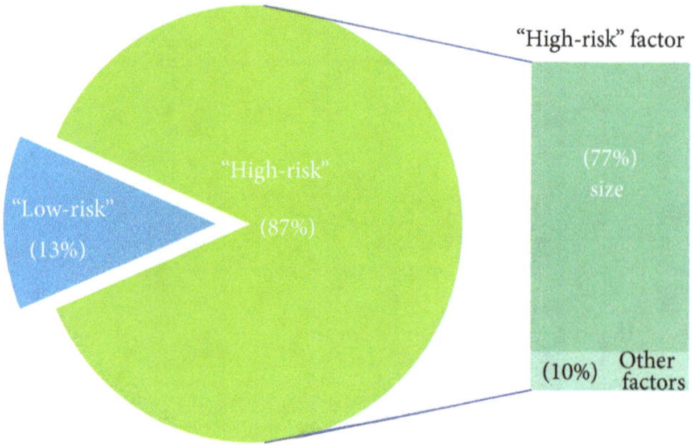

FIGURE 3: Proportion of "high-risk" versus "low-risk" tumors by NCCN guidelines.

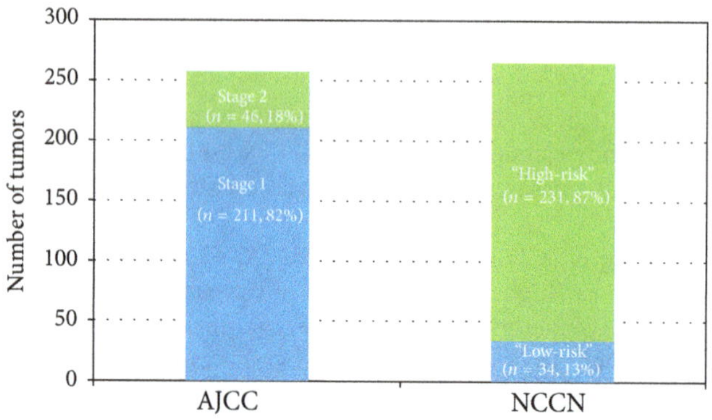

FIGURE 4: Proportions of "high-risk" and "low-risk" cSCCs by AJCC criteria versus NCCN guidelines.

nervous system tumors use alternate systems as the TNM criteria cannot be employed rationally in these cancers [4]. Likewise, it can be awkward to apply the TNM criteria to cSCC.

The omission of established cSCC "high-risk" factors, such as host immunosuppression and tumor recurrence, from the current AJCC staging criteria (AJCC 7th edition) is worthy of discussion. As mentioned above, as a rule the AJCC staging utilizes primary tumor characteristics only and does not permit host factors to be considered. To blindly adhere to these restrictions (which do not allow for the consideration of "immunosuppression" or "recurrence" as "high-risk" factors) appears short-sighted as the exclusion of these important clinical factors may lead to inaccurate prognostic estimates. Like Breuninger et al. [6], the authors believe that a relevant staging system should estimate the risk of metastasis. Hence, when creating a possible new cSCC staging system, Breuninger et al. considered all factors associated with increased metastatic risk and recommended that history of "immunosuppression" should be recorded despite the fact that it was "not a tumor factor" [6].

If the ultimate goal of the AJCC staging system is the "analysis of the care of patients with similar prognosis" [4], then the inclusion of "immunosuppression" and "recurrence" as factors that influence stage determination is apropos and can be considered. The AJCC 7th edition already allows clinically significant "nonanatomic" predictors to be used for staging when the factor's prognostic accuracy has been sufficiently validated [4]. For example, the Féderation Internationale de Gynécologie et d'Obstétrique (FIGO) prognostic score (which is based on 8 factors including patient characteristics/history such as age, antecedent pregnancy, serum human chorionic gonadotropin (hcG) level, and response to chemotherapy) is employed in the staging of gestational trophoblastic tumors [4].

On initial review, there appears to be enough corroborating data to support the use of host "immunosuppression" as a determinant of AJCC stage; its association with increased metastasis has been reported in a number of studies [7–10]. However, a statistically significant association between "immunosuppression" and "metastasis" has not been consistently demonstrated in multivariable analyses. Brantsch et al. [11] found that immunosuppressive status was a significant predictor, while Peat et al., Karia et al., and Jambusaria-Pahlajani et al. did not [12–14]. Jambusaria-Pahlajani et al. acknowledged that although their analysis was based on a large cohort ($n = 523$), the study was underpowered to draw any conclusions on the association between immunosuppression and metastasis [14]. Another possible reason for the exclusion of "immunosuppression" within the AJCC staging criteria may be due to the fact that "immunosuppression" itself is a broad category and may include patients with rheumatoid arthritis on long-term low dose methotrexate, patients with liver or kidney transplants, and patients with chronic lymphocytic leukemia (CLL) or heart or lung transplants on voriconazole. Because cSCC outcomes likely vary widely between these patient cohorts, the AJCC is likely correct to exclude "immunosuppression" as a risk factor required for staging at this time.

While it is still hazy as to what constitutes "immunosuppression," it is clear that a patient history of "immunosuppression" does figure into a clinician's assessment of metastatic risk. A recent survey of Mohs surgeons showed that more than half of them (55%) thought that "immunosuppression" was an AJCC risk factor [15]. In view of this, we think that even if it is not included as a risk factor required for staging, information regarding "immunosuppression" should be documented on the AJCC staging form. In their critique of the 6th edition of AJCC staging system (AJCC 6th edition), Dinehart and Peterson highlighted "immunosuppression" as a "marquee variable" and recommended that the letter "I" be placed in front of the stage or a separate "H" category (for "host") be developed to reflect immune status [16]. In their appraisal of the AJCC 7th edition, Warner and Cockerell called the lack of documentation regarding immunosuppressive status "a shortcoming" of the system and advocated for its mandatory documentation [17]. We agree that it is important to document the presence or absence of "immunosuppression" on the cSCC staging form. In order to mirror the staging forms of other cancers, we recommend that a patient's immune status be collected as a "clinically significant prognostic factor," which allows the data to be recorded even if it is not incorporated into staging calculation. The host factor of "profound immunosuppression" is a "clinically significant prognostic factor" used in the staging of Merkel cell carcinoma (MCC) [18]. The cohorts of patients (e.g., history of HIV/AIDS, CLL, or solid organ transplantation) that are considered to be treated with "profound immunosuppression" in MCC are the same as those that are found to have increased rates of metastasis in cSCC. Therefore, it seems sensible to suggest that "profound immunosuppression" should be added to the AJCC cSCC staging form as a "clinically significant prognostic factor."

Currently, the TNM classification examines characteristics of primary tumors; as such, "recurrence" by definition cannot be included as a factor for staging. Many analyses aimed at identifying risk factors for cSCC metastasis have found that "recurrent" tumors are more likely to be metastatic than primary tumors [12, 19]. On the other hand, studies focused on evaluating the cSCC AJCC staging system have excluded "recurrence" as a risk factor for metastasis to reflect the standard method of defining metastatic risk based on the attributes of a primary tumor only; consequently, there is no data regarding "recurrent" tumors and its impact on AJCC staging classification. If it is decided that AJCC stage should pertain to primary tumors only, we think that information regarding whether or not a tumor is "recurrent" at the time of treatment should still be recorded on the staging form, either as a "clinically significant prognostic factor" or by placing the letter "r" before the stage as suggested by Dinehart and Peterson [16].

Besides the addition of new factors, we think that the AJCC staging system could be improved by revising the existing T-stage categories. The inadequacy of the AJCC 7th edition cSCC criteria is evidenced by the fact that the T-classification from the European counterpart to the AJCC, the Union for International Cancer Control (UICC), is quite different for cSCC whereas, for most cancers, the AJCC and UICC systems are essentially, if not completely the same [20]. In fact, the UICC T-classification may share more in common with the outdated AJCC 6th edition than the current AJCC 7th edition.

In both the AJCC (6th and 7th editions) and the UICC systems (Table 4), a 2 cm cutoff is used to distinguish between T1 and T2 [4, 20, 21]. When applied to our cohort, the 2 cm size cutoff had important implications. While the majority of tumors were T1 (82%) by AJCC 7th edition, almost all T2 tumors (45 of 46) were T2 due to size alone. In addition, like Breuninger et al. [6], we observed that the expansion of AJCC 7th edition T2 criteria to include tumors of any size that possess two or more "high-risk" features did not significantly change the proportion of T1 and T2 tumors. In our cohort, only 1 of 211 tumors that measured <2 cm had enough risk factors to be "upstaged" to T2.

There were no AJCC 7th edition T3 (tumor with invasion of maxilla, mandible, orbit, or temporal bones) or T4 (tumor with invasion of skeleton (axial or appendicular) or perineural invasion of skull base) tumors in this cohort. The data evaluated here was derived from patients that were initially seen by dermatology, and thus, our study set may be comprised of less aggressive tumors than those examined in other recent studies. However, similar findings to ours (very few T3/T4 tumors) were reported by Breuninger et al. [6] and Jambusaria-Pahlajani et al. [14]. In fact, the lack of T3/T4 tumors in their cohort (4 of 523) led Jambusaria-Pahlajani et al. to conclude that AJCC 7th edition T3 or T4 tumors are so rare that they are unlikely to affect prognostic results [14].

Appreciating that T3/T4 tumors were extremely uncommon and that almost all tumors (98%) were T1/T2, Jambusaria-Pahlajani et al. proposed an "alternative" tumor staging system to improve T-stage stratification [14]. The method, now called the Brigham and Women's Hospital (BWH) system, reportedly provides improved distinctiveness (outcome differences between stages), homogeneity (outcome similarity within stages), and monotonicity (outcome worsening with increasing stage) compared to the AJCC or UICC staging systems [22]. The major differences between BWH system and AJCC 7th edition are as follows: (1) in BWH, size is not the primary determinant of T-stage but one of several prognostic factors (i.e., tumor diameter 2 cm, poorly differentiated histology, perineural invasion 0.1 mm, or tumor invasion beyond fat) that are used in its calculation and (2) T2 is subdivided into T2a and T2b (Table 4). We commend Karia et al. for improving T-stage classification with the BWH system, but think further enhancements can still be made. The factors included in the BWH system were primarily based on the narrow list of AJCC "high-risk" features. Consequently, there may be additional factors (e.g. some factors from the broad list of the NCCN "high-risk" factors) which have not been considered yet and merit inclusion.

As in the BWH system [22], in the system proposed by Peat et al. [12], Breslow depth and Clark level as well as other histopathologic features (e.g., moderate or poor differentiation and/or perineural invasion) were validated by multivariable analyses before inclusion into the staging criteria. Given the strength of the data, it seems reasonable to suggest that BD and CL should be recorded for each tumor. In the present study, we did not collect information on the depth of invasion unless it was recorded on the initial biopsy report. This missing histopathologic data can be considered to be a limitation of our study as the lack of BD or CL (recorded in only 2 of 269 tumors) likely impacted the categorization of tumors as high- or low-risk. It was a deliberate choice of the authors not to perform additional dermatopathologic review as our analysis was intended to demonstrate how staging and classification would apply to data that is routinely recorded during clinical practice. Given the sheer number of SCCs, with estimates ranging from 419,543 to more than 700,000 cases per year in USA, it may not be feasible to require a detailed histopathologic synopsis for cSCC as the one in place for melanoma [23, 24]. In addition, the collection of some histopathologic information like BD or CL which is straightforward to determine for melanomas is challenging or not feasible for cSCCs. For example, collecting precise information on the "true" depth of the tumor is difficult for cSCCs, which may be treated in a variety of ways including Mohs surgery, electrodessication, and curettage or topical 5-fluorouracil, where it may be difficult or impossible to obtain an accurate measurement of tumor depth. However, reliance on a depth reported from the initial biopsy report is also problematic since cSCC diagnosis is usually based on

TABLE 4: Summary of the AJCC 6th edition, AJCC 7th edition, UICC, and BWH tumor- (T-) stage systems.

T-stage	AJCC 6th	AJCC 7th	UICC	T-stage	BWH
T1	Tumor 2 cm or less in greatest dimension	Tumor <2 cm in greatest dimension with fewer than two "high-risk" features[*]	Tumor ≤2 cm in largest horizontal size	T1	0 high-risk factors[‡]
T2	Tumor more than 2 cm but not more than 5 cm in greatest dimension	Tumor >2 cm in greatest dimension or tumor any size with two or more "high-risk" features[*]	Tumor >2 cm in largest horizontal size	T2a	1 high-risk factor[‡]
				T2b	2-3 high risk factors[‡]
T3	Tumor more than 5 cm in greatest dimension	Tumor with invasion of orbit, maxilla, mandible, or temporal bones	Deep infiltration (skeleton muscle, cartilage, or bone)	T3	≥4 high risk factors[‡]
T4	Tumor invades deep extradermal structures (i.e., cartilage, skeleton muscle, or bone)	Tumor with invasion of skeleton (axial or appendicular) or perineural invasion of skull base	Infiltration of base of skull or vertebra	T4	n/a

[*] AJCC high-risk factors include >2 mm thickness, Clark level ≥IV, perineural invasion, primary site ear, primary site non-hair-bearing lip, or poorly differentiated histology.

[‡] BWH "high-risk" factors include tumor diameter ≥2 cm, poorly differentiated histology, perineural invasion ≥0.1 mm, or tumor invasion beyond fat (excluding bone invasion which automatically upgrades tumor to BWH stage T3).

a partial biopsy of the tumor using the shave technique. As the AJCC staging system continues to be refined, it is important that the factors required for staging be not only statistically sound, but also ones that are realistic to collect on a large scale. If the factors are too time consuming to record for every cSCC, classifying tumors with incomplete data may lead to erroneous staging assignment and flawed prognostic estimates.

In contrast to the AJCC staging system which endeavors to stratify patients of similar outcomes and provide prognostic estimates, the NCCN guidelines are intended to direct tumor treatment and management. Using the NCCN classification, almost 90% of the same cohort of tumors analyzed by the AJCC staging system was deemed to be "high-risk," suggesting that the NCCN's definition of "high-risk" cSCC may be too inclusive. The primary focus in the creation of the NCCN definition of "high-risk" in the 2012 cSCC NCCN guidelines was developing a list of "high-risk" factors for recurrence; identifying risk factors specifically for metastasis (which may overlap with those associated with tumor recurrence) was a secondary concern. Consequently, the "high-risk" criteria used in 2012 NCCN cSCC guidelines may have been kept intentionally broad so as to encompass all factors that have been reported to be associated with a higher rate of recurrence [5].

It is worth mentioning that the list of "high-risk" factors in the 2014 cSCC NCCN guidelines [25] indicates that these factors are "high-risk" for local recurrence OR metastasis; this list is almost exactly the same as the 2012 list of "high-risk" factors which were labeled as "high-risk" for recurrence only [5]. The difference between the two lists is that moderately differentiated histology is no longer considered a "high-risk" factor in the 2014 guidelines. This modification resulted in a negligible change in the percentage of "high-risk" tumors—85.6% (2014) versus 87% (2012)—with only 4 "high-risk" tumors by 2012 NCCN guidelines switching groups when the 2014 NCCN guidelines were applied.

Since only 1 of 12 high-risk factors is needed to for a tumor to be categorized as "high-risk," tumors with vastly different metastatic potential are all grouped together as "high-risk." In the current 2014 NCCN guidelines, a tumor that has 4 risk factors (e.g., poorly differentiated 2 cm tumor on the ear invading cartilage with perineural invasion) is considered to be the same as a 6 mm cSCC on the nose, which is considered "high-risk" based on its size and location alone. Even when analyzing tumors that each possess only 1 risk factor (e.g., 5 mm cSCC on the arm in a liver transplant patient maintained on low-dose immunosuppression or a 2 cm well-differentiated tumor on the lateral canthus), the current NCCN guidelines do not distinguish between these two tumors with different levels of metastatic risk.

In summary, our analysis revealed that there is discordance between the AJCC and NCCN definitions of "high-risk" cSCCs. Though the two guidelines are based on different methodologies and serve different purposes, the definitions of "high-risk" cSCC and the cohort they describe should be more similar. When evaluating the AJCC staging system and NCCN cSCC guidelines, it is important to recognize that the cSCC guidelines are still in their infancy as it was not until 2010 that cSCC received a separate set of NCCN guidelines and its own AJCC staging system (in the most recent 7th edition). All in all, the AJCC 7th edition and the NCCN guidelines represent significant progress in the classification and management of cSCCs. Nevertheless, prospective multicenter studies are still needed to determine the role of individual risk factor and the impact of multiple risk factors to generate a unified definition of "high-risk" cSCC in order to develop appropriate treatment guidelines and staging systems that are both practical to implement and accurate in order to optimize the care of our patients.

References

[1] L. Lansbury, J. Leonardi-Bee, W. Perkins, T. Goodacre, J. A. Tweed, and F. J. Bath-Hextall, "Interventions for non-metastatic squamous cell carcinoma of the skin," *Cochrane Database of Systematic Reviews*, vol. 4, Article ID CD007869, 2010.

[2] F. Bath-Hextall, J. Leonardi-Bee, N. Somchand, A. Webster, J. Delitt, and W. Perkins, "Interventions for preventing non-melanoma skin cancers in high-risk groups," *Cochrane Database of Systematic Reviews*, no. 4, Article ID CD005414, 2007.

[3] N. D. L. S. Brougham, E. R. Dennett, R. Cameron, and S. T. Tan, "The incidence of metastasis from cutaneous squamous cell carcinoma and the impact of its risk factors," *Journal of Surgical Oncology*, vol. 106, no. 7, pp. 811–815, 2012.

[4] "Cutaneous squamous cell carcinoma and other cutaneous carcinomas," in *AJCC Cancer Staging Manual*, S. B. Edge, D. R. Byrd, C. C. Compton et al., Eds., pp. 301–314, Springer, New York, NY, USA, 7th edition, 2010.

[5] "NCCN Guidelines version 01.2012 Basal Cell and Squamous Cell Skin Cancers," National Comprehensive Cancer Network, 2012.

[6] H. Breuninger, K. Brantsch, T. Eigentler, and H.-M. Häfner, "Comparison and evaluation of the current staging of cutaneous carcinomas," *Journal der Deutschen Dermatologischen Gesellschaft*, vol. 10, no. 8, pp. 579–586, 2012.

[7] J. A. Carucci, J. C. Martinez, N. C. Zeitouni et al., "In-transit metastasis from primary cutaneous squamous cell carcinoma in organ transplant recipients and nonimmunosuppressed patients: clinical characteristics, management, and outcome in a series of 21 patients," *Dermatologic Surgery*, vol. 30, part 2, no. 4, pp. 651–655, 2004.

[8] S. M. Dinehart, D. Z. J. Chu, A. W. Maners, and S. V. Pollack, "Immunosuppression in patients with metastatic squamous cell carcinoma from the skin," *Journal of Dermatologic Surgery and Oncology*, vol. 16, no. 3, pp. 271–274, 1990.

[9] J.-C. Martinez, C. C. Otley, T. Stasko et al., "Defining the clinical course of metastatic skin cancer in organ transplant recipients: a multicenter collaborative study," *Archives of Dermatology*, vol. 139, no. 3, pp. 301–306, 2003.

[10] J. O'Hara, A. Ferlito, R. P. Takes et al., "Cutaneous squamous cell carcinoma of the head and neck metastasizing to the parotid gland—a review of current recommendations," *Head and Neck*, vol. 33, no. 12, pp. 1789–1795, 2011.

[11] K. D. Brantsch, C. Meisner, B. Schönfisch et al., "Analysis of risk factors determining prognosis of cutaneous squamous-cell carcinoma: a prospective study," *The Lancet Oncology*, vol. 9, no. 8, pp. 713–720, 2008.

[12] B. Peat, P. Insull, and R. Ayers, "Risk stratification for metastasis

from cutaneous squamous cell carcinoma of the head and neck," *ANZ Journal of Surgery*, vol. 82, no. 4, pp. 230–233, 2012.

[13] P. S. Karia, J. Han, and C. D. Schmults, "Cutaneous squamous cell carcinoma: Estimated incidence of disease, nodal metastasis, and deaths from disease in the United States, 2012," *Journal of the American Academy of Dermatology*, vol. 68, no. 6, pp. 957–966, 2013.

[14] A. Jambusaria-Pahlajani, P. A. Kanetsky, P. S. Karia et al., "Evaluation of AJCC tumor staging for cutaneous squamous cell carcinoma and a proposed alternative tumor staging system," *JAMA Dermatology*, vol. 149, no. 4, pp. 402–410, 2013.

[15] K. G. Leblanc Jr. and G. D. Monheit, "Understanding and use of the american joint committee on cancer seventh edition guidelines for cutaneous squamous cell carcinoma: a survey of dermatologic surgeons," *Dermatologic Surgery*, vol. 40, no. 5, pp. 505–510, 2014.

[16] S. M. Dinehart and S. Peterson, "Evaluation of the American Joint Committee on Cancer staging system for cutaneous squamous cell carcinoma and proposal of a new staging system," *Dermatologic Surgery*, vol. 31, no. 11, part 1, pp. 1379–1384, 2005.

[17] C. L. Warner and C. J. Cockerell, "The new seventh edition American joint committee on cancer staging of cutaneous non-melanoma skin cancer: a critical review," *American Journal of Clinical Dermatology*, vol. 12, no. 3, pp. 147–154, 2011.

[18] "Merkel cell carcinoma," in *AJCC Cancer Staging Manual*, S. B. Edge, D. R. Byrd, C. C. Compton et al., Eds., pp. 315–324, Springer, New York, NY, USA, 7th edition, 2010.

[19] M. J. Veness, C. E. Palme, and G. J. Morgan, "High-risk cutaneous squamous cell carcinoma of the head and neck: results from 266 treated patients with metastatic lymph node disease," *Cancer*, vol. 106, no. 11, pp. 2389–2396, 2006.

[20] "Carcinoma of skin," in *UICC International Union Against Cancer TNM Classification of Malignant Tumors*, L. Tobin, M. Gospodarowicz, and C. Wittekind, Eds., pp. 165–168, Wiley-Blackwell, West Sussex, UK, 7th edition, 2009.

[21] "Carcinoma of the skin," in *AJCC Cancer Staging Manual*, F. L. Greene, D. L. Page, I. D. Fleming et al., Eds., pp. 203–208, Springer, New York, NY, USA, 6th edition, 2002.

[22] P. S. Karia, A. Jambusaria-Pahlajani, D. P. Harrington, G. F. Murphy, A. A. Qureshi, and C. D. Schmults, "Evaluation of American Joint Committee on Cancer, International Union Against Cancer, and Brigham and Women's Hospital tumor staging for cutaneous squamous cell carcinoma," *Journal of Clinical Oncology*, vol. 32, no. 4, pp. 327–334, 2014.

[23] P. S. Karia, J. Han, and C. D. Schmults, "Cutaneous squamous cell carcinoma: estimated incidence of disease, nodal metastasis, and deaths from disease in the United States, 2012," *Journal of the American Academy of Dermatology*, vol. 68, no. 6, pp. 957–966, 2013.

[24] M. R. Donaldson and B. M. Coldiron, "No end in sight: the skin cancer epidemic continues," *Seminars in Cutaneous Medicine and Surgery*, vol. 30, no. 1, pp. 3–5, 2011.

[25] "NCCN Guidelines version 02.2014 Basal and Squamous Cell Skin Cancers," National Comprehensive Cancer Network, 2014.

2

Characterization of the Merkel Cell Carcinoma miRNome

Matthew S. Ning,[1] Annette S. Kim,[2] Nripesh Prasad,[3,4] Shawn E. Levy,[4] Huiqiu Zhang,[5] and Thomas Andl[1]

[1] *Division of Dermatology, Department of Medicine, Vanderbilt University Medical Center, Medical Center North, Room A2310A, 1161 21st Avenue South, Nashville, TN 37232-2600, USA*
[2] *Department of Pathology, Microbiology, and Immunology, Vanderbilt University Medical Center, Nashville, TN 37232-2600, USA*
[3] *Department of Biological Sciences, University of Alabama in Huntsville, Huntsville, AL 35805, USA*
[4] *HudsonAlpha Institute for Biotechnology, Huntsville, AL 35806, USA*
[5] *OrioR Lab, LLC, Rockville, MD 20852, USA*

Correspondence should be addressed to Thomas Andl; thomas.andl@vanderbilt.edu

Academic Editor: S. Ugurel

MicroRNAs have been implicated in various skin cancers, including melanoma, squamous cell carcinoma, and basal cell carcinoma; however, the expression of microRNAs and their role in Merkel cell carcinoma (MCC) have yet to be explored in depth. To identify microRNAs specific to MCC (MCC-miRs), next-generation sequencing (NGS) of small RNA libraries was performed on different tissue samples including MCCs, other cutaneous tumors, and normal skin. Comparison of the profiles identified several microRNAs upregulated and downregulated in MCC. For validation, their expression was measured via qRT-PCR in a larger group of MCC and in a comparison group of non-MCC cutaneous tumors and normal skin. Eight microRNAs were upregulated in MCC: miR-502-3p, miR-9, miR-7, miR-340, miR-182, miR-190b, miR-873, and miR-183. Three microRNAs were downregulated: miR-3170, miR-125b, and miR-374c. Many of these MCC-miRs, the miR-183/182/96a cistron in particular, have connections to tumorigenic pathways implicated in MCC pathogenesis. *In situ* hybridization confirmed that the highly expressed MCC-miR, miR-182, is localized within tumor cells. Furthermore, NGS and qRT-PCR reveal that several of these MCC-miRs are highly expressed in the patient-derived MCC cell line, MS-1. These data indicate that we have identified a set of MCC-miRs with important implications for MCC research.

1. Introduction

Merkel cell carcinoma (MCC) is a primary neuroendocrine carcinoma of the skin of uncertain origin. Although not as prevalent as other skin cancers, MCC is aggressive and has a high mortality rate, with an overall five-year survival of sixty percent [1]. Median survival for patients with and without regional lymph node involvement at presentation is thirteen and forty months, respectively [2], and up to fifty percent of patients eventually develop systemic disease with metastases to liver, bone, and brain [3].

Unfortunately, while the incidence of MCC increases, our knowledge of these tumors remains limited. Several factors are implicated in its pathogenesis, including UV radiation exposure, an associated polyomavirus (MCPyV), and immunosuppression [4, 5], but the lack of effective treatment options available for MCC reflects our limited knowledge. In an attempt to expand our understanding, we focus our attention on microRNAs, small single-stranded RNA molecules that participate in the negative regulation of gene expression.

With average lengths of roughly twenty-two nucleotides, these molecules serve as guides of the RNA-induced silencing complex (RISC). MicroRNAs regulate the expression of genes by binding to partially complementary target sites in mRNA transcripts and inhibiting their translation [6]. A wealth of data has accumulated in recent years implicating microRNAs as significant modulators of gene expression, and through their unique role in posttranscriptional regulation, they can function as important regulators of tumor growth and metastasis.

The study of microRNAs holds much promise for improving the diagnosis and treatment of cancer. Recent progress in

Table 1: MCC sample data. Clinical information corresponding to each of the FFPE MCC samples utilized in qRT-PCR analysis.

#	Age (yrs)	Sex	Race	P/M	Metastasis/invasion/recurrence	Clinical information
1	57	F	W	P	6/9 axillary LNs+, distant LN+	N/A
2	57	F	W	P	Soft tissue involvement, 2/6 LNs+, distant LN+	N/A
3	63	M	W	P	Lumbar spinal cord involvement highly suspected based on FDG-PET/CT imaging	Immunosuppression regimen for renal transplant: mycophenolate mofetil, prednisone, tacrolimus
4	64	M	W	P	N/A	Immunosuppression regimen for renal transplant 2° granulomatosis with polyangiitis: mycophenolate mofetil, prednisone, tacrolimus; history of multiple SCC
5	65	M	W	M	Submandibular gland with soft tissue involvement, 6/24 LNs+, local recurrence	N/A
6	70	M	W	M	Distant (supraclavicular) LN+	History of renal cancer
7	71	M	W	M	Parotid gland with intraparotid LN involvement, local recurrence	N/A
8	72	M	W	P	Local recurrence	History of colon cancer
9	72	M	W	M	Thyroid, parotid gland involvement, 3/23 LNs+	Concurrent papillary thyroid carcinoma
10	76	M	W	P	Distant (cervical) LN+	Concurrent SCC, history of lung cancer
11	76	M	W	P	6/37 axillary LNs+	N/A
12	78	M	W	P	Parotid gland involvement, 9/28 LNs+, local recurrence	N/A
13	79	M	W	P	N/A	History of bladder cancer
14	79	M	W	M	Salivary gland, deep soft tissue surrounding large arteries and skeletal muscle involvement, 14/20 LNs+	N/A
15	80	F	W	M	Multifocal extranodal tumor invasion, soft tissue, and sternocleidomastoid muscle involvement, 11/15 LNs+	History of chronic lymphocytic leukemia
16	82	M	W	P	Parotid gland involvement, distant LN+	History of colon cancer, laryngeal cancer, multiple SCC
17	82	F	W	P	Parotid gland involvement, 2/5 LNs+	History of breast cancer
18	82	M	W	M	Parotid gland with invasion of right upper neck soft tissue, 2/11 LNs+, distant LN+	History of colon cancer, laryngeal cancer, multiple SCC
19	85	M	W	P	N/A	History of acute myeloid leukemia, in remission
20	85	M	W	M	Rectum involvement	History of rectal cancer, prostate cancer

LN: lymph node; M: metastasis; P: primary; W: white.

our understanding of the role of microRNAs in disease has excited oncology. An effective antiviral therapy was recently developed based on microRNA biology, and microRNAs are promising new tools and targets in cancer research [7].

Indeed, microRNAs have been demonstrated to play significant roles in the pathogenesis of other skin cancers, such as squamous cell carcinoma (SCC) and melanoma [6]. They have also been implicated in basal cell carcinoma (BCC) and may even be employed in the accurate identification of cancer subtype, as demonstrated for melanoma and cutaneous T-cell lymphoma (CTCL) [6]. However, despite the volume of literature on microRNAs in skin cancer, little is yet known about the role that these molecules play in MCC. Thus, we set out to close this knowledge gap and define the microRNAs involved in MCC biology.

2. Methods

2.1. Samples. Frozen tissue samples of various skin cancers (MCC, melanoma, SCC, and BCC), normal skin, and normal lymph node were obtained from the Cooperative Human Tissue Network (CHTN) and stored at −80°C. Formalin-fixed paraffin-embedded (FFPE) tissue samples of various skin cancers (MCC, melanoma, SCC, and BCC) and normal skin were obtained from Vanderbilt Pathology and Dermatopathology (Nashville, TN). Clinical information corresponding to the FFPE MCC samples is provided (Table 1).

2.2. Cell Lines. All cell lines were cultured in DMEM with 10% FCS and Pen-Strep.

2.3. RNA Isolation. Total RNA, including microRNAs, was isolated from frozen tissue and cell culture with the miRNeasy Mini Kit and from FFPE tissue with the miRNeasy FFPE Kit (Qiagen; Hilden, Germany), according to the manufacturer's protocols. The concentration and integrity of the extracted total RNA were estimated by Qubit 2.0 Fluorometer (Invitrogen, Carlsbad, CA, USA) and Agilent 2100 Bioanalyzer (Applied Biosystems, Carlsbad, CA, USA), respectively. RNA samples with a RNA Integrity Number (RIN) value of at least 7.0 or higher was used for further processing.

2.4. Small RNA (miRNA) Library Preparation and Sequencing. Approximately 1 μg of total RNA from each sample was taken into small RNA library preparation protocol using NEBNext Small RNA Library Prep Set for Illumina (New England BioLabs Inc., Ipswich, MA, USA) according to manufacturer's protocol. Briefly, 3′ adapters were ligated to total input RNA followed by hybridization of multiplex SR RT primers and ligation of multiplex 5′ SR adapters. Reverse transcription (RT) was done using SuperScript III RT (Life Technologies, Grand Island, NY, USA) for 1 hour at 50°C. Immediately after RT reaction, PCR amplification was performed for 15 cycles using LongAmp Taq 2X master mix. Illumina indexed primers were added to uniquely barcode each sample. Post-PCR material was purified using QIAquick PCR purification kit (Qiagen Inc., Valencia, CA, USA). Post-PCR yield and concentration of the prepared libraries were assessed using Qubit 2.0 Fluorometer and DNA 1000 chip on Agilent 2100 Bioanalyzer. Size selection of small RNA with a target size range of 140 bp was done by running samples on a 6% PAGE gel for 1 hour at 120 V. Accurate quantification for sequencing applications was performed using the qPCR-based KAPA Biosystems Library Quantification kit. Each library was diluted to a final concentration of 12.5 nM and pooled in equimolar ratios prior to clustering. Cluster generation was carried out on a cBot v1.4.36.0 using Illumina's Truseq Single Read (SR) Cluster Kit v3.0. Single End (SE) sequencing was performed to generate at least 15 million reads per sample on an Illumina HiSeq2000, running HiSeq Control Software (HCS) v1.5.15.1, using a 50-cycle TruSeq SBS HS v3 reagent kit. The clustered flowcells were sequenced for 56 cycles, consisting of a 50-cycle read, followed by a 6-cycle index read. Image analysis and base calling was performed using the standard Illumina Pipeline consisting of Real time Analysis (RTA) version v1.13 and demultiplexed using bcl2fastq converter with default settings.

2.5. Processing of Small RNA-Seq Reads. At least 15 million, 50 bp, SE reads were generated from each sample. Further downstream analysis of the sequenced reads from each sample was performed as per our unique in-house pipeline. Briefly, quality control checks on raw sequence data from each sample will be performed using FastQC (Babraham Bioinformatics, London, UK). Raw reads were then imported on a commercial data analysis platform CLCbio (CLCbio, MA, USA). Adapter trimming was done to remove ligated adapter from 3′ end of the sequenced reads with only one mismatch allowed; poorly aligned 3′ ends were also trimmed. Sequences shorter than 15 nucleotides length were excluded from further analysis. Trimmed Reads were then used to extract and count the small RNA which were then annotated with microRNAs in miRBase release 18 database. Samples were grouped as per their types identifiers and quantification of miRNA abundance was done. Differential expression of miRNA was calculated on the basis of their fold change (default cut-off $\geq\pm2.0$) between mapped counts observed between individual groups.

2.6. Quantitative Real-Time Reverse Transcription Polymerase Chain Reaction (qRT-PCR). To validate the NGS data, the expression of microRNAs was analyzed via quantitative real-time reverse transcription polymerase chain reaction (qRT-PCR) with the Rotor-Gene SYBR Green PCR Kit, miScript Primer Assays, and miScript Universal Primer, following reverse transcription of total RNA with the miScript II RT Kit (Qiagen; Hilden, Germany).

The qRT-PCR analysis was performed in technical replicates according to the manufacturer's instructions using the Rotor-Gene SYBR Green PCR Master Mix (Qiagen; Hilden, Germany). The packaged operating software was utilized for instrument control, data acquisition, and raw data analysis. The plates were run in relative quantification ($\Delta\Delta C_t$) mode with triplicate measurements.

Amplification curves were analyzed using the packaged operating software, and assays were inspected for distinct melting curves. In addition, only assays detected with $C_t < 35$ were included in the data analysis. To calculate the relative expression levels of target microRNAs, the $\Delta\Delta C_t$ algorithm method was utilized. miR-423-3p and miR-423-5p were stably expressed across all samples, thus the average of their C_ts in each sample was used as the normalization factor. Assays were calibrated to the same normal skin sample.

2.7. In Situ Hybridization (ISH). In situ detection of miR-182 was carried out using the AccuRISH service of OrioR Lab, LLC (Rockville, MD). An RNAse-free tissue sectioning environment was created by treating the microtome, blades, water bath, ice bucket, forceps, and slide tray with RNaseZap, followed by RNase-free water. Each 5-μm tissue section was dewaxed, rehydrated, and demasked, and protease treatment was optimized for each tissue block with GAPDH probe and differing concentrations of Protease K. After treatment, tumor and normal tissue sections were stained side-by-side using an anti-miR-182 oligonucleotide probe of same concentration with same hybridization and stringent washing temperature of 55–60°C. The final color development for all sections of each batch was terminated together after ninety minutes. All pictures were taken using an Olympus DP70 digital camera with the same setting.

3. Results

3.1. Differential MicroRNA Expression Based on High-Throughput Sequencing Data. Sequencing of small RNA libraries was performed for the following frozen tissue samples: three MCCs, one melanoma, one SCC, one BCC, and one normal skin. The MCC and melanoma were lymph node metastases, while the SCC and BCC were primary

TABLE 2: MCC-miR candidates identified via NGS. Lists of top fifteen microRNAs upregulated and downregulated in MCC ($n = 3$) versus other tissues (1 melanoma, 1 SCC, 1 BCC, and 1 normal skin sample) and list of fifteen microRNAs expressed in MS-1, based on NGS data.

Upregulated in MCC versus other skin cancers[1]		Upregulated in MCC versus normal skin[1]		Downregulated in MCC versus all other samples[1]		Highly expressed in MS-1	
microRNA	Fold change[2]	microRNA	Fold change[2]	microRNA	Fold change[2]	microRNA	RPKM
miR-885	234.3	miR-183	54.6	miR-455	−100.0	miR-182	441,774
miR-1252	159.4	miR-182	44.3	miR-146a	−33.3	miR-183	406,019
miR-190b	72.3	miR-96	26.4	miR-125b-2	−16.7	miR-10b	368,383
miR-876	69.7	miR-7-2	9.0	miR-224	−16.7	miR-30d	354,071
miR-873	62.2	miR-7-1	8.4	miR-125b-1	−16.7	let-7i	302,976
miR-1468	42.5	miR-769	6.0	miR-452	−12.5	miR-30a	256,918
miR-3065	33.8	miR-708	5.8	miR-27a	−8.3	miR-21	231,060
miR-3074	19.9	miR-93	5.7	miR-503	−6.7	miR-26a	230,375
miR-1250	15.6	miR-106b	5.7	miR-34a	−5.3	miR-9-2	152,761
miR-502	15.2	miR-9-2	4.7	miR-378d-2	−4.8	miR-20a	118,839
miR-660	14.4	miR-532	4.7	miR-24-2	−4.0	miR-532	109,596
miR-501	9.3	miR-9-3	4.7	miR-193a	−4.0	miR-93	108,909
miR-708	9.2	miR-9-1	4.7	miR-378i	−3.6	miR-340	89,562
miR-532	8.2	miR-340	4.0	miR-22	−3.0	miR-7-1	73,329
miR-500a	7.6	miR-192	3.5	miR-34c	−2.9	miR-96a	60,009

[1]Inclusion criteria: >100 reads in all MCC samples; [2]Fold change (default cut-off $\geq \pm 2.0$) between mapped counts observed between individual groups.

cutaneous lesions. Comparison of the sequencing profiles identified several microRNAs upregulated and downregulated in MCC versus other tissues (Table 2).

3.2. Confirmation of MCC-miRs via qRT-PCR. To validate the next generation sequencing (NGS) data, several microRNAs were evaluated via qRT-PCR in larger cohorts of FFPE tissue samples. The MCC cohort consisted of a mixture of primary cutaneous lesions and metastases (Table 1). The tumor group consisted of primary cutaneous lesions of melanoma, SCC, and BCC (Figure 1). The qRT-PCR results confirmed the upregulation (≥2-fold) of eight microRNAs in MCC: miR-502-3p, miR-9, miR-7, miR-340, miR-182, miR-190b, miR-873, and miR-183. In addition, three microRNAs were found to be downregulated (≥2-fold) in MCC: miR-3170, miR-125b, and miR-374c. The data also identified the slight upregulation (≥1.5-fold) of miR-96a, another member of the miR-183/96/182 cluster.

To assess whether these microRNAs are specific tumor markers for MCC, the expression of each of the eight MCC-miRs was evaluated via qRT-PCR in several frozen MCC lymph node metastases and compared to a human tissue panel consisting of twelve different organs (Figure 2). Three of the MCC-miRs demonstrated higher expression (≥2-fold) in the MCC cohort versus all other organs: miR-183, miR-182, and miR-190b.

3.3. MCC-miRs Are Highly Expressed in the MCC Cell Line, MS-1. To assess the potential of these findings for future functional studies, NGS of small RNA libraries was performed for the patient derived MCPyV-positive cell line, MS-1 (Table 2). Several of the same MCC-miRs found to be upregulated in the tissue samples also demonstrated high absolute expression values in MS-1. Thus, the expression of each of the MCC-miRs was evaluated via qRT-PCR in MS-1 and compared to that of various non-MCC cell lines (Figure 3). The following MCC-miRs were confirmed to be elevated (≥2-fold) in MS-1 versus a set of sixteen non-MCC cell lines: miR-183, miR-182, miR-340, and miR-190b—interestingly, the same microRNAs were found to be upregulated in MCC versus the tissue panel. Together, these data indicate that we have identified a set of high quality MCC-miRs.

The expression of each of the four microRNAs was also evaluated via qRT-PCR in the MCPyV-negative cell line, MCC13, but with different results (Figure 3). In contrast to MS-1, the four microRNAs, miR-183, miR-182, miR-340, and miR190b demonstrated low expression levels in MCC13. The levels of these microRNAs were instead comparable to that of the other cell lines. Explanations for this discrepancy are provided in the discussion.

3.4. In Situ Hybridization (ISH) Confirms miR-182 Expression in MCC Cells. To support the notion that these microRNAs play a role in the actual tumor cells in lieu of the surrounding tissue, ISH was performed for one of the more highly expressed MCC-miRs, miR-182, on a sample of MCC of the cheek and on a sample of normal skin (Figure 4). As expected, miR-182 was localized to MCC cells, and, as expected from the qRT-PCR data, expression in surrounding tissue and normal skin was low compared to that in MCC cells.

4. Discussion

MCC remains one of the least understood cancers of the skin. MicroRNAs are a relatively young field of biomedical

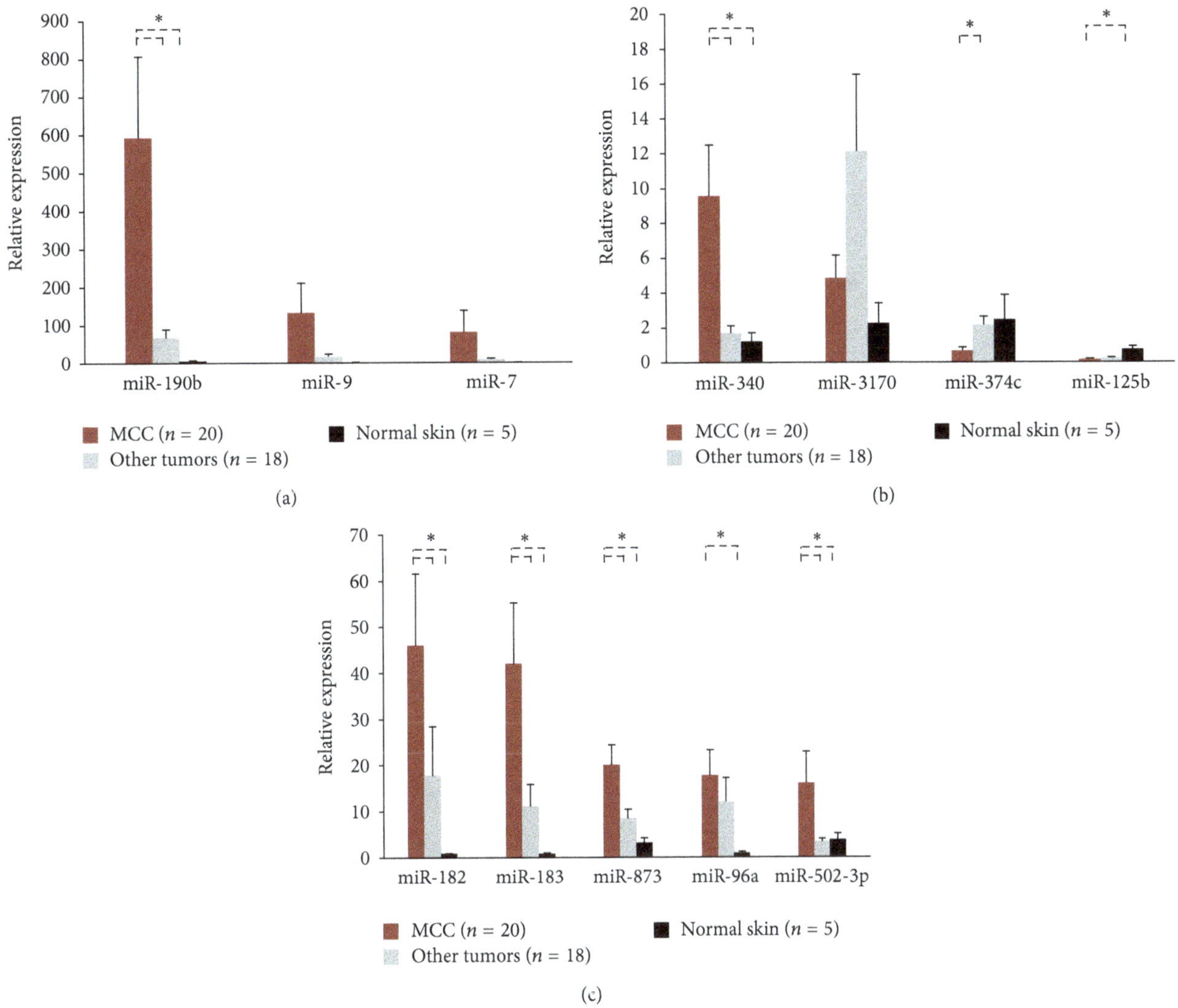

FIGURE 1: Validation of MCC-miRs via qRT-PCR. Eight microRNAs were confirmed to be upregulated in MCC versus other tumors and normal skin: miR-190b, miR-9, miR-7, miR-182, miR-183, miR-873, miR-502-3p, and miR-340. The tumor group consists of melanoma ($n = 5$), SCC ($n = 6$), and BCC ($n = 7$). Error bars refer to SEM. *Welch's t-test: $P < 0.05$.

research, born in 2000 with the detection of let-7 in humans, with potential for applications in other pathologies [6, 7]. We believe this will hold true in MCC as well, for which we have identified eight upregulated and three downregulated microRNAs. These MCC-miRs have several implications for the future of MCC research.

4.1. MCC-miRs in Cancer: miR-182-183-96. While these MCC-miRs are highly expressed in MCC, some of them have been demonstrated to play significant roles in the pathogenesis of other cancers as well. In particular, the miR-183/96/182 cluster, at chromosomal locus 7q32, is expressed in a diversity of cancers and may contribute to their pathogenesis by targeting multiple components of the cell cycle, DNA damage response, and homologous recombination pathways, and by enriching pathways associated with metastasis, migration, and epithelial mesenchymal transition [8]. Here we review significant findings in the literature concerning this cluster.

Regarding skin cancer, the miR-183 cluster is frequently overexpressed in melanoma. Our work confirms this observation, inasmuch as miR-182 and miR-183 were upregulated in melanoma versus SCC, BCC, and normal skin (although still not as highly expressed as in MCC). In melanoma, overexpression of miR-182 promotes survival, migration, and metastasis by directly repressing the tumor suppressors FOXO3 and microphthalmia-associated transcription factor-M; and expression of miR-182 increases with progression from primary to metastatic melanoma [9]. This correlation between miR-182 level and aggressiveness is interesting, when noting that MCC, in general, is widely considered to be a tumor with a similar level of aggressiveness as melanoma. It is tempting to entertain the notion that a common pathway may perhaps exist within the two and that a greater dysregulation of said pathway in MCC could account for its high rate of metastasis, morbidity, and mortality. Downregulation of FOX transcription factors is a common theme of this cluster, as

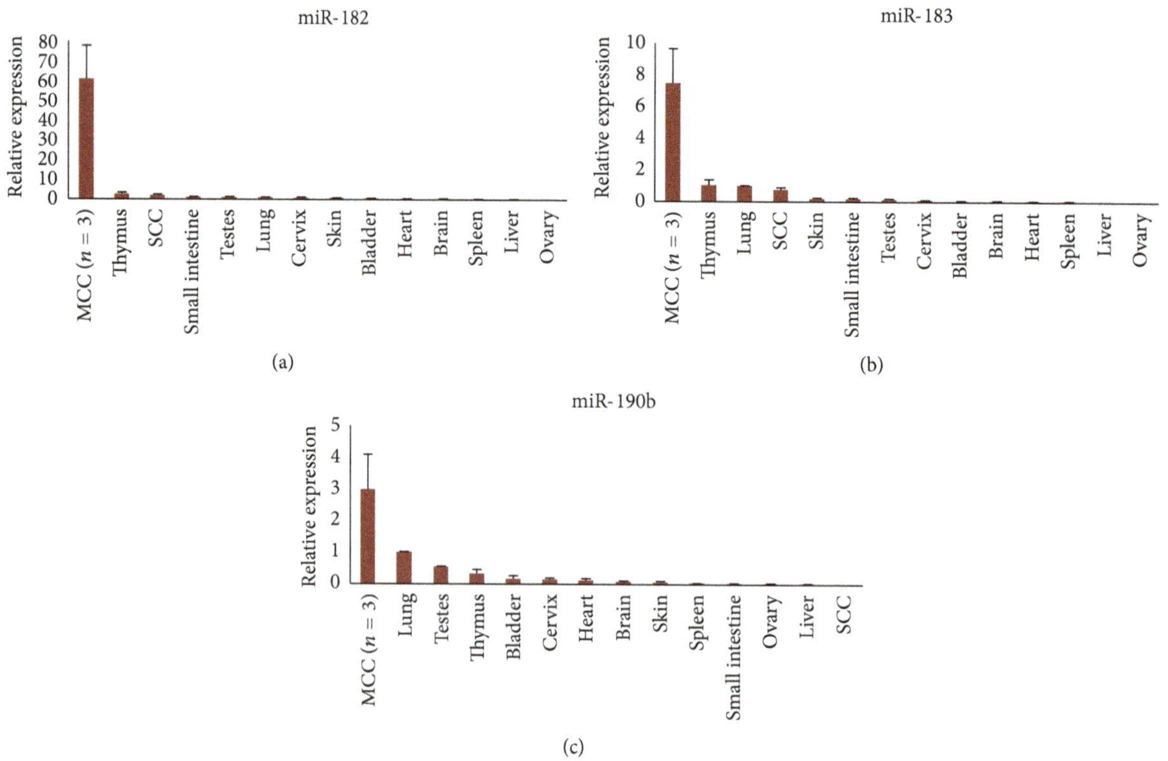

FIGURE 2: MCC-miRs are specific for MCC. Three MCC-miRs were confirmed via qRT-PCR to be upregulated in frozen MCC samples versus a human tissue panel consisting of twelve different body organs: miR-182, miR-183, and miR-190b. Error bars refer to SEM.

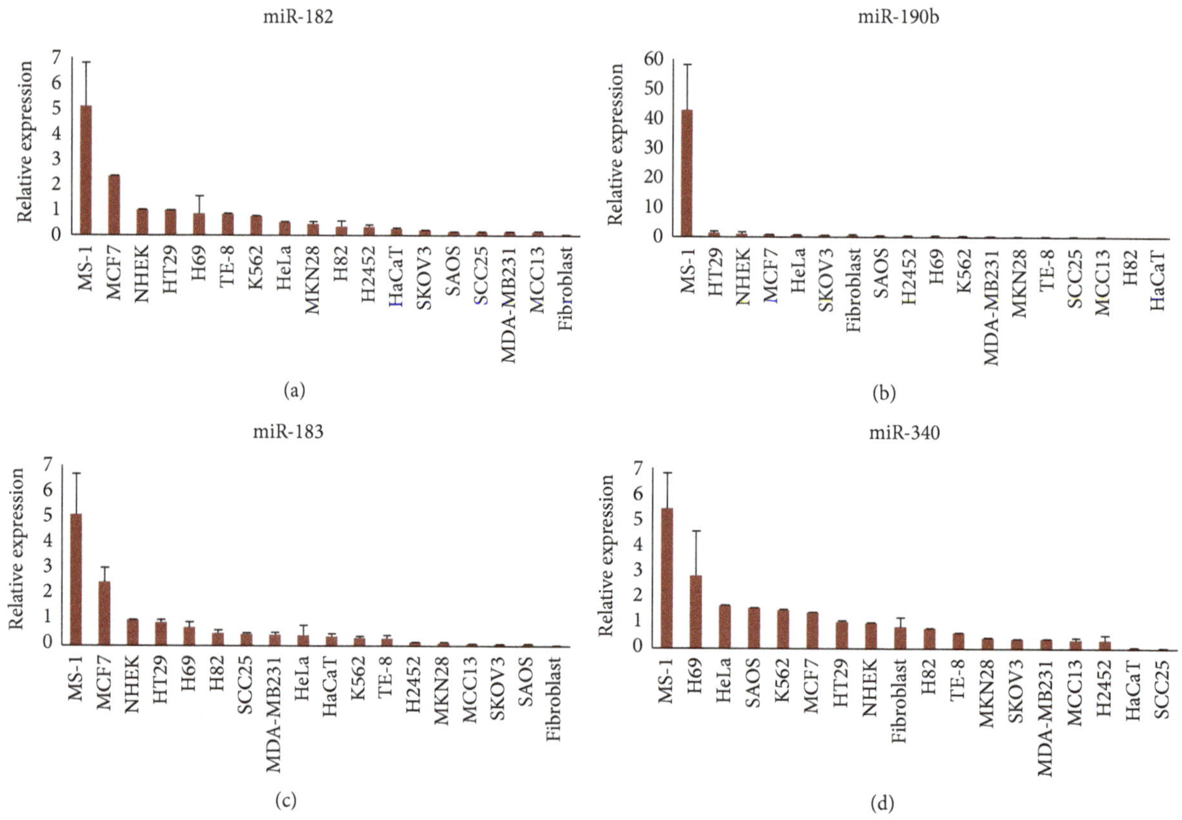

FIGURE 3: MCC-miRs are highly expressed in MS-1. Four MCC-miRs were confirmed via qRT-PCR to be upregulated in the MCC cell line, MS-1, versus sixteen other non-MCC cell lines: miR-182, miR-183, miR-190b, and miR-340. Error bars refer to SEM.

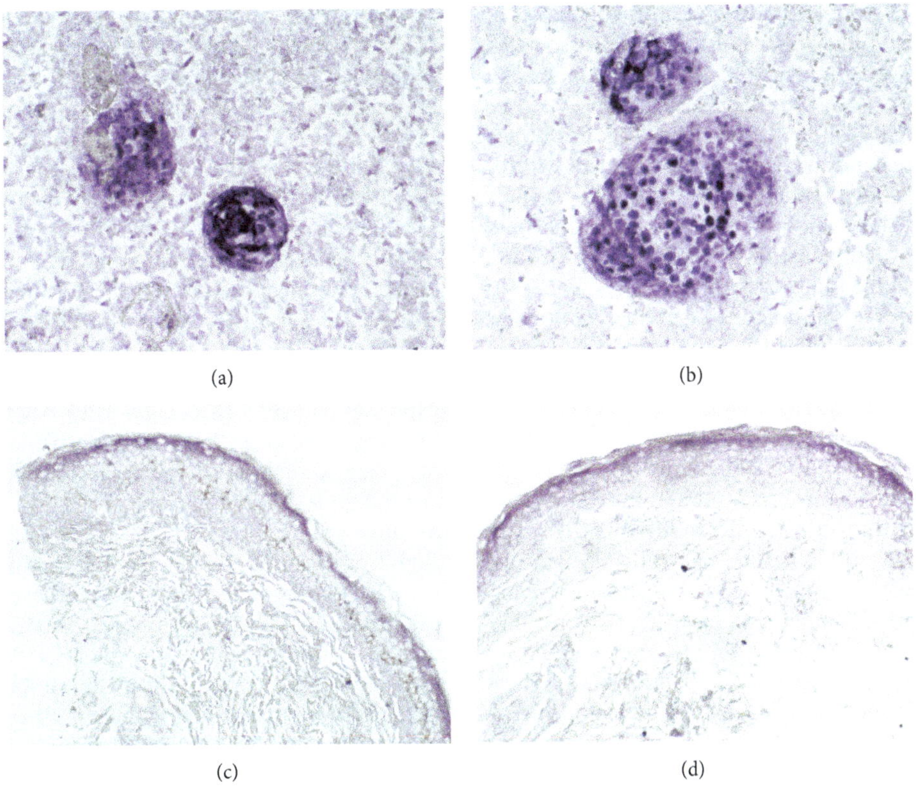

FIGURE 4: *In situ* hybridization (ISH) confirms that miR-182 is localized to MCC tumor cells. Panels (a) and (b) demonstrate that miR-182 is highly expressed in MCC cells versus the surrounding tissue in a sample of MCC of the cheek; original magnification ×200. Panels (c) and (d) demonstrate that miR-182 expression is low compared to that in MCC cells in a sample of normal skin; original magnification ×200.

miR-183/96/182 have been demonstrated to inhibit FOXO1 in classical Hodgkin lymphoma [10] and in endometrial cancer as well, resulting in decreased G1 cell cycle arrest and cell death [11]. Aberrations of FOX transcription factors have yet to be evaluated in MCC and may be an avenue worth exploring, considering this new information.

The miR-183/96/182 cluster serves essential functions in various noncutaneous carcinomas as well, with much research focused on its role in breast cancer, particularly with invasion and metastasis. For example, in mammary ductal carcinoma *in situ*, both miR-182 and miR-183 have been demonstrated to target CBX7, a regulator of E-cadherin expression [12]. miR-182, activated by β-catenin, also targets the matrix metalloproteinase inhibitor RECK, resulting in increased MMP-9 activity [13], as well as MIM, which normally suppresses metastasis by inhibition of RHOA. Dysregulation of these pathways shares the common result of increasing tumor motility and colony formation, and indeed, overexpression of miR-182 in breast cancer cell xenografts results in increased pulmonary colonization by cancer cells [14].

4.2. miR-183/96/182: Potential Target Genes Relevant to MCC. The molecular pathways altered in MCC pathogenesis have yet to be fully characterized, but a literature review reveals that some connections to well-known tumorigenic pathways have been made. For example, multiple research groups have discovered that the PI3K/AKT/mTOR pathway is activated, independent of MCPyV-status, in the majority of human MCCs, identifying it as a potential new therapeutic target [15, 16]. Interestingly, the miR-183/96/182 cluster has been demonstrated to enhance PI3K/AKT/mTOR signaling and promote cell migration in medulloblastoma, with the majority of this effect attributed to miR-182. Knockdown of the full cluster in medulloblastoma cells results in dysregulation of the PI3K/AKT/mTOR signaling axis and enhancement of genes related to apoptosis [17]; thus, the miR-183/96/182 cluster again appears as an attractive target for potential therapeutic applications in MCC.

As an additional note, data also suggest that inactivation of PTEN may play a role in MCC pathogenesis; however, mutation and homozygous deletion screening of the PTEN gene in tumor samples reveals nonsense mutations and homozygous deletions in only a small subset of patients [18]. This suggests that alternative mechanisms may exist leading to the inhibition of PTEN. The miR-183/96/182 cluster may provide an explanation to this puzzle, inasmuch as miR-183 has been demonstrated to target the tumor suppressor gene, EGR1, and participate in a miR-183-EGR1-PTEN network that promotes tumorigenesis and cell migration in synovial sarcoma, rhabdomyosarcoma, and colon cancer [19].

4.3. Diagnostic Markers: miR-190b, miR-182, and miR-183. Furthermore, some of these MCC-miRs, when employed in combination, could be potentially useful in the diagnosis of MCC. Misdiagnosis is high on the list of issues associated with this cancer; however, unlike BCC, for which it may often be confused [20–22], a delay in diagnosis could prove to be fatal. Cytokeratin (CK) 20 has demonstrated its usefulness in the immunohistochemical (IHC) diagnosis of this cancer; however, there have been reports of CK20−/CK7+ variants of MCC [23, 24]; thus, another tumor marker may aid pathologists. We have demonstrated, via ISH, that miR-182 is indeed localized to the tumor cells (Figure 4).

Recently, Renwick et al. demonstrated that multicolor microRNA FISH can be utilized to effectively differentiate between MCC and BCC in FFPE tissues. The researchers employed miR-205 and miR-375, which were shown to be tumor-specific for BCC and MCC, respectively [25]. Similar methods could be applied with other microRNAs highly expressed in MCC, for example miR-182 and the other identified MCC-miRs in this work, in order to increase the specificity of such a diagnostic test. Although miR-375 was not identified in our study, our MCC-miRs were identified using a larger cohort of MCC samples and have greater versatility as diagnostic markers, inasmuch as they were measured in a wider range of tumors, cell lines, and normal tissues. Thus, they would complement miR-375 well in a multicolor microRNA FISH assay.

In addition, our results from the tissue panel demonstrate that the MCC-miRs could also potentially serve as markers for tumor metastasis (Figure 2). Since baseline levels of these microRNAs are relatively low in target organs such as liver, bone, and brain, among other sites of metastatic involvement, they could potentially serve as markers for MCC cells disseminated in these tissues.

Employing microRNA signatures as diagnostic tools has been successfully carried out for other skin cancers. In 2011, Ralfkiaer et al. developed a qRT-PCR-based classifier consisting of three microRNAs capable of differentiating CTCL from other cutaneous pathologies with high accuracy [26]. As another example, Poliseno et al. developed a microRNA signature that differentiates between superficial and nodular spreading melanoma [27]. These examples demonstrate that microRNA classifiers can potentially function as straightforward disease markers. Perhaps this notion may be practically applied in the context of MCC.

4.4. Functional Studies: MS-1. Finally, we demonstrated that several of these MCC-miRs are highly expressed in the patient-derived MCC cell line, MS-1. The same findings were not demonstrated with the MCPyV-negative cell line, MCC13; however, we are not the first to experience such findings. In their previously mentioned study, Renwick et al., upon clustering samples via comparison of microRNA profiles, found that MCPyV-positive cell lines (MS-1, MKL-1, MKL-2) clustered in the MCC group, while MCPyV-negative cell lines (MCC13, MCC26, UISO) clustered in the non-MCC group [25]. Their findings, in addition to ours, support the notion that intrinsic miRNome differences exist between the two cell lines.

This raises the question of which cell line, MS-1 or MCC13, holds more validity as a surrogate of MCC *in vivo.* To address this problem, we refer to the recent work of Guastafierro et al. [28], which characterizes the intrinsic cellular, immunohistochemical, and virological differences between MS-1 and MCC13 in detail. Morphologically, MS-1 and other MCPyV-positive cell lines (MKL-1, MKL-2) grow as floating aggregates in suspension, while MCC13 and other MCPyV-negative cell lines (UISO, MCC26) grow as adherent monolayers in culture. Immunohistochemically, MS-1 is positive for the traditional MCC-markers, CK20 and synaptophysin, and negative for CK7, but in contrast, MCC13 is the exact opposite: negative for CK20 and synaptophysin and positive for CK7. And virologically, MS-1 harbors the integrated viral sequence within its genome and consequently expresses antigens associated with MCPyV-infection and tumorigenesis (e.g., large T antigen), while MCC13 does neither. Taking these differences into account, Guastafierro et al. raise the legitimate question of whether or not the MCPyV-negative cell lines (MCC13, UISO, MCC26, and MaTi) even stem from accurately diagnosed MCC tumors [28].

Based upon these findings, we believe that our results in the MS-1 and MCC13 cell lines corroborate the existing literature that suggests that only the MCPyV-positive cell lines truly mimic MCC. Its cellular, immunohistochemical, and virological features, along with its high expression of MCC-miRs, showcase MS-1 as an attractive candidate for future studies. Further evaluation of the miRNomes of other MCPyV-positive cell lines (MKL-1, MKL-2) would be valuable in supporting this notion.

Acknowledgments

Support of this work by the American Skin Association via the Medical Student Grant Targeting Melanoma and Skin Cancer Research is gratefully acknowledged. This work was also supported by the Meharry-Vanderbilt-TSU Cancer Research Partnership (NIH/NCI U54 CA91405-10) and by CTSA Award no. UL1TR000445 from the National Center for Advancing Translational Sciences. Its contents are solely the responsibility of the authors and do not necessarily represent official views of the National Center for Advancing Translational Sciences or the National Institutes of Health. In addition, The authors are indebted to Dr. Lloyd E. King, Jr., M.D., Ph.D. of Vanderbilt University Medical Center, for providing them with several of the MCC samples utilized in this study. The authors also thank the Chang-Moore Laboratory at the University of Pittsburgh for providing them with the MS-1 cell line.

References

[1] *Merkel Cell Carcinoma. AJCC Staging Manual*, Springer, New York, NY, USA, 2009.

[2] W. H. Morrison, L. J. Peters, E. G. Silva, C. D. Wendt, K. Kian Ang, and H. Goepfert, "The essential role of radiation therapy in securing locoregional control of Merkel cell carcinoma," *International Journal of Radiation Oncology Biology Physics*, vol. 19, no. 3, pp. 583–591, 1990.

[3] P. J. Allen, W. B. Bowne, D. P. Jaques, M. F. Brennan, K. Busam, and D. G. Coit, "Merkel cell carcinoma: prognosis and treatment of patients from a single institution," *Journal of Clinical Oncology*, vol. 23, no. 10, pp. 2300–2309, 2005.

[4] M. Heath, N. Jaimes, B. Lemos et al., "Clinical characteristics of Merkel cell carcinoma at diagnosis in 195 patients: the AEIOU features," *Journal of the American Academy of Dermatology*, vol. 58, no. 3, pp. 375–381, 2008.

[5] H. Feng, M. Shuda, Y. Chang, and P. S. Moore, "Clonal integration of a polyomavirus in human Merkel cell carcinoma," *Science*, vol. 319, no. 5866, pp. 1096–1100, 2008.

[6] M. S. Ning and T. Andl, "Control by a hair's breadth: the role of microRNAs in the skin," *Cellular and Molecular Life Sciences*, vol. 70, no. 7, pp. 1149–1169, 2013.

[7] K. M. Nelson and G. J. Weiss, "MicroRNAs and cancer: past, present, and potential future," *Molecular Cancer Therapeutics*, vol. 7, no. 12, pp. 3655–3660, 2008.

[8] K. Krishnan, A. L. Steptoe, H. C. Martin et al., "MicroRNA-182-5p targets a network of genes involved in DNA repair," *RNA*, vol. 19, no. 2, pp. 230–242, 2013.

[9] M. F. Segura, D. Hanniford, S. Menendez et al., "Aberrant miR-182 expression promotes melanoma metastasis by repressing FOXO3 and microphthalmia-associated transcription factor," *Proceedings of the National Academy of Sciences of the United States of America*, vol. 106, no. 6, pp. 1814–1819, 2009.

[10] L. Xie, A. Ushmorov, F. Leithauser et al., "FOXO1 is a tumor suppressor in classical Hodgkin lymphoma," *Blood*, vol. 119, no. 15, pp. 3503–3511, 2012.

[11] S. S. Myatt, J. Wang, L. J. Monteiro et al., "Definition of microRNAs that repress expression of the tumor suppressor gene FOXO1 in endometrial cancer," *Cancer Research*, vol. 70, no. 1, pp. 367–377, 2010.

[12] B. N. Hannafon, P. Sebastiani, A. de las Morenas, J. Lu, and C. L. Rosenberg, "Expression of microRNA and their gene targets are dysregulated in preinvasive breast cancer," *Breast Cancer Research*, vol. 13, no. 2, article R24, 2011.

[13] C. H. Chiang, M. F. Hou, and W. C. Hung, "Up-regulation of miR-182 by β-catenin in breast cancer increases tumorigenicity and invasiveness by targeting the matrix metalloproteinase inhibitor RECK," *Biochimica Et Biophysica Acta*, vol. 1830, no. 4, pp. 3067–3076, 2013.

[14] R. Lei, J. Tang, X. Zhuang et al., "Suppression of MIM by microRNA-182 activates RhoA and promotes breast cancer metastasis," *Oncogene*, 2013.

[15] V. Nardi, Y. Song, J. A. Santamaria-Barria et al., "Activation of PI3K signaling in merkel cell carcinoma," *Clinical Cancer Research*, vol. 18, no. 5, pp. 1227–1236, 2012.

[16] C. Hafner, R. Houben, A. Baeurle et al., "Activation of the PI3K/AKT pathway in merkel cell carcinoma," *PLoS ONE*, vol. 7, no. 2, Article ID e31255, 2012.

[17] S. D. Weeraratne, V. Amani, N. Teider et al., "Pleiotropic effects of miR-183~96~182 converge to regulate cell survival, proliferation and migration in medulloblastoma," *Acta Neuropathologica*, vol. 123, no. 4, pp. 539–552, 2012.

[18] M. van Gele, J. Helen Leonard, N. van Roy, A. L. Cook, A. de Paepe, and F. Speleman, "Frequent allelic loss at 10Q23 but low incidence of PTEN mutations in merkel cell carcinoma," *International Journal of Cancer*, vol. 92, no. 3, pp. 409–413, 2001.

[19] A. L. Sarver, H. Li, and S. Subramanian, "MicroRNA miR-183 functions as an oncogene by targeting the transcription factor EGR1 and promoting tumor cell migration," *Cancer Research*, vol. 70, no. 23, pp. 9570–9580, 2010.

[20] C. D. Shipkov, J.-M. Dumollard, A. Mojallal, and P. Seguin, "Merkel cell carcinoma vs. basal cell carcinoma: histopathologic challenges," *Journal of Cutaneous Pathology*, vol. 35, no. 8, pp. 789–790, 2008.

[21] S. Thakur, K. Chalioulias, M. Hayes, and A. While, "Bilateral primary Merkel cell carcinoma of the upper lid misdiagnosed as basal cell carcinoma," *Orbit*, vol. 27, no. 2, pp. 139–141, 2008.

[22] N. J. Ball and G. Tanhuanco-Kho, "Merkel cell carcinoma frequently shows histologic features of basal cell carcinoma: a study of 30 cases," *Journal of Cutaneous Pathology*, vol. 34, no. 8, pp. 612–619, 2007.

[23] L. Pilloni, C. Manieli, G. Senes, D. Ribuffo, and G. Faa, "Merkel cell carcinoma with an unusual immunohistochemical profile," *European Journal of Histochemistry*, vol. 53, no. 4, p. e33, 2009.

[24] K. B. Calder, S. Coplowitz, S. Schlauder, and M. B. Morgan, "A case series and immunophenotypic analysis of CK20−/CK7+ primary neuroendocrine carcinoma of the skin," *Journal of Cutaneous Pathology*, vol. 34, no. 12, pp. 918–923, 2007.

[25] N. Renwick, P. Cekan, P. A. Masry et al., "Multicolor microRNA FISH effectively differentiates tumor types," *The Journal of Clinical Investigation*, vol. 123, no. 6, pp. 2694–2702, 2013.

[26] U. Ralfkiaer, P. H. Hagedorn, N. Bangsgaard et al., "Diagnostic microRNA profiling in cutaneous T-cell lymphoma (CTCL)," *Blood*, vol. 118, no. 22, pp. 5891–5900, 2011.

[27] L. Poliseno, A. Haimovic, M. F. Segura et al., "Histology-specific microRNA alterations in melanoma," *Journal of Investigative Dermatology*, vol. 132, no. 7, pp. 1860–1868, 2012.

[28] A. Guastafierro, H. Feng, M. Thant et al., "Characterization of an early passage Merkel cell polyomavirus-positive Merkel cell carcinoma cell line, MS-1, and its growth in NOD scid gamma mice," *Journal of Virological Methods*, vol. 187, no. 1, pp. 6–14, 2013.

3

Mycosis Fungoides in Iranian Population: An Epidemiological and Clinicopathological Study

Farahnaz Fatemi Naeini,[1] Bahareh Abtahi-Naeini,[1,2] Hamidreza Sadeghiyan,[2] Mohammad Ali Nilforoushzadeh,[3] Jamshid Najafian,[4] and Mohsen Pourazizi[5]

[1] *Skin Diseases and Leishmaniasis Research Center, Department of Dermatology, Isfahan University of Medical Sciences, Isfahan, Iran*
[2] *Students' Research Committee, Isfahan University of Medical Sciences, Isfahan, Iran*
[3] *Skin and Stem Cell Research Center, Tehran University of Medical Sciences, Tehran, Iran*
[4] *Cardiovascular Research Center, Cardiovascular Research Institute, Isfahan University of Medical Sciences, Isfahan, Iran*
[5] *Students' Research Committee, Semnan University of Medical Sciences, Semnan, Iran*

Correspondence should be addressed to Mohsen Pourazizi; m.pourazizi@yahoo.com

Academic Editor: Iris Zalaudek

Background. Mycosis fungoides (MF) is the most common subtype of cutaneous T-cell lymphoma. Extensive studies on Iranian MF patients are absent. The present study aimed to produce updated clinical information on Iranian MF patients. *Methods.* This was a retrospective, descriptive, single-center study, including all cases of MF seen in the Department of Dermatology, University Hospital of Isfahan, Iran, between 2003 and 2013. Data systematically recorded for each patient included clinical, biological, histological, and molecular findings. *Results.* Eighty-six patients with clinical and histologic diagnosis of MF were included in the study. Thirty-nine patients (45.3%) were male. Female predominance was observed in patients (male : female ratio is 1 : 1.2). Patients were between 7 and 84 years of age (median: 41). The interval from disease onset to diagnosis ranged from 0 to 55 years (median: 1 year). Eighteen cases (20.9%) had unusual variants of MF. The most common types included hypopigmented and poikilodermatous MF. Childhood cases of MF constituted 5.8% (5/86) of all patients. The early stages were seen in 82 cases (95.34%). *Conclusion.* The major differences in epidemiologic characteristics of MF in Iran are the lack of male predominance and the lower age of patients at the time of diagnosis.

1. Introduction

Mycosis fungoides (MF) is the most common subtype of cutaneous T-cell lymphoma (CTCL). MF differs from other primary CTCLs by virtue of unique clinical features and histopathology [1, 2]. Patients with MF commonly present with persistent and/or slowly progressive skin lesions of varying size and shape [3].

The natural history of MF is characterized by an indolent progression through four stages: patch, plaque, tumor, and visceral involvement, but this progression is not necessarily seen in all patients [4]. Many variants of this lymphoma substantially differ from "classic" MF and are therefore sometimes referred to as "atypical" forms of the disease [4]. Atypical forms of MF include hypopigmented, hyperpigmented, ichthyosiform, pityriasis lichenoides-like, granulomatous, folliculotropic, bullous, palmoplantar, pagetoid reticulosis, and granulomatous slack skin [3, 4].

The peak age at presentation is in excess of 55 to 60 years, with a 2 : 1 male : female ratio [5, 6]. Although MF is a disease mainly seen in older patients, it can be seen in patients under the age of 35 with similar clinical findings [7, 8].

Extensive studies on Iranian MF patients are absent. The present study thus aimed to produce updated clinical information on Iranian MF patients, including epidemiology, patient characteristics, clinicopathologic features, and treatment.

2. Methods

Between 2003 and 2013, patients with MF from single-center resident training hospitals had been retrospectively enrolled into the study.

A diagnosis of MF was confirmed according to International Society for Cutaneous Lymphoma (ISCL)/EORTC criteria [1, 9] and, if necessary, based on the proposed algorithm for early phase disease [10].

The analyzed clinical data included the age of the patients at the time of diagnosis, the age of the patients at the time of initiation, the cutaneous lesion, sex, and the status of disease at the last follow-up examination. Hematoxylin and eosin-stained slides, immunohistochemical stains for basic B- and T-cell markers (CD20 and CD3 and/or CD45RO), and additional immunostaining, including CD4, CD8, CD30, and CD5, were histologically evaluated by an expert dermatopathologist. Polymerase chain reaction analyses of T-cell receptors (TCR) b or c and immunoglobulin heavy chain gene rearrangement were reviewed.

In all the patients, the presence of extracutaneous disease at the time of diagnosis had been excluded by standard staging procedures.

Stage workup (chest radiology, bone marrow biopsy, computed tomography scan of chest, abdomen, and pelvis) and overall survival were obtained by reviewing the clinical records.

To determine the stage of MF, the tumor-node-metastasis (TNM) system was used [11]. The clinical staging was performed as proposed by Olsen et al. [12].

After data collection, statistical analysis was performed by the SPSS software version 19.

3. Results

Eighty-six patients with clinical and histologic diagnosis of MF were included in the study.

Table 1 summarizes the demographic profiles and basic data of the 86 patients in our study with MF (Table 1). 45.3% patients (39 cases) were male. Female predominance was observed in the patients (male : female ratio is 1 : 1.2). All patients were Iranian. The patients with MF were between 7 and 84 years of age (median: 41). The mean ± standard deviation (SD) age at the time of skin lesion initiation was 45.02 ± 17.47 and 38.80 ± 16.02 for males and females, respectively.

The interval from disease onset to diagnosis ranged from 0 to 55 years (median: 1 year).

Table 2 summarizes the clinical and histologic variants of the patients with MF (Table 2). At the time of diagnosis, the most prevalent skin lesions were an erythematous scaly patch (Figure 1).

From 68 patients with classic MF, 42 patients presented with the patch, 21 with plaque, 4 with a tumor, and only one with erythroderma (Table 2). From 86 patients with MF, 18 cases (20.9%) had unusual variants. The most common types included hypopigmented MF (Figure 1(b)) and poikilodermatous MF (Figure 1(c)). Other clinical types of MF

Table 1: Demographic profile and basic data of 86 patients with mycosis fungoides.

Age (years)	
Range	7–84
Median	41
Mean (±SD)	41.51 ± 16.85
Sex	
Male	39 (45.3%)
Female	47 (54.7%)
Latent period (years)	
Range	0–55
Median	1
Mean (±SD)	4.67 ± 8.70
Type of MF	
Classic	68 (79.06%)
Variant	18 (20.94%)
TNM stage	
IA	36 (41.9%)
IB	43 (50%)
IIA	1 (1.2%)
IIB	5 (5.8%)
IIIA	1 (1.2%)
IVA1	0
IVA2	0
IVB	0

including pityriasis lichenoides-like lesions, syringotropic, ichthyosiform, and bullous variant were not observed in our patients. Hypopigmented skin lesions were seen in 5 (5.8%) patients and included a pure hypopigmented variant in three patients, whereas others had hypopigmented lesions mixed with other types. This group included 4 women and one man, 15–34 years of age, at diagnosis (Table 2). The patients with hypopigmented MF were observed to have a younger mean age at diagnosis (25.60 ± 7.30 years) as compared with other MF cases (42.52 ± 16.80 years).

Only one patient had folliculotropic MF (Figure 1(d)). One patient had lymphomatoid papulosis accompanying MF. Three patients (3.5%) had a solitary MF lesion, whereas others had multiple lesions (Table 2).

Childhood cases of MF (younger than 18 years) constituted 5.8% (5/86) of all the MF patients. There were two male and three female patients (male : female ratio is 1 : 1.5).

There was no familial clustering. None of the patients had HIV or other forms of immunosuppression.

According to the TNM classification, among 86 cases of MF, the early stage (stage I + IIA) included 82 cases (95.34%) and the advanced stage (stage IIB + III + IV) included four cases (4.66%). One female patient had a large cell transformation during the course of disease. Progression to the late stages of MF is not seen in childhood/juvenile-onset MF patients.

Immunophenotypic analysis demonstrated that 77.6% of the patients with MF were CD4 positive. CD20 was negative in all patients. In our patients, the conventional T-helper

TABLE 2: Clinical characteristics of patients based on the different clinical variants of mycosis fungoides.

Classification	Number of cases (%)	Sex		Age, year median (range)	Latent period, year median (range)	Staging	
		M	F			Early	Advanced
Classic type of MF ($n = 68$)							
(i) Patch	42 (48.8)	19	23	42 (7–82)	1 (0–27)	42	0
(ii) Plaque	21 (24.4)	11	10	48 (19–84)	1 (0–30)	21	0
(iii) Tumoral	4 (4.7)	3	1	55 (31–59)	7 (3–25)	2	2
(iv) Generalized erythroderma	1 (1.2)	1	0	45	1	0	1
Variant type of MF ($n = 18$)							
(i) Hypopigmented	5 (5.8)	1	4	28 (15–34)	3 (1–10)	5	0
(ii) Poikilodermic	5 (5.8)	2	3	44 (23–62)	1 (0–55)	5	0
(iii) Solitary	3 (3.5)	2	1	31 (30–38)	0 (0–6)	3	0
(iv) Hyperpigmented	2 (2.3)	0	2	32 (23–41)	0	2	0
(v) Folliculotropic	1 (1.2)	0	1	45	1	0	1
(vi) Pigmented purpura-like lesion	1 (1.2)	0	1	26	0	1	0
(vii) Hyperkeratotic	1 (1.2)	0	1	18	0	1	0

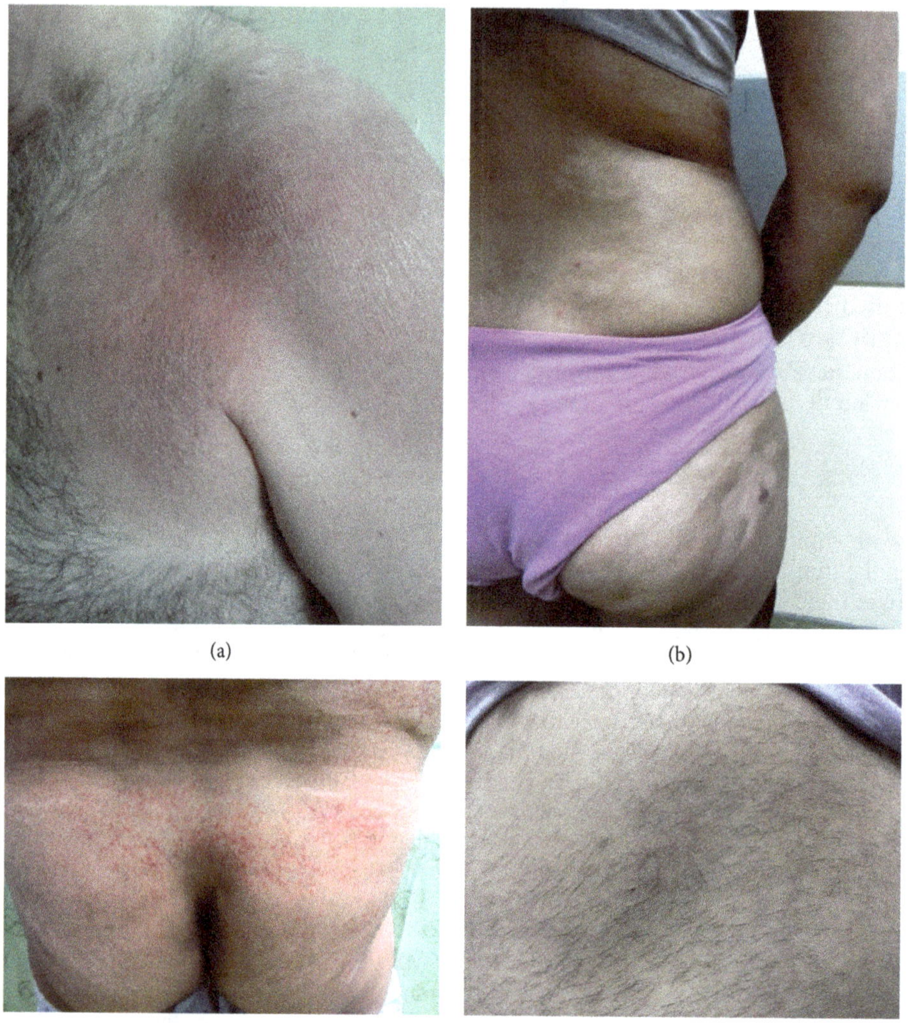

FIGURE 1: (a) Classic mycosis fungoides. Erythematous mildly scaly patch in the upper trunk. (b) Hypopigmented mycosis fungoides. Multiple hypopigmented and ill-defined to well-defined patches were seen on the back and thigh. (c) Poikilodermatous mycosis fungoides. The lesions are characterized by hypopigmentation and hyperpigmentation with atrophy and telangiectasia. (d) Folliculotropic mycosis fungoides. Diffuse perifollicular inflammatory papules coalescing into plaques.

TABLE 3: T-helper phenotype in 86 Iranian patients.

T-helper phenotype	Frequency	Percent (%)
CD4+/CD8+	13	15.5
CD4−/CD8−	4	4
CD4+/CD8−	54	63
CD4−/CD8+	15	17.5

TABLE 4: Treatment modalities used for mycosis fungoides in 86 Iranian patients[a].

Treatment modality	Number (%)
Topical corticosteroids	7 (8.1)
Topical carmustine (BCNU)	37 (43)
Topical nitrogen mustard	1 (1.2)
Narrow-band UVB (NBUVB)	33 (38.4)
Oral psoralen plus UVA (PUVA)	23 (26.7)
Local radiotherapy	3 (3.5)
Chemotherapy (systemic)	1 (1.2)
Methotrexate	1 (1.2)
Interferon	3 (3.5)

[a]Many patients had more than one treatment modality at different periods of their disease.

phenotype (CD4+/CD8−) was the most common one (63% of patients) (Table 3).

A clonal T-cell receptor rearrangement was detected in the skin biopsy in 9 patients (36%) from a total of 25 patients in whom T-cell receptor analysis was possible.

Antibodies to HTLV-1 were not detected in the sera of any patients with MF by ELISA. Seven patients (8.1%) had abnormal lactate dehydrogenase (LDH). None of the patients died during the study period in the early stages.

Table 4 summarizes the different treatment modalities used (Table 4). Thirteen patients (15.3%) of the whole achieved complete clearance.

4. Discussion

The major differences in the epidemiologic characteristics of MF in Isfahan, Iran, are lack of male predominance and the lower age of patients at the time of diagnosis in those reported from the West. It was reported that the incidence rate of MF in Isfahan is the same as that in other parts of Iran, which is largely similar to the data of other countries [7].

MF is generally rare among Asians and it has a higher incidence rate in blacks [13, 14]; it can be concluded that immunogenetics or interactions of genetic susceptibility and the environment may have a role in MF incidence [5].

There is a male predominance in almost all studies on CTCLs and MF, with a male : female ratio of 1.3 : 1 to 2 : 1 [15–17].

The proportion of our patients complaining on the onset of their disease before 21 years was much higher, similar to the epidemiological study in Kuwait [18]. The occurrence of MF in younger patients in Isfahan, Iran, may be related to some ethnic or genetic variations, but the environmental and occupational factors need to be determined.

Some studies have found an increased incidence of CTCL among workers in chemical science, transportation, and manufacturing industries, whereas other studies have not [19].

Hydrocarbons and petrochemical exposure have been reported to carry an increased MF risk [20, 21]. Whether a greater exposure to chemical agents has some contribution to the course of MF in this region remains to be determined.

In the Iran-Iraq War (1980–1988), it is not known whether chemical weapons by Iraq contained Sulfur mustard (SM), a DNA alkylation, and a well-known carcinogenic agent [22]. This hypothesis can be considered for relatively younger ages of diagnosis among the population in Kuwait. The exposure to burning oil during the war contributed to environmental pollution [18]. To evaluate a possibility of pollutants playing a role in the etiology of CTCL, more data needs to be addressed as potential confounders in future studies.

The prevalence of childhood MF among different studies has varied between 2.7% and 16.6% [23, 24]. In the present study, about 6% of cases were younger than 18 years at the time of diagnosis. Thus, our study is compatible with these reports. There was no significant difference in gender in our study in childhood MF.

Among the atypical forms of MF, hypopigmentation is one of the most prevalent forms in Asians [25]. Hypopigmented MF is overwhelming in Asians, with only 16 cases reported as of 2012 in Caucasians [3]. Compared with other clinical manifestations of MF, the hypopigmented MF is more prevalent in young age groups [18, 25]. The reason for the relative high frequency of hypopigmented MF in young patients is not known [26, 27]. In agreement with our study, the mean age at diagnosis is lower in the hypopigmented compared with the classic variant [28, 29]. On the other hand, the hypopigmented variant was noted in 79% of patients less than 18 years old [30].

Our data is compatible with the study of Quaglino et al. [31] in the fact that the current study showed a minority of patients were found to have tumor lesions or erythroderma and extracutaneous involvement. The definitive diagnosis of MF, particularly early stage of disease, is challenging as many of its clinical and pathologic features are nonspecific.

The median time from symptom onset to diagnosis in retrospective studies is 3-4 years, but it may exceed four decades [14, 32, 33].

The current study differs from that of Quaglino et al. in the fact that the median time from the onset of cutaneous lesions to diagnosis was 2 years [31].

In the present study, the mean time from symptom onset to definite diagnosis was about 5–10 years, which is significantly different in male and female patients.

Several studies have shown that nearly all patients with MF are HTLV-1 seronegative [34]. Our findings do not support an association between HTLV-1 infections and showed that MF does not correlate with HTLV-1 infections in Isfahan, Iran.

Usually, MF is characterized by an infiltrate of T-helper memory lymphocytes (CD3+, CD4+, CD5+, CD8−, and

CD45RO+) [1]. However, in a minority of cases the neoplastic cells exhibit a T-cytotoxic (CD4−/CD8+) or a CD4/CD8 double-negative phenotype that shows no clinical and/or prognostic differences [35]. de Marchi et al. showed that the coexpression of CD4 and CD8 in patients with MF is associated with a slightly lower rate of progressive disease compared with patients with conventional CD4+/CD8− phenotype. These findings raise the possibility that the coexpression of CD4 and CD8 in cutaneous lesions may confer a better prognosis in MF [36]. The lower tendency of progression of the disease in our patients with the coexpression of CD4 and CD8 might be related to the increased activity of antitumor CD8+ lymphocytes infiltrating the lesions [36].

5. Conclusions

Although the group of this study is really not very large and also the number of the patients with more advanced disease is small, it may be the starting point for a larger multicenter study in Iran. Whether the occurrence of MF in younger patients in Iran is related to some ethnic or genetic variations or to environmental factors needs to be determined. A prospective multicenter study on a larger population of patients with a longer follow-up might be useful to confirm the possible causes of these epidemiological differences.

Acknowledgments

The authors would like to thank Dr. Mina Saber (dermatologist) and Dr. Maryam Gholami (dermatologist) for their help with using the photoclinical databank.

References

[1] R. Willemze, E. S. Jaffe, G. Burg et al., "WHO-EORTC classification for cutaneous lymphomas," *Blood*, vol. 105, no. 10, pp. 3768–3785, 2005.

[2] R. S. Siegel, T. Pandolfino, J. Guitart, S. Rosen, and T. M. Kuzel, "Primary cutaneous T-cell lymphoma: review and current concepts," *Journal of Clinical Oncology*, vol. 18, no. 15, pp. 2908–2925, 2000.

[3] M. S. Jang, D. Y. Kang, J. B. Park, S. T. Kim, and K. S. Suh, "Cutaneous T-cell lymphoma in asians," *ISRN Dermatology*, vol. 2012, Article ID 575120, 8 pages, 2012.

[4] D. V. Kazakov, G. Burg, and W. Kempf, "Clinicopathological spectrum of mycosis fungoides," *Journal of the European Academy of Dermatology and Venereology*, vol. 18, no. 4, pp. 397–415, 2004.

[5] V. D. Criscione and M. A. Weinstock, "Incidence of cutaneous T-cell lymphoma in the United States, 1973–2002," *Archives of Dermatology*, vol. 143, no. 7, pp. 854–859, 2007.

[6] N. S. Agar, E. Wedgeworth, S. Crichton et al., "Survival outcomes and prognostic factors in mycosis fungoides/Sézary syndrome: validation of the revised International Society for Cutaneous Lymphomas/European Organisation for Research and Treatment of Cancer staging proposal," *Journal of Clinical Oncology*, vol. 28, no. 31, pp. 4730–4739, 2010.

[7] M. Salehi, Z. Azimi, F. Fatemi, P. Rajabi, M. Kazemi, and G. Amini, "Incidence rate of mycosis fungoides in Isfahan (Iran)," *The Journal of Dermatology*, vol. 37, no. 8, pp. 703–707, 2010.

[8] F. F. Naeini, H. Sadeghiyan, M. Pourazizi, J. Najafian, and B. Abtahi-Naeini, "Characteristics of primary cutaneous T-cell lymphoma in Iran: a 10-year retrospective study," *International Scholarly Research Notices*, vol. 2014, Article ID 820921, 5 pages, 2014.

[9] R. Willemze, H. Kerl, W. Sterry et al., "EORTC classification for primary cutaneous lymphomas: a proposal from the cutaneous lymphoma study group of the European organization for research and treatment of cancer," *Blood*, vol. 90, no. 1, pp. 354–371, 1997.

[10] N. Pimpinelli, E. A. Olsen, M. Santucci et al., "Defining early mycosis fungoides," *Journal of the American Academy of Dermatology*, vol. 53, no. 6, pp. 1053–1063, 2005.

[11] J. J. Scarisbrick, "Staging and management of cutaneous T-cell lymphoma," *Clinical and Experimental Dermatology*, vol. 31, no. 2, pp. 181–186, 2006.

[12] E. Olsen, E. Vonderheid, N. Pimpinelli et al., "Revisions to the staging and classification of mycosis fungoides and Sézary syndrome: a proposal of the International Society for Cutaneous Lymphomas (ISCL) and the cutaneous lymphoma task force of the European Organization of Research and Treatment of Cancer (EORTC)," *Blood*, vol. 110, no. 6, pp. 1713–1722, 2007.

[13] E. S. T. Tan, M. B. Y. Tang, and S. H. Tan, "Retrospective 5-year review of 131 patients with mycosis fungoides and Sézary syndrome seen at the National Skin Centre, Singapore," *Australasian Journal of Dermatology*, vol. 47, no. 4, pp. 248–252, 2006.

[14] R. van Doorn, C. W. van Haselen, P. C. V. V. Vader et al., "Mycosis fungoides: disease evolution and prognosis of 309 Dutch patients," *Archives of Dermatology*, vol. 136, no. 4, pp. 504–510, 2000.

[15] B. Tahmasebi, M. Mahmoudi, Y. Yahyapour, M. Jamshidi, and N. K. Holakouei, "Determination and comparison of incidence rate and trend of morbidity of leukemia and lymphoma in Mazandaran province (1376–1382)," *Journal of Mazandaran University of Medical Sciences*, vol. 16, no. 54, pp. 87–89, 2006.

[16] S. Babazadeh, A. R. Andalib, J. Emami et al., "Epidemiology of cancers in Isfahan province: a retrospective study (1981–1996)," *Journal of Research in Medical Sciences*. In press.

[17] R. A. Wilcox, "Cutaneous T-cell lymphoma: 2014 update on diagnosis, risk-stratification, and management," *The American Journal of Hematology*, vol. 89, pp. 837–851, 2014.

[18] Q. A. Alsaleh, A. Nanda, H. Al-Ajmi et al., "Clinicoepidemiological features of mycosis fungoides in Kuwait, 1991–2006," *International Journal of Dermatology*, vol. 49, no. 12, pp. 1393–1398, 2010.

[19] J. F. Moreau, J. M. Buchanich, J. Z. Geskin, O. E. Akilov, and L. J. Geskin, "Non-random geographic distribution of patients with cutaneous T-cell lymphoma in the Greater Pittsburgh Area," *Dermatology Online Journal*, vol. 20, no. 7, 2014.

[20] M. H. Greene, N. A. Dalager, S. I. Lamberg, C. E. Argyropoulos, and J. F. Fraumeni Jr., "Mycosis fungoides: epidemiologic observations," *Cancer Treatment Reports*, vol. 63, no. 4, pp. 597–606, 1979.

[21] M. M. Morales-Suárez-Varela, J. Olsen, P. Johansen et al., "Occupational sun exposure and mycosis fungoides: a european multicenter case-control study," *Journal of Occupational and Environmental Medicine*, vol. 48, no. 4, pp. 390–393, 2006.

[22] J. S. Graham and B. A. Schoneboom, "Historical perspective on effects and treatment of sulfur mustard injuries," *Chemico-Biological Interactions*, vol. 206, no. 3, pp. 512–522, 2013.

[23] E. Tan, Y. K. Tay, and Y. C. Giam, "Profile and outcome of childhood mycosis fungoides in Singapore," *Pediatric Dermatology*, vol. 17, no. 5, pp. 352–356, 2000.

[24] A. Nanda, Q. A. Alsaleh, H. Al-Ajmi et al., "Mycosis fungoides in arab children and adolescents: a report of 36 patients from Kuwait," *Pediatric Dermatology*, vol. 27, no. 6, pp. 607–613, 2010.

[25] R. Akaraphanth, M. C. Douglass, and H. W. Lim, "Hypopigmented mycosis fungoides: treatment and a 6(1/2)-year follow-up of 9 patients," *Journal of the American Academy of Dermatology*, vol. 42, no. 1, part 1, pp. 33–39, 2000.

[26] R. Fink-Puches, A. Chott, M. Ardigó et al., "The spectrum of cutaneous lymphomas in patients less than 20 years of age," *Pediatric Dermatology*, vol. 21, no. 5, pp. 525–533, 2004.

[27] P. Quaglino, A. Zaccagna, A. Verrone, F. Dardano, and M. G. Bernengo, "Mycosis fungoides in patients under 20 years of age: report of 7 cases, review of the literature and study of the clinical course," *Dermatology*, vol. 199, no. 1, pp. 8–14, 1999.

[28] U. Khopkar, B. R. Doshi, A. M. Dongre, and S. Gujral, "A study of clinicopathologic profile of 15 cases of hypopigmented mycosis fungoides," *Indian Journal of Dermatology, Venereology and Leprology*, vol. 77, no. 2, pp. 167–173, 2011.

[29] K. M. AlGhamdi, M. M. Arafah, L. A. Al-Mubarak, A. Khachemoune, and F. M. Al-Saif, "Profile of mycosis fungoides in 43 Saudi patients," *Annals of Saudi Medicine*, vol. 32, no. 3, pp. 283–287, 2012.

[30] P. M. Laws, N. H. Shear, and E. Pope, "Childhood mycosis fungoides: experience of 28 patients and response to phototherapy," *Pediatric Dermatology*, vol. 31, no. 4, pp. 459–464, 2014.

[31] P. Quaglino, N. Pimpinelli, E. Berti et al., "Time course, clinical pathways, and long-term hazards risk trends of disease progression in patients with classic mycosis fungoides: a multicenter, retrospective follow-up study from the Italian Group of Cutaneous Lymphomas," *Cancer*, vol. 118, no. 23, pp. 5830–5839, 2012.

[32] Y. H. Kim, H. L. Liu, S. Mraz-Gernhard, A. Varghese, and R. T. Hoppe, "Long-term outcome of 525 patients with mycosis fungoides and Sézary syndrome: clinical prognostic factors and risk for disease progression," *Archives of Dermatology*, vol. 139, no. 7, pp. 857–866, 2003.

[33] S. O. Arulogun, H. M. Prince, J. Ng et al., "Long-term outcomes of patients with advanced-stage cutaneous T-cell lymphoma and large cell transformation," *Blood*, vol. 112, no. 8, pp. 3082–3087, 2008.

[34] G. P. Taylor, "The epidemiology and clinical impact of HTLV infections in Europe," *AIDS Reviews*, vol. 1, no. 4, pp. 195–204, 1999.

[35] A. D. Tosca, A. G. Varelzidis, J. Economidou, and J. D. Stratigos, "Mycosis fungoides: evaluation of immunohistochemical criteria for the early diagnosis of the disease and differentiation between stages," *Journal of the American Academy of Dermatology*, vol. 15, no. 2, pp. 237–245, 1986.

[36] S. U. de Marchi, G. Stinco, E. Errichetti, S. Bonin, N. di Meo, and G. Trevisan, "The influence of the coexpression of CD4 and CD8 in cutaneous lesions on prognosis of mycosis fungoides: a preliminary study," *Journal of Skin Cancer*, vol. 2014, Article ID 624143, 4 pages, 2014.

4

Surgical Excision with Forehead Flap as Single Modality Treatment for Basal Cell Cancer of Central Face: Single Institutional Experience of 50 Cases

Jagdeep Rao[1] and Harsh Deora[2]

[1] *Department of Plastic Surgery, Sawai Man Singh Medical College, Jaipur, Rajasthan 300204, India*
[2] *Department of General Surgery, Sawai Man Singh Medical College, Jaipur, Rajasthan 300204, India*

Correspondence should be addressed to Harsh Deora; demo5601@gmail.com

Academic Editor: Arash Kimyai-Asadi

Basal cell carcinoma (BCC) is the most common skin cancer worldwide. The WHO has defined it as "a locally invasive, slowly spreading tumor which rarely metastasizes, arising in the epidermis or hair follicles and in which the peripheral cells usually simulate the basal cells of the epidermis." Here we discuss the management of BCCs of central face with surgical excision and reconstruction with forehead flap as single modality treatment. *Material and Methods.* This is a retrospective review of 50 patients who underwent surgical excision of BCC involving the facial region followed by primary reconstruction using forehead flaps at a single institution. There were 20 males and 30 females, mean age of 59 years. *Results.* No recurrence at primary site was observed during the follow-up of 1–4 yrs. There was no ectropion or exposure sequela. However, epiphora was evident. Size of lesions ranged from 2 to 6 cm. Keloid formation was seen in 2 (4%) patients. Functional and cosmetic outcomes were satisfactory. *Conclusion.* For the face, the best reconstructive effort eventually fails in the face of tumor recurrence. The forehead flap represents one of the best methods for repair of extensive facial defects. Complete tumor extirpation, the primary event, is the key.

1. Introduction

Basal cell carcinoma (BCC) is the most common skin cancer worldwide [1]. The World Health Organization Committee defined it based on the histological typing of skin tumors as "a locally invasive, slowly spreading tumor which rarely metastasizes, arising in the epidermis or hair follicles and in which, in particular, the peripheral cells usually simulate the basal cells of the epidermis" [2]. BCC constitutes approximately 75% of nonmelanoma skin cancers. It is usually observed in older patients, especially in those frequently and intensively exposed to ultraviolet radiation during their lives. The most typical site of BCC is uncovered skin directly exposed to the sun. Thus, BCC is often observed in head and neck areas, especially the eyelid and nose. It occurs chiefly in the elderly and is more common in males. Generally speaking, the tumor grows slowly and behaves in a nonaggressive fashion. BCC may be treated by surgery, cryotherapy, radiotherapy, and curettage and electrodessication [3]. Other less frequently used treatment modalities include the topical application of 5-fluorouracil (5-FU) ointment, laser treatment, and systemic chemotherapy [4]. To achieve a favorable outcome, it is important to recognize the histological subtypes, identify the anatomic locations that can increase the risk of spread, and understand the limitations of all available treatment modalities. If surgical defects are repaired, it is necessary to carefully plan the reconstruction after the tumor margins have been cleared. The forehead flap is an axial flap based on supraorbital/supratrochlear blood vessels. The flap has been used extensively in nasal reconstruction [5]. This paper discusses the management of basal cell carcinomas of the facial region with surgical excision and reconstruction with forehead flap as single modality treatment.

2. Patients and Methods

This is a retrospective review of 50 patients who underwent surgical excision of BCC involving the facial region followed

Table 1: Distribution of lesions on face.

Malar region	15
Nose	13
Eyelids	7
Cheeks	7
Forehead	4
Lips	2
Others	2
Total	50

Table 2: Size of lesions.

2-3 cm	28
3-4 cm	15
4-5 cm	5
5-6 cm	2

by primary reconstruction using forehead flaps. Patients who underwent reconstruction without forehead flaps were excluded. There were a total of 50 patients treated over a period of 3 years (2009–2012). There were 20 males and 30 females with a mean age of 59 years (range 50–71 years). In all patients, the diagnosis of BCC was confirmed by an incisional biopsy prior to definitive management. None of the patients had evidence of regional or distant metastasis (Table 1). This work was carried out in the Department of Plastic Surgery, Sawai Man Singh Medical College, Jaipur. The duration of follow-up ranged from 1 to 4 yrs.

2.1. Surgical Procedure. The forehead flap is a 2-stage procedure, and patients should receive preoperative counselling concerning their appearance between the first and second stages of the procedure. Thorough preoperative planning, including assessment of the defect, hairline height, and forehead laxity, is important. Patients should be given wound care instructions and realistic goals about the final outcome of their reconstruction. The lesion gross outline was marked by dots, and then about 5 mm free healthy margin was marked by a continuous line. The proposed reconstruction flap was marked at the same time. The defects following excision ranged from 3 × 4 cm to 5 × 7 cm in size (Table 2). In all cases, excision of the lesion included periosteum and, hence, bare bone was evident at the base of the defects.

2.2. Surgical Reconstruction. In all cases, the median or paramedian pedicled forehead flap was the main method of surgical reconstruction. For difficult areas such as those involving the medial canthus or the eyelids, the flap was rotated toward the defect for repair of the medial canthus, anterior lamella of the lower eyelid, and the side of the nose. Mucosal or skin grafts were sutured to the undersurface of the flap to reconstruct the conjunctiva. No cartilage grafts were used (to reconstruct the tarsal plate) because the flaps were "stiff" enough to provide self-support. Whenever possible (especially with defects extending to the nasolabial fold), primary closure of the edge of the defect was done. Lacrimal

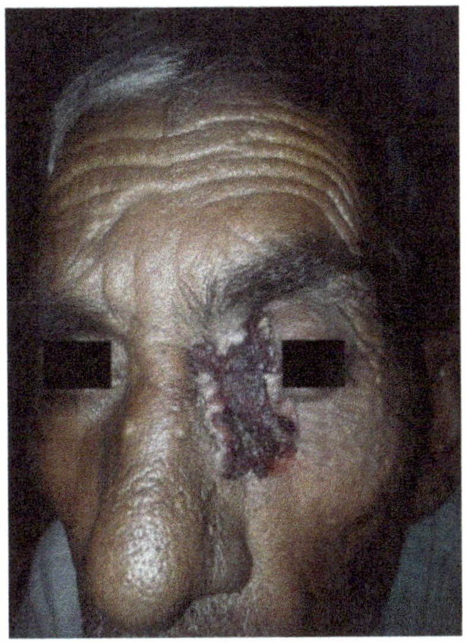

Figure 1: Preoperative image of BCC face involving medial canthus.

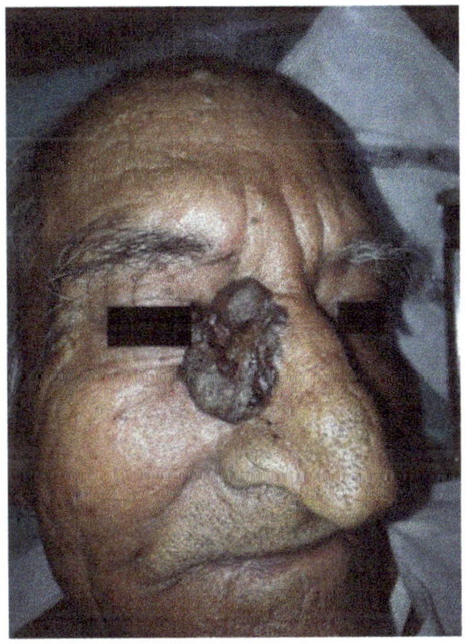

Figure 2: Preoperative image of BCC face.

system reconstruction was not performed in any of the patients. The donor sites of the forehead flaps were covered using split thickness skin grafts in 20 patients and primary closure using skin advancement in the remaining 30 patients. Forehead flaps were divided 3 weeks later. The pedicles were returned back to their donor sites in the forehead after excision of the skin grafts. Demonstrative examples are shown (Figures 1 and 2).

Patients are discharged home after surgery or kept overnight for observation and wound care. It has been our experience that most patients who undergo extensive nasal reconstruction appreciate an overnight admission to aid in wound care and to ensure adequate intravenous hydration. Prescriptions at discharge include a broad-spectrum antibiotic, which is to be taken for 7 to 10 days. A mild pain reliever, such as diclofenac sodium, and an antiemetic are often

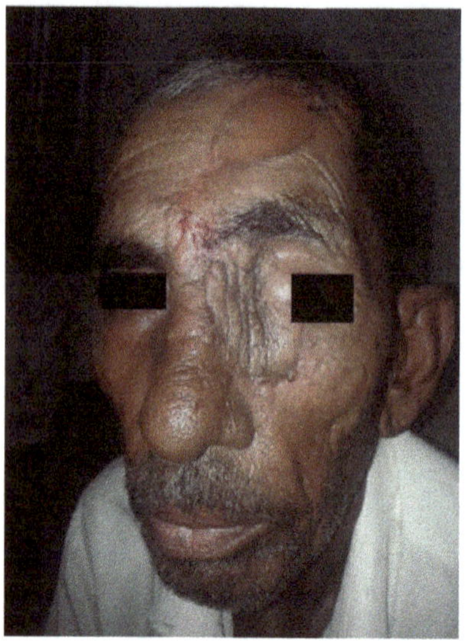

Figure 3: Reconstruction using forehead flap with SSG closure.

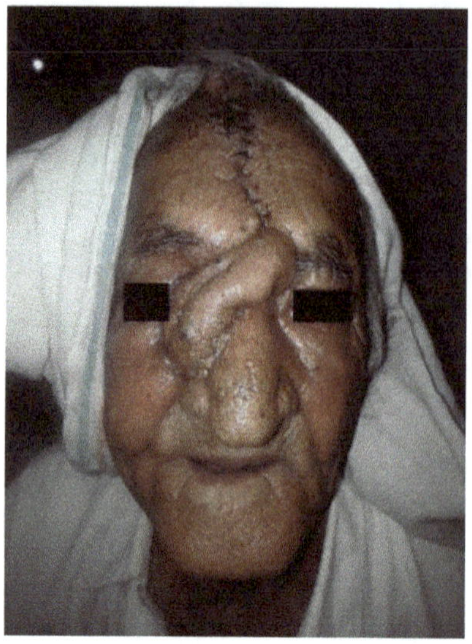

Figure 4: Reconstruction using forehead flap with primary closure.

prescribed. Postoperative wound care consists of twice daily cleansing of the suture lines with spirit and application of an antibiotic ointment or petroleum jelly.

3. Results

All patients tolerated the surgical procedures well with no systemic or anesthesia-related complications. There were no infections or hematomas. All flaps survived completely and there were no instances of skin/mucosal graft loss (Figures 3 and 4).

Follow-up ranged from 1 to 4 years (mean of 3 years). Tumor recurrence was not seen in any of the patients, during this period. Functionally, whenever the eyelid was involved, there was no ectropion and the margin was well aligned and stable. Eyelid closure was adequate and there were no exposure sequelae. However, epiphora was evident since lacrimal system reconstruction was not performed.

Cosmetically, there were some color mismatch and no eyelashes. All patients required debulking of the flaps because of the bulky appearance. Debulking was done 3–6 months following the reconstructive procedures. In 30 patients, the entire forehead donor site was closed at the time of primary reconstruction. In the rest of the 20 patients, partial graft loss was observed in 5 of them which was later excised at the time of dressing and was allowed to heal secondarily. Keloid formation was seen in 2 patients (4%). All patients were satisfied with the functional and cosmetic outcomes (Figure 5).

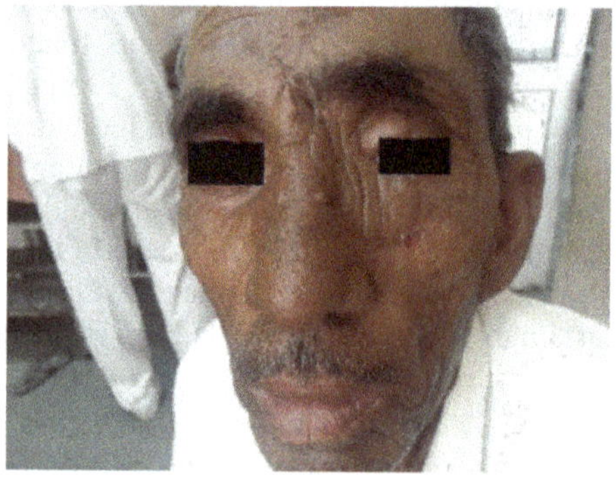

Figure 5: Final result at follow-up.

4. Discussion

Basal cell carcinoma grows slowly and is painless. A lesion that bleeds easily or does not heal well may be suspected for BCC. The majority of these cancers occur on areas of skin that are regularly exposed to sunlight or other ultraviolet radiation as in the midface [6]. They may also appear on the scalp. All managed cases gave in the history long duration of exposure to the sunlight due to either their occupations (farmers) or social hobbies (swimming for long duration in summer vacations). All cases had lesions on the midface, where exposure to sun is intense.

Basal cell skin cancer used to be more common in people over age of 40 [7]. In our series all cases (100%) were senile and over age of 50 years, as long period and repeated exposure to sunlight are required to introduce the malignant changes in the skin.

Basal cell skin cancers almost never spread, but metastatic cases have been reported. If left untreated, it may grow into surrounding areas and destroy nearby tissues and bone [8, 9]. We have not recorded metastases in our cases. Multiple lesions on the face are common, and new lesions may appear during various years of follow-up, as the predisposing factors cause wide and diffuse skin changes which are not localized to one site [10]. In our series, no patient had multiple lesions on the face on initial presentation. The rate of recurrence is reported to vary and between 6 and 10% [11]. In this study, in the duration of follow-up, no patient developed recurrence at sites of previous resections. Excision of large facial malignant ulcer with forehead flap based on the supratrochlear artery or the frontal branch of a side superficial temporal artery in a 1-stage operation [12] has also been reported but the series is usually small and a two-stage reconstruction offers a better uptake, especially in older patients.

The criterion for surgical treatment varies depending on the size, depth, and location of the lesions. The aim was to excise the tumor radically with gross 5 mm free margins and to reconstruct the defect with the least cosmetic deformity, taking into consideration putting the line of resection in or parallel to normal skin creases.

Periocular reconstruction following the excision of cutaneous malignancy includes providing stable eyelid margin, providing reasonable symmetry with smooth internal surfaces, providing adequate eyelid closure to avoid exposure sequelae, restoring normal tension, and providing sufficient horizontal and vertical eyelid dimensions for maximal function [13, 14]. Although various local flaps have been used for the reconstruction of medial canthus/adjacent eyelid defects [15, 16], we find the forehead flap to be the most suited for these defects. In fact, we believe it should be considered as the flap of choice in large defects mainly because it satisfies the principles of periocular reconstruction. The proximity of the flap and the arc of its rotation make it easier to provide a stable eyelid margin. The flap is an axial type with rich blood supply and, hence, it could be of sufficient size to ensure adequate reconstruction of large defects without tension or vertical eyelid deficiency. The rich blood supply at the distal end of the flap also ensures good take of the mucosal or skin grafts which provide conjunctival reconstruction in full thickness eyelid defects.

For nasal reconstructions, the midline forehead skin flap can serve as a cover for any nasal reconstruction from severe tip and ala loss to a total nasal defect. Using this flap, aesthetic and functional reconstruction can be achieved by creating a nose that blends well with the face. The seagull-shaped flap is based on one of the supratrochlear vessel bundles. Its vertical axis is placed over the midline of the forehead, and the wings are designed to lie in natural transverse creases. The forehead flap is elevated and transposed 180° to cover the new nose. The body of the seagull lies along the bridge, the wings curl at the ala and turn into the nostril sills, and the seagull head and neck create the tip and columella [17].

Despite all these advantages, some disadvantages when using forehead flaps should be mentioned, which include the two-stage procedure, the color mismatch, the bulkiness of the flap, and the donor site scar.

There are also few rare complications such as sepsis and necrosis which are avoided by gentle care of flaps, antibiotics, plenty of fluid intake, wide pedicle covered with petroleum gauze, and avoidance of excess torsion at base [18].

5. Conclusion

The face is one of the most common locations for skin cancer and frequently represents a significant challenge for reconstruction after surgical excision. Reconstruction of defects created by removal of cancer represents the secondary event in successful skin cancer treatment. Complete tumor extirpation, the primary event, is the key. The best reconstructive effort eventually fails in the face of tumor recurrence. The forehead flap represents one of the best methods for repair of extensive facial defects. Outstanding functional and cosmetic results can be achieved. Proper execution requires considerable technical skill and experience. Preoperative counseling is vitally important. Also, a thorough understanding of anatomy and aesthetics is required.

References

[1] H.-Y. Lin, C.-Y. Cheng, W.-M. Hsu, W. H. L. Kao, and P. Chou, "Incidence of eyelid cancers in Taiwan. A 21-year review," *Ophthalmology*, vol. 113, no. 11, pp. 2101–2107, 2006.

[2] G. H. Jacobs, J. J. Rippey, and M. Altini, "Prediction of aggressive behavior in basal cell carcinoma," *Cancer*, vol. 49, no. 3, pp. 533–537, 1982.

[3] M. T. Lalloo and S. Sood, "Head and neck basal cell carcinoma: treatment using a 2-mm clinical excision margin," *Clinical Otolaryngology and Allied Sciences*, vol. 25, no. 5, pp. 370–373, 2000.

[4] Y. Ö. Tiftikcioğlu, Ö. Karaaslan, H. M. Aksoy, B. Aksoy, and U. Koçer, "Basal cell carcinoma in Turkey," *Journal of Dermatology*, vol. 33, no. 2, pp. 91–95, 2006.

[5] A. C. Paddack, R. W. Frank, H. J. Spencer, J. M. Key, and E. Vural, "Outcomes of paramedian forehead and nasolabial interpolation flaps in nasal reconstruction," *Archives of Otolaryngology—Head and Neck Surgery*, vol. 138, no. 4, pp. 367–371, 2012.

[6] American Academy of Pediatrics, "Policy statement—ultraviolet radiation: a hazard to children and adolescents," *Pediatrics*, vol. 127, no. 3, pp. 588–597, 2011.

[7] American Cancer Society, *Facts & Figures 2011*, American Cancer Society, Atlanta, Ga, USA, 2011.

[8] M. Akinci, S. Aslan, F. Markoç, B. Cetin, and A. Cetin, "Metastatic basal cell carcinoma," *Acta Chirurgica Belgica*, vol. 108, no. 2, pp. 269–272, 2008.

[9] A. Vu and D. Laub Jr., "Metastatic basal cell carcinoma: a case report and review of the literature," *Eplasty*, vol. 11, article ic8, 2011.

[10] P. Mohanty, L. Mohanty, and B. P. Devi, "Multiple cutaneous malignancies in xeroderma pigmentosum," *Indian Journal of Dermatology, Venereology and Leprology*, vol. 67, no. 2, pp. 96–97, 2001.

[11] N. M. Mc Loone, J. Tolland, M. Walsh, and O. M. Dolan, "Follow-up of basal cell carcinomas: an audit of current practice," *Journal of the European Academy of Dermatology and Venereology*, vol. 20, no. 6, pp. 698–701, 2006.

[12] X. F. Xiang, B. Cheng, J. B. Tang, Y. H. Wu, M. Xuan, and Y. Peng, "The scalping forehead flap for 1-stage reconstruction of large facial defects after tumor resection," *The Journal of Craniofacial Surgery*, vol. 24, no. 4, pp. e346–e347, 2013.

[13] S. M. Hayano, K. M. Whipple, B. S. Korn, and D. O. Kikkawa, "Principles of periocular reconstruction following excision of cutaneous malignancy," *Journal of Skin Cancer*, vol. 2012, Article ID 438502, 6 pages, 2012.

[14] C. N. Czyz, K. V. Cahill, J. A. Foster, K. S. Michels, C. M. Clark, and N. E. Rich, "Reconstructive options for the medial canthus and eyelids following tumor excision," *Saudi Journal of Ophthalmology*, vol. 25, no. 1, pp. 67–74, 2011.

[15] S. G. J. Ng, C. F. Inkster, and B. Leatherbarrow, "The rhomboid flap in medial canthal reconstruction," *British Journal of Ophthalmology*, vol. 85, no. 5, pp. 556–559, 2001.

[16] J. Yan, L. Liu, and J. Qian, "Reconstruction of upper eyelid and medial canthus following basal cell carcinoma resection: a successful one-stage repair with three local flaps," *International Journal of Dermatology*, vol. 52, no. 5, pp. 611–613, 2013.

[17] D. R. Millard, "Midline forehead skin flap," in *Grabb's Encyclopedia of Flaps*, S. Berish, Ed., vol. 1, pp. 99–100, Lippincott Williams & Wilkins, Philadelphia, Pa, USA, 2009.

[18] H. T. Hoffman and S. R. Baker, "Nasal reconstruction with the rapidly expanded forehead flap," *Laryngoscope*, vol. 99, no. 10 I, pp. 1096–1098, 1989.

5

Merkel Cell Carcinoma of the Head and Neck: A Single Institutional Experience

G. Morand,[1] D. Vital,[1] T. Pézier,[1] D. Holzmann,[1] M. Roessle,[2] A. Cozzio,[3] and G. F. Huber[1]

[1] *Division of Otolaryngology, Head and Neck Surgery, University Hospital Zurich, Frauenklinikstraße 24, 8091 Zurich, Switzerland*
[2] *Institute of Surgical Pathology, University Hospital Zurich, Frauenklinikstraße 24, 8091 Zurich, Switzerland*
[3] *Division of Dermatology, University Hospital Zurich, Frauenklinikstraße 24, 8091 Zurich, Switzerland*

Correspondence should be addressed to G. Morand; gregoire.morand@usz.ch

Academic Editor: Boban M. Erovic

Merkel cell carcinoma (MCC) is a rare cutaneous malignancy occurring mostly in older immunocompromized Caucasian males. A growing incidence of MCC has been reported in epidemiological studies. Treatment of MCC usually consists of surgical excision, pathological lymph node evaluation, and adjuvant radiotherapy. This paper reports the experience of a single tertiary center institution with 17 head and neck Merkel cell carcinoma patients. Median followup for the cohort was 37.5 months. After five years, recurrence-free survival, disease specific survival, and overall survival were 85%, 90%, and 83%, respectively. Our limited data support the use of adjuvant radiotherapy. We also report two cases of MCC located at the vestibule of the nose and two cases of spontaneous regression after diagnostic biopsy. About 40% of our patients were referred to our center for surgical revision and pathological lymph node evaluation. Increased awareness of MCC and an interdisciplinary approach are essential in the management of MCC.

1. Introduction

In 1875, Merkel, professor of anatomy at the University of Rostock, Germany, for the first time described "Tastzellen" (touch cells)—later known as Merkel cells—in the epidermis of domestic animals and humans [1]. In 1972, Toker first reported a case series of five patients with "trabecular carcinoma" and recognized a "distinct pathological entity," with a "capricious clinical behaviour" [2]. It took Tang and Toker another six years to determine that trabecular carcinoma "most probably" derives from Merkel cells [3].

More recently, in 2008, a previously unknown polyomavirus was found to be integrated in Merkel cell carcinoma (MCC) [4]. Now known as Merkel Cell polyomavirus (MCV), this virus is indeed thought to be a causative agent in MCC [5, 6] and has been associated with about 80% of MCC cases [4, 7–10]. A previous study from our institution reported similar prevalence of MCV in MCC [11]. Conflicting evidence exists about the prognostic value of MCV status [7, 8, 12–14].

Important differential diagnoses of MCC are basal cell carcinoma, small cell melanoma, lymphoma, small blue round cell tumours, and especially metastatic small cell lung carcinoma [15]. A thorough histo- or cytopathological workup including immunohistochemistry (e.g., CK20, TTF-1, and neuroendocrine markers) [16] combined with entire examination and clinical history usually allows to differentiate the above mentioned entities.

A recent study by Smith et al. [17] drawn from an US-population based database (SEER) with over 4,300 MCC patients showed that 48% of all MCC are primarily located in the head and neck area (HN-MCC), with men representing about 61% of the patient population. The overwhelming majority of patients were Caucasian.

Hodgson [18] reported a incidence of Merkel cell carcinoma of 0.44/100,000/year in 2001 from the same database. Interestingly, there seems to be a sharp increase in the number of cases being reported. Hodgson performed a comparative analysis and showed an 8% estimated annual percentage change (EAPC) in MCC incidence from 1986 until 2001. This change was attributed to the ageing of population and the growing prevalence of immunocompromized patients, two known risk factors for MCC [18–22]. Furthermore, the authors noted that this change might also result from increased awareness and reporting of MCC [18]. A further risk factor for MCC is UVB exposure, as shown in epidemiological studies [23] and mutations analysis of TP53 [24]. Expression of p53 has been correlated to MCV-negative MCC [13, 14, 25], thus suggesting a different pathogenesis in MCV-positive and MCV-negative MCC.

The authors of another epidemiological study from The Netherlands [19] reported similar incidence trends of MCC with an EAPC of 8%. For the same period, the EAPC for melanoma and squamous cell carcinoma of the skin were 4% and about 2%, respectively.

The prognosis of MCC remains poor, with a 5-year relative survival for local, regional, and metastatic disease of about 75%, 50%, and 20%, respectively [19]. Smith et al. reported a 5-year disease specific survival for pN0, pN1, and M1 in HN-MCC patients of 83.3%, 58.3%, and 31.3%, respectively [17]. Epidemiological analyses have established several prognostic factors in HN-MCC [17]: male sex, >T2-primaries, N-positive, M-positive, and tumour location at the lip were shown to be independent negative risk factors. Unlike for nonhead and neck-MCC (NHN-MCC), increasing tumour size was not a prognostic factor for HN-MCC [17].

Lemos et al. have shown the critical impact of pathological lymph node evaluation for MCC patients [26]. For example, in the management of cutaneous melanoma, sentinel lymph node biopsy (SLNB) is now a standard of care [27]. Analogically, SLNB has gained popularity in the past years in the management of MCC, currently being recommended as standard treatment [28], independently of the size of the primary tumour [29–32], as SLNB permits a pathological lymph node evaluation with less morbidity compared to elective neck dissection [33, 34]. SLNB studies have shown that about 30% of cN0 MCC patients harbour occult metastasis [35, 36], with up to 20% false negative rate [37, 38].

Prophylactic irradiation is usually accepted as an alternative in the management of the clinically negative neck [39].

The superiority of adjuvant radiotherapy in local and regional control has been shown in a meta-analysis of observational studies [40]. A recent multicentric prospective randomized controlled trial conducted in France again showed improved locoregional control [41]. Both studies could not prove a significant advantage of adjuvant radiotherapy on disease specific survival.

For inoperable patients, an in-field control rate of 75% has been reported with radiotherapy alone, with 55 Gy as a minimum dose for macroscopic disease [42]. Other studies also show acceptable results for radiotherapy alone [43, 44].

The aim of this study was to report the experience of a single institution tertiary center in Switzerland.

2. Methods

After local ethics committee approval, we performed a retrospective chart review of all patients treated for a Merkel cell carcinoma in the department for Otorhinolaryngology—Head and Neck Surgery—at the University Hospital of Zurich, Switzerland, between January 1990 and August 2012. We searched our electronic patient database using the following keywords: "Merkel cell carcinoma," "Merkel cell," and the ICD-10-Code for Merkel cell carcinoma (C44.*). A single reviewer (GM) was responsible for sorting the eligible patients out of the generated list.

Inclusion criteria were confirmed histopathological diagnosis of Merkel cell carcinoma and location of the primary tumour in the head and neck. Only patients treated at our department were included. Patients treated by other departments (e.g., plastic surgery) were not included.

For each patient, the following parameters were assessed: tumour site, age, sex, immunosuppression, TNM-stadium (AJCC, 7th Edition 2010 [39]), treatment modality of local and regional disease, location of primary tumour, surgical margins, recurrence-free survival (RFS), disease specific survival (DSS), and overall survival (OS).

Descriptive statistics were performed using Microsoft Excel 2007. Kaplan Meier estimates were calculated using IBM SPSS 19 and the survival functions were compared by log rank tests.

3. Results

3.1. Demographics, Tumour Location, Staging, and Risk Factors. Seventeen patients (4 male, 13 female, ratio 1 : 3.3) met the inclusion criteria (Table 1). The mean age was 71 y (SD 15.8, median 73, range 40–89). Ten primaries (58%) were located on the cheek, two on the external ear (12%), two in the vestibule of the nose (12%), one at the lower lip (6%), one at the eyelid (6%), and one at the glabella (6%). Diabetes was reported for one patient (6%); HIV/AIDS or immunosuppression after organ transplant was not reported for any patients.

According to AJCC, 7th Edition 2010 [45], stage Ia was present in four cases (24%); stage Ib in one (6%); stage IIa in two (12%); stage IIb in two (12%); stages IIc and IIIa in zero; stage IIIb in four (24%); and stage IV in zero cases. In four patients (24%), tumour stage was not available because of missing data.

Median followup for the cohort was 37.5 months (mean 62, SD 72, range 5–288). One patient (6%) died of Merkel cell carcinoma, three (18%) of other causes. After five years, recurrence-free survival (RFS), disease specific survival (DSS), and overall survival (OS) were 85%, 90%, and 83%, respectively (Figure 1).

3.2. Treatment Options, Surgical Margins, Pathological Lymph Node Evaluation. Sixteen patients (94%) underwent primary surgical resection. One patient (6%) underwent primary radiotherapy, as surgical excision would have resulted in complete removal of the nose, which was unacceptable to the patient. This patient was excluded from further analysis.

In three out of sixteen patients (19%), surgical excision margins of 2 cm were reported and in two cases margins of 1 cm (13%). In one case (6%), Mohs surgery was used.

In three cases (19%), margins smaller than 1 cm were used, twice because the surgeon did not consider MCC in the

Table 1: Summary of patients characteristics.

∘	Age	Sex	Location	Side	T	N	M	Therapy	Recurrence	Followup	Outcome
1	73	f	Cheek	Right	pT2	cN0	M0	Excision only	No	170	MCC unrelated death
2	81	f	Cheek	Left	pT2	pN0 (0/31)	M0	Excision + ND + RT	No	9	RFS
3	52	f	Vestibule of nose	Right	pT1	pN0 (sn 0/4)	M0	Excision + SLNB	No	18	RFS
4	88	f	Glabella	Middle	pT1	cN0	M0	Excision only	Yes[§]	27	disease specific death
5	86	f	Pinna	left	pTx	cN0	M0	Excision + RT[*]	No	0	lost to followup
6	64	m	Cheek	Right	pT1	pN0 (sn 0/1)	M0	Excision + SLNB + RT	No	72	RFS
7	57	f	Cheek	Right	pT1	pN0 (sn 0/3)	M0	Excision + SLNB	No	66	RFS
8	73	f	Lower lid	Left	pTx	pN0 (sn 0/1)	M0	Excision + SLNB	Yes[‡]	74	MCC unrelated death
9	86	m	Cheek	Left	pT2	pN0 (0/23)	M0	Excision + ND + RT[**]	No	36	RFS
10	65	f	Cheek	Left	pTx	pN0 (sn 0/2)	M0	Excision + SLNB + RT	No	39	RFS
11	40	f	Cheek	Left	pT1	pN1b (4/26)	M0	Excision + ND + RT	No	21	RFS
12	62	f	Cheek	Right	pT1	pN0 (0/40)	M0	Excision + ND + RT	No	24	RFS
13	86	m	Pinna	Right	pT1	pN2 (3/21)	M0	Excision + ND + RT	No	11	MCC unrelated death
14	51	f	Cheek	Right	pTx	cN0	M0	Excision + RT	No	288	RFS
15	72	m	Lower lip	Middle	pTx	pN1b (3/28)[$]	M0	Excision + ND + RT	No	63	RFS
16	77	f	Cheek	Right	pT2	pN1b (1/25)	M0	Excision + ND + RT	No	72	RFS
17	89	f	Vestibule of nose	Left	cT2	cN0	M0	Radiotherapy only	No	5	RFS

Age in years; f: female; m: male. TNM stadium according to AJCC, 7th Edition, 2010. RT: radiotherapy. [$]bilateral neck dissection, left 3/14, right 0/14. [*]RT refused by patient. [**]RT could not be performed because of wound healing problems. [§]regional recurrence after 11 months. [‡]local recurrence after 12 months. Followup in months. SLNB: sentinel lymph node biopsy. ND: neck dissection. RFS: recurrence-free survival. MCC: Merkel cell carcinoma.

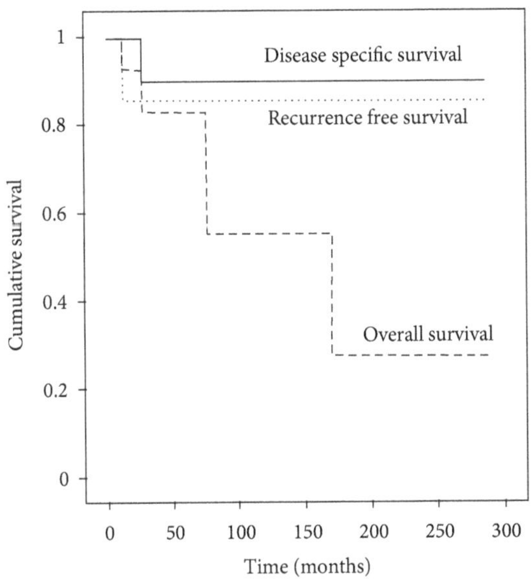

Figure 1: Survival analysis.

clinical differential diagnosis. For the remaining case, a two-step surgery was chosen, with the use of artificial skin graft, whilst a definitive histological margin was performed which led to a further excision a week later.

In seven cases (44%), surgical margins were not available; all these patients were referred to our institution after having primary surgery elsewhere.

All of the patients who had planned 2 cm excision margins had clear histological margins. One of the two patients with a planned 1 cm margin had to undergo a second operation to obtain clear histological margins. This patient (number 8) did not receive adjuvant radiotherapy as the primary was located at the lower lid and concerns were raised about the irradiation of the eye. He suffered a local recurrence one year later and had to undergo extended resection with orbital exenteration, free flap reconstruction, and adjuvant radiotherapy.

Of the patients who were initially operated in other hospitals and for those with planned excision margins of <1 cm, nine out of ten (90%) had to undergo at least one second surgical intervention. Data is incomplete for the last patient.

There was not statistical relation between surgical margins and recurrence-free survival ($P = 0.47$).

Of the sixteen patients who underwent primary surgical excision, sentinel lymph node biopsy was performed in five patients (31%) and was always negative. Mean number of sentinel nodes was 2.2 (range 1–4).

Two patients (12%) underwent therapeutic selective neck dissection for clinically positive neck disease (patients 11 and 13).

Five patients (31%) had elective selective neck dissections, showing regional disease in two cases (12%).

Five patients (31%) underwent, in addition to neck dissection, superficial parotidectomy, due to the localisation of the primary tumour and the expected lymphatic drainage. No disease was found in any of the parotid specimens.

Five patients (31%) did not have any pathological node evaluation, in one case because of the patient comorbidities. This patient (number 4) went on to develop regional recurrence 11 months later. He could not undergo salvage neck dissection and was treated with locoregional radiotherapy.

A few months later, he had distant metastatic disease and died twenty-six months after the initial surgery.

3.3. Recurrence, Radiotherapy, and Outcome. Two patients (12%) developed the locoregional recurrence. Patient 8 had a primary at the lower eyelid with a local recurrence 12 months after primary surgery. Patient 4 showed a regional recurrence, as discussed above. These patients received radiotherapy after locoregional recurrence.

In eleven patients (69%), adjuvant radiotherapy was recommended. One patient (6%) refused and another patient could not undergo radiotherapy because of severe wound healing problems.

Three patients (31%) did not have any radiation. Two of them underwent excision biopsy outside our clinic and were referred for revision surgery and pathological node evaluation. For both patients, the revision specimens and SLNB were free of tumour in the histopathological analysis. Adjuvant radiotherapy was therefore not performed.

Of the nine patients who had adjuvant radiotherapy following surgery, none suffered recurrence. Without adjuvant radiotherapy following surgery, two of six patients (33%) developed locoregional recurrence. There was a trend to a better RFS in patients who underwent adjuvant radiation ($P = 0.051$, log rank test).

Mean adjuvant radiation dose was 62.4 Gy (SD 4.8, median 62, range 54–70).

4. Discussion

MCC is a rare malignancy, occurring mostly in older immunocompromized Caucasian males. As the population in most Western countries continues ageing [46] and the prevalence of immunosuppression increases [47], epidemiological studies have shown an increase in MCC incidence.

The growing incidence of MCC has led to an increased awareness and reporting of MCC. Searching for "Merkel cell carcinoma" in PubMed database reveals a steady increase in results by year, with about 40 publications per year in the 90s, to over 160 publications for the year 2010 or 2011.

We report here a single institution retrospective analysis. The demographics of our patient cohort differ from other retrospective reports, as do our survival rates [17, 48–51]. The mean age is slightly lower than in other larger reports [17] and we have a predominance of women and no immunosuppressed patients, which could be explained by our relatively small patient cohort.

Considering a cohort with elderly patients, a difference between the OS and the DSS can be explained by comorbidities. We had in fact more disease unrelated deaths as disease specific deaths in the follow-up period.

In comparison to other reports [26, 40, 52], our favourable DSS and DFS could be explained by high rate of combined therapy, high rate of pathological lymph node dissection, low rate of distant disease at diagnosis, a predominance of women [17], and lack of immunosuppressed patients [22]. Our results must however been interpreted in light of the small cohort size.

As reported elsewhere [53], we did not find surgical margins to significantly affect recurrence-free survival. This is consistent with the fact that clear histological margins were obtained for every patient, independently of the surgical excision margins chosen initially. For HN-MCC, we recommend margins of 1 cm, or nonfeasible, two-step or Mohs surgery [28, 54, 55].

We observed a trend supporting the use of adjuvant radiotherapy. Although not significant, this result complies with stronger evidence [40, 41].

We report two cases of MCC occurring in the vestibule of the nose. This location has been reported very rarely in the literature [56]. One patient was treated using Mohs surgery. For the other patient, primary radiotherapy was chosen because an ablation of the nose would have been necessary to obtain clear surgical margins.

We also report two cases of surgical revision after external excision biopsy with lack of MCC cells in the revision specimen and SLNB, thus who either had been fully excised surgically or with spontaneous regression following biopsy, as already described in many other reports [56–61].

Analogically, MCC of unknown primary has also been described [62, 63]. Although the mechanism of regression is not known, immune infiltration has been proposed [64]. However, in a recent study with 37 patients, no significant increase in intratumoral CD8 T-cell infiltration after biopsy could be found [65].

As seven out of seventeen of the patients (41%) in this study were referred to surgical revision and pathological lymph node evaluation, we think that continuing education is essential, particularly for house physicians and general practitioners, who need to be aware of this rare but increasing malignancy, usually gentle in presentation [66, 67].

Our results should be interpreted cautiously, as biased by missing data and heterogeneous population. Our statistical analysis lacks power due to our low number of patientS and events. As a tertiary center, we also suffer referral bias. Nevertheless, bearing these caveats in mind, we believe that a few lessons can be learned from this paper.

In conclusion, we believe that increased awareness of MCC is essential to ensure an optimal initial management. Failure to do so can lead to a higher number of surgical interventions and missing or incomplete pathological staging.

Surgical removal of HN-MCC should assure oncological sufficient treatment, while preserving cosmetic or functional essential structure. An alternate surgical technique should be used, as appropriate.

To overcome these challenges, we strongly believe that a multidisciplinary approach and collaboration is essential. In accordance with the available literature, in Zurich, we have established an internal guideline, with a systematic assessing of several variables, thus allowing high quality data for further studies.

References

[1] F. Merkel, "Tastzellen und Tastkörperchen bei den Hausthieren und beim Menschen," *Archiv für Mikroskopische Anatomie*, vol. 11, no. 1, pp. 636–652, 1875.

[2] C. Toker, "Trabecular carcinoma of the skin," *Archives of Dermatology*, vol. 105, no. 1, pp. 107–110, 1972.

[3] C. K. Tang and C. Toker, "Trabecular carcinoma of the skin. An ultrastructural study," *Cancer*, vol. 42, no. 5, pp. 2311–2321, 1978.

[4] H. Feng, M. Shuda, Y. Chang, and P. S. Moore, "Clonal integration of a polyomavirus in human Merkel cell carcinoma," *Science*, vol. 319, no. 5866, pp. 1096–1100, 2008.

[5] R. Houben, J. Grimm, C. Willmes et al., "Merkel cell carcinoma and Merkel cell polyomavirus: evidence for hit-and-run oncogenesis," *The Journal of Investigative Dermatology*, vol. 132, no. 1, pp. 254–256, 2012.

[6] X. Sastre-Garau, M. Peter, M. F. Avril et al., "Merkel cell carcinoma of the skin: pathological and molecular evidence for a causative role of MCV in oncogenesis," *Journal of Pathology*, vol. 218, no. 1, pp. 48–56, 2009.

[7] K. M. Garneski, A. H. Warcola, Q. Feng, N. B. Kiviat, J. H. Leonard, and P. Nghiem, "Merkel cell polyomavirus is more frequently present in North American than Australian Merkel cell carcinoma tumors," *The Journal of Investigative Dermatology*, vol. 129, no. 1, pp. 246–248, 2009.

[8] H. Sihto, H. Kukko, V. Koljonen, R. Sankila, T. Böhling, and H. Joensuu, "Clinical factors associated with merkel cell polyomavirus infection in merkel cell carcinoma," *Journal of the National Cancer Institute*, vol. 101, no. 13, pp. 938–945, 2009.

[9] Y. L. Tolstov, D. V. Pastrana, H. Feng et al., "Human Merkel cell polyomavirus infection II. MCV is a common human infection that can be detected by conformational capsid epitope immunoassays," *International Journal of Cancer*, vol. 125, no. 6, pp. 1250–1256, 2009.

[10] J. C. Becker, R. Houben, S. Ugurel, U. Trefzer, C. Pföhler, and D. Schrama, "MC polyomavirus is frequently present in Merkel cell carcinoma of European patients," *The Journal of Investigative Dermatology*, vol. 129, no. 1, pp. 248–250, 2009.

[11] J. Mangana, P. Dziunycz, K. Kerl et al., "Prevalence of Merkel cell polyomavirus among Swiss Merkel cell carcinoma patients," *Dermatology*, vol. 221, no. 2, pp. 184–188, 2010.

[12] D. Schrama, W. K. Peitsch, M. Zapatka et al., "Merkel cell polyomavirus status is not associated with clinical course of merkel cell carcinoma," *Journal of Investigative Dermatology*, vol. 131, no. 8, pp. 1631–1638, 2011.

[13] H. Higaki-Mori, S. Kuwamoto, T. Iwasaki et al., "Association of Merkel cell polyomavirus infection with clinicopathological differences in Merkel cell carcinoma," *Human Pathology*, vol. 43, no. 12, pp. 2282–2291, 2012.

[14] H. Sihto, H. Kukko, V. Koljonen et al., "Merkel cell polyomavirus infection, large T antigen, retinoblastoma protein and outcome in Merkel cell carcinoma," *Clinical Cancer Research*, vol. 17, no. 14, pp. 4806–4813, 2011.

[15] C. Andres, U. Puchta, and M. J. Flaig, "Detection of merkel cell polyomavirus DNA in atypical fibroxanthoma in correlation to clinical features," *American Journal of Dermatopathology*, vol. 32, no. 8, pp. 799–803, 2010.

[16] M. Bobos, P. Hytiroglou, I. Kostopoulos, G. Karkavelas, and C. S. Papadimitriou, "Immunohistochemical distinction between Merkel cell carcinoma and small cell carcinoma of the lung," *American Journal of Dermatopathology*, vol. 28, no. 2, pp. 99–104, 2006.

[17] V. A. Smith, E. R. Camp, and E. J. Lentsch, "Merkel cell carcinoma: identification of prognostic factors unique to tumors located in the head and neck based on analysis of SEER data," *The Laryngoscope*, vol. 122, no. 6, pp. 1283–1290, 2012.

[18] N. C. Hodgson, "Merkel cell carcinoma: changing incidence trends," *Journal of Surgical Oncology*, vol. 89, no. 1, pp. 1–4, 2005.

[19] B. A. Reichgelt and O. Visser, "Epidemiology and survival of Merkel cell carcinoma in the Netherlands. A population-based study of 808 cases in 1993-2007," *European Journal of Cancer*, vol. 47, no. 4, pp. 579–585, 2011.

[20] J. F. Buell, J. Trofe, M. J. Hanaway et al., "Immunosuppression and merkel cell cancer," *Transplantation Proceedings*, vol. 34, no. 5, pp. 1780–1781, 2002.

[21] U. Wieland, S. Silling, N. Scola et al., "Merkel cell polyomavirus infection in HIV-positive men," *Archives of Dermatology*, vol. 147, no. 4, pp. 401–406, 2011.

[22] J. Kaae, A. V. Hansen, R. J. Biggar et al., "Merkel cell carcinoma: incidence, mortality, and risk of other cancers," *Journal of the National Cancer Institute*, vol. 102, no. 11, pp. 793–801, 2010.

[23] R. W. Miller and C. S. Rabkin, "Merkel cell carcinoma and melanoma: etiological similarities and differences," *Cancer Epidemiology Biomarkers and Prevention*, vol. 8, no. 2, pp. 153–158, 1999.

[24] M. Van Gele, M. Kaghad, J. H. Leonard et al., "Mutation analysis of P73 and TP53 in Merkel cell carcinoma," *British Journal of Cancer*, vol. 82, no. 4, pp. 823–826, 2000.

[25] M. Waltari, H. Sihto, H. Kukko et al., "Association of Merkel cell polyomavirus infection with tumor p53, KIT, stem cell factor, PDGFR-alpha and survival in Merkel cell carcinoma," *International Journal of Cancer*, vol. 129, no. 3, pp. 619–628, 2011.

[26] B. D. Lemos, B. E. Storer, J. G. Iyer et al., "Pathologic nodal evaluation improves prognostic accuracy in Merkel cell carcinoma: analysis of 5823 cases as the basis of the first consensus staging system," *Journal of the American Academy of Dermatology*, vol. 63, no. 5, pp. 751–761, 2010.

[27] C. M. Balch, D. L. Morton, J. E. Gershenwald et al., "Sentinel node biopsy and standard of care for melanoma," *Journal of the American Academy of Dermatology*, vol. 60, no. 5, pp. 872–875, 2009.

[28] O. Boccara, C. Girard, L. Mortier et al., "Guidelines for the diagnosis and treatment of Merkel cell carcinoma—Cutaneous Oncology Group of the French Society of Dermatology," *European Journal of Dermatology*, vol. 22, no. 3, pp. 375–379, 2012.

[29] J. L. Schwartz, K. A. Griffith, L. Lowe et al., "Features predicting sentinel lymph node positivity in Merkel cell carcinoma," *Journal of Clinical Oncology*, vol. 29, no. 8, pp. 1036–1041, 2011.

[30] S. Asioli, A. Righi, D. de Biase et al., "Expression of p63 is the sole independent marker of aggressiveness in localised (stage I-II) Merkel cell carcinomas," *Modern Pathology*, vol. 24, no. 11, pp. 1451–1461, 2011.

[31] J. B. Stokes, K. S. Graw, L. T. Dengel et al., "Patients with Merkel cell carcinoma tumors ≤ 1.0 cm in diameter are unlikely to harbor regional lymph node metastasis," *Journal of Clinical Oncology*, vol. 27, no. 23, pp. 3772–3777, 2009.

[32] A. A. Sarnaik, J. S. Zager, L. E. Cox, T. M. Ochoa, J. L. Messina, and V. K. Sondak, "Routine omission of sentinel lymph node biopsy for merkel cell carcinoma ≤ 1 cm is not justified," *Journal of Clinical Oncology*, vol. 28, no. 1, article e7, 2010.

[33] K. Murer, G. F. Huber, S. R. Haile et al., "Comparison of morbidity between sentinel node biopsy and elective neck dissection for treatment of the n0 neck in patients with oral squamous cell carcinoma," *Head & Neck*, vol. 33, no. 9, pp. 1260–1264, 2011.

[34] C. S. Landry, K. M. McMasters, and C. R. Scoggins, "The evolution of the management of regional lymph nodes in melanoma," *Journal of Surgical Oncology*, vol. 96, no. 4, pp. 316–321, 2007.

[35] R. C. Fields, K. J. Busam, J. F. Chou et al., "Recurrence and survival in patients undergoing sentinel lymph node biopsy for merkel cell carcinoma: analysis of 153 patients from a single institution," *Annals of Surgical Oncology*, vol. 18, no. 9, pp. 2529–2537, 2011.

[36] S. G. Gupta, L. C. Wang, P. F. Peñas, M. Gellenthin, S. J. Lee, and P. Nghiem, "Sentinel lymph node biopsy for evaluation and treatment of patients with Merkel cell carcinoma. The Dana-Farber experience and meta-analysis of the literature," *Archives of Dermatology*, vol. 142, no. 6, pp. 685–690, 2006.

[37] V. Koljonen, T. Böhling, and S. Virolainen, "Tumor burden of sentinel lymph node metastasis in Merkel cell carcinoma," *Journal of Cutaneous Pathology*, vol. 38, no. 6, pp. 508–513, 2011.

[38] J. Howle and M. Veness, "Sentinel lymph node biopsy in patients with Merkel cell carcinoma: an emerging role and the Westmead hospital experience," *The Australasian Journal of Dermatology*, vol. 53, no. 1, pp. 26–31, 2012.

[39] S. Miller, *NCCN Clinical Practice Guidelines in Oncology (NCCN Guidelines): Merkel Cell Carcinoma*, 10th edition, 2012.

[40] K. G. Lewis, M. A. Weinstock, A. L. Weaver, and C. C. Otley, "Adjuvant local irradiation for Merkel cell carcinoma," *Archives of Dermatology*, vol. 142, no. 6, pp. 693–700, 2006.

[41] T. Jouary, C. Leyral, B. Dreno et al., "Adjuvant prophylactic regional radiotherapy versus observation in stage I Merkel cell carcinoma: a multicentric prospective randomized study," *Annals of Oncology*, vol. 23, no. 4, pp. 1074–1080, 2012.

[42] M. Veness, M. Foote, V. Gebski, and M. Poulsen, "The role of radiotherapy alone in patients with merkel cell carcinoma: reporting the australian experience of 43 patients," *International Journal of Radiation Oncology Biology Physics*, vol. 78, no. 3, pp. 703–709, 2010.

[43] E. Pape, N. Rezvoy, N. Penel et al., "Radiotherapy alone for Merkel cell carcinoma: a comparative and retrospective study of 25 patients," *Journal of the American Academy of Dermatology*, vol. 65, no. 5, pp. 983–990, 2011.

[44] C. S. L. Koh and M. J. Veness, "Role of definitive radiotherapy in treating patients with inoperable Merkel cell carcinoma: the Westmead Hospital experience and a review of the literature," *Australasian Journal of Dermatology*, vol. 50, no. 4, pp. 249–256, 2009.

[45] S. B. Edge and C. C. Compton, "The american joint committee on cancer: The 7th edition of the AJCC cancer staging manual and the future of TNM," *Annals of Surgical Oncology*, vol. 17, no. 6, pp. 1471–1474, 2010.

[46] A. C. Ezeh, J. Bongaarts, and B. Mberu, "Global population trends and policy options," *Lancet*, vol. 380, no. 9837, pp. 142–148, 2012.

[47] C. Ulrich, T. Schmook, M. M. Sachse, W. Sterry, and E. Stockfleth, "Comparative epidemiology and pathogenic factors for nonmelanoma skin cancer in organ transplant patients," *Dermatologic Surgery*, vol. 30, no. 4, pp. 622–627, 2004.

[48] A. E. Brissett, K. D. Olsen, J. L. Kasperbauer et al., "Merkel cell carcinoma of the head and neck: a retrospective case series," *Head and Neck*, vol. 24, no. 11, pp. 982–988, 2002.

[49] A. L. Dancey, S. S. Rayatt, C. Soon, A. Ilchshyn, I. Brown, and S. Srivastava, "Merkel cell carcinoma: a report of 34 cases and literature review," *Journal of Plastic, Reconstructive and Aesthetic Surgery*, vol. 59, no. 12, pp. 1294–1299, 2006.

[50] A. C. Hui, A. L. Stillie, M. Seel, and J. Ainslie, "Merkel cell carcinoma: 27-year experience at the Peter Maccallum cancer centre," *International Journal of Radiation Oncology Biology Physics*, vol. 80, no. 5, pp. 1430–1435, 2011.

[51] K. C. Wong, F. Zuletta, S. J. Clarke, and P. J. Kennedy, "Clinical management and treatment outcomes of Merkel cell carcinoma," *Australian and New Zealand Journal of Surgery*, vol. 68, no. 5, pp. 354–358, 1998.

[52] H. Medina-Franco, M. M. Urist, J. Fiveash, M. J. Heslin, K. I. Bland, and S. W. Beenken, "Multimodality treatment of merkel cell carcinoma: case series and literature review of 1024 cases," *Annals of Surgical Oncology*, vol. 8, no. 3, pp. 204–208, 2001.

[53] A. M. Gillenwater, A. C. Hessel, W. H. Morrison et al., "Merkel cell carcinoma of the head and neck: effect of surgical excision and radiation on recurrence and survival," *Archives of Otolaryngology*, vol. 127, no. 2, pp. 149–154, 2001.

[54] W. J. O'Connor, R. K. Roenigk, and D. G. Brodland, "Merkel cell carcinoma: comparison of Mohs micrographic surgery and wide excision in eighty-six patients," *Dermatologic Surgery*, vol. 23, no. 10, pp. 929–933, 1997.

[55] B. E. Pennington and D. J. Leffell, "Mohs micrographic surgery: established uses and emerging trends," *Oncology*, vol. 19, no. 9, pp. 1165–1171, 2005.

[56] P. D. Karkos, A. Sastry, S. Hampal, and M. Al-Jafari, "Spontaneous regression of Merkel cell carcinoma of the nose," *Head and Neck*, vol. 32, no. 3, pp. 411–414, 2010.

[57] C. Ciudad, J. A. Avilés, F. Alfageme, M. Lecona, R. Suárez, and P. Lázaro, "Spontaneous regression in merkel cell carcinoma: report of two cases with a description of dermoscopic features and review of the literature," *Dermatologic Surgery*, vol. 36, no. 5, pp. 687–693, 2010.

[58] S. J. Hassan, M. Knox, M. Griffin, and M. J. Kennedy, "Spontaneous regression of metastatic merkel cell carcinoma," *Irish Medical Journal*, vol. 103, no. 1, pp. 21–22, 2010.

[59] Y. Yagi, A. Fujisawa, M. Makiura, and K. Morita, "Spontaneous regression of Merkel cell carcinoma after biopsy," *Journal of Dermatology*, vol. 36, no. 5, pp. 312–313, 2009.

[60] M. J. Vesely, D. J. Murray, P. C. Neligan et al., "Complete spontaneous regression in Merkel cell carcinoma," *Journal of Plastic, Reconstructive & Aesthetic Surgery*, vol. 61, no. 2, pp. 165–171, 2008.

[61] A. G. Richetta, M. Mancini, A. Torroni et al., "Total spontaneous regression of advanced merkel cell carcinoma after biopsy: review and a new case," *Dermatologic Surgery*, vol. 34, no. 6, pp. 815–822, 2008.

[62] G. F. Huber, M. Khalil, V. Falck, T. W. Matthews, and J. C. Dort, "Merkel cell carcinoma with solitary parotid metastasis: diagnostic dilemma in the absence of a primary site," *The Journal of Otolaryngology*, vol. 36, no. 5, pp. E70–E72, 2007.

[63] J. L. Deneve, J. L. Messina, S. S. Marzban et al., "Merkel cell carcinoma of unknown primary origin," *Annals of Surgical Oncology*, vol. 19, no. 7, pp. 2360–2366, 2012.

[64] T. Inoue, K. Yoneda, M. Manabe, and T. Demitsu, "Spontaneous regression of Merkel cell carcinoma: a comparative study of TUNEL index and tumor-infiltrating lymphocytes between spontaneous regression and non-regression group," *Journal of Dermatological Science*, vol. 24, no. 3, pp. 203–211, 2000.

[65] S. Koba, K. G. Paulson, K. Nagase et al., "Diagnostic biopsy does not commonly induce intratumoral CD8 T cell infiltration

in Merkel cell carcinoma," *PloS ONE*, vol. 7, no. 7, Article ID e41465, 2012.

[66] T. Jaeger, J. Ring, and C. Andres, "Histological, immunohistological, and clinical features of merkel cell carcinoma in correlation to merkel cell polyomavirus status," *Journal of Skin Cancer*, vol. 2012, Article ID 983421, 5 pages, 2012.

[67] M. Heath, N. Jaimes, B. Lemos et al., "Clinical characteristics of Merkel cell carcinoma at diagnosis in 195 patients: the AEIOU features," *Journal of the American Academy of Dermatology*, vol. 58, no. 3, pp. 375–381, 2008.

6

Treatment Patterns in Patients with Metastatic Melanoma

Zhongyun Zhao, Song Wang, and Beth L. Barber

Amgen Inc., Thousand Oaks, CA 91320, USA

Correspondence should be addressed to Zhongyun Zhao; zhongyun@amgen.com

Academic Editor: Giuseppe Argenziano

Objective. To describe treatment patterns and factors influencing treatment in a real-world setting of US patients with metastatic melanoma (MM). *Methods.* This was a retrospective claims-based study among patients with MM diagnosed between 2005 and 2010 identified from MarketScan databases. *Results.* Of 2546 MM patients, 66.8% received surgery, 44.7% received radiation, 38.7% received systemic therapies, and 17.7% received all modalities. Patients with lung, brain, liver, or bone metastases were less likely to undergo surgery (all $P < 0.0001$); patients with lung ($P = 0.04$), brain ($P < 0.001$), or liver metastases ($P = 0.03$) were more likely to receive systemic therapies; patients with brain ($P < 0.0001$) or bone metastases ($P < 0.0001$) were more likely to receive radiation therapy. Oncologists were more likely to recommend systemic therapy ($P < 0.0001$) or radiation ($P < 0.0001$), while dermatologists were more likely to recommend surgery ($P = 0.002$). Monotherapy was the dominant systemic therapy (82.4% patients as first-line). *Conclusions.* Only 39% of MM patients received systemic therapies, perhaps reflecting efficacy and safety limitations of conventional systemic therapies for MM. Among those receiving systemic therapy, monotherapy was the most common approach. Sites of metastases and physician speciality influenced treatment patterns. This study serves as a baseline against which future treatment pattern studies, following approval of new agents, can be compared.

1. Introduction

Melanoma has the fastest rising incidence rate compared with that of any other malignancy [1]. Metastatic melanoma (MM) is the most aggressive form of skin cancer and generally has a poor prognosis with a median overall survival of 6–10 months and a 5-year survival of 5–10%, depending on the location of the metastasis [2], compared with 5-year survival rates of 98.2% and 62.4% for localised and regional melanoma, respectively [3].

Prior to the approval of ipilimumab and vemurafenib in 2011, only two therapies were approved by the US Food and Drug Administration for treatment of MM, dacarbazine and high-dose interleukin-2 (HD IL-2). Since its approval in the 1970s, dacarbazine monotherapy has been commonly used for the treatment of MM [4], although its use is limited by a low response rate [5, 6] as well as a lack of an overall survival benefit and significant toxicity [7]. HD IL-2 is associated with durable responses in only a small percentage of carefully selected patients [8] and is limited by severe toxicities [9].

Prior to the introduction of the newer agents, treatment guidelines recommended resection, observation, or systemic therapy for patients with resectable stage IV melanoma. For those with unresectable stage IV disease, palliative resection and/or radiation for symptomatic patients or best supportive care can be considered; some of these patients can be treated with systemic therapy or enrolled into a clinical trial [10–12]. This lack of preferred conventional treatments most likely reflects the lack of efficacy of conventional MM therapies [10, 11], and is likely to change as experience with newer agents increases and additional agents become available.

It is therefore increasingly important to understand the factors that influence treatment decisions in patients with MM. No study has explored administrative data from a real-world clinical setting to characterise treatment patterns in this population. To identify the factors that influence treatment choices, we examined retrospective claims data prior to the introduction of the newer agents from the commercially insured population to document real-world treatment patterns in patients with MM in the USA. This study provides a baseline for comparison to future analyses as new agents become available.

2. Patients and Methods

2.1. Data Source. This was a retrospective claims-based study of patients with MM using administrative claims (medical and pharmacy) taken from the Thomson Reuters MarketScan Commercial Claims and Encounter database and the Medicare Supplemental and Coordination of Benefits database, between 1 January 2005 and 30 June 2010. These data included the full continuum of care under a variety of plan types across all settings (physician office visits, emergency room visits, inpatient hospital stays, outpatient visits, and outpatient pharmacy claims). The study population had a similar overall age distribution to that of a nationally representative population in Medical Expenditure Panel Survey.

2.2. Study Population. Patients who were eligible for inclusion in the study were those with at least two outpatient (or at least one inpatient) melanoma diagnoses (ICD-9-CM: 172.xx, V10.82) and at least two outpatient (or at least one inpatient) diagnoses for metastases (ICD-9-CM: 197.xx, 198.xx). Thus, patients who were included in this study would have distant metastases. If patients were identified based on outpatient diagnoses, the two outpatient diagnoses for melanoma and the two diagnoses for metastases were required to be at least 30 days apart. The first metastasis date should be no more than 30 days prior to, or any time after, the first date of melanoma diagnosis, and the index date was the first date of diagnosis of metastases. Patients who had other primary malignant tumours prior to diagnosis of melanoma, those who were younger than 18 years old at the index, and those with a preindex period of <6 months were excluded from the analysis.

2.3. Study Measures. The main study measures included identification of the percentage of patients who received cancer-related surgery, radiation, or systemic therapy for the treatment of MM. The type of surgery includes incision, excision, repair, shaving, removal, and destruction, etc., and the sites of surgery include skin, soft tissue, lymph nodes, lung, liver, and brain. Systemic drug treatments were identified using the Healthcare Common Procedure Coding System, the International Classification of Diseases (9th Revision), Clinical Modification (ICD-9-CM) procedure codes, or National Drug Code for any of the drug agents in postindex and included Bacillus Calmette-Guérin, carboplatin, carmustine, cisplatin, dacarbazine, docetaxel, granulocyte-macrophage colony-stimulating factor (GM-CSF), IL-2, interferon alfa-2b, paclitaxel, temozolomide, and vinblastine.

Further analysis of patients receiving systemic therapy was performed to identify the type of systemic drugs used by lines of therapy and the duration of therapy. Here, a treatment regimen was defined as one or more agents administered within a 4-day period, with the condition that all elements were administered more than once within 28 days. In the event that a new drug was added to a regimen within 28 days of the start of a line of therapy, this was considered an addition to the existing treatment regimen rather than a new line of therapy. The end of a given line of therapy was defined as either a 90-day gap in treatment or initiation of a new regimen that was not merely the addition of a new drug to the existing regimen.

Other study measures included demographic factors (such as age, gender, and region), type of health insurance plan, baseline Charlson comorbidities, metastatic site at index date, and speciality of treating physician within 90 days after index date. Each patient was followed from index date to death, termination of health insurance, or until end of database availability (30 June 2010), whichever occurred first.

2.4. Statistical Analysis. Factors influencing use of surgery, systemic therapy, or radiation were assessed by logistic regressions. Mean and standard deviation (SD) were calculated for continuous variables, while percentages were calculated for categorical variables for patient demographic and clinical characteristics. Treatment patterns for systemic therapies including percentage of patients receiving each drug of interest and duration of therapy were presented descriptively by graphs. All data were analysed using SAS programs (SAS Institute Inc., Cary, NC, USA) organised under UNIX using SAS version 9.2.

3. Results

3.1. Patient Demographics. A total of 2546 patients with MM were identified in the MarketScan databases with a mean age at index of 60.6 (±14.0) years, 6.8% of whom were 18–<40 years old, 58.5% were 40–<65 years old, and 34.7% were 65 years and older. The main sites of metastases were lung (21.2%), brain (18.7%), distant areas of skin (11.4%), bone (11.2%), liver (10.0%), and other sites (27.5%). Other sites include gastrointestinal tract, adrenal gland, genital, kidney, and ovary. The mean length of follow-up (SD) was 322.4 days (356.3) (Table 1).

3.2. Overall Patterns of Care. Overall, 66.8% of patients received cancer-related surgery, 44.7% received radiation, 38.7% received systemic drug therapies, and 17.7% of patients received all three treatments.

As shown in Table 2, a number of factors appear to influence treatment decisions in patients with MM. These include site of metastases, speciality of treating physician, and type of health insurance. Specifically, patients with lung, brain, liver, or bone metastases were significantly less likely to undergo surgery (all $P < 0.0001$), whereas patients with lung, brain, or liver metastases were more likely to receive systemic therapy ($P = 0.04$, $P < 0.001$, and $P = 0.03$, resp.), and patients with brain or bone metastases were significantly more likely to receive radiation therapy ($P < 0.0001$). In addition, patients who were treated by oncologists were significantly more likely to receive systemic therapy ($P < 0.0001$) or radiation ($P < 0.0001$), whilst those treated by dermatologists were more likely to receive surgery

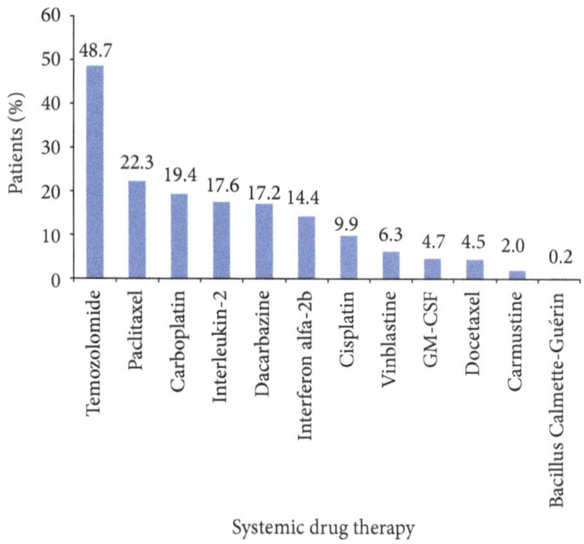

FIGURE 1: Treatment patterns among patients who received systemic drug treatment.

(P = 0.002). Finally, patients with comprehensive medical insurance were more likely to receive radiation (P = 0.031) than those with insurance provided by a Health Maintenance Organization (HMO), the Preferred Provider Organization (PPO), or those with a Point-of-Service Plan (POS).

3.3. Treatment Patterns in Patients Receiving Systemic Drug Therapy. The treatment patterns in patients receiving systemic drug therapy across all lines of therapy are summarised in Figure 1. Among the 985 patients who received systemic drug therapy, the most prevalent agent was temozolomide (48.7%), followed by paclitaxel (22.3%), carboplatin (19.4%), IL-2 (17.6%), and dacarbazine (17.2%). The site of metastases influenced the type of systemic regimen received; for example, patients with brain metastasis were more likely to receive temozolomide and did not receive treatment with IL-2.

Further examination of the treatment patterns by lines of systemic drug demonstrated 82.4% of patients received monotherapy as the first documented therapy after diagnosis, with temozolomide (38.5%) and dacarbazine (8.2%) being the most commonly used chemotherapy agents. IL-2 (14.3%) and interferon α-2b (11.4%) were the predominant immunotherapies, and carboplatin + paclitaxel was the most common combination therapy (9.4%) (Figure 2).

The mean duration of treatment in the first-line setting was 63 days, ranging from 32 days on IL-2 to 124 days on GM-CSF (Figure 3). Of the 985 patients who received first-line therapy, 287 (29.1%) patients subsequently received second-line treatment. In this setting, temozolomide (26.8%) was again the most commonly used agent, followed by carboplatin + paclitaxel (16.7%), IL-2 (11.9%), dacarbazine (10.5%), and paclitaxel (8.4%), with the majority of patients receiving monotherapy (68.0%) (Figure 2). The mean duration of treatment was 70.7 days, ranging from 19 days on cisplatin to 238 days on GM-CSF (Figure 3).

TABLE 1: Patient demographic and clinical characteristics.

	Total (n = 2546)
Age, mean (SD)	60.6 (14.0)
18–<40, %	6.8
40–<65, %	58.5
65 and older, %	34.7
Female, %	36.5
Health insurance plan, %	
Comprehensive	20.9
HMO	12.3
POS	6.7
PPO	56.1
Other plans	4.0
Medicare beneficiaries, %	33.0
Regions, %	
North east	10.5
North central	29.1
South	41.6
West	18.8
Metastasis site at index, %	
Lung	21.2
Brain	18.7
Distant part of skin	11.4
Bone	11.2
Liver	10.0
Other sites	27.5
Charlson comorbidity index (excluding cancer), mean (SD)	0.82 (1.17)
Specialty of treating physician within 90 days after index, %	
Oncologist	52.1
Dermatologist	15.0
Length of follow-up, mean days (SD)	322.4 (356.3)

Of the 287 patients who received second-line treatment, 71 (24.7%) went on to receive third-line therapy. In this setting, monotherapy was also predominant (63.4%), with patients receiving single-agent chemotherapy with temozolomide (21.1%), paclitaxel (18.3%), or dacarbazine (5.6%) (Figure 2). Combination of carboplatin + paclitaxel was used in 19.7% of patients and single-agent immunotherapy with IL-2 was used in 8.5% of patients. The mean duration of treatment was 68.5 days, ranging from 7 days on interferon α-2b to 105 days on docetaxel (Figure 3).

4. Discussion

Analysis of administrative claims data allows examination of treatment patterns in the real-world setting, reflecting the diversity of the agents used in clinical practice. This study

Table 2: Logistic regression of factors influencing systemic therapy, surgery, and radiation.

	Systemic therapy			Surgery			Radiation		
	Odds ratio	*P* value	95% confidence interval	Odds ratio	*P* value	95% confidence interval	Odds ratio	*P* value	95% confidence interval
Age at index	0.970	<0.0001	[0.961, 0.980]	0.986	0.013	[0.976, 0.997]	0.984	0.001	[0.974, 0.994]
Female	0.787	0.008	[0.658, 0.939]	0.887	0.216	[0.734, 1.073]	0.727	0.001	[0.607, 0.870]
Type of insurance plan									
Comprehensive	1.168	0.529	[0.720, 1.897]	1.160	0.563	[0.701, 1.918]	1.721	0.031	[1.050, 2.281]
HMO	1.105	0.688	[0.679, 1.799]	0.676	0.134	[0.404, 1.129]	1.190	0.500	[0.718, 1.973]
POS	0.805	0.423	[0.474, 1.368]	0.981	0.946	[0.558, 1.725]	1.543	0.120	[0.894, 2.663]
PPO	1.041	0.858	[0.673, 1.610]	1.053	0.827	[0.665, 1.667]	1.489	0.084	[0.948, 2.338]
Medicare beneficiary	0.755	0.071	[0.557, 1.025]	0.902	0.537	[0.651, 1.250]	0.850	0.301	[0.624, 1.157]
Region									
Northeast	0.898	0.528	[0.643, 1.254]	1.541	0.020	[1.069, 2.222]	1.044	0.806	[0.742, 1.469]
North central	1.026	0.843	[0.793, 1.328]	1.040	0.783	[0.786, 1.377]	1.019	0.889	[0.782, 1.328]
South	0.857	0.214	[0.672, 1.093]	1.044	0.748	[0.803, 1.356]	1.070	0.594	[0.835, 1.371]
Metastasis site at index									
Lung	1.292	0.039	[1.013, 1.647]	0.418	<0.0001	[0.319, 0.548]	0.920	0.498	[0.723, 1.171]
Brain	1.598	0.000	[1.239, 2.062]	0.498	<0.0001	[0.377, 0.658]	6.388	<0.0001	[4.851, 8.412]
Distant part of skin	1.054	0.730	[0.782, 1.420]	0.867	0.451	[0.598, 1.257]	0.929	0.628	[0.691, 1.250]
Bone	0.830	0.245	[0.606, 1.136]	0.302	<0.0001	[0.219, 0.417]	2.628	<0.0001	[1.966, 3.512]
Liver	1.426	0.026	[1.044, 1.946]	0.280	<0.0001	[0.201, 0.391]	0.624	0.005	[0.451, 0.865]
Charlson comorbidity index (removed cancer)	0.985	0.683	[0.918, 1.058]	1.155	0.000	[1.068, 1.250]	1.065	0.084	[0.992, 1.143]
Specialty of treating physician within 90 days after index									
Oncologist	1.534	<0.0001	[1.288, 1.828]	1.051	0.606	[0.870, 1.269]	1.581	<0.0001	[1.324, 1.887]
Dermatologist	0.902	0.406	[0.708, 1.150]	1.586	0.002	[1.181, 2.129]	0.808	0.089	[0.632, 1.033]
Length of follow-up	1.001	<0.0001	[1.001, 1.001]	1.003	<0.0001	[1.002, 1.003]	1.000	0.163	[1.000, 1.000]

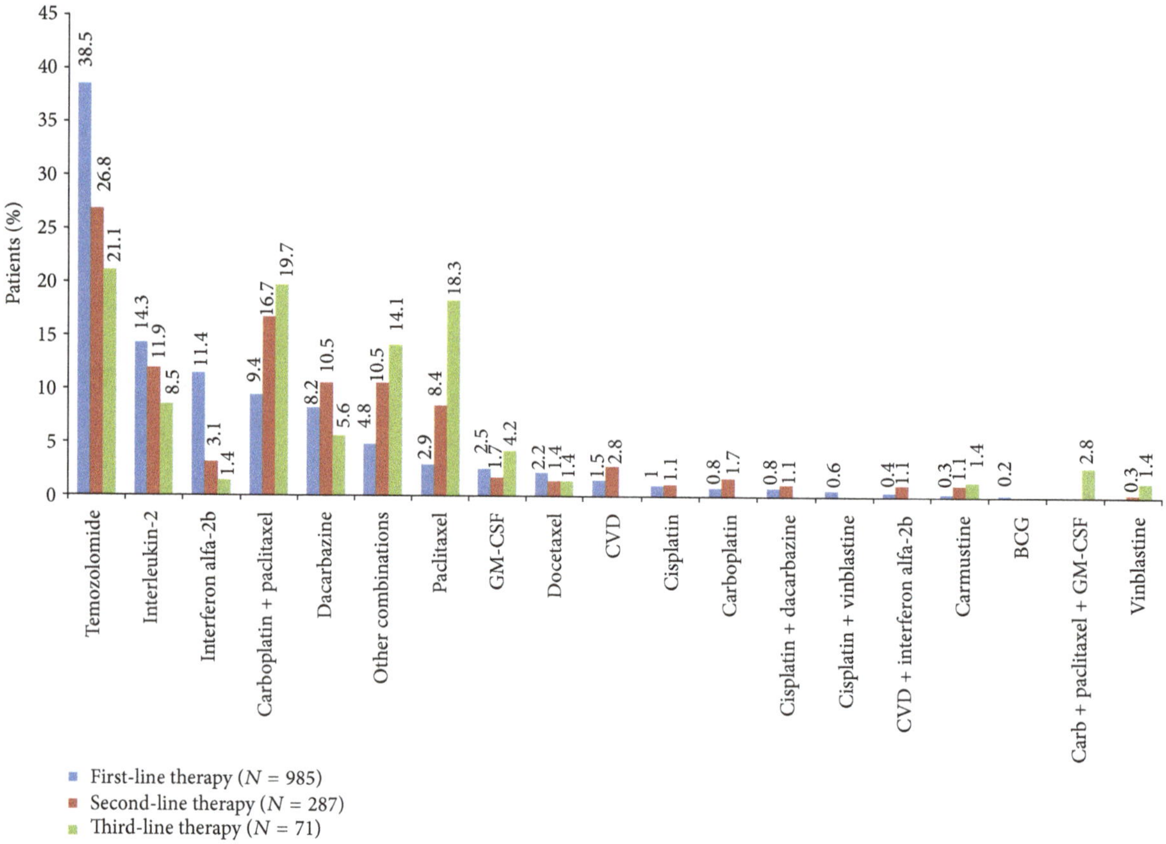

FIGURE 2: Treatment patterns by line of therapy.

therefore aimed to document real-world treatment patterns in patients with MM, with a focus on the types of systemic drug therapies used in first-, second-, and third-line therapy. The large study population of 2546 patients provided a robust data set with which to examine these aims.

Examination of MarketScan databases revealed that the majority of patients with MM received cancer-related surgery (66.8%). Only a relatively low proportion of patients (38.7%) received systemic drug therapy, perhaps reflecting the lack of efficacy with conventional treatment agents. The current study also identifies a number of factors, including sites of metastases, speciality of the treating physician, and the type of insurance held, which appear to influence whether a patient receives surgery, systemic drug therapy, or radiation.

As expected, given the lack of consensus on the effective use of conventional systemic drugs in MM, examination of the patterns of systemic drug therapy revealed that a variety of chemotherapy agents were used, with off-label temozolomide monotherapy being the most prevalent agent among patients who received drug treatment (48.7%). The increased use of temozolomide over dacarbazine (17.2%) observed in this study is likely to be a result of the greater ease of administration of temozolomide due to its oral availability and its ability to cross the blood-brain barrier [13], with neither showing overall survival benefit. As expected, other commonly used treatments consisted of immunotherapies, such as IL-2 and interferon alfa-2b, and single-agent chemotherapy with paclitaxel or carboplatin. Given that conventional chemotherapy agents are associated with poor response rates [5, 6] or, in the case of IL-2, significant toxicity [9, 14], these findings represent an unmet need for more effective treatment alternatives in patients with MM.

When the types of agents used were categorised according to lines of treatment, off-label temozolomide monotherapy remained the most common approach across all three lines of treatment (first-, second-, and third-line). It is interesting to note that monotherapy in general was prevalent across all three lines of therapy, reflecting that although combination chemotherapy and biochemotherapy have been shown to improve objective response rates in some cases, they tend not to extend survival and are associated with greater toxicity [4, 7, 15]. While GM-CSF was not the most frequently used treatment option, it was associated with the longest duration of treatment in first- and second-line. The long treatment duration with GM-CSF might be because it has a tolerable safety profile and patients who received GM-CSF likely were young and had low baseline comorbid disease burden [16].

It is important to acknowledge some limitations of the study, including its reliance on administrative claims submitted solely for the purposes of medical reimbursement. The databases for the commercially insured patient population are not necessarily representative of all patients with MM in the USA. The analysis of specific systemic agents used is also limited by the varying detail with which systemic therapies

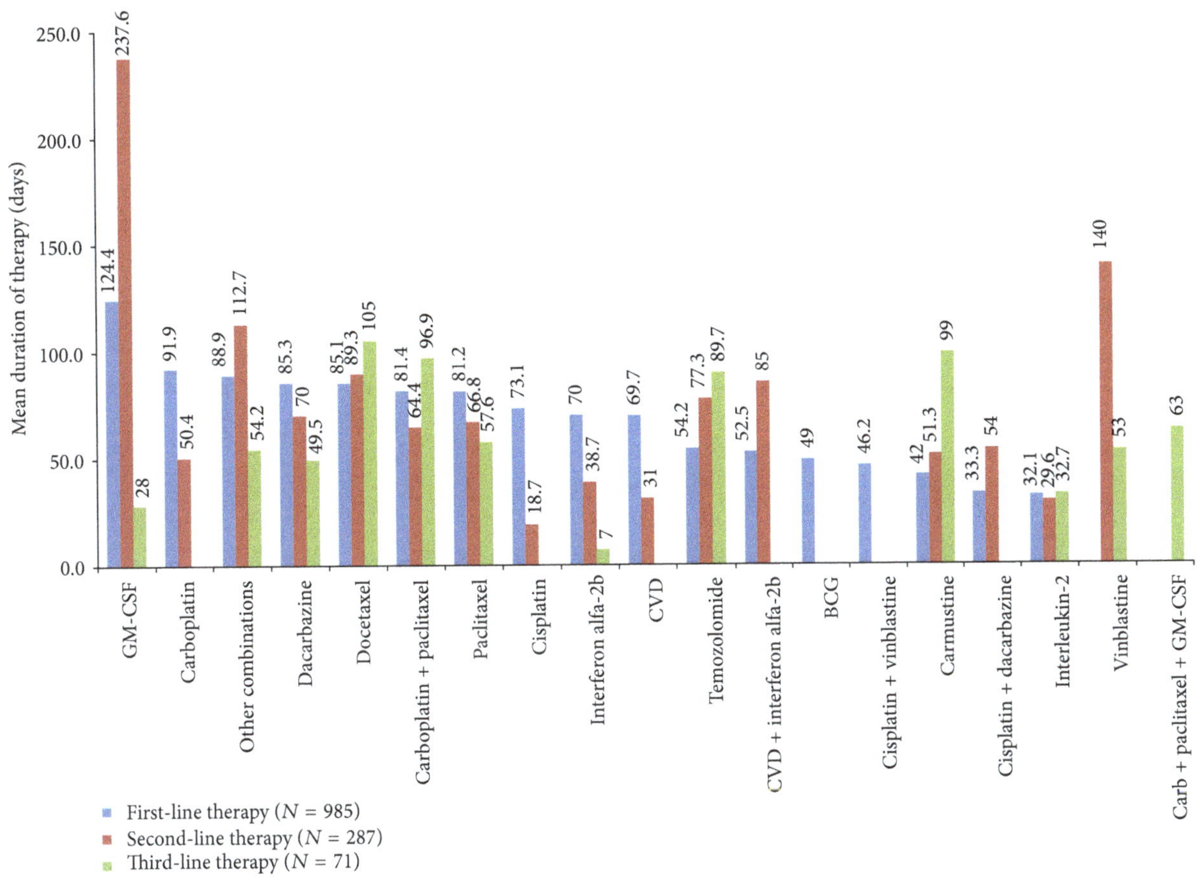

FIGURE 3: Treatment duration by line of therapy.

are coded for purposes of medical care reimbursement. The impact of potential misclassification bias stemming from analyses of claims data has been described previously [17, 18]. In addition, the number of patients identified as receiving systemic drug therapy may be underrepresented since information was not recorded for patients enrolled in clinical trials. Also, in the analysis of subsequent treatments observed, patients with a short follow-up period might not have had their second or third line of therapy captured and so the percentage of second- and third-line therapy might be underestimated. Finally, the relevance of this study will depend on the success of agents that have recently come to market, including ipilimumab and vemurafenib. These are likely to pave the way for the next generation of targeted therapies and therefore may change the way MM is treated in the future. As such, it would be interesting to assess how real-world treatment patterns in MM change over the coming years.

5. Conclusions

This study described the treatment patterns in patients with MM in the USA, showing the variety of systemic agents that were used during the study period. These findings demonstrate the need for more efficacious and tolerable treatment alternatives for MM. Furthermore, this study provides an overview of how patients with MM were managed before the newer agents were approved and serves as a baseline for future studies of this type to assess how newer agents are adopted into clinical practice in real-world settings and how they influence the treatment patterns of patients with MM.

Authors' Contribution

Zhongyun Zhao and Beth L. Barber contributed to concept development, analysis plan, and paper development. Song Wang contributed to concept development, analysis plan, and execution of analysis. All authors agree to take responsibility of the whole paper.

Acknowledgment

Medical writing assistance was provided by ApotheCom Scope Medical Ltd., funded by Amgen Inc.

References

[1] J. Manola, M. Atkins, J. Ibrahim, and J. Kirkwood, "Prognostic factors in metastatic melanoma: a pooled analysis of Eastern

Cooperative Oncology Group trials," *Journal of Clinical Oncology*, vol. 18, no. 22, pp. 3782–3793, 2000.

[2] A. M. Leung, D. M. Hari, and D. L. Morton, "Surgery for distant melanoma metastasis," *The Cancer Journal*, vol. 18, no. 2, pp. 176–184, 2012.

[3] "National Cancer Institute statistics," 2012, http://seer.cancer.gov/statfacts/html/melan.html.

[4] J. Fricker, "New era in metastatic melanoma," *Molecular Oncology*, vol. 4, pp. 91–97, 2010.

[5] P. B. Chapman, A. Hauschild, C. Robert et al., "Improved survival with vemurafenib in melanoma with BRAF V600E mutation," *The New England Journal of Medicine*, vol. 364, no. 26, pp. 2507–2516, 2011.

[6] A. Hauschild, J. J. Grob, L. V. Demidov et al., "Dabrafenib in BRAF-mutated metastatic melanoma: a multicentre, open-label, phase 3 randomised controlled trial," *The Lancet*, vol. 380, no. 9839, pp. 358–365, 2012.

[7] S. Bhatia, S. S. Tykodi, and J. A. Thompson, "Treatment of metastatic melanoma: an overview," *Oncology*, vol. 23, no. 6, pp. 488–496, 2009.

[8] S. Jang and M. B. Atkins, "Which drug, and when, for patients with BRAF-mutant melanoma?" *The Lancet Oncology*, vol. 14, no. 2, pp. e60–e69, 2013.

[9] A. C. Buzaid and M. Atkins, "Practical guidelines for the management of biochemotherapy-related toxicity in melanoma," *Clinical Cancer Research*, vol. 7, no. 9, pp. 2611–2619, 2001.

[10] "National Comprehensive Cancer Network (NCCN) Guidelines for Melanoma, Version 1," 2014, http://www.nccn.org/professionals/physician_gls/pdf/melanoma.pdf.

[11] C. Fellner, "Ipilimumab, (yervoy) prolongs survival in advanced melanoma: serious side effects and a hefty price tag may limit its use," *Pharmacy and Therapeutics*, vol. 37, no. 9, pp. 503–530, 2012.

[12] C. Garbe, K. Peris, A. Hauschild et al., "Diagnosis and treatment of melanoma. European consensus-based interdisciplinary guideline—update 2012," *European Journal of Cancer*, vol. 48, no. 15, pp. 2375–2390, 2012.

[13] I. Quirt, S. Verma, T. Petrella, K. Bak, and M. Charette, "Temozolomide for the treatment of metastatic melanoma," *Current Oncology*, vol. 14, no. 1, pp. 27–33, 2007.

[14] A. M. Menzies, G. V. Long, and R. Murali, "Dabrafenib and its potential for the treatment of metastatic melanoma," *Drug Design, Development and Therapy*, vol. 6, pp. 391–405, 2012.

[15] C. Garbe, T. K. Eigentler, U. Keilholz, A. Hauschild, and J. M. Kirkwood, "Systematic review of medical treatment in melanoma: current status and future prospects," *Oncologist*, vol. 16, no. 1, pp. 5–24, 2011.

[16] Z. Zhao, S. Wang, B. Barber, and V. Wagner, "DTIC and GM-CSF in the treatment of patients with metastatic melanoma," *Journal of Clinical Oncolology*, vol. 30, supplement, 2012, abstract no. e19045.

[17] E. Losina, J. Barrett, J. A. Baron, and J. N. Katz, "Accuracy of Medicare claims data for rheumatologic diagnoses in total hip replacement recipients," *Journal of Clinical Epidemiology*, vol. 56, no. 6, pp. 515–519, 2003.

[18] R. Newcomer, T. Clay, J. S. Luxenberg, and R. H. Miller, "Misclassification and selection bias when identifying Alzheimer's disease solely from Medicare claims records," *Journal of the American Geriatrics Society*, vol. 47, no. 2, pp. 215–219, 1999.

7

Melanoma Development and Progression are Associated with Rad6 Upregulation and β-Catenin Relocation to the Cell Membrane

Karli Rosner,[1,2,3] Darius R. Mehregan,[2,4] Evangelia Kirou,[1,2] Judith Abrams,[5,6] Seongho Kim,[5,6] Michelle Campbell,[4] Jillian Frieder,[1] Kelsey Lawrence,[1] Brittany Haynes,[6] and Malathy P. V. Shekhar[6,7,8]

[1] *Laboratory for Molecular Dermatology, Barbara Ann Karmanos Cancer Institute, 110 East Warren Avenue, Detroit, MI 48201, USA*
[2] *Department of Dermatology, School of Medicine, Wayne State University, Detroit, MI 48201, USA*
[3] *Center for Molecular Medicine and Genetics, School of Medicine, Wayne State University, Detroit, MI 48201, USA*
[4] *Pinkus Dermatopathology Laboratory, Monroe, MI 48162, USA*
[5] *Biostatistics, Barbara Ann Karmanos Cancer Institute, Detroit, MI 48201, USA*
[6] *Department of Oncology, School of Medicine, Wayne State University, Detroit, MI 48201, USA*
[7] *Department of Pathology, School of Medicine, Wayne State University, Detroit, MI 48201, USA*
[8] *Barbara Ann Karmanos Cancer Institute, Detroit, MI 48201, USA*

Correspondence should be addressed to Karli Rosner; krosner@med.wayne.edu and Malathy P. V. Shekhar; shekharm@karmanos.org

Academic Editor: Selma Ugurel

We have previously demonstrated that Rad6 and β-catenin enhance each other's expression through a positive feedback loop to promote breast cancer development/progression. While β-catenin has been implicated in melanoma pathogenesis, Rad6 function has not been investigated. Here, we examined the relationship between Rad6 and β-catenin in melanoma development and progression. Eighty-eight cutaneous tumors, 30 nevi, 29 primary melanoma, and 29 metastatic melanomas, were immunostained with anti-β-catenin and anti-Rad6 antibodies. Strong expression of Rad6 was observed in only 27% of nevi as compared to 100% of primary and 96% of metastatic melanomas. β-Catenin was strongly expressed in 97% of primary and 93% of metastatic melanomas, and unlike Rad6, in 93% of nevi. None of the tumors expressed nuclear β-catenin. β-Catenin was exclusively localized on the cell membrane of 55% of primary, 62% of metastatic melanomas, and only 10% of nevi. Cytoplasmic β-catenin was detected in 90% of nevi, 17% of primary, and 8% of metastatic melanoma, whereas 28% of primary and 30% of metastatic melanomas exhibited β-catenin at both locations. These data suggest that melanoma development and progression are associated with Rad6 upregulation and membranous redistribution of β-catenin and that β-catenin and Rad6 play independent roles in melanoma development.

1. Introduction

The Wnt/β-catenin pathway has been implicated in the development and progression of melanoma and a wide range of cancer types, including colorectal cancer, breast cancer, esophageal carcinoma, and liver cancer [1–3]. Under normal conditions, intracellular β-catenin levels are kept low through a multiprotein system that mediates β-catenin degradation [4]. Increases in expression and binding of certain Wnt ligands to Frizzled receptor or mutations in specific components of the β-catenin degradation assembly deactivate this regulatory mechanism. Consequently, β-catenin accumulates in the cytoplasm and translocates to the nucleus. Nuclear β-catenin stimulates transcription of a large number of TCF/β-catenin responsive genes that include cyclin D1, c-myc [5, 6], and the melanocyte-specific gene, microphthalmia-associated transcription factor MITF-M [7]. Thus, accumulation of nuclear β-catenin as observed in several cancer types is considered a marker of canonical Wnt/β-catenin pathway deregulation and unfavorable prognosis [3, 8].

Previous studies have reported an association between nuclear β-catenin accumulation and melanoma progression and suggested nuclear β-catenin to be a marker of poor prognosis [1, 7]. However, recent studies have shown that contrary to breast and colon cancer, metastatic progression of melanoma is associated with decreases in nuclear and cytoplasmic β-catenin expression [9, 10]. Moreover, clinical, genetic, and histological studies suggest that nuclear and cytoplasmic β-catenin may be used as biomarkers of good prognosis in melanoma [11–14].

Recently, HHR6, a human homologue of the yeast Rad6 gene and a principal component of the postreplication DNA repair pathway, has been identified as an important regulator of canonical Wnt/β-catenin signaling [15, 16]. HHR6, referred hereafter as Rad6, stabilizes β-catenin by polyubiquitin modifications that render β-catenin resistant to 26S proteasomal degradation [16]. Furthermore, Rad6 is a transcriptional target of β-catenin [17], thus revealing a positive feedback loop between β-catenin-mediated activation of Rad6 gene expression and Rad6-induced β-catenin stabilization.

Rad6 expression is low in normal breast tissues; however, increases in Rad6 protein expression are detected in hyperplastic, ductal carcinoma *in situ* (DCIS) and invasive breast carcinomas [15]. We have previously demonstrated a role for Rad6 in breast cancer progression through its regulatory effect on the canonical Wnt/β-catenin pathway [18]. Since the decrease/loss of nuclear β-catenin [9, 10], rather than increases as in breast cancer, is linked to melanoma progression, it is not known whether Rad6 and β-catenin work in concert to promote melanoma pathogenesis. Furthermore, Rad6 expression in the skin has not been investigated, and there are no data on the role of Rad6 in the pathogenesis of benign (nevi) and malignant (melanoma) melanocytic lesions. It is important to address this gap in knowledge because of the unmet medical need for new effective antimelanoma therapies and because Rad6 and β-catenin have been identified as therapeutic targets [19, 20].

In this study, we examined Rad6 and β-catenin expressions in serial sections of nevi, primary, and metastatic melanomas to determine their potential roles in melanoma development and metastatic progression. Our data suggest that membranous relocation of β-catenin and upregulation of Rad6 are independent markers of melanoma development and progression. We also offer a hypothesis that explains the role of membranous β-catenin relocation and decreasing cytoplasmic β-catenin in melanoma development, a phenomenon that has been linked to unfavorable prognosis [9, 21, 22].

2. Materials and Methods

2.1. Patients and Specimens. Cases were retrieved from the files of the Pinkus Dermatopathology Laboratory (PDL), a private dermatopathology laboratory located in Monroe, MI. Preserved paraffin-embedded tissue specimens collected for each case were assigned an accession code that excluded patient identifier information. Nevus and primary melanoma cases were selected for study using random numbers generated by a uniform random number generator (Stata/MP 13.1). The study groups consisted of 30 cases of melanocytic nevi, 29 cases of primary cutaneous melanoma, and 29 cases of metastatic cutaneous melanoma. The melanoma and melanocytic nevus subtypes are listed in Table 1. The study includes all metastatic cutaneous melanoma samples that were archived between 2010 and 2012. The number of cases for each nevus and primary melanoma subtype was determined to reflect the lesion's relative representation in cases obtained at the PDL during the above period. Atypical nevi were diagnosed using criteria originally proposed by Clark and lesion architecture as reviewed by Roth et al. [23]. This study was approved by the Wayne State University Human Investigation Committee.

2.2. Antibodies. Primary antibodies used in the study are as follows: (i) anti-β-catenin (IS702) was purchased from Dako (Glostrup, Denmark) and used in an undiluted form; and (ii) anti-Rad6 (ab31917) was purchased from Abcam (Cambridge, MA) and used at a 1 : 500 dilution. In humans, the yeast homologous Rad6 gene is duplicated and the proteins encoded by the two genes HHR6A (or Rad6A) and HHR6B (Rad6B) from chromosomes Xq24-q25 and 5q23-q31, respectively, share 95% identical amino acid residues [24]. Neither ab31917, our own Rad6 antibody [15], nor any other commercially available anti-Rad6 antibody is currently able to distinguish between Rad6A and Rad6B proteins. Therefore, rather than referring as Rad6A or Rad6B, we refer to the protein detected by the antibody as Rad6.

2.3. Immunohistochemistry Staining. Immunohistochemistry was performed as previously described [25]. Briefly, five-micrometer sections were deparaffinized in xylene and rehydrated in graded ethanol. For antigen retrieval, sections were microwaved in citrate buffer pH 6.0 (BioGenex, San Ramon, CA, USA) for 12 min at 95°C and cooled for 30 min prior to immunostaining. Sections were incubated with 3% hydrogen peroxide for 15 min, followed by incubation with primary antibody for 60 min. An automated immunostainer (i6000; BioGenex) was utilized for subsequent incubation steps: sections were incubated in MultiLink biotinylated anti-IgG for 20 min, horseradish peroxidase conjugated secondary antibody for 20 min, followed by development with 3-amino-9-ethyl-carbazole for 10 min (BioGenex). Sections were then counterstained with hematoxylin. All incubation steps were performed at room temperature, and sections were washed with Tris-buffered saline between incubations.

2.4. Controls. Lung and colon cancer tissues were included as positive controls for immunostaining with anti-β-catenin antibody, and breast cancer tissues were included as positive controls for staining with anti-Rad6 antibody. Tissue sections incubated without primary antibody served as negative controls.

Table 1: Association of melanocytic nevi and melanoma with demographic characteristics of the patients.

Melanocytic tumor type and subtype		No. Cases		Gender		Age
		n	Total N	M	F	Median (Range)
Nevi	Junctional nevus	5	30	11	19	43 (33–53)
	Intradermal nevus	7				
	Compound nevus	10				
	Atypical nevus	8				
PM	SSMM	17	29	14	15	58 (48–68)
	Nodular Melanoma	7				
	Lentigo Malignant Melanoma	5				
MM	Metastatic Melanoma	29	29	19	10	67 (58–76)
	significance			$P = 0.08$		$P = 0.00025$

M: male; F: female; CI: confidence interval; PM: primary melanoma; MM: metastatic melanoma; SSM: superficial spreading melanoma.

2.5. Cell Enumeration. Stained sections were independently enumerated by two coauthors (D. R. Mehregan and M. Campbell), who were blinded to patient medical records for each case. Blinded enumeration was performed under light microscopy at 400x magnification, and an ocular grid consisting of a simple square lattice of 100 test points was utilized to count the number of positively and negatively stained melanomas or nevus cells for each section. Per section, the total number of positively and negatively stained cells was counted for each of three sequential horizontal fields. The mean value of the three fields was used to estimate the relative density of cells in a specimen. To increase assessment accuracy, all positively and negatively stained melanomas or nevus cells in a visual field were individually counted as opposed to being graded as ranges of percentages. Enumeration data were reviewed independently by each evaluator. When independent readings for positively stained cells differed by 20% for a given section, both evaluators reviewed the section together to establish a consensus reading. A specimen was considered negative if less than 4% of the cells were immunostained for Rad6 or β-catenin. A tumor was considered to be stained with high intensity if >50% of the cells in a specimen expressed Rad6 or β-catenin, similar to the criteria used by Mineta et al. [26].

2.6. Statistical Analysis. Kruskal-Wallis tests were used to compare groups on the basis of continuous variables such as age and percent positive cells. Chi-square tests for differences in proportions were used to compare groups on the basis of categorical variables such as gender and β-catenin localization. Spearman's rank correlation was used to assess the pairwise association between age and percent of Rad6 positive and β-catenin positive cells. Multinomial logistic regression was used to assess the simultaneous association of Rad6 and age with diagnostic group. Adjustments were made for multiple comparisons using Wilcoxon rank sum tests with Bonferroni correction for pairwise comparisons.

3. Results

Our analysis included 30 individuals diagnosed with nevi, 29 with primary melanoma, and 29 with metastatic melanoma (Table 1). These groups differed marginally with respect to gender ($P = 0.08$) and significantly in age ($P = 0.0001$). Significant age differences were observed between individuals with nevi and those with either primary melanomas ($P = 0.02$) or metastatic melanomas ($P = 0.0001$). In contrast, no age difference is observed between individuals with primary and metastatic melanomas ($P = 0.27$). Significant differences in age were also observed between groups defined by β-catenin localization ($P = 0.007$). Individuals with β-catenin localized in the cytoplasm were significantly younger than individuals with β-catenin localization at the cell membrane ($P = 0.02$) and marginally younger than individuals with β-catenin localization at both the cytoplasm and the cell membrane ($P = 0.05$). When age was categorized as <50, 50–60, and >60 years, there were statistically significant differences in Rad6 expression between the groups ($P = 0.0008$), although there is substantial variability (Table 2). Median Rad6 is greater in the group of people older than 60 years compared to the 50–60 years old group ($P = 0.04$) and <50 years old group ($P = 0.001$). A 20% discrepancy of positively stained cells between the two evaluators was observed in fewer than 5% of the cases, and these cases were evaluated together to establish a consensus reading.

Table 2: Rad6 positive cells by age groups.

Age (years)	N	Rad6 Percent Median (IQR)
<50	31	65 (0, 96)
50–60	16	86 (24, 95)
>60	38	96 (88, 100)

N: number of patients, IQR: interquartile range.

3.1. β-Catenin Immunostaining. Melanoma development and progression were not associated with significant changes in percentage of specimens expressing β-catenin. β-Catenin staining was observed in 97% of nevi and in all primary and metastatic melanomas. Also, the percentages of nevi (93%), primary melanoma (97%), and metastatic melanoma (93%) that expressed β-catenin in more than 50% of the cells did not differ significantly (Figures 1, 2, and 3). However, significant differences were observed between the percentages of nevi

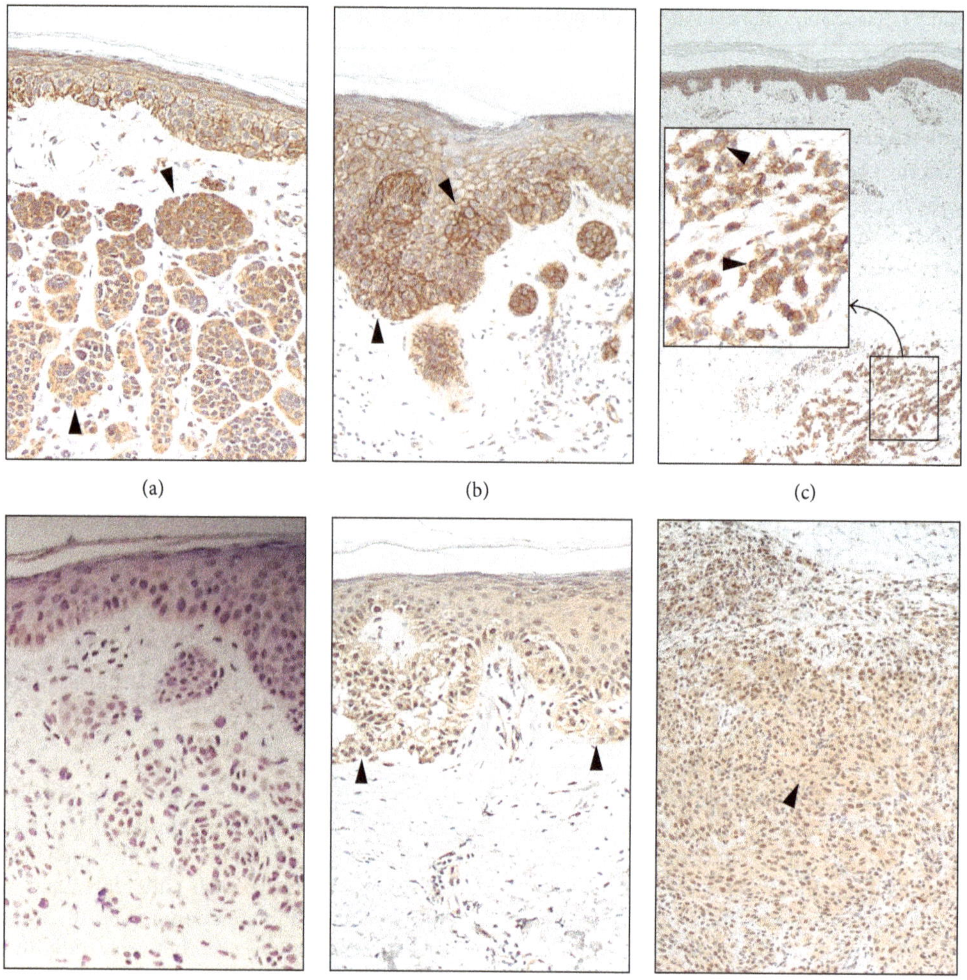

FIGURE 1: Representative pictures of β-catenin ((a)–(c)) and Rad6 ((d)–(f)) staining in nevus ((a), (d)), primary melanoma ((b), (e)), and metastatic melanoma ((c), (f)). Closed arrowheads point to positively immunostained cells. The highlighted square in panel (c) is magnified. Original magnification ×400.

(59%), primary melanoma (90%), and metastatic melanoma (56%) that expressed β-catenin in more than 90% of the cells ($P = 0.02$; Figure 2). These differences were greatly impacted by the percentage of primary melanomas (48%) that expressed β-catenin in 100% of the cells, which was approximately twofold higher than the percentages of nevi (21%) or metastatic melanoma (26%) (data not shown).

3.2. Intracellular Localization of β-Catenin. None of the nevi or melanomas expressed β-catenin in the nucleus (Figure 1). The percentage of tumors that expressed membranous β-catenin increased dramatically from nevi (10%) to primary and metastatic melanomas (83% and 93%, resp.; $P < 0.0001$; Figure 4). Concurrently with this increase, the percentage of tumors that expressed cytoplasmic β-catenin decreased from nevi (90%) to primary and metastatic melanomas (45% and 38%, resp.; $P < 0.0001$; Figure 4). In contrast, no significant differences were observed between the percentages of primary and metastatic melanomas that expressed β-catenin at either the membrane (83% and 93%, resp.; $P = 0.289$) or the cytoplasm (45% and 38%, resp.; $P = 0.633$; Figure 4). While all four nevi types (junctional, intradermal, compound, and atypical) expressed β-catenin in the cytoplasm, only junctional and atypical nevi expressed β-catenin at the plasma membrane. As opposed to nevi types, the three primary melanoma types examined (superficial spreading, nodular, and lentigo maligna) did not differ in β-catenin localization as β-catenin was localized at the plasma membrane, in the cytoplasm, or in both (Figure 4).

3.3. Rad6 Immunostaining. The majority of nevi (63%) did not express Rad6. Conversely, all primary melanomas (100%) and the majority of metastatic melanomas (96%) exhibited greater than 50% Rad6 expression. The increase in tumor populations expressing Rad6 from 37% of nevi to 100% of primary and metastatic melanomas was significant ($P = 0.0001$; Figures 1, 2, and 3). Melanoma progression from primary to metastatic disease was not associated with changes

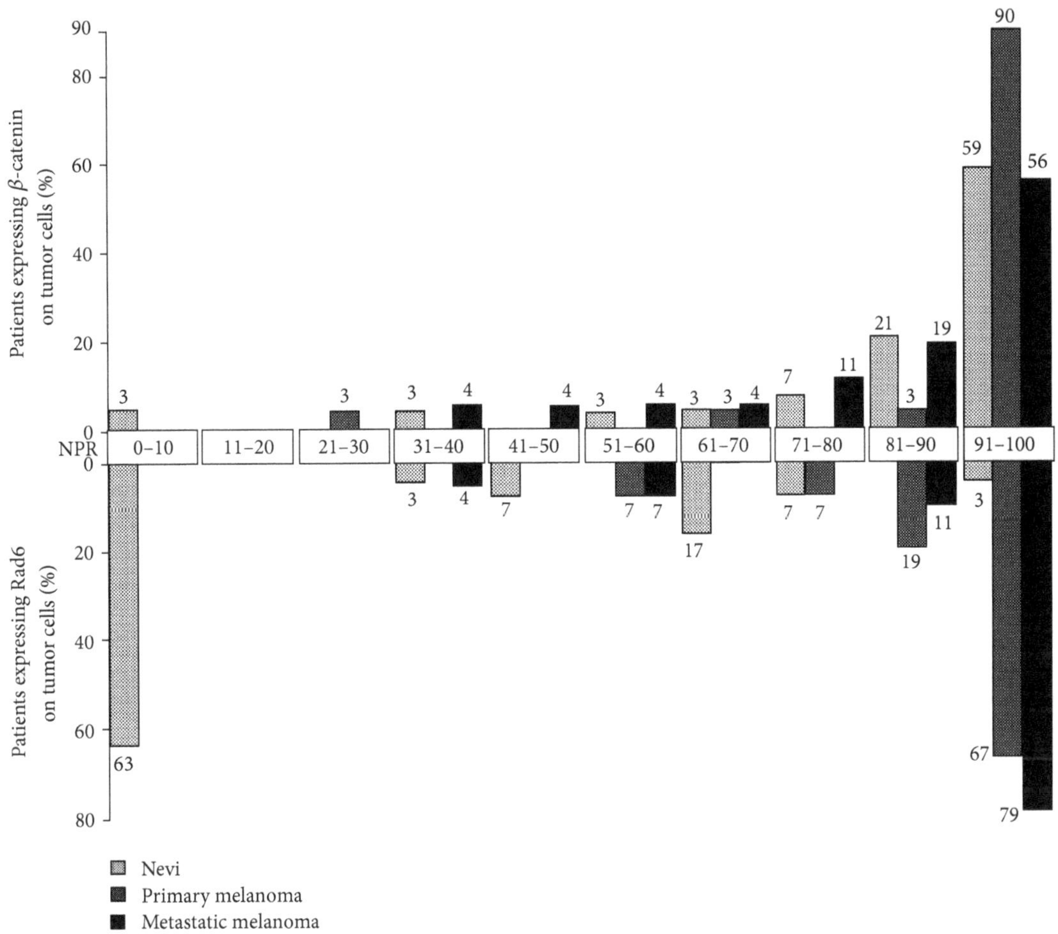

FIGURE 2: Percentages of nevi, primary melanomas, and metastatic melanomas with Rad6 and β-catenin positive cells shown in increments of 10 percentage points.

in the (i) percentage of melanomas expressing Rad6 (100% of primary and metastatic melanomas), or (ii) percentage of melanomas expressing Rad6 in more than 50% of the tumor cells (100% and 96% of primary and metastatic melanomas, resp.). The increase in proportion of tumor populations, expressing Rad6 in more than 50% of the cells in primary melanoma (67%) versus metastatic melanoma (79%) was not significant ($P = 0.37$; Figure 2). This study was not designed to test whether the distribution of the tumor cells positive for Rad6 is the same between the subtypes of nevi. However, the percentages of benign tumors that lacked Rad6 were similar between atypical nevi (62%) and the group of other three nevi types (59%).

3.4. Rad6 as a Putative Biomarker for Differentiating Nevi from Melanoma. Interestingly, only one of the 30 nevi (atypical nevus, 3%) expressed Rad6 in >80% of the cells, and none of the primary and metastatic melanomas expressed Rad6 in <40% of the cells (Figure 2). These results prompted us to examine whether Rad6 expression can serve as a marker for histological diagnosis of melanoma. Using a multiple logistic regression model, we found that the strength of Rad6 expression is a strong predictor of melanoma ($P < 0.001$) even when age group ($P = 0.65$) and gender ($P = 0.24$) are included in the model. The model predicts that every 1% increase in Rad6 expression results in a 9% increase in the probability that a lesion is melanoma. If we assume that a predicted probability of >0.5 indicates melanoma, the model with only Rad6 has sensitivity of 93% and specificity of 80%. These results are very encouraging; however, they need to be validated in a larger study.

3.5. Correlation between β-Catenin and Rad6. The expression profiles of β-catenin and Rad6 differed considerably in nevi. Approximately 93% of nevi expressed β-catenin in more than 50% of the cells, whereas only 27% of the same population of nevi expressed Rad6 (Figure 2). β-Catenin and Rad6 expressions in nevi were not significantly correlated ($r = 0.06$; $P = 0.77$). There is a 2.7-fold difference in the percentage of primary melanomas (100%) expressing Rad6 compared to nevi (37%) and virtually no difference in β-catenin expression between primary and metastatic melanomas (100%). Accordingly, Rad6 and β-catenin expressions in primary melanoma were not correlated ($r < 0.001, P > 0.99$). A significant correlation between Rad6 and β-catenin positive cells was observed in metastatic melanoma ($r = 0.45$, $P = 0.02$).

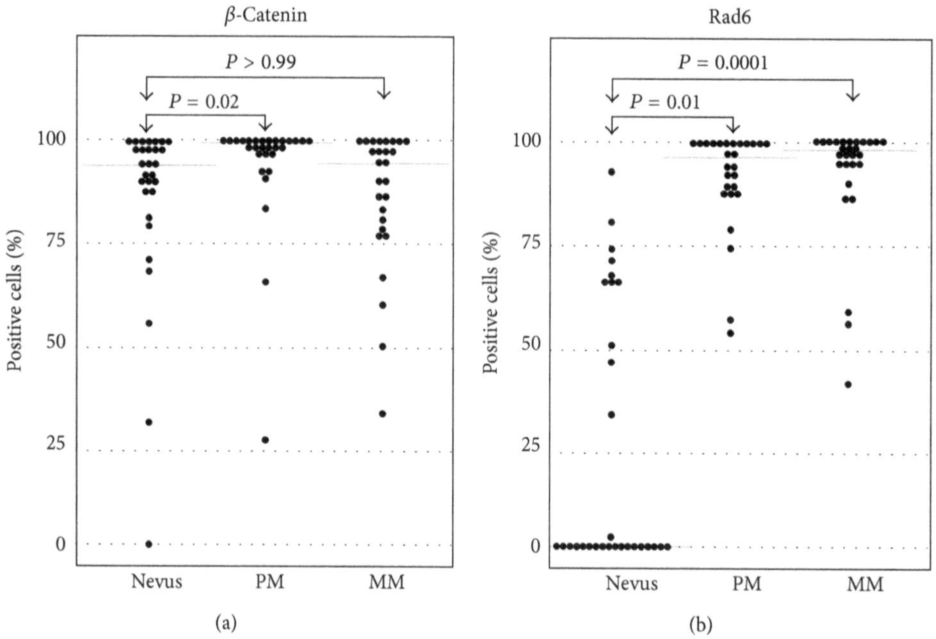

FIGURE 3: Boxplots of Rad6 and β-catenin positive cells in nevi, primary melanoma (PM), and metastatic melanoma (MM). Kruskal-Wallis tests showed that there are significantly more Rad6 positive cells in primary and metastatic melanomas as compared to nevi. Median values are indicated by gray horizontal lines.

However, this association diminished ($r = 0.40$, $P = 0.05$) following the exclusion of two observations which are disproportionally influential (one with <50% positive Rad6 and one with <50% positive β-catenin).

4. Discussion

This is the first study to characterize Rad6 expression in cutaneous benign and malignant melanocytic tumors. In this study, we examined the association between Rad6 and β-catenin expressions in benign and malignant melanocytic tumors to determine whether Rad6 works in concert with β-catenin to influence melanoma development and progression. Rad6 and β-catenin positively regulate each other in breast cancer [15, 18]. However, while β-catenin has been implicated in the pathogenesis of melanoma and other cancer types, data about the role of Rad6 in cancer pathogenesis are mostly limited to breast cancer. Approximately 30% of melanomas develop in preexisting benign melanocytic neoplasms (nevi) [27]. Therefore, we hypothesized that comparison of Rad6 and β-catenin expressions in the same nevi and melanoma tumors would help determine whether these two signals collaborate to promote melanoma development and progression as they do in breast cancer [15, 28].

4.1. The Percentage of Samples Expressing β-Catenin Was Equally High in Nevi and Melanoma and Does Not Support a Central Role for β-Catenin Level in Melanoma Initiation and Progression. Accumulation of nuclear and cytoplasmic β-catenin has been implicated in driving the development and progression of several cancer types (e.g., colon and ovarian cancers) [29–31]. However, our results show that the expression levels of β-catenin do not contribute to melanoma initiation and progression since no difference in β-catenin levels was found between nevi, primary melanoma, and metastatic melanoma (93%–97% of all samples expressed β-catenin in >50% of the tumor cells). The high expression levels of β-catenin are in line with the crucial role of β-catenin in differentiation and proliferation of both normal melanocytes and metastatic melanoma cells [32]. Also, our findings are in agreement with previous reports of positive β-catenin staining in nevi (100%) and primary melanoma (95%, 94%) but are higher than reported in metastatic melanoma (75%, 68%) [9, 21]. The variation in expression of β-catenin levels in metastatic melanomas between the studies can be attributed to differences in the type of metastatic tissues. While we studied only melanoma metastases to the skin, other studies either obtained 58% of their specimens from lymph nodes, tonsil, and liver or did not identify the anatomical site of their metastases [9, 21]. Furthermore, different anatomical sites may regulate dissimilar antigen expressions in metastases that originate from the same primary tumor in the same patient [33, 34].

4.2. Nuclear β-Catenin Was Absent from All Nevi and Melanomas, Indicating Its Low Usefulness as a Prognostic Marker in Melanoma. Previous studies have shown higher percentages of nuclear β-catenin in nevi than in melanoma (84% versus 33%, and 44% versus 15%) [9, 22]. Those observations provided the basis for the currently held concept that loss of nuclear and cytoplasmic β-catenin suggest poor prognosis and decreased overall survival of melanoma patients [12, 22]. In light of these data, the absence of nuclear β-catenin in all the nevi and melanomas analyzed in our study was surprising. Usage of different anti-β-catenin antibodies may explain in part the discrepancy in nuclear β-catenin expression observed between the studies. However, our results are consistent with the lack of nuclear β-catenin reported in four studies which comprised 57 nevi, more than 55 primary melanomas, and 20 metastatic melanomas [21, 35–37]. Moreover, nuclear β-catenin was not found in either the nevus portion or the melanoma portion of 15 cutaneous lesions and was absent in additional 42 primary melanomas [38]. In another study of 70 primary melanomas, nuclear β-catenin was reported in only 6.4% of the melanomas [39]. Finally, in a study of 230 primary and metastatic melanomas, nuclear β-catenin was reported in only 13 cases (5.6%) and therefore those cases were excluded from analysis [21]. Taken together, the absence or negligible amount of nuclear β-catenin detected in the aforementioned studies as well as ours suggests possible extranuclear roles for β-catenin in nevi and melanoma. This notion is supported by a role for cytoplasmic β-catenin to execute functions that do not require nuclear translocation (e.g., activation of MAP kinase p38 and NF-kB) [37, 40].

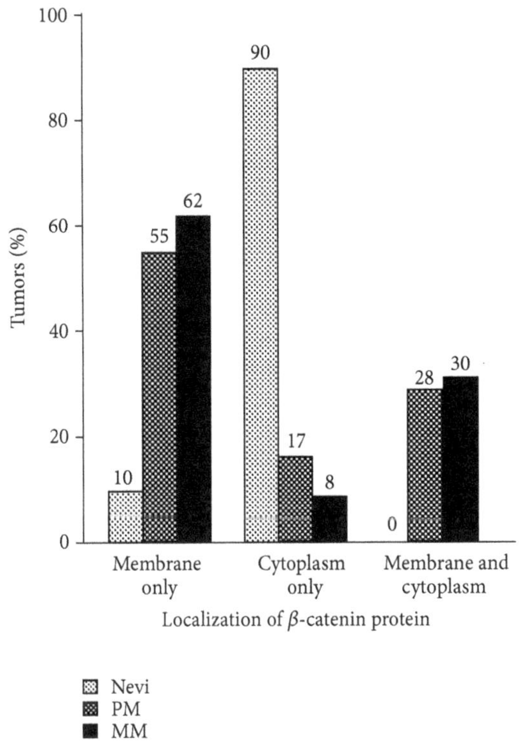

Figure 4: Subcellular localization of β-catenin in nevi, primary melanomas (PM), and metastatic melanomas (MM). Percentages of tumors expressing β-catenin exclusively in the cytoplasm or on cell membrane, or in both compartments.

4.3. Nevus to Melanoma Progression Is Associated with Cytoplasmic to Membranous Translocation of β-Catenin. A major finding of this study is the association between melanoma development and intracellular redistribution of β-catenin. The percentage of cases that expressed β-catenin on the cell membrane increased dramatically from 10% in nevi to 83% and 93% in primary and metastatic melanomas, respectively. Concurrently, the percentage of cases that expressed cytoplasmic β-catenin decreased from 90% in nevi to 45% and 39% in primary and metastatic melanomas, respectively (Figure 4). We hypothesize that the relocation of β-catenin from the cytoplasm to the cell membrane may serve as a deactivating mechanism of canonical Wnt/β-catenin signaling and that the resulting reduction in cytoplasmic β-catenin level may contribute to the malignant transformation of melanocytic nevi. The proposed hypothesis is supported by the following observations: (i) as in our study, Bachmann et al. also reported an association between nevus to melanoma development and relocation of β-catenin to the cell membrane [22]. Nevertheless, the authors of that study did not offer an explanation for their observation; (ii) our analysis of the data of Kagashita et al. showed β-catenin decrease in the cytoplasm and increase at the cell membrane and that these changes in β-catenin distribution corresponded with the malignant transition of nevi [9]; (iii) Wnt4 signal has been identified as a mechanism that can drive β-catenin relocation from cytoplasm to cell membrane [41]; and (iv) β-catenin relocation from cytoplasm to cell membrane has been reported to block β-catenin signaling in a human embryonic kidney (HEK293) cell line [41]. Of note, this hypothesis can explain how despite the abundant β-catenin expression in melanoma [1, 7], cytoplasmic β-catenin is selectively decreased, a phenomenon that has been associated with unfavorable melanoma prognosis [9, 21, 22]. Our current efforts are directed towards determining if the increases in membranous β-catenin observed in primary and metastatic melanomas result from relocation of existing molecules in the cytoplasm or deposition of newly generated β-catenin at the membranous site.

4.4. Rad6 Plays a Role in Melanoma Development and Progression, but Not in Nevi Formation. Rad6 has been implicated in early breast cancer development since an increase in Rad6 levels is observed in adenosis and benign hyperplasias as compared to normal tissue [15]. In contrast, our findings do not support Rad6 to play a similar role in nevus formation as in benign breast neoplasia, since 63% of the nevi were negative for Rad6. Rad6 has also been implicated in breast cancer progression because Rad6 levels increase with progression from ductal carcinoma *in situ* to invasive primary carcinoma and metastatic cancer [15, 28]. In accordance with the upregulation of Rad6 in early stages of breast cancer development as compared to benign hyperplasia [15, 17], we observed a striking increase in Rad6 expression in primary melanoma when compared to nevi. While all primary melanomas displayed strong Rad6 staining (>50% of the tumor cells), Rad6 was negative in 63% of the nevi. These findings suggest that Rad6 may play a role in malignant transformation of nevi as in breast cancer. Progression of melanoma from primary to metastatic disease was not significantly associated with further changes in the percentage of tumors expressing Rad6 or Rad expression intensity as >50% of tumor cells stained positively in 100% and 96% of primary melanomas and metastatic melanomas, respectively. These findings suggest that Rad6 may play a sustained role in melanoma metastasis as it does in melanoma development.

4.5. Correlation between β-Catenin and Rad6. In benign and malignant breast tumors, Rad6 stabilizes β-catenin, and, in turn, β-catenin positively upregulates Rad6 transcription [15–17]. However, this direct positive correlation between β-catenin and Rad6 expression does not appear to be conserved in melanoma as the expression profiles of β-catenin and Rad6 differed considerably in nevi. Approximately 93% of nevi expressed β-catenin compared to only 27% of nevi that expressed Rad6 in more than 50% of their cells (Figure 2). These observations suggest that the high β-catenin expression in nevi is likely driven by regulators other than Rad6. At first glance, it would appear that β-catenin and Rad6 expressions are correlated in primary melanoma because these proteins were coexpressed in approximately all primary melanomas. Also, these findings correspond to the 80% correlation between Rad6 and β-catenin expressions in primary breast cancer [17]. However, it is unlikely that the high Rad6 expression in primary melanoma is driven by the concurrent high β-catenin expression, because Rad6 expression is low in nevi despite the presence of high cytoplasmic β-catenin expression that is comparable to primary melanoma. This notion is confirmed by lack of statistical correlation between Rad6 and β-catenin expressions in primary melanoma. β-Catenin is not the only activator of Rad6; for instance, Rad6 is activated by nerve growth factor in nervous tissue [42]. Therefore, it is conceivable that, in primary melanoma, Rad6 expression is regulated by yet unidentified activators. We also demonstrated that further progression of melanoma from primary to metastatic disease is not associated with a correlation between the β-catenin and Rad6 expressions. Taken together, our study does not support a direct positive interaction between β-catenin and Rad6 in either benign or malignant melanocytic tumors.

5. Conclusion

We characterized for the first time Rad6 expression in cutaneous benign and malignant melanocytic tumors. We are showing a striking upregulation of Rad6 from a negative expression in most benign melanocytic tumors to 100% of primary and metastatic melanomas. These findings strongly suggest a role for Rad6 in the development of primary melanoma and metastatic disease. We show that in contrast to Rad6, β-catenin is expressed in more than 50% of the tumor cells in almost all nevi and melanoma tumors. Taken together, in contrast to the Rad6 β-catenin positive relationship in breast cancer [15–17], our study does not support a similar positive interaction between β-catenin and Rad6 in benign or malignant melanocytic tumors. Finally, our findings suggest a role for the cytoplasmic to membrane translocation of β-catenin in the development of primary melanoma. Future studies will determine whether newly generated β-catenin at the membranous site coincide with β-catenin translocation from the cytoplasm.

Abbreviations

HHR6: Human homologue of the yeast Rad6
DCIS: Ductal carcinoma *in situ*
PDL: Pinkus Dermatopathology Laboratory.

Acknowledgments

This work was supported by Startup Funds from Wayne State University and a Grant from NIH (R21CA178117-01). The Biostatistics Core is supported, in part, by NIH Center Grant P30 CA022453 to the Karmanos Cancer Institute at Wayne State University.

References

[1] D. L. Rimm, K. Caca, G. Hu, F. B. Harrison, and E. R. Fearon, "Frequent nuclear/cytoplasmic localization of β-catenin without exon 3 mutations in malignant melanoma," *American Journal of Pathology*, vol. 154, no. 2, pp. 325–329, 1999.

[2] C.-T. Yeh, C.-J. Yao, J.-L. Yan et al., "Apoptotic cell death and inhibition of Wnt/β-catenin signaling pathway in human colon cancer cells by an active fraction (hs7) from taiwanofungus camphoratus," *Evidence-based Complementary and Alternative Medicine*, vol. 2011, Article ID 750230, 2011.

[3] G. Zulehner, M. Mikula, D. Schneller et al., "Nuclear β-catenin induces an early liver progenitor phenotype in hepatocellular carcinoma and promotes tumor recurrence," *American Journal of Pathology*, vol. 176, no. 1, pp. 472–481, 2010.

[4] B. Bellei, A. Pitisci, C. Catricalà, L. Larue, and M. Picardo, "Wnt/β-catenin signaling is stimulated by α-melanocyte-stimulating hormone in melanoma and melanocyte cells: Implication in cell differentiation," *Pigment Cell and Melanoma Research*, vol. 24, no. 2, pp. 309–325, 2011.

[5] L. Larue and V. Delmas, "Secrets to developing Wnt-age melanoma revealed," *Pigment Cell and Melanoma Research*, vol. 22, no. 5, pp. 520–521, 2009.

[6] T. Yaguchi, Y. Goto, K. Kido et al., "Immune suppression and resistance mediated by constitutive activation of Wnt/β-catenin signaling in human melanoma cells," *The Journal of Immunology*, vol. 189, no. 5, pp. 2110–2117, 2012.

[7] H. R. Widlund, M. A. Horstmann, E. Roydon Price et al., "β-Catenin-induced melanoma growth requires the downstream target Microphthalmia-associated transcription factor," *Journal of Cell Biology*, vol. 158, no. 6, pp. 1079–1087, 2002.

[8] S. C. C. Wong, E. S. F. Lo, K. C. Lee, J. K. C. Chan, and W. L. W. Hsiao, "Prognostic and diagnostic significance of β-catenin nuclear Immunostaining in colorectal cancer," *Clinical Cancer Research*, vol. 10, no. 4, pp. 1401–1408, 2004.

[9] T. Kageshita, C. V. Hamby, T. Ishihara, K. Matsumoto, T. Saida, and T. Ono, "Loss of β-catenin expression associated with disease progression in malignant melanoma," *British Journal of Dermatology*, vol. 145, no. 2, pp. 210–216, 2001.

[10] A. Demunter, L. Libbrecht, H. Degreef, C. De Wolf-Peeters, and J. J. Van den Oord, "Loss of membranous expression β-catenin is associated with tumor progression in cutaneous melanoma

and rarely caused by exon 3 mutations," *Modern Pathology*, vol. 15, no. 4, pp. 454–461, 2002.

[11] O. M. Lucero, D. W. Dawson, R. T. Moon, and A. J. Chien, "A re-evaluation of the "oncogenic" nature of Wnt/β-catenin signaling in melanoma and other cancers," *Current Oncology Reports*, vol. 12, no. 5, pp. 314–318, 2010.

[12] B. E. G. Rothberg, A. J. Berger, A. M. Molinaro et al., "Melanoma prognostic model using tissue microarrays and genetic algorithms," *Journal of Clinical Oncology*, vol. 27, no. 34, pp. 5772–5780, 2009.

[13] I. Arozarena, H. Bischof, D. Gilby, B. Belloni, R. Dummer, and C. Wellbrock, "In melanoma, beta-catenin is a suppressor of invasion," *Oncogene*, vol. 30, no. 45, pp. 4531–4543, 2011.

[14] A. J. Chien, E. C. Moore, A. S. Lonsdorf et al., "Activated Wnt/β-catenin signaling in melanoma is associated with decreased proliferation in patient tumors and a murine melanoma model," *Proceedings of the National Academy of Sciences of the United States of America*, vol. 106, no. 4, pp. 1193–1198, 2009.

[15] M. P. V. Shekhar, A. Lyakhovich, D. W. Visscher, H. Heng, and N. Kondrat, "Rad6 overexpression induces multinucleation, centrosome amplification, abnormal mitosis, aneuploidy, and transformation," *Cancer Research*, vol. 62, no. 7, pp. 2115–2124, 2002.

[16] M. P. V. Shekhar, B. Gerard, R. J. Pauley, B. O. Williams, and L. Tait, "Rad6B is a positive regulator of β-catenin stabilization," *Cancer Research*, vol. 68, no. 6, pp. 1741–1750, 2008.

[17] M. P. V. Shekhar, L. Tait, and B. Gerard, "Essential role of T-cell factor/β-catenin in regulation of Rad6B: a potential mechanism for Rad6B overexpression in breast cancer cells," *Molecular Cancer Research*, vol. 4, no. 10, pp. 729–745, 2006.

[18] B. Gerard, L. Tait, P. Nangia-Makker, and M. P. V. Shekhar, "Rad6B acts downstream of Wnt signaling to stabilize β-catenin: implications for a novel Wnt/β-catenin target," *Journal of Molecular Signaling*, vol. 6, article 6, 2011.

[19] M. P. V. Shekhar, L. A. Biernat, N. Pernick, L. Tait, J. Abrams, and D. W. Visscher, "Utility of DNA postreplication repair protein Rad6B in neoadjuvant chemotherapy response," *Medical Oncology*, vol. 27, no. 2, pp. 466–473, 2010.

[20] S. Dihlmann and M. Von Knebel Doeberitz, "Wnt/β-catenin-pathway as a molecular target for future anti-cancer therapeutics," *International Journal of Cancer*, vol. 113, no. 4, pp. 515–524, 2005.

[21] G. M. Mælandsmo, R. Holm, J. M. Nesland, Ø. Fodstad, and V. A. Flørenes, "Reduced β-catenin expression in the cytoplasm of advanced-stage superficial spreading malignant melanoma," *Clinical Cancer Research*, vol. 9, no. 9, pp. 3383–3388, 2003.

[22] I. M. Bachmann, O. Straume, H. E. Puntervoll, M. B. Kalvenes, and L. A. Akslen, "Importance of P-cadherin, β-catenin, and Wnt5a/Frizzled for progression of melanocytic tumors and prognosis in cutaneous melanoma," *Clinical Cancer Research*, vol. 11, no. 24, pp. 8606–8614, 2005.

[23] M. E. Roth, J. M. Grant-Kels, A. B. Ackerman et al., "The histopathology of dysplastic nevi: continued controversy," *American Journal of Dermatopathology*, vol. 13, no. 1, pp. 38–51, 1991.

[24] A. Lyakhovich and M. P. V. Shekhar, "RAD6B overexpression confers chemoresistance: RAD6 expression during cell cycle and its redistribution to chromatin during DNA damage-induced response," *Oncogene*, vol. 23, no. 17, pp. 3097–3106, 2004.

[25] K. Rosner, D. R. Mehregan, D. Moussai, J. Abrams, G. Tromp, and D. A. Mehregan, "WT1 marker is not sufficient for distinguishing between melanoma and melanocytic nevi," *Journal of Cutaneous Pathology*, vol. 36, no. 10, pp. 1077–1082, 2009.

[26] H. Mineta, K. Miura, S. Takebayashi et al., "Cyclin D1 overexpression correlates with poor prognosis in patients with tongue squamous cell carcinoma," *Oral Oncology*, vol. 36, no. 2, pp. 194–198, 2000.

[27] D. C. Whiteman, W. J. Pavan, and B. C. Bastian, "The melanomas: a synthesis of epidemiological, clinical, histopathological, genetic, and biological aspects, supporting distinct subtypes, causal pathways, and cells of origin," *Pigment Cell and Melanoma Research*, vol. 24, no. 5, pp. 879–897, 2011.

[28] B. Gerard, M. A. Sanders, D. W. Visscher, L. Tait, and M. P. Shekhar, "Lysine 394 is a novel RAD6B-induced ubiquitination site on beta-catenin," *Biochimica et Biophysica Acta*, vol. 1823, no. 10, pp. 1686–1696, 2012.

[29] T. Oyama, Y. Yamada, K. Hata et al., "Further upregulation of β-catenin/Tcf transcription is involved in the development of macroscopic tumors in the colon of $Apc^{\mathrm{Min}/+}$ mice," *Carcinogenesis*, vol. 29, no. 3, pp. 666–672, 2008.

[30] P. J. Morin, A. B. Sparks, V. Korinek et al., "Activation of β-catenin-Tcf signaling in colon cancer by mutations in β-catenin or APC," *Science*, vol. 275, no. 5307, pp. 1787–1790, 1997.

[31] J. Palacios and C. Gamallo, "Mutations in the β-catenin gene (CTNNB1) in endometrioid ovarian carcinomas," *Cancer Research*, vol. 58, no. 7, pp. 1344–1347, 1998.

[32] T. Sinnberg, M. Menzel, D. Ewerth et al., "β-catenin signaling increases during melanoma progression and promotes tumor cell survival and chemoresistance," *PLoS ONE*, vol. 6, no. 8, Article ID e23429, 2011.

[33] X. Zhang, C. Morrissey, S. Sun et al., "Androgen receptor variants occur frequently in castration resistant prostate cancer metastases," *PLoS ONE*, vol. 6, no. 11, Article ID e27970, 2011.

[34] C. G. J. M. Hilders, I. M. Munoz, Y. Nooyen, and G. J. Fleuren, "Altered HLA expression by metastatic cervical carcinoma cells as a factor in impaired immune surveillance," *Gynecologic Oncology*, vol. 57, no. 3, pp. 366–375, 1995.

[35] D. S. A. Sanders, K. Blessing, G. A. R. Hassan, R. Bruton, J. R. Marsden, and J. Jankowski, "Alterations in cadherin and catenin expression during the biological progression of melanocytic tumours," *Journal of Clinical Pathology, Molecular Pathology*, vol. 52, no. 3, pp. 151–157, 1999.

[36] R. Silye, A. J. Karayiannakis, K. N. Syrigos et al., "E-cadherin/catenin complex in benign and malignant melanocytic lesions.," *The Journal of Pathology*, vol. 186, no. 4, pp. 350–355, 1998.

[37] S. Kuphal and A. K. Bosserhoff, "Phosphorylation of β-catenin results in lack of β-catenin signaling in melanoma," *International Journal of Oncology*, vol. 39, no. 1, pp. 235–243, 2011.

[38] G. De Panfilis, D. Ferrari, S. Santoro et al., "Cytoplasmic β-catenin is lacking in a subset of melanoma-associated naevi, but is detectable in naevus-associated melanomas: potential implications for melanoma tumorigenesis?" *British Journal of Dermatology*, vol. 160, no. 3, pp. 600–608, 2009.

[39] N. Pećina-Slaus, M. Zigmund, V. Kusec, T. N. Martić, M. Cacić, and M. Slaus, "E-cadherin and β-catenin expression patterns in malignant melanoma assessed by image analysis," *Journal of Cutaneous Pathology*, vol. 34, no. 3, pp. 239–246, 2007.

[40] S. Kuphal, I. Poser, C. Jobin, C. Hellerbrand, and A. K. Bosserhoff, "Loss of E-cadherin leads to upregulation of NFκB

activity in malignant melanoma," *Oncogene*, vol. 23, no. 52, pp. 8509–8519, 2004.

[41] P. Bernard, A. Fleming, A. Lacombe, V. R. Harley, and E. Vilain, "Wnt4 inhibits β-catenin/TCF signalling by redirecting β-catenin to the cell membrane," *Biology of the Cell*, vol. 100, no. 3, pp. 167–177, 2008.

[42] P. Kavakebi, B. Hausott, A. Tomasino, S. Ingorokva, and L. Klimaschewski, "The N-end rule ubiquitin-conjugating enzyme, HR6B, is up-regulated by nerve growth factor and required for neurite outgrowth," *Molecular and Cellular Neuroscience*, vol. 29, no. 4, pp. 559–568, 2005.

8

Targeted Therapies Compared to Dacarbazine for Treatment of BRAF^{V600E} Metastatic Melanoma: A Cost-Effectiveness Analysis

Vanessa Shih, Renske M. ten Ham, Christine T. Bui, Dan N. Tran, Jie Ting, and Leslie Wilson

Department of Clinical Pharmacy, University of California, San Francisco, 3333 California Street, Laurel Heights, San Francisco, CA 94143, USA

Correspondence should be addressed to Leslie Wilson; wilsonl@pharmacy.ucsf.edu

Academic Editor: Lionel Larue

Purpose. Two BRAF^{V600E} targeted therapies, dabrafenib and vemurafenib, have received US approval for treatment of metastatic melanoma in BRAF^{V600E} patients, a mutation that affects ~50% of patients. We evaluated the cost-effectiveness of BRAF inhibitors and traditional chemotherapy for treatment of metastatic melanoma. *Methods*. A Markov model was developed using a societal perspective. Transition probabilities were derived from two Phase III registration trials comparing each BRAF inhibitor against dacarbazine. Costs were obtained from literature, national databases, and Medicare fee schedules. Utilities were obtained from published literature. Deterministic and probabilistic sensitivity analyses were run to test the impact of uncertainties. *Results*. The incremental cost-effectiveness ratio of dabrafenib was $149,035/QALY compared to dacarbazine. Vemurafenib was dominated by dabrafenib. Probabilistic sensitivity analysis showed that, at a willingness-to-pay (WTP) threshold of ≤$100,000/QALY, dacarbazine was the optimal treatment in ~85% of simulations. At a WTP threshold of ≥$150,000/QALY, dabrafenib was the optimal treatment. *Conclusion*. Compared with dacarbazine, dabrafenib and vemurafenib were not cost-effective at a willingness-to-pay threshold of $100,000/QALY. Dabrafenib is more efficient compared to vemurafenib. With few treatment options, dabrafenib is an option for qualifying patients if the overall cost of dabrafenib is reduced to $30,000–$31,000 or a WTP threshold of ≥$150,000/QALY is considered. More comparative data is needed.

1. Introduction

Malignant melanoma continues to increase dramatically in incidence worldwide [1]. In 2013, an estimated 76,690 people in the US were diagnosed with melanoma of the skin, of whom about 9,480 will die of the disease [2]. The prognosis of patients with metastatic melanoma is very poor with the one-year survival rate ranging from 33 to 62%, depending on disease stage [3]. In patients diagnosed with melanoma, about 40–60% carry mutations in BRAF [4], which can lead to increased cellular proliferation and increased oncogenic cell activity [5]. Among these patients, 80–90% have the amino acid valine replaced with glutamic acid at codon 600 (BRAF^{V600E}) [4, 6].

Until 2011, dacarbazine, a chemotherapeutic alkylating agent, was the standard of care for patients with metastatic melanoma despite its lack of survival benefit [7, 8]. However, due to improved knowledge on the molecular biology of melanoma and the discovery of oncogenic mutations contributing to disease progression, two novel therapies were developed [9]. In 2011, the US Food and Drug Administration (FDA) approved the BRAF kinase inhibitor vemurafenib (Zelboraf, Genentech, South San Francisco, CA) for treatment of metastatic melanoma in patients with the BRAF^{V600E} mutation. A second BRAF inhibitor, dabrafenib (Tafinlar, GlaxoSmithKline, Brentford, UK), was approved in 2013 for the same indication. Compared with palliative chemotherapy, BRAF inhibition demonstrated overall survival improvement and produced a response rate of nearly 50% in clinical trials [9, 10]. Additionally, BRAF inhibitors are oral agents and provide an improved side effect profile compared to chemotherapy.

However, BRAF inhibitor responses are not durable with development of resistance commonly occurring [11].

Furthermore, BRAF inhibitors come with a high cost burden so the question remains if these novel therapies provide value. The purpose of this study was to perform a cost-effectiveness analysis of the newly available oral targeted therapies vemurafenib and dabrafenib compared to each other and to dacarbazine in patients with unresectable stage III or stage IV metastatic melanoma positive for the $BRAF^{V600E}$ mutation. To our knowledge, this is the first study to assess the comparative economic value of these therapies and results from this analysis may be used to inform decision making processes.

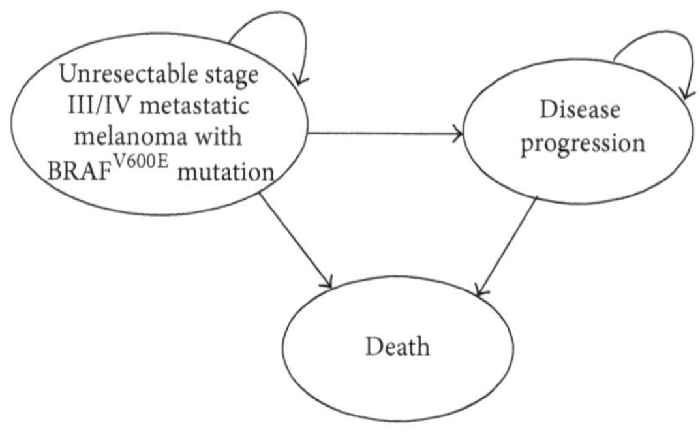

FIGURE 1: Markov structure diagramming progression of patients through health states.

2. Methods

2.1. Study Population. Our study population was patients from two published Phase III clinical trials with unresectable stage III or stage IV metastatic melanoma positive for the $BRAF^{V600E}$ mutation [4, 6]. Both were multicenter, randomized trials enrolling patients from twelve countries across Europe, North America, and Australia. The vemurafenib trial assigned 675 patients to either vemurafenib (n = 337, median age 56 years) or dacarbazine (n = 338, median age 52 years). We used the trial overall survival data results that were used by the FDA for drug approval and were available at the time of our study, begun in October 2013. Median follow-up time for the vemurafenib group was 3.8 months and the dacarbazine group 2.3 months. The dabrafenib trial assigned 250 patients to receive dabrafenib (n = 187, median age 53 years) or dacarbazine (n = 63, median age 50 years) and had a median time on study of 4.9 months. In both trials, patient populations had similar patient characteristics, disease severity, and disease progression. We did not use the results of the extended follow-up analysis published later because the longer follow-up time was longer for vemurafenib (12.5 months) and made the dabrafenib study noncomparable [21].

2.2. Model Overview. A Markov model was constructed to compare the cost-effectiveness of dabrafenib, vemurafenib, and dacarbazine using TreeAge Pro 2013 (TreeAge Software, Williamstown, MA, USA) for treatment of patients with stage IV or unresectable stage III metastatic melanoma with the $BRAF^{V600E}$ mutation. This model was from a US societal perspective over the patient's remaining lifetime. We used 2013 USD and a societal willingness-to-pay (WTP) threshold of $100,000 per quality-adjusted life year (QALY).

Each monthly cycle of the model simulated the disease progression of a patient cohort through three discrete health states: stable disease, progression, and death (Figure 1). All patients started in stable disease and could remain with stable disease, move to progression, or die. Patients in the progression state could remain in progression or die (absorbing state).

Model outcomes were total treatment costs measured in 2013 US dollars and effect measured in QALY. Cost-effectiveness of each treatment was compared from least to most expensive using the incremental cost-effectiveness ratio (ICER) as defined by $(\text{Cost}_{\text{treatment1}} - \text{Cost}_{\text{treatment2}})/(\text{QALY}_{\text{treatment1}} - \text{QALY}_{\text{treatment2}})$.

2.3. Model Inputs. Model inputs were clinical inputs including monthly health state transition probabilities, monthly side effect probabilities, and health state utilities to obtain QALYs, as well as cost inputs. Progression-free survival (PFS) for vemurafenib was derived from the published Phase III pivotal trial, while overall survival (OS) was obtained from the FDA summary basis for approval which was available at the time of this study [4, 22]. PFS and OS for dabrafenib were derived from the published Phase III pivotal trial [6]. Probability of death was 1-OS and probability of disease progression was OS-PFS. Dacarbazine was used as the comparator drug in both Phase III pivotal trials. Since patient characteristics of the dacarbazine treatment arms in both Phase III studies were similar, PFS and OS for dacarbazine were derived by averaging probabilities from both trials. The Declining Exponential Approximation of Life Expectancy (DEALE) method was used to extend the survival curves to represent a lifetime horizon (Figure 2) [23, 24]. DEALE is a good approximation when survival is short such as in these trials (10 months for vemurafenib and 9 months for dabrafenib). The hazard rate (HR) was calculated from the probability of overall survival and progression-free survival at month 8 in both trials and was then used to model mortality for the patient's remaining lifetime, assuming a constant HR.

Adverse event probabilities were obtained from published Phase III trials [4, 6]. All Grade III and Grade IV adverse events were included in the model along with Grade I and Grade II adverse events that were costly to treat or occurred with high frequency (Table 1). Adverse events included in the model fell into three categories: (i) hematological complications including neutropenia, thrombocytopenia, and leukopenia which occurred primarily in patients on dacarbazine; (ii) gastrointestinal adverse events including nausea, vomiting, and diarrhea which occurred across all treatment groups; (iii) skin adverse events including hyperkeratosis, skin papillomas, nonmelanoma skin cancers, and palmar plantar erythrodysesthesia (PPE) which affected primarily patients on dabrafenib and vemurafenib. Adverse events were assumed to need treatment independently of each other with

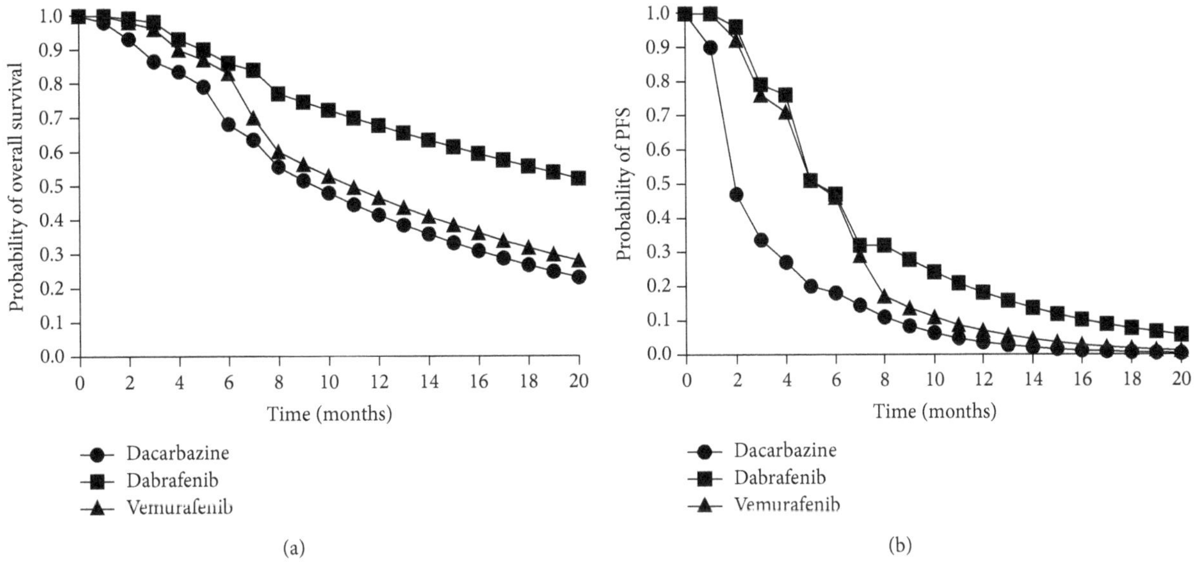

FIGURE 2: (a) Kaplan-Meier Overall Survival Curve. (b) Kaplan-Meier Progression-Free Survival Curve. (The probabilities from 0–8 months are from clinical trial data. The probabilities from 8 months to end of life are modeled using the DEALE method.)

the exception of nausea and vomiting which were assumed to occur together and require overlapping treatments.

Health utilities were included for quality adjustment expressed by QALYs. A drug-specific utility was calculated for both the stable disease and progression health states taking into account drug-specific rates of adverse events obtained from trial data (Table 1) [4, 6]. The proportion of the cohort experiencing each set of adverse events was multiplied by the utility weights for the adverse event states and summed to obtain the expected value of the utility for the health state specific to each drug. Utilities for melanoma health states were obtained from a published study that elicited utilities for metastatic melanoma specific health states from healthy volunteers in the United Kingdom and Australia [25]. Utilities for skin-related adverse event health states were taken from a catalog of dermatology utilities [26]. Utilities for non-skin-related adverse event states were obtained from other published studies [27]. A recent analysis demonstrating improved quality of life on dabrafenib compared with dacarbazine was not used as it did not provide real utilities required in a cost-effectiveness comparison [28].

Cost inputs included direct drug costs and costs of treating adverse events (Table 1). Drug costs were obtained from Redbook Online (Truven Health Analytics) and for dacarbazine this included costs for a prophylactic antiemetic regimen per National Comprehensive Cancer Network (NCCN) guidelines [12, 13]. In the dabrafenib trial, patients in the comparator arm could cross over to the treatment arm per protocol [6]. The vemurafenib trial protocol was later amended to allow for crossover as well [4]. To account for the crossover in the treatment costs, an additional cost equal to the cost of dabrafenib was included for all patients in the progression state in the dacarbazine treatment arm. Adverse event costs were obtained from literature [17, 29, 30], the Centers for Medicare and Medicaid Services (CMS) reimbursement fee schedules using Current Procedural Treatment (CPT) codes for physician procedural costs [15], and the Healthcare Cost and Utilization Project (HCUP) database for hospitalization costs [14].

2.4. Sensitivity Analysis. To evaluate the impact of drug cost on cost-effectiveness, a one-way sensitivity analysis was performed on the cost of dabrafenib and the cost of vemurafenib. Probabilistic sensitivity analysis on all variables was performed with a Monte Carlo simulation, randomly sampling 10,000 iterations, using confidence intervals where available, beta distributions for probabilities, and gamma distributions for costs. Using the Monte Carlo simulations, the cost-effectiveness acceptability curve was constructed plotting the percentage of iterations where each therapy was cost-effective against a range of WTP thresholds along the x-axis. The percentage of cost-effective iterations was calculated for each therapy by first calculating the net monetary benefit (NMB) at each WTP threshold (λ) using the equation NMB = $\lambda \times$ (Total Effect − Total Cost) [31]. Then, for each treatment at each WTP threshold, the proportion of iterations where the treatment had the highest NMB provided the percentage of cost-effective iterations.

3. Results

3.1. Cost-Effectiveness Analysis. Total cost represents drug costs and toxicity management costs accrued over the patients' entire remaining lifetime. Drug costs were applied during all cycles in which patients were alive and side effect management costs, weighted by probability of occurring, were applied during each cycle in which patients received drug. Total cost was lowest for the dacarbazine treatment arm ($15,221), followed by dabrafenib ($38,547) and then vemurafenib ($49,937). Effectiveness of dacarbazine, vemurafenib,

TABLE 1: Model inputs.

	Vemurafenib	Dabrafenib	Dacarbazine
Base case adverse event probabilities by drug [4, 6]			
Vomiting, nausea, Grades 1, 2	0.0023	0.0009	0.0106
Vomiting, nausea, Grades 3, 4	0.0010	0	0.0007
Diarrhea, Grades 1, 2	0.0230	0	0.0006
Diarrhea, Grades 3, 4	0.0005	0	0.0001
Hyperkeratosis, Grades 1, 2	0.0172	0.0113	0
Hyperkeratosis, Grades 3, 4	0.0010	0.0009	0
Skin papilloma, Grades 1, 2	0.0169	0	0
Skin papilloma, Grades 3, 4	0	0	0
Squamous cell carcinoma, Grades 1, 2	0	0.0018	0
Squamous cell carcinoma, Grades 3, 4	0.0105	0.0036	0
Keratoacanthoma, Grades 1, 2	0.0051	0	0
Keratoacanthoma, Grades 3, 4	0	0	0
Neutropenia, Grades 1, 2	0.0002	0	0.0019
Neutropenia, Grades 3, 4	0.0002	0.0004	0.0086
PPE, Grades 1, 2	0	0.0055	0
PPE, Grades 3, 4	0	0.0018	0
Leukopenia, Grades 1, 2	0	0	0.0013
Leukopenia, Grades 3, 4	0	0	0.0007
Thrombocytopenia, Grades 1, 2	0	0	0
Thrombocytopenia, Grades 3, 4	0	0	0.0020

	Base case value	Sensitivity analysis		Distribution
		Lower value	Upper value	
Drug-specific utility values for each health state including side effects				
Stable disease, dacarbazine	0.69	0	1	Beta
Progression, dacarbazine	0.45	0	1	Beta
Stable disease, dabrafenib	0.79	0	1	Beta
Progression, dabrafenib	0.52	0	1	Beta
Stable disease, vemurafenib	0.73	0	1	Beta
Progression, vemurafenib	0.49	0	1	Beta
Monthly drug costs (2013 USD)				
Dacarbazine cost per month, assuming one cycle per month and including administration and prophylactic antiemetic treatment costs [12–14]	$988.86	$678.29	$1356.85	Gamma
Dabrafenib monthly cost [6, 13]	$7569.60	$5677.20	$9462.00	Gamma
Vemurafenib monthly cost [4, 13]	$10807.40	$8105.55	$13509.25	Gamma
Toxicity management costs per month on treatment				
Hyperkeratosis, Grades 1, 2 [13, 15, 16]	$126.66	$114.26	$424.95	Gamma
Hyperkeratosis, Grades 3, 4 [13, 15, 16]	$1082.84	$1070.84	$1706.93	Gamma
Squamous cell carcinoma [15, 17]	$1595	$1128	$3408	Gamma
Nausea, vomiting BRAF inhibitor, Grades 1, 2 [12, 13]	$274.58	$274.58	$419.54	Gamma
Nausea, vomiting BRAF inhibitor, Grades 3, 4 [12–14]	$6855.76	$4480.05	$8009.39	Gamma
Diarrhea, Grades 1, 2 [13, 18]	$5.81	$5.81	$45.89	Gamma
Diarrhea, Grades 3, 4 [13–15, 18]	$7404.11	$3550.28	$7845	Gamma
Keratoacanthoma, Grades 1, 2 [6, 13, 15]	$113.67	$66.72	$181.31	Gamma
Skin papilloma, Grades 2, 3 [15]	$73	$61	$97	Gamma
PPE [13, 15, 19, 20]	$113.67	$113.67	$178.62	Gamma
Nausea, vomiting, dacarbazine, Grades 1, 2 [12, 13]	$84.66	$2.78	$4485.98	Gamma
Nausea, vomiting, dacarbazine, Grades 3, 4 [12–14]	$6665.84	$4208.25	$12075.84	Gamma

TABLE 2: Cost-effectiveness of dabrafenib relative to dacarbazine and vemurafenib relative to dabrafenib.

	Total cost	Total effectiveness	Incremental cost	Incremental effectiveness	ICER
Dacarbazine	$15,221	0.1820 QALYs			
Dabrafenib	$38,547	0.3385 QALYs	$23,325	0.1565 QALYs	$149,042
Vemurafenib	$49,938	0.2905 QALYs	Dominated	Dominated	Dominated

QALYs: quality-adjusted life years; ICER: incremental cost-effectiveness ratio.
Note: comparisons are to the next least costly alternative.

TABLE 3: Base case cost-effectiveness of vemurafenib relative to dacarbazine.

	Total cost	Total effectiveness	Incremental cost	Incremental effectiveness	ICER
Dacarbazine	$15,221	0.1820 QALYs			
Vemurafenib	$49,938	0.2905 QALYs	$34,717	0.1085 QALYs	$319,972

QALYs: quality-adjusted life years; ICER: incremental cost-effectiveness ratio.
Note: comparison is to the chemotherapy drug option.

and dabrafenib was 0.1820, 0.2905, and 0.3385 QALYs, respectively (Table 2).

Dacarbazine was the least costly, but also least effective (Table 2). However, the ICER of dabrafenib, the next more costly option, relative to dacarbazine, was high, $149,035/QALY. This is not considered cost-effective, exceeding the current average US societal WTP of $100,000/QALY. Vemurafenib was dominated by dabrafenib because it was more costly than dabrafenib and less effective, demonstrating a strong preference for dabrafenib over vemurafenib for cost-effectiveness. In addition, the ICER of vemurafenib over dacarbazine chemotherapy was $319,972/QALY, clearly higher than any acceptable WTP threshold (Table 3).

3.2. Sensitivity Analysis

3.2.1. Deterministic Sensitivity Analysis. One-way sensitivity analyses were performed on the cost of dabrafenib and vemurafenib in order to determine the effect of drug cost on cost-effectiveness. Using a WTP threshold of $100,000/QALY gained, dabrafenib only became a cost-effective option compared to dacarbazine when its cost was decreased to below $5,259/month, a ~30% decrease in monthly price. Vemurafenib was dominated by dabrafenib and was not cost-effective compared with dacarbazine.

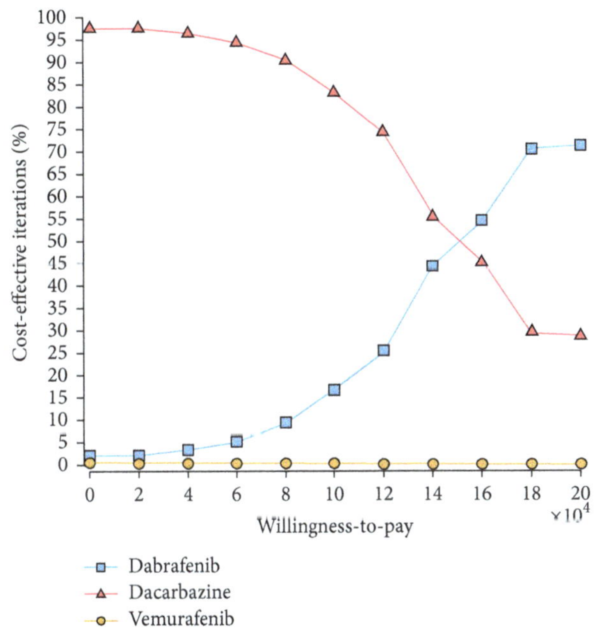

FIGURE 3: Cost-effectiveness acceptability curve. This acceptability curve shows, for each drug, which percentage of 10,000 Monte Carlo iterations is cost-effective over a range of WTP thresholds.

3.2.2. Probabilistic Sensitivity Analysis. At a WTP threshold of $100,000/QALY, dacarbazine was the optimal treatment in about 85% of simulations while dabrafenib was the optimal treatment in about 15% of simulations (Figure 3). Thus, at this threshold, dacarbazine was the most cost-effective treatment despite its lower survival. At WTP threshold of ≥$150,000/QALY, dabrafenib became the optimal treatment, being cost-effective in the majority of iterations.

4. Discussion

We found that, at a societal WTP threshold of ≤$100,000/QALY, dacarbazine was the optimal treatment. At this threshold, neither dabrafenib nor vemurafenib was cost-effective relative to dacarbazine. The ICER high for dabrafenib and even higher for vemurafenib compared to dacarbazine was likely due to a large incremental cost for the two BRAF inhibitors with only a mild but important increase in QALY of about two months. The large incremental costs are primarily attributable to differences in drug costs; dabrafenib and vemurafenib are eight- and tenfold more expensive than dacarbazine even when including a prophylactic antiemetic regimen with dacarbazine. However, we also found that dabrafenib dominates vemurafenib, indicating strongly that dabrafenib is the more cost-effective choice between the two targeted therapies, which are becoming standard treatment.

A recently published study compared the cost-effectiveness of three treatment strategies, vemurafenib, ipilimumab, and dacarbazine [32]. They found an ICER for vemurafenib compared to dacarbazine of $353,993/QALY, which is comparable to our ICER for vemurafenib compared to dacarbazine of $319,972/QALY. Our study adds to the literature by comparing the two BRAF inhibitors and demonstrating superiority of dabrafenib over vemurafenib in terms of value.

Cost-effectiveness analysis (CEA) results may be used as indicators of appropriate drug pricing or as the basis of price negotiations between drug manufacturers and payers based on implicit thresholds which indicate a society's WTP for improvements in health given a fixed budget. In the US, commonly cited thresholds for coverage range from $50,000 to $100,000/QALY while benchmarking approaches suggest threshold values ranging from $20,000 to $358,000/QALY [33]. This threshold has not been obtained by appropriately ranking the ICERs of all treatments until a fixed budget is reached. Instead, ICERs are used to add new favorable interventions, under the thresholds, but without removing those above the thresholds. Therefore the best threshold is uncertain and should vary by each budget under consideration. If we use the WHO threshold of two to three times the per capita annual income, the US threshold would be between $110,000/QALY and $160,000/QALY [34]. Others who account for inflation in health care spending suggest a threshold of $200,000/QALY and $300,000/QALY [34]. It has been argued that this threshold should be increased for end-of-life treatments [35]. In the UK where coverage of new therapies is linked to a demonstration of cost-effectiveness under a £30,000/QALY threshold, new guidelines from NICE have allowed for approval of previously cost-inefficient therapies for treatments meeting the following criteria: for patients with a short life expectancy, extension of life by at least three months compared to the current NHS standard, and for a small patient population [36]. Approval is also appropriate if the appraisal committee believes the QALY weight that will drop the ICER below £30,000/QALY accurately represents public preferences [36].

From a US payer perspective, high drug costs create incentives to restrict use, but, from a provider perspective, these therapies provide life-extending opportunities and these benefits have been realized with one study demonstrating coverage of vemurafenib in at least 50% of plans examined when it was the only targeted therapy [37]. Nationally, this need has been recognized with the mandate from CMS that Medicare drug plans cover "all or substantially all" drugs in specific therapeutic classes, including anticancer agents [38]. Although our ICER for dabrafenib compared to dacarbazine is not cost-effective at that price under the traditional WTP threshold, as an end-of-life treatment for a disease state with few options, there is evidence to suggest that, at negotiated prices within specific health plans, it is within acceptable limits to US payers and can be recommended as a treatment option with value [35]. This acceptance reflects the recent editorial reviewing ICER thresholds which suggests using between $100,000/QALY and $150,000/QALY [34].

While novel targeted therapies may have a place in treatment algorithms, strategies to minimize their ICER and the subsequent budget impact on payers will increase the value of these products. Our sensitivity analyses also demonstrated that 30% price cuts are necessary to reduce the ICER of dabrafenib compared to dacarbazine to below the current WTP threshold holding all other factors constant. This highlights the need for price negotiations as well as patient assistance programs from the manufacturer to further increase these therapies' value proposition. Our study also demonstrated for the first time that if targeted therapies are chosen over chemotherapy, dabrafenib is clearly the cost-effective choice, dominating vemurafenib.

Our study has a few limitations. First, the sample size of the vemurafenib trial was three times larger than the sample size of the dabrafenib trial, potentially biasing the results in favor of dabrafenib by potentially presenting a lower incidence of adverse events. However, the large difference in drug cost between the two targeted therapies supports that the difference in adverse event probabilities and subsequently the difference in costs due to adverse events would not be the primary driver of differences in costs between dabrafenib and vemurafenib. Second, a recent study published the extended OS results of the Phase III vemurafenib trial which included the protocol amendment allowing crossover to a treatment arm as patients on dacarbazine progressed [21]. However, this was written into the protocol from the beginning for the dabrafenib trial and patients were analyzed per intent to treat. The crossover would likely lead to an overestimation of the effectiveness of dacarbazine and, in reality, we should see a larger incremental QALY for the targeted therapies. Considering this limitation, a larger incremental QALY may have resulted in a lower ICER. It would take an incremental effect of 0.2333 QALYs to bring the ICER to under the cost-effective threshold. Finally, our study did not include utilities for drug formulation which, if included, may lower the ICER of the oral targeted therapies. A previous study found that patients in the palliative care setting preferred oral chemotherapy to intravenous therapy [39] and this preference for oral treatment has been cited as a main driver for the increase in oral chemotherapy agents available [40]. Inclusion of these utilities would decrease the ICER for targeted therapies, potentially bringing them closer to the societal WTP threshold.

In conclusion, this analysis demonstrated that, at a strict WTP threshold of $100,000/QALY, dacarbazine is the most cost-effective treatment and that dabrafenib dominates vemurafenib. Since society has demonstrated a willingness to accept higher value thresholds in general and particularly for end of life treatments, we consider dabrafenib to have value in this disease state with very few options, especially after pricing negotiations specific to each healthcare system. These pioneer treatments come at a high cost for payers and determining the cost-effectiveness of these therapies will be paramount from a payer and provider perspective in order to make coverage as well as treatment decisions. This CEA is the first step in generating the evidence to support the clinically based NCCN recommendations of dabrafenib as first line treatment if a fixed budget and societal preference allow a WTP threshold of $150,000. Future studies should update this study with real-world comparative data on the effectiveness of these drugs as well as comparing the cost-effectiveness of combination treatment approaches which are now being considered.

Disclosure

Poster presentation was presented at the ISPOR 19th Annual International Meeting, 5/31/2014–6/4/2014 at the Palais des Congres in Montreal, Quebec, Canada.

References

[1] E. Linos, S. M. Swetter, M. G. Cockburn, G. A. Colditz, and C. A. Clarke, "Increasing burden of melanoma in the United States," *Journal of Investigative Dermatology*, vol. 129, no. 7, pp. 1666–1674, 2009.

[2] R. Siegel, D. Naishadham, and A. Jemal, "Cancer statistics, 2013," *CA: A Cancer Journal for Clinicians*, vol. 63, no. 1, pp. 11–30, 2013.

[3] C. M. Balch, J. E. Gershenwald, S.-J. Soong et al., "Final version of 2009 AJCC melanoma staging and classification," *Journal of Clinical Oncology*, vol. 27, no. 36, pp. 6199–6206, 2009.

[4] P. B. Chapman, A. Hauschild, C. Robert et al., "Improved survival with vemurafenib in melanoma with BRAF V600E mutation," *New England Journal of Medicine*, vol. 364, no. 26, pp. 2507–2516, 2011.

[5] C. Greenman, P. Stephens, R. Smith et al., "Patterns of somatic mutation in human cancer genomes," *Nature*, vol. 446, pp. 153–158, 2007.

[6] A. Hauschild, J.-J. Grob, L. V. Demidov et al., "Dabrafenib in BRAF-mutated metastatic melanoma: a multicentre, open-label, phase 3 randomised controlled trial," *The Lancet*, vol. 380, no. 9839, pp. 358–365, 2012.

[7] NCCN, *National Comprehensive Cancer Network Clinical Practice Guidelines: Melanoma (Version 4.2014)*, 2014, http://www.nccn.org/professionals/physician_gls/pdf/melanoma.pdf.

[8] S. Bhatia, S. S. Tykodi, and J. A. Thompson, "Treatment of metastatic melanoma: an overview," *Oncology*, vol. 23, no. 6, pp. 488–496, 2009.

[9] S. Jang and M. B. Atkins, "Which drug, and when, for patients with BRAF-mutant melanoma?" *The Lancet Oncology*, vol. 14, no. 2, pp. e60–e69, 2013.

[10] F. Sabbatino, Y. Wang, X. Wang, S. Ferrone, and C. R. Ferrone, "Emerging BRAF inhibitors for melanoma," *Expert Opinion on Emerging Drugs*, vol. 18, no. 4, pp. 431–443, 2013.

[11] J. J. Luke and F. S. Hodia, "Ipilimumab, vemurafenib, dabrafenib, and trametinib: synergistic competitors in the clinical management of BRAF mutant malignantmelanoma," *The Oncologist*, vol. 18, no. 6, pp. 717–725, 2013.

[12] National Comprehensive Cancer Network (NCCN), *National Comprehensive Cancer Network Clinical Practice Guidelines in Oncology: Antiemesis (Version 2.2014)*, National Comprehensive Cancer Network (NCCN), Philadelphia, Pa, USA, 2014, http://www.nccn.org/professionals/physician_gls/pdf/antiemesis.pdf.

[13] Red Book Online, http://www.thomsonhc.com.

[14] AHRQ, Agency for Healthcare Research and Quality: Healthcare Cost and Utilization Project (HCUP) Database, http://www.ahrq.gov/research/data/hcup/index.html.

[15] J. B. Davis, *Medical Fees*, Practice Management Information Corporation, Los Angeles, Calif, USA, 2013.

[16] J. E. Battley, E. Lenihan, H. P. Redmond, M. Murphy, and D. G. Power, "Treatment of BRAF inhibitor-induced hyperkeratosis," *Acta Oncologica*, vol. 52, no. 4, pp. 874–877, 2013.

[17] L. S. Wilson, M. Pregenzer, R. Basu et al., "Fee comparisons of treatments for nonmelanoma skin cancer in a private practice academic setting," *Dermatologic Surgery*, vol. 38, no. 4, pp. 570–584, 2012.

[18] H. L. DuPont, "Guidelines on acute infectious diarrhea in adults. The Practice Parameters Committee of the American College of Gastroenterology," *The American Journal of Gastroenterology*, vol. 92, no. 11, pp. 1962–1975, 1997.

[19] P. Gomez and M. E. Lacouture, "Clinical presentation and management of hand-foot skin reaction associated with sorafenib in combination with cytotoxic chemotherapy: experience in breast cancer," *The Oncologist*, vol. 16, no. 11, pp. 1508–1519, 2011.

[20] J. D. Webster-Gandy, C. How, and K. Harrold, "Palmar-plantar erythrodysesthesia (PPE): a literature review with commentary on experience in a cancer centre," *European Journal of Oncology Nursing*, vol. 11, no. 3, pp. 238–246, 2007.

[21] G. A. McArthur, P. B. Chapman, C. Robert et al., "Safety and efficacy of vemurafenib in BRAFV600E and BRAFV600K mutation-positive melanoma (BRIM-3): extended follow-up of a phase 3, randomised, open-label study," *The Lancet Oncology*, vol. 15, no. 3, pp. 323–332, 2014.

[22] USFDA, "Zelboraf—Summary Basis for Approval," 2011.

[23] J. R. Beck, J. P. Kassirer, and S. G. Pauker, "A convenient approximation of life expectancy (the 'DEALE'). I. validation of the method," *The American Journal of Medicine*, vol. 73, no. 6, pp. 883–888, 1982.

[24] E. Keeler and R. Bell, "New DEALEs: other approximations of life expectancy," *Medical Decision Making*, vol. 12, no. 4, pp. 307–311, 1992.

[25] K. M. Beusterien, S. M. Szabo, S. Kotapati et al., "Societal preference values for advanced melanoma health states in the United Kingdom and Australia," *British Journal of Cancer*, vol. 101, no. 3, pp. 387–389, 2009.

[26] S. C. Chen, A. M. Bayoumi, S. L. Soon et al., "A catalog of dermatology utilities: a measure of the burden of skin diseases," *Journal of Investigative Dermatology Symposium Proceedings*, vol. 9, no. 2, pp. 160–168, 2004.

[27] A. Lloyd, B. Nafees, J. Narewska, S. Dewilde, and J. Watkins, "Health state utilities for metastatic breast cancer," *British Journal of Cancer*, vol. 95, no. 6, pp. 683–690, 2006.

[28] J. J. Grob, M. M. Amonkar, S. Martin-Algarra et al., "Patient perception of the benefit of a BRAF inhibitor in metastatic melanoma: quality-of-life analyses of the BREAK-3 study comparing dabrafenib with dacarbazine," *Annals of Oncology*, vol. 25, no. 7, pp. 1428–1436, 2014.

[29] D. Weycker, J. Malin, J. Edelsberg, A. Glass, M. Gokhale, and G. Oster, "Cost of neutropenic complications of chemotherapy," *Annals of Oncology*, vol. 19, no. 3, pp. 454–460, 2008.

[30] L. S. Elting, S. B. Cantor, C. G. Martin et al., "Cost of chemotherapy-induced thrombocytopenia among patients with lymphoma or solid tumors," *Cancer*, vol. 97, no. 6, pp. 1541–1550, 2003.

[31] G. R. Barton, A. H. Briggs, and E. A. L. Fenwick, "Optimal cost-effectiveness decisions: the role of the cost-effectiveness acceptability curve (CEAC), the cost-effectiveness acceptability frontier (CEAF), and the expected value of perfection information (EVPI)," *Value in Health*, vol. 11, no. 5, pp. 886–897, 2008.

[32] P. Curl, I. Vujic, L. J. van 't Veer, S. Ortiz-Urda, J. G. Kahn, and A. T. Slominski, "Cost-effectiveness of treatment strategies for BRAF-mutated metastatic melanoma," *PLoS ONE*, vol. 9, no. 9, 2014.

[33] C. Evans, M. Tavakoli, and B. Crawford, "Use of quality adjusted life years and life years gained as benchmarks in economic evaluations: a critical appraisal," *Health Care Management Science*, vol. 7, no. 1, pp. 43–49, 2004.

[34] P. J. Neumann, J. T. Cohen, and M. C. Weinstein, "Updating cost-effectiveness—the curious resilience of the $50,000-per-QALY threshold," *The New England Journal of Medicine*, vol. 371, no. 9, pp. 796–797, 2014.

[35] V. Barzey, M. B. Atkins, L. P. Garrison, Y. Asukai, S. Kotapati, and J. R. Penrod, "Ipilimumab in 2nd line treatment of patients with advanced melanoma: a cost-effectiveness analysis," *Journal of Medical Economics*, vol. 16, no. 2, pp. 202–212, 2013.

[36] M. Collins and N. Latimer, "NICE's end of life decision making scheme: impact on population health," *British Medical Journal*, vol. 346, no. 7905, Article ID f1363, 2013.

[37] American Cancer Society, *Cancer Drug Coverage in Health Insurance Marketplace Plans*, 2014, http://www.acscan.org/content/wp-content/uploads/2014/03/Marketplace_formularies_whitepaper.pdf.

[38] Center for Medicare Advocacy, *Part D/Prescription Drug Benefits*, Center for Medicare Advocacy, 2014, http://www.medicareadvocacy.org/medicare-info/medicare-part-d/.

[39] G. Liu, E. Franssen, M. I. Fitch, and E. Warner, "Patient preferences for oral versus intravenous palliative chemotherapy," *Journal of Clinical Oncology*, vol. 15, no. 1, pp. 110–115, 1997.

[40] S. N. Weingart, P. B. Bach, K. Eng et al., "NCCN task force report: oral chemotherapy," *Journal of the National Comprehensive Cancer Network*, vol. 6, supplement 3, pp. S1–S14, 2008.

9

Merkel Cell Carcinoma: The Past, the Present, and the Future

Inamaria Erovic[1] and Boban M. Erovic[2]

[1] *Medical University of Vienna, 1090 Vienna, Austria*
[2] *Medical University of Vienna, Department of Otolaryngology, Head and Neck Surgery, 1090 Vienna, Austria*

Correspondence should be addressed to Boban M. Erovic; boban.erovic@meduniwien.ac.at

Academic Editor: Justin Lee

Since the first description of the Merkel cell carcinoma by Cyril Toker in 1972, the number of studies has significantly increased over the last 4 decades. In this review, we will illustrate the historical background of the Merkel cell carcinoma beginning with the 19th century, the first description of the Merkel cell to the finding of the CK20 as a highly specific diagnostic marker and finally to the recently detected Merkel cell polyomavirus (MCPyV). Moreover, we will highlight the beginning of adjuvant therapeutic regimens with radiotherapy and chemotherapy and discuss the diagnostic work-up including imaging and histology of patients with Merkel cell carcinoma. Another very rapidly growing and interesting field of research is the development of patients' specific and tailored targeted therapy, in particular in patients with distant metastatic disease.

1. Introduction

Since the first description of the Merkel cell carcinoma by Cyril Toker in 1972, the number of studies has significantly increased over the last 4 decades. In this review, we will illustrate the historical background of the Merkel cell carcinoma beginning with the 19th century, the first description of the Merkel cell to the finding of the CK20 as a highly specific diagnostic marker and finally to the recently detected Merkel cell polyomavirus (MCPyV).

Moreover, we will highlight the beginning of adjuvant therapeutic regimens with radiotherapy and chemotherapy and discuss the diagnostic work-up including imaging and histology of patients with Merkel cell carcinoma.

Another very rapidly growing and interesting field of research is the development of patients'-specific and tailored targeted therapy, in particular in patients with distant metastatic disease.

2. Finding the Merkel Cell

Friedrich Sigmund Merkel was born on April 5, 1845 and died on May 28, 1919. He was a German anatomist and histopathologist who first described the so-called *Tastzellen* or touch cells in the skin [1] (Figure 1). Interestingly, three years later the term Merkel cell was born, by a young anatomist Robert Bonnet (1851–1921) who later worked with Dr. Merkel.

In mammals, Merkel cells are localized in the basal layer of the skin and mucosa [2] either as single cells or in clusters (in german *haarscheiben*). Clusters contain about 50 cells (touch domes) and are in close neighborhood to nerve terminals forming mechanoreceptors [2]. There are other cells called "Merkel-cell-like" cells, also in the skin and mucosa but without contact with nerve terminals. They are probably part of a diffuse neuroendocrine system and do not function as mechanoreceptors. Probably, these cells, rather than those acting as mechanoreceptors, are the origin of the highly malignant Merkel cell carcinoma. Recent studies could show that Merkel cells originate from the neural crest [3] and are found in the skin and parts of the mucosa that are derived from the ectoderm.

2.1. Structure of Merkel Cells. With the introduction of the electron microscopy in medicine in the 1960s, new significant knowledge in regard to cellular anatomy was gained. Particularly, in 1965 and 1969 Munger, Iggo and Muir showed that Merkel cells are clear and oval cells,

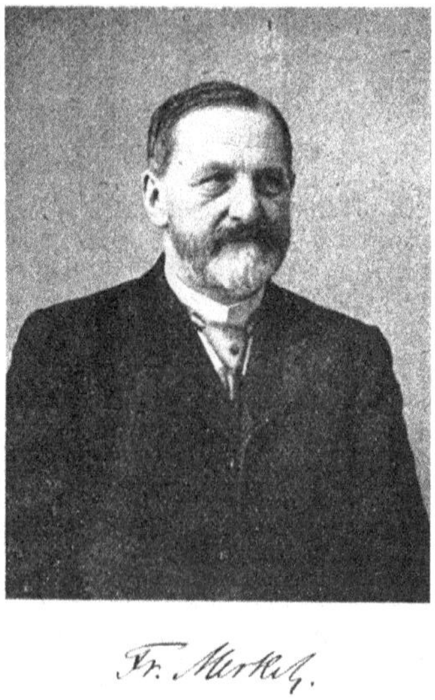

FIGURE 1: Friedrich Sigmund Merkel (1845–1919).

measuring approximately 10–15 μm in the long axis having lobulated nuclei that contain intermediate cytokeratin and neurofilaments [4, 5]. Moreover, Merkel cells have spike-like protrusions that enable them to interdigitate with the surrounding keratinocytes. The nerve terminals of the Merkel cells are packed with mitochondria and optically clear vesicles [4].

2.2. Protein Expression in Merkel Cells. The most interesting fact in regard to the protein expression profile is that epithelial proteins like cytokeratins but also neuroendocrine markers like neuron-specific enolase can be found in Merkel cells [2]. In particular, cytokeratin 20 is of significant value as a highly specific marker for Merkel cells in normal squamous epithelium [6]. Besides neuron-specific enolase, protein gene product 9.5, synaptophysin, and chromogranin A are found immunohistochemically in Merkel cells as well [2].

2.3. First Description of the Merkel Cell Carcinoma. In 1972, Toker first described a trabecular carcinoma of the skin [7]. In those days, he was a pathologist at the Mount Sinai School of Medicine, City University of New York and later Professor of Pathology and Head of the Division of Surgical Pathology at the University of Maryland Hospital and Medical School in Baltimore, MD, USA. He analyzed five cases and described clinical and histomorphological aspects. In particular, tumor cells displayed large, oval nuclei with vesicular chromatin and prominent nucleoli. The tumor growth pattern was trabecular and column-like infiltrating between dermal bundles. In regard to the origin of the trabecular carcinoma, Dr. Toker hypothesized that the carcinoma cells derived from epithelial structures are capable of forming primitive sudoriferous structures, that is, early fetal sweat glands.

Six years later, in 1978 Tang and Toker found dense-core granules in three of the original tumors by electron microscopy [8]. Merkel cells are the only cells in the skin that have dense-core granules. This fact led subsequently to the hypothesis that this trabecular skin carcinoma arises from Merkel cells. Further electron microscope studies showed that both Merkel cells and Merkel cell carcinoma cells have overlapping electron microscopic features. On the protein level, immunohistochemical expression of Cytokeratin 20 supports the hypothesis that the Merkel cell is the cellular origin of this aggressive skin tumor [6]. However, to date there is a controversy going on regarding the origin of the Merkel cell carcinoma. Some authors believe that the Merkel cell carcinoma derives from pluripotent stem cells from the skin. Our research group could show as well that Bmi-1, a stem cell marker, was homogenously and highly positive in all Merkel cell carcinoma samples [9]. Therefore, throughout the last decades Merkel cell carcinoma has been described under trabecular carcinoma of the skin, cutaneous neuroendocrine carcinoma, and Merkel cell carcinoma. The name Merkel cell carcinoma was first proposed by De Wolff-Peeters in 1980 and remains the most used and accepted term [10].

However, whether the Merkel cell carcinoma truly derives from the Merkel cell is still to date very controversially discussed. Without any doubt, more studies are needed to elucidate the origin of Merkel cell carcinoma because systemic therapy in patients with disseminated disease would probably have a significant higher impact on survival and disease-free rates due to modifications based on the origin of the cancer cells.

2.4. CK20 as the Key Diagnostic Marker for Merkel Cell Carcinoma. In the decades following its initial discovery, reports on the pathogenesis, course, and treatment of Merkel cell carcinoma were scarce attributing to its rarity as a disease entity, lack of biomarkers for diagnosis, and nonunified staging classifications. In 1992, Dr. Moll and colleagues recognized that Cytokeratin 20 (CK20) expression was highly specific for Merkel cell carcinoma [6]. In this study, 15 specimens with Merkel cell carcinoma were tested for CK20 using the immunoblotting and immunohistochemistry technique. All cases for CK20 were significantly positive, and the authors proposed that this marker is highly specific for Merkel cell carcinoma. Moreover, CK20 helps to distinguish between Merkel cell and small-cell lung carcinoma cells since both tumors are morphologically similar [6].

In the following years, new studies showed that approximately 5% of all Merkel cell carcinoma specimens lack CK20 expression [11]. As a consequence, Jaeger showed in a recently published review that besides CK20 expression neuron-specific-enolase (NSE) and neurofilament protein (NFP) is specific for Merkel cell carcinoma [12]. Another very important tumor marker is thyroid transcription factor-1 (TTF-1). TTF-1 is a very reliable and accurate diagnostic marker for small-cell lung carcinoma but it is not expressed by Merkel cell carcinoma [13]. Other "negative" markers are leucocyte common antigen (LCA) and cytokeratin-7 (CK7) that are positive in lymphoma [14, 15] and small-cell carcinoma of the lung (SCLC), respectively [16]. Differentiating malignant melanoma and Merkel cell carcinoma is based on CK20 positivity in Merkel cell carcinoma but negativity for HBM45, NKI/C3, and S-100 [17].

3. Prognostic and Predictive Factors in Merkel Cell Carcinoma

In a recently published study, it could be shown that immunosupression and advanced-stage disease was a significant predictor for decreased survival in 240 patients with Merkel cell carcinoma [18]. Interestingly, tumor size had no impact on survival [18]. Touzé and colleagues found that high antibody titers of MCPyV were a significant predictor for progression-free survival [19]. Another study performed by Poulsen and colleagues showed that again stage was a significant prognostic factor for better survival but that intratumoral CD8+ lymphocyte invasion was shown to be a significant biomarker for improved survival in MCC patients as well [20]. This observation could be underlined by the study performed by Sihto et al. This study group could show that in 116 patients that besides intratumor infiltration with CD8+ cells high CD3+ tumor count has a significant impact on patients' overall survival [21].

Clinical factors like tumor thickness, size, sex, and age are shown to not be a reliable prognostic factor for overall and disease-free survival [18, 20, 22].

3.1. Finding of the Merkel Cell Carcinoma Polyomavirus. In 2008, Feng and coworkers found novel viral sequences in four Merkel cell carcinoma tumor tissues [23]. After sequence analysis, it could be shown that they encoded for a polyomavirus which was subsequently named as Merkel cell polyomavirus. Further studies showed a prevalence of 40% to 100% of the MCPyV in Merkel cell carcinoma specimens [24].

In particular, polyomaviruses encode for large and small T-antigens which bind to host proteins facilitating (i) viral replication and (ii) inactivation of tumor suppressor proteins p53 and pocket retinoblastoma (pRb). Feng and colleagues observed a monoclonal viral integration 5 out of 10 (50%) patient samples and interestingly primary and metastatic MCC tissues from the same patient showed an identical viral integration pattern, indicating that the integration of MCV preceded the metastatic spreading of the cancer [23].

The number of studies dealing with the MCPyV expression significantly increased over the last 3 years [11, 25]. In particular, in a large Australian cohort Paik and colleagues could show that the MCPyV large T protein was only detected in 7% of the specimens localized in the head and neck area and in 24% from other anatomic sites [11]. Since the expression of MCPyV large T-protein in Merkel cell carcinoma specimens in patients with less sun exposure is unknown, our group recently conducted a study and showed that MCPyV large T-protein was highly expressed in primary as well as metastatic lesions [25]. This observation is highly clinically relevant in two points: firstly MCPyV large T-protein can be easily and cost-effectively detected by CM2B4, a highly sensitive and specific mouse monoclonal antibody, in specimens that lack CK20 immunoreactivity.

Secondly, since the expression of MCPyV large T-protein is homogenously overexpressed in primary and more important in metastatic lymph nodes it can be used as a target protein for systemic therapy in patients with disseminated disease with very poor outcome [26, 27].

3.2. Management of Patients with Merkel Cell Carcinoma

3.2.1. Surgery and Postoperative Radiotherapy. The first retrospective study in regard to treatment and management of Merkel cell carcinoma patients was conducted at the MD Anderson Cancer Center [28]. Between 1966 and 1983, 41 patients with Merkel cell carcinoma were treated. It could be shown that wide surgical resection of the primary lesion with neck dissection and adjuvant radiotherapy is the best treatment for controlling locoregional disease [28]. The first and still to date solemn prospective trial was performed in 2003 by the TASMAN group [29]. Interestingly, this study showed that adjuvant radiotherapy significantly prolonged locoregional disease-free survival whereas radiation had no impact on patients' overall survival [29].

3.2.2. Mohs Surgery. Mohs micrographic surgery was introduced by Dr. Frederic Mohs in the 1930s and became over the decades a reliable technique for resection of cutaneous tumors particular at delicate sites. In case of Merkel cell carcinoma, only a few reports are available. A retrospective study conducted by Gollard and colleagues presented excellent results with no recurrence rate after 3 years. However, only 8 patients were included in this study. Another paper including 45 patients with Merkel cell carcinoma showed that Mohs surgery is a reliable and cost-effective technique [30]. The authors compared the outcome of two groups: one with Mohs surgery alone and one with adjuvant radiotherapy. In the first group only 1 (4%) marginal recurrence and 3 in transit-metastasis could be observed whereas in the second group none recurrent disease were observed in the radiation group. Nevertheless, in both groups, overall and disease-free survival were not significantly different between treatment groups. The authors conclude that radiotherapy is beside surgical resection a key factor for successful management of patients with Merkel cell carcinoma [30].

3.2.3. Radiotherapy. Merkel cell carcinoma is a highly radiosensitive skin tumor [10]. Studies could show that adjuvant radiotherapy to the primary site and the nodal basins significantly improves locoregional control and overall survival [23, 24]. In patients where no surgical treatment, due to low medical performance, can be offered, primary treatment with radiation shows an excellent outcome and locoregional control rates [28, 29]. Controversies still exist regarding the treatment of the neck. The majority of the cancer centers worldwide prefer doing a selective a neck dissection with adjuvant radiotherapy [31]. However, numerous studies showed that radiotherapy alone to the neck has comparable locoregional control rates to surgery [32–34].

Since the discovery of the MCPyV, future studies are showing whether its expression is able to stratify patients either to primary radiotherapy or surgery plus adjuvant radiotherapy treatment. Such stratification has already taken place in squamous cell carcinoma of the oropharynx. In these patients, the human papilloma virus status decides whether patients will undergo primary radiotherapy or surgery with adjuvant radiotherapy [35].

3.2.4. Chemotherapy. In the mid-eighties, several studies were conducted to evaluate the efficacy of chemotherapy in patients with disseminated Merkel cell carcinoma disease [31, 36].

For the first attempts to treat MCC metastases, regimens were chosen similar to those used for small-cell lung carcinomas because of its neuroendocrine differentiation and histopathologic features [31]. George and colleagues introduced carboplatin and reported a positive effect on patients' progression-free survival [31]. In the following years, a huge number of case series were published presenting therapeutic outcome after single or combined treatment with radiotherapy [37–42]. Agents like carboplatin, cisplatin, 5-FU, cyclophosphamide, doxorubicin (or epirubicin), vincristine plus or minus prednisone, and etoposide were used with the hope to improve significantly patients outcome. In fact etoposide was better tolerated and showed a significant response in one study [43]. Unfortunately, still to date there is no first-line chemotherapy established for Merkel cell carcinoma patients. In fact, chemotherapy is used either in advanced-stage disease or in patients with recurrent, nonresectable, or disseminated disease. Therefore, the outcome is very controversially discussed in the literature. In particular, in a retrospective analysis including a huge number of patients' adjuvant chemotherapy was linked to a worse overall survival compared to patients who did not received chemotherapy [44].

Without doubt new systemic therapeutic strategies are needed for patients with Merkel cell carcinomas. One of such new strategies is termed as targeted anticancer therapies. Such therapies are shown to be very promising options in treating different types of cancer, that is, gastrointestinal tumors [45] or renal cell carcinomas [46]. Due to the rareness of the disease, a very limited number of studies are available. The first studies showed that c-kit, a receptor tyrosine kinase, is in 15–90% expressed by Merkel cell carcinoma cells. Recently, we conducted a study looking at a distinct panel of target proteins and we could find that therapeutically useful targets c-kit, Bmi-1, Mcl-1, VEGF-A and VEGF-C, VEGF-R2, PDGF-α and PDGF-β were expressed in Merkel cell carcinoma [9]. Another recently published study showed that survivin was a promising candidate for a new target therapy in Merkel cell carcinoma [47]. Looking at these studies the results are very promising and validate further clinical studies on the use of multitargeted tyrosine kinase inhibitors and antisense oligonucleotides in Merkel cell carcinoma [9].

Recently two studies showed that targeting MCPyV can be a promising option in patients with Merkel cell carcinoma [26, 27].

4. Imaging

For patients with Merkel cell carcinomas, imaging and subsequently staging of the tumor are of utmost importance. Since the introduction of ultrasonography in the late seventies, sonography of the neck is a key staging tool for patients with Merkel cell carcinoma. First reports on sonography and Merkel cell carcinoma were published in the late 90s [48]. Beyond ultrasonography, CT and MRI scanning are important for determining tumor size, location, and eventual bone invasion [48, 49]. In the late nineties, octreotide scanning in Merkel cell carcinoma patients was proposed to show a reliable detecting rate compared to CT and MRI imaging [50]. In the following years, however, it was shown that the octreotide scan has a low sensitivity and specificity [50]. Another whole body imaging technique, FDG-PET and PET-CT scanning showed highly reliable and accurate images in Merkel cell carcinoma patients with metastatic disease [49].

Sentinel node biopsy was introduced by Cabanas in 1977 in patients with penile carcinoma [51] enabling detection of micrometastasis in lymph nodes. This technique gains more and more importance in the management of patients with Merkel cell carcinoma since studies showed that patients with negative neck nodes have a risk of 30% to harbor micrometastasis in the neck nodes [52]. Another significant benefit of sentinel node imaging and mapping is an option to avoid the morbidity of an elective neck dissection in sentinel node negative patients [52–58].

5. Perspectives

Since the discovery of the Merkel cell in the skin in the 19th century and the description of the Merkel cell carcinoma in the early 70s, many new implementations in medicine with regard to diagnosis, imaging, and treatment have been introduced.

However, the management of patients with Merkel cell carcinoma is a tremendous challenge for the clinician as well as the patient and their families. The first step for optimal treatment is clinical investigation and proper diagnostic work-up of the patient including determination of the histology, either by excision biopsy or fine needle biopsy, imaging of the tumor and any metastatic disease, and finally determination of the therapeutic plan within a multidisciplinary setting.

In particular, diagnosis of Merkel cell carcinoma is based upon the CK20 positivity determined by immunohistochemistry whereas staging relies on ultrasonography, sentinel node, and CT/MRI and PET-CT scanning. Primary treatments including surgical resection and radiotherapy are currently the treatment of choice. In patients with recurrent either locoregional or distant metastasis, treatment options are very limited. In the case of resectable locoregional disease, surgical resection is an accurate way of treatment and for most of the patients it is unfortunately the only therapeutic option. However, in the presence of distant metastatic disease, there are no established systemic therapeutic regimens. The number of studies focusing on the development of new targeted anticancer therapy is steadily rising, and thus there is hope that new drug regimes for patients with distant and systemic Merkel cell carcinoma disease will be available in the near future. In particular, many study groups are looking for new strategies to target the Merkel cell polyoma virus either to prevent infection or to inhibit viral-induced carcinogenesis.

References

[1] F. Merkel, "Tastzellen und Tastkörperchen bei den Hausthieren und beim Menschen," *Archiv für Mikroskopische Anatomie*, vol. 11, no. 1, pp. 636–652, 1875.

[2] Z. Halata, M. Grim, and K. I. Bauman, "Friedrich Sigmund Merkel and his "Merkel cell", morphology, development, and physiology: review and new results," *Anatomical Record Part A*, vol. 271, no. 1, pp. 225–239, 2003.

[3] V. Szeder, M. Grim, Z. Halata, and M. Sieber-Blum, "Neural crest origin of mammalian Merkel cells," *Developmental Biology*, vol. 253, no. 2, pp. 258–263, 2003.

[4] B. L. Munger, "The intraepidermal innervation of the snout skin of the opossum. A light and electron microscope study, with observations on the nature of Merkel's Tastzellen," *Journal of Cell Biology*, vol. 26, no. 1, pp. 79–97, 1965.

[5] A. Iggo and A. R. Muir, "The structure and function of a slowly adapting touch corpuscle in hairy skin," *Journal of Physiology*, vol. 200, no. 3, pp. 763–796, 1969.

[6] R. Moll, A. Löwe, J. Laufer, and W. W. Franke, "Cytokeratin 20 in human carcinomas: a new histodiagnostic marker detected by monoclonal antibodies," *American Journal of Pathology*, vol. 140, no. 2, pp. 427–447, 1992.

[7] C. Toker, "Trabecular carcinoma of the skin," *Archives of Dermatology*, vol. 105, no. 1, pp. 107–110, 1972.

[8] C. K. Tang and C. Toker, "Trabecular carcinoma of the skin. An ultrastructural study," *Cancer*, vol. 42, no. 5, pp. 2311–2321, 1978.

[9] M. Brunner, D. Thurnher, J. Pammer et al., "Expression of VEGF-A/C, VEGF-R2, PDGF-α/β, c-kit, EGFR, Her-2/Neu, Mcl-1 and Bmi-1 in Merkel cell carcinoma," *Modern Pathology*, vol. 21, no. 7, pp. 876–884, 2008.

[10] C. De Wolf-Peeters, K. Marien, J. Mebis, and V. Desmet, "A cutaneous APUDoma or Merkel cell tumor? A morphologically recognizable tumor with a biological and histological malignant aspect in contrast with its clinical behavior," *Cancer*, vol. 46, no. 8, pp. 1810–1816, 1980.

[11] J. Y. Paik, G. Hall, A. Clarkson et al., "Immunohistochemistry for Merkel cell polyomavirus is highly specific but not sensitive for the diagnosis of Merkel cell carcinoma in the Australian population," *Human Pathology*, vol. 42, pp. 1385–1390, 2011.

[12] T. Jaeger, J. Ring, and C. Andres, "Histological, immunohistological, and clinical features of merkel cell carcinoma in correlation to merkel cell polyomavirus status," *Journal of Skin Cancer*, vol. 2012, Article ID 983421, 5 pages, 2012.

[13] A. L. Dancey, S. S. Rayatt, C. Soon, A. Ilchshyn, I. Brown, and S. Srivastava, "Merkel cell carcinoma: a report of 34 cases and literature review," *Journal of Plastic, Reconstructive and Aesthetic Surgery*, vol. 59, no. 12, pp. 1294–1299, 2006.

[14] J. C. Becker, C. S. Kauczok, S. Ugurel, S. Eib, E. B. Bröcker, and R. Houben, "Merkel cell carcinoma: molecular pathogenesis, clinical features and therapy," *Journal of the German Society of Dermatology*, vol. 6, no. 9, pp. 709–720, 2008.

[15] J. Becker, C. Mauch, R. D. Kortmann et al., "Short German guidelines: Merkel cell carcinoma," *Journal of the German Society of Dermatology*, vol. 6, pp. S15–S16, 2008.

[16] M. Bobos, P. Hytiroglou, I. Kostopoulos, G. Karkavelas, and C. S. Papadimitriou, "Immunohistochemical distinction between Merkel cell carcinoma and small cell carcinoma of the lung," *American Journal of Dermatopathology*, vol. 28, no. 2, pp. 99–104, 2006.

[17] G. J. Kontochristopoulos, P. G. Stavropoulos, K. Krasagakis, S. Goerdt, and C. C. Zouboulis, "Differentiation between Merkel cell carcinoma and malignant melanoma: an immunohistochemical study," *Dermatology*, vol. 201, no. 2, pp. 123–126, 2000.

[18] T. I. Tarantola, L. A. Vallow, M. Y. Halyard et al., "Prognostic factors in Merkel cell carcinoma: analysis of 240 cases," *Journal of the American Academy of Dermatology*, vol. 68, pp. 425–432, 2013.

[19] A. Touzé, E. Le Bidre, H. Laude et al., "High levels of antibodies against merkel cell polyomavirus identify a subset of patients with merkel cell carcinoma with better clinical outcome," *Journal of Clinical Oncology*, vol. 29, no. 12, pp. 1612–1619, 2011.

[20] K. G. Paulson, J. G. Iyer, A. R. Tegeder et al., "Transcriptome-wide studies of merkel cell carcinoma and validation of intratumoral cd8+ lymphocyte invasion as an independent predictor of survival," *Journal of Clinical Oncology*, vol. 29, no. 12, pp. 1539–1546, 2011.

[21] H. Sihto, T. Böhling, H. Kavola et al., "Tumor infiltrating immune cells and outcome of Merkel cell carcinoma: a population-based study," *Clinical Cancer Research*, vol. 18, pp. 2872–2881, 2012.

[22] R. Gollard, R. Weber, M. P. Kostky et al., "Merkel cell carcinoma: review of 22 cases with surgical, pathologic, and therapeutic considerations," *Cancer*, vol. 88, pp. 1842–1851, 2000.

[23] H. Feng, M. Shuda, Y. Chang, and P. S. Moore, "Clonal integration of a polyomavirus in human Merkel cell carcinoma," *Science*, vol. 319, no. 5866, pp. 1096–1100, 2008.

[24] M. Agelli, L. X. Clegg, J. C. Becker, and D. E. Rollison, "The etiology and epidemiology of merkel cell carcinoma," *Current Problems in Cancer*, vol. 34, pp. 14–37, 2010.

[25] B. M. Erovic, A. Al Habeeb, L. Harris, D. P. Goldstein, D. Ghazarian, and J. C. Irish, "Significant overexpression of the Merkel cell polyomavirus (MCPyV) large T antigen in Merkel cell carcinoma," *Head & Neck Surgery*, vol. 35, no. 2, pp. 184–189, 2013.

[26] R. Arora, Y. Chang, and P. S. Moore, "MCV and Merkel cell carcinoma: a molecular success story," *Current Opinion in Virology*, vol. 2, pp. 489–498, 2012.

[27] Q. Zeng, B. P. Gomez, R. P. Viscidi et al., "Development of a DNA vaccine targeting Merkel cell polyomavirus," *Vaccine*, vol. 30, pp. 1322–1329, 2012.

[28] H. Goepfert, D. Remmler, E. Silva, and B. Wheeler, "Merkel cell carcinoma (endocrine carcinoma of the skin) of the head and neck," *Archives of Otolaryngology*, vol. 110, no. 11, pp. 707–712, 1984.

[29] M. Poulsen, D. Rischin, E. Walpole et al., "High-risk Merkel cell carcinoma of the skin treated with synchronous carboplatin/etoposide and radiation: a Trans-Tasman Radiation Oncology Group Study-TROG 96:07," *Journal of Clinical Oncology*, vol. 21, no. 23, pp. 4371–4376, 2003.

[30] J. D. Boyer, J. A. Zitelli, D. G. Brodland, and G. D'Angelo, "Local control of primary Merkel cell carcinoma: review of 45 cases treated with Mohs micrographic surgery with and without adjuvant radiation," *Journal of the American Academy of Dermatology*, vol. 47, no. 6, pp. 885–892, 2002.

[31] T. K. George, A. Di Sant'Agnese, and J. M. Bennett, "Chemotherapy for metastatic Merkel cell carcinoma," *Cancer*, vol. 57, pp. 178–182, 1986.

[32] B. D. Lawenda, M. G. Arnold, V. A. Tokarz et al., "Analysis of radiation therapy for the control of Merkel cell carcinoma head and neck based on 36 cases and a literature review," *Ear, Nose and Throat Journal*, vol. 87, no. 11, pp. 634–643, 2008.

[33] L. Mortier, X. Mirabel, C. Fournier, F. Piette, and E. Lartigau, "Radiotherapy alone for primary Merkel cell carcinoma," *Archives of Dermatology*, vol. 139, pp. 1587–1590, 2003.

[34] L. C. Fang, B. Lemos, J. Douglas, J. Iyer, and P. Nghiem, "Radiation monotherapy as regional treatment for lymph node-positive merkel cell carcinoma," *Cancer*, vol. 116, no. 7, pp. 1783–1790, 2010.

[35] A. M. Chen, J. Li, L. A. Beckett et al., "Differential response rates to irradiation among patients with human papillomavirus positive and negative oropharyngeal cancer," *Laryngoscope*, vol. 123, no. 1, pp. 152–157, 2013.

[36] J. H. Raaf, C. Urmacher, and W. K. Knapper, "Trabecular (Merkel cell) carcinoma of the skin. Treatment of primary, recurrent, and metastatic disease," *Cancer*, vol. 57, no. 1, pp. 178–182, 1986.

[37] J. Redmond III, J. Perry, P. Sowray, S. J. Vukelja, and N. Dawson, "Chemotherapy of disseminated merkel-cell carcinoma," *American Journal of Clinical Oncology*, vol. 14, no. 4, pp. 305–307, 1991.

[38] M. Azagury, B. Chevallier, D. Atlan, Y. Graic, J. P. Dayot, and E. Thomine, "VP-16, cisplatin, doxorubicin, and bleomycin in metastatic Merkel cell carcinoma," *American Journal of Clinical Oncology*, vol. 16, no. 2, pp. 102–104, 1993.

[39] E. Bajetta, L. Rimassa, C. Carnaghi et al., "5-Fluorouracil, dacarbazine, and epirubicin in the treatment of patients with neuroendocrine tumors," *Cancer*, vol. 83, pp. 372–378, 1998.

[40] T. Y. Eng, M. Naguib, C. D. Fuller, W. E. Jones, and T. S. Herman, "Treatment of recurrent merkel cell carcinoma: an analysis of 46 cases," *American Journal of Clinical Oncology*, vol. 27, no. 6, pp. 576–583, 2004.

[41] E. R. Kokoska, M. S. Kokoska, B. T. Collins, D. R. Stapleton, and T. P. Wade, "Early aggressive treatment for merkel cell carcinoma improves outcome," *American Journal of Surgery*, vol. 174, no. 6, pp. 688–693, 1997.

[42] E. Voog, P. Biron, J. P. Martin, and J. Y. Blay, "Chemotherapy for patients with locally advanced or metastatic Merkel cell carcinoma," *Cancer*, vol. 85, pp. 2589–2595, 1999.

[43] M. Schlaak, T. Podewski, W. Von Bartenwerffer et al., "Induction of durable responses by oral etoposide monochemotherapy in patients with metastatic Merkel cell carcinoma," *European Journal of Dermatology*, vol. 22, pp. 187–191, 2012.

[44] P. J. Allen, W. B. Bowne, D. P. Jaques, M. F. Brennan, K. Busam, and D. G. Coit, "Merkel cell carcinoma: prognosis and treatment of patients from a single institution," *Journal of Clinical Oncology*, vol. 23, no. 10, pp. 2300–2309, 2005.

[45] R. P. DeMatteo, R. G. Maki, S. Singer, M. Gonen, M. F. Brennan, and C. R. Antonescu, "Results of tyrosine kinase inhibitor therapy followed by surgical resection for metastatic gastrointestinal stromal tumor," *Annals of Surgery*, vol. 245, no. 3, pp. 347–352, 2007.

[46] R. J. Motzer, B. I. Rini, R. M. Bukowski et al., "Sunitinib in patients with metastatic renal cell carcinoma," *Journal of the American Medical Association*, vol. 295, no. 21, pp. 2516–2524, 2006.

[47] R. Arora, M. Shuda, A. Guastafierro et al., "Survivin is a therapeutic target in Merkel cell carcinoma," *Science Translational Medicine*, vol. 4, Article ID 133ra56, 2012.

[48] O. Catalano, G. Catalano, and A. Nunziata, "The echographic and computed radiographic findings in 2 cases of Merkel-cell carcinoma," *Radiologia Medica*, vol. 94, no. 5, pp. 529–530, 1997.

[49] P. Peloschek, C. Novotny, C. Mueller-Mang et al., "Diagnostic imaging in Merkel cell carcinoma: lessons to learn from 16 cases with correlation of sonography, CT, MRI and PET," *European Journal of Radiology*, vol. 73, no. 2, pp. 317–323, 2010.

[50] D. J. Kwekkeboom, A. M. Hoff, S. W. J. Lamberts, H. Yoe Oei, and E. P. Krenning, "Somatostatin analogue scintigraphy: a simple and sensitive method for the in vivo visualization of Merkel cell tumors and their metastases," *Archives of Dermatology*, vol. 128, no. 6, pp. 818–821, 1992.

[51] R. M. Cabanas, "An approach for the treatment of penile carcinoma," *Cancer*, vol. 39, no. 2, pp. 456–466, 1977.

[52] M. Loyo, J. Schussel, E. Colantuoni et al., "Detection of Merkel cell virus and correlation with histologic presence of Merkel cell carcinoma in sentinel lymph nodes," *British Journal of Cancer*, vol. 106, pp. 1314–1319, 2012.

[53] J. H. Leonard, J. R. Ramsay, J. H. Kearsley, and G. W. Birrell, "Radiation sensitivity of Merkel cell carcinoma cell lines," *International Journal of Radiation Oncology Biology Physics*, vol. 32, no. 5, pp. 1401–1407, 1995.

[54] P. Mojica, D. Smith, and J. D. I. Ellenhorn, "Adjuvant radiation therapy is associated with improved survival in merkel cell carcinoma of the skin," *Journal of Clinical Oncology*, vol. 25, no. 9, pp. 1043–1047, 2007.

[55] M. J. Veness, L. Perera, J. McCourt et al., "Merkel cell carcinoma: improved outcome with adjuvant radiotherapy," *ANZ Journal of Surgery*, vol. 75, no. 5, pp. 275–281, 2005.

[56] C. S. L. Koh and M. J. Veness, "Role of definitive radiotherapy in treating patients with inoperable Merkel cell carcinoma: the Westmead Hospital experience and a review of the literature," *Australasian Journal of Dermatology*, vol. 50, no. 4, pp. 249–256, 2009.

[57] M. J. Veness, C. E. Palme, and G. J. Morgan, "Merkel cell carcinoma: a review of management," *Current Opinion in Otolaryngology and Head and Neck Surgery*, vol. 16, no. 2, pp. 170–174, 2008.

[58] R. E. Warner, M. J. Quinn, G. Hruby, R. A. Scolyer, R. F. Uren, and J. F. Thompson, "Management of Merkel cell carcinoma: the roles of lymphoscintigraphy, sentinel lymph node biopsy and adjuvant radiotherapy," *Annals of Surgical Oncology*, vol. 15, no. 9, pp. 2509–2518, 2008.

10

AP1 Transcription Factors in Epidermal Differentiation and Skin Cancer

Richard L. Eckert,[1,2,3] Gautam Adhikary,[1] Christina A. Young,[1] Ralph Jans,[1] James F. Crish,[4] Wen Xu,[1] and Ellen A. Rorke[5]

[1] *Department of Biochemistry and Molecular Biology, University of Maryland, School of Medicine, 108 North Greene Street, Rm 103, Baltimore, MD 21201, USA*
[2] *Department of Dermatology, University of Maryland, School of Medicine, Baltimore, MD 21201, USA*
[3] *Department of Obstetrics and Genecology and Reproductive Sciences, University of Maryland, School of Medicine, Baltimore, MD 21201, USA*
[4] *Department of Cell Biology, Cleveland Clinic Foundation, Cleveland, OH 44106, USA*
[5] *Department of Microbiology and Immunology, University of Maryland, School of Medicine, Baltimore, MD 21201, USA*

Correspondence should be addressed to Richard L. Eckert; reckert@umaryland.edu

Academic Editor: Deric L. Wheeler

AP1 (jun/fos) transcription factors (*c-jun, junB, junD, c-fos, FosB, Fra-1, and Fra-2*) are key regulators of epidermal keratinocyte survival and differentiation and important drivers of cancer development. Understanding the role of these factors in epidermis is complicated by the fact that each protein is expressed, at different levels, in multiple cells layers in differentiating epidermis, and because AP1 transcription factors regulate competing processes (i.e., proliferation, apoptosis, and differentiation). Various *in vivo* genetic approaches have been used to study these proteins including targeted and conditional knockdown, overexpression, and expression of dominant-negative inactivating AP1 transcription factors in epidermis. Taken together, these studies suggest that individual AP1 transcription factors have different functions in the epidermis and in cancer development and that altering AP1 transcription factor function in the basal versus suprabasal layers differentially influences the epidermal differentiation response and disease and cancer development.

1. Introduction

Keratinocytes are the major cell type responsible for the structure of the epidermis. They begin as stem cells in the basal epidermal layer and hair follicles [1–3]. During differentiation, as the cells migrate to the surface, cell division ceases and morphological changes ensue to produce the spinous, granular, transition, and cornified layers. Spinous layer cells are distinguished by the presence of desmosomal connections, whereas granular layer cells are characterized by the presence of granules that contain the products of keratinocyte differentiation. Differentiation of the granular layer cells results in the formation of the transition zone which separates the dead from living epidermal layers. It is in this zone that the cellular constituents are extensively enzymatically remodeled. This remodeling results in the covalent crosslinking of proteins to produce terminally differentiated corneocytes that form the skin surface [4, 5]. Achieving these morphological alterations relies on executing a preset program of differentiation that requires tight regulation of gene transcription [6].

The process of activation and suppression of gene transcription is controlled by a diverse family of regulators called transcription factors. Transcription factors mediate the final steps in the relay of information from the cell surface to the nucleus and the gene. This is accomplished by the interaction of the transcription factor with specific DNA elements that are usually located immediately upstream of the sequence that encodes the gene. DNA elements are generally a short DNA sequence of 8–20 nucleotides that encode a specific consensus sequence. A host of transcription factors has been implicated in control of epidermal differentiation and function, including activator protein 1 (AP1), AP2, Sp1, POU domain proteins, and CCAAT enhancer binding proteins [7]. AP1 transcription factors are among the most interesting and important regulators in epidermis [7]. Members of this family (c-fos, fosB, Fra-1, Fra-2, c-jun, junB, and junD) are expressed in specific epidermal layers and control multiple key functions [8]. This review focuses on summarizing interesting animal-based studies designed to identify the impact of perturbing AP1 transcription factor function on epidermal homeostasis and cancer.

2. MAPK and AP1 Transcription Factors Are Key Regulators of Keratinocyte Differentiation

The mitogen-activated protein kinases (MAPK) comprise major signaling cascades that regulate differentiation-associated gene expression in epidermis [9–14]. Each MAPK cascade consists of three kinase modulates which include an MEK kinase (MEKK), a mitogen-activate protein kinase/extracellular signal regulated kinase (MEK), and a mitogen-activated protein kinase (MAPK) [15–18]. Activated MEKK phosphorylates MEK which phosphorylates the MAPK. Activated MAPKs phosphorylate a variety of target proteins including transcription factors [10, 19–21]. The most extensively studied MAPKs are the ERK kinases (ERK1, ERK2), the c-jun N-terminal kinases (JNK1, JNK2), and the p38 kinases (p38α, β, δ, and γ). Figure 1 presents a schematic of the p38δ MAPK pathway which regulates expression of differentiation-associated genes during keratinocyte differentiation [7, 11]. The cascade consists of upstream regulator proteins (novel protein kinase c and Ras), an MAPK module (MEKK1, MEK3, and p38δ) and AP1 transcription factors. Activation of this cascade by a differentiation stimulus causes sequential phosphorylation and activation of kinases in the MAPK module which leads to increased AP1 transcription factor level and binding to the DNA response element in the target gene. This leads to increased target gene transcription [10–14, 22].

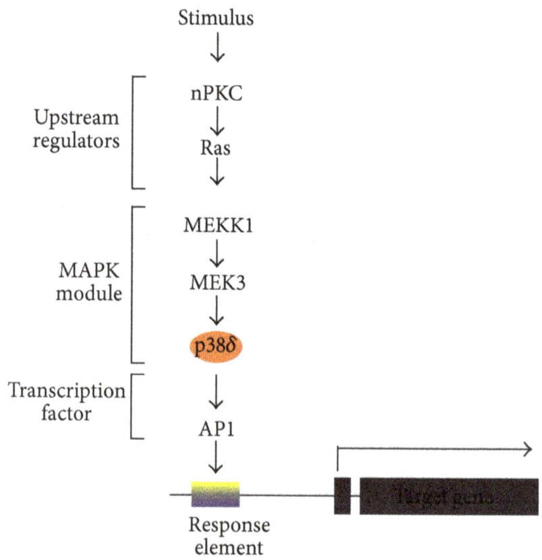

Figure 1: MAPK and AP1 transcription factor control of gene expression. The p38δ MAPK cascade that controls the expression of differentiation-associated genes in epidermis is depicted [10]. The three kinases of the MAPK module include MEKK1, MEK3, and p38δ MAPK. A differentiation stimulus activates upstream regulatory proteins, in this case novel protein kinase c (nPKC) and the Ras small GTPase. These events lead to phosphorylation and activation of MEKK1 which phosphorylates MEK3 which phosphorylates p38δ MAPK. Ultimately p38δ MAPK increases AP1 transcription factor expression and activity and the AP1 transcription factors bind to the response element on the target gene promoter to increase transcription.

AP1 transcription factors are key downstream targets of MAPK signaling in keratinocytes [12–14, 22–24]. Activator protein one (AP1) transcription factors include jun (c-jun, junB, junD) and fos (c-fos, FosB, Fra-1, Fra-2) family members [25–28]. They form jun-jun and jun-fos dimers that interact with specific AP1 transcription factor consensus DNA binding elements in target genes to regulate expression. They control keratinocyte proliferation [29–31], differentiation [10, 11, 32], and apoptosis [23, 33] and are important in tumor progression and disease development [9–11, 14, 22, 23, 34–38]. As an example, increased p38δ MAPK activity results in increased AP1 transcription factor level, increased AP1 transcription factor binding to DNA elements on the involucrin promoter, and increased involucrin gene transcription via a scheme similar to that shown in Figure 1 [8, 39]. The major AP1 factors that interact with the promoter are JunB, JunD, and Fra-1. Moreover, TAM67, a dominant-negative mutant of c-jun that inhibits the activity of all AP1 transcription factors [40], inhibits p38δ-dependent involucrin promoter activation [13]. MAPK activation by p38δ also results in increased C/EBPα and Sp1 binding to DNA binding sites in the involucrin gene promoter [41–43]. Thus, a PKC, Ras, MEKK1, MEK3 pathway activates p38δ MAPK and p38δ, in turn, acts to increase binding of selected AP1, Sp1, and C/EBP factors to the hINV promoter to increase promoter activity. However, the AP1 transcription factors are the most important family of regulators. In fact, it would be difficult to envision a more important family of transcriptional regulatory proteins in epidermal keratinocytes.

AP1 action in epidermis is complicated for several reasons. First, multiple AP1 family members are expressed in epidermis and form multiple dimer pairs. AP1 transcription factors can theoretically form eighteen different homo- and heterodimers, and work in other systems show that the particular dimer that is formed influences activity. For example, coexpression of c-fos with c-jun, leading to c-fos:c-jun dimer formation, enhances the transforming capacity of c-jun, whereas pairing c-jun with junB inhibits c-jun transforming capacity [44–46]. These differences may be related to the higher DNA binding and transcriptional activity of c-jun:c-fos heterodimer in comparison to c-jun:junB heterodimer [47]. Thus, it is safe to assume that the dimer that is formed influences activity in differentiating keratinocytes. Second, the expression level of most AP1 family members changes during keratinocyte differentiation [8, 48]. This means that different pairing combinations exist in the basal versus suprabasal layers and that this is likely to drive differences in activity and target gene selection. Third, covalent modification of individual AP1 transcription factors (e.g., phosphorylation) influences activity [49, 50]. For example, c-jun undergoes transient N-terminal phosphorylation as cells exit the G2 phase of the cell cycle, and this state is maintained until the cells complete mitosis [45]. An important lesson from these studies is that the composition of AP1 transcription factors in the tissue and the posttranslational modification state can influence biological activity. The fact that each AP1 transcription factor forms multiple hetero- and homodimers indicates that manipulating the level of one AP1 transcription factor, either by overexpression or knockout, will modify the function of other members. These features must be considered when interpreting the results of studies that alter AP1 transcription factor level or function in epidermis.

3. Animal Models of AP1 Transcription Factor Function

A number of laboratories have used *in vivo* mouse genetic models to study AP1 transcription factor function [34, 51, 52, 52–55]. These include embryonic knockout [54, 56–64], conditional knockout, inducible knockdown, expression of mutant dominant-negative AP1 proteins [65, 65–71], and targeted expression of intact wild-type proteins [72–74, 74–76]. These studies have targeted a variety of tissues, including the epidermis, liver, mammary gland, heart, bone, and blood [77]. The first lesson from these studies is that appropriate AP1 transcription factor expression is required for survival. For example, c-jun knockout mice die at embryonic day E13 due to defects in liver and heart development [78]. Likewise, junB null mice display extraembryonic tissue defects and die at embryonic E9.5 [56]. Fra-1 null mice survive only till embryonic day E9.5, and death is associated with defects in the yolk sac and placenta [54]. JunD knockout mice are born but fail to reproduce due to defects in spermatogenesis and reproduction [64]. These studies indicate that AP1 factors are essential for embryonic survival and are necessary for sustained development and reproduction. This is consistent with a central role for this family of proteins in maintaining tissue and organ homeostasis [77].

AP1 transcription factors also have tissue-specific effects. An *in vivo* example of this is that transgenic re-expression of junB in junB-null embryos rescues the mice from embryonic death. This is associated with normalization of most tissues; however, the junB transgene is silenced by an epigenetic mechanism in the myeloid lineage, and so these mice develop progressive myeloid leukemia [79]. This is also true in the context of tumor formation where AP1 transcription factors can function as oncogenes or tumor suppressors. For example, junD promotes cell survival by protecting cells from p53-dependent senescence and apoptosis [80, 81]. In contrast, JunD can also antagonize ras-mediated transformation [82]. Fra-1 has a complex role in that it enhances breast cancer cell chemosensitivity by driving cancer stem cells from dormancy [83]. In addition, Fra-1 deficient embryonic fibroblasts are resistant to peroxide-induced cell death, presumably because Fra-1 attenuates Nrf2-driven antioxidant responses [84]. Moreover, Fra-1 is increased in breast cancer where it functions as an oncogene to enhance tumor cell migration [85]. Thus, Fra-1 has multiple roles depending upon the tumor type and conditions.

4. AP1 Transcription Factors in Epidermis Knockout and Overexpression Studies

4.1. c-Jun and JunB—an Epidermal Oncogene and a Tumor Suppressor. Altering AP1 transcription factor expression changes epidermal function. Mice in which c-jun is conditionally knocked out in the epidermis develop normal skin, but epidermal growth factor receptor (EGFR) level is reduced in the eyelids leading to open eyes at birth [86]. This mimics the phenotype observed in EGFR- or TNFα-null mice [87–90]. In addition, in the absence of c-jun, the tumor-prone K5-SOS-F transgenic mice develop smaller epidermal papilloma, suggesting that c-jun is required for tumor formation [86], and it has been noted that c-jun expression is increased in tumors, and overexpression of c-jun in an oncogenic Ras background enhances tumor formation [91]. These findings suggest that c-jun functions as an oncogene in keratinocytes.

Mice lacking junB in keratinocytes are born with a normal epidermis. However, the epidermis is not completely normal, as epidermal JunB knockout mice display delayed wound healing [51] and develop systemic lupus erythematosus, an autoimmune disease that influences multiple tissues [92]. This phenotype is associated with increased secretion of epidermis-produced interleukin 6 (IL-6) that is associated with loss of JunB-dependent suppression IL-6 gene expression. IL-6 appears to play an essential role in phenotype development, as the phenotype is alleviated when epidermal JunB-null mice are bred to IL-6 deficient mice [92]. Absence of JunB in the epidermis also results in the release of large quantities of epidermis-derived granulocyte-colony stimulating factor (G-CSF) which is associated with skin ulceration, myeloproliferative disease, and low bone mass [93]. G-CSF appears to be essential for phenotype appearance, as breeding JunB null mice into a G-CSF null background reverses the myeloproliferative phenotype [93]. In addition, simultaneous conditional deletion of c-jun and JunB in the epidermis produces a psoriasis-like phenotype [94]. This is associated with increased production of tumor necrosis factor-alpha (TNFα) and increased epidermal S100A8/S100A9 expression [52]. Chemokine/cytokine production in epidermis presumably recruits immune cells to the epidermis to produce the psoriatic phenotype. Tissue inhibitor of metalloproteinase-3 (TIMP3) level is reduced in junB/c-jun null epidermis. As TIMP3 is an inhibitor of TNFα converting enzyme (TACE), loss of TIMP3 leads to enhanced epidermal TNFα cleavage and release [95]. TNFα is a key regulator in this context, as the biological phenotype can be mitigated by breeding these mice into a TNFα-null background [95]. Moreover, vascular endothelial growth factor (VEGF) also influences this phenotype, as anti-VEGF antibody treated junB/c-jun null mice show a pronounced reduction of inflammatory cells within the dermis and more normal epidermal differentiation [94]. JunB absence also increases tumor forming potential [91]. Tumor formation in Ras-activated cancer cells is inhibited by overexpression of JunB, an effect that requires the JunB transactivation domain [91]. Moreover, expression of dominant-negative JunB in this model, which inhibits JunB function, increases tumor formation [91].

4.2. c-Fos Acts as an Oncogene in Epidermis. JunB and c-jun are the most heavily studied AP1 transcription factors, but information is also available regarding the role of c-fos. Challenge of v-H-ras positive mice with DMBA (7,12-dimethylbenz[a]anthracene) and TPA (12-O-tetradecanoylphorbol-13-acetate), in the two-stage carcinogenesis protocol, increases skin tumor formation. However, tumor formation is attenuated in the absence of c-fos [34] which is associated with increased p53 expression [96]. The higher than normal level of p53 leads to epidermal tumor cell differentiation and suppression of skin tumor formation, in part due to p53-dependent transcriptional activation of TNFα converting enzyme [96].

4.3. Activating Transcription Factor 2 (ATF2) Suppresses Skin Tumor Formation. Activating transcription factor 2 (ATF2) is a stress-regulated transcription factor, and ATF2 transcriptional activity requires leucine zipper-dependent heterodimerization with members of the AP1 family, including c-jun [97, 98]. Expression of an inactive mutant form of ATF2 (lacking the DNA binding and leucine zipper domains) in the basal epidermis results in reduced tumor formation. When subjected to a two-stage DMBA/TPA skin carcinogenesis protocol, mice expressing the inactive ATF2 display increased tumor formation, and keratinocytes derived from these mice display enhanced anchorage-independent growth [99]. The resulting tumors display enhanced β-catenin and cyclin D1 and reduced Notch1 expression. This is consistent with the observation of reduced ATF2 and increased β-catenin in human squamous and basal cell carcinoma samples [99] and suggests that ATF2 suppresses epidermal carcinogenesis.

5. AP1 Transcription Factors in Epidermis-Dominant-Negative c-Jun (TAM67)

We have hypothesized that AP1 transcription factors perform different functions in the basal (proliferating) versus suprabasal (differentiating) epidermis [11]. However, testing this hypothesis is complicated by the fact that virtually all of the AP1 family members are expressed, at some level, in both the basal and suprabasal compartments [8, 25, 48]. Thus, we sought a model system where we could achieve complete suppression of AP1 transcription factor function in specific epidermal layers. This goal is difficult to achieve using gene knockout strategies, since knockout normally obviates expression of the targeted gene in all epidermal layers. Thus, we turned to targeted expression of dominant-negative c-jun (TAM67) in specific epidermal layers. In our case, we targeted TAM67 expression to the upper epidermal layers to achieve inactivation of AP1 transcription factor function in the suprabasal epidermis [66]. These studies follow a strategy developed by Nancy Colburn and associates where they targeted TAM67 to the basal epidermal layers using the K14 promoter [100]. This strategy has several advantages. First, TAM67 interferes with the function of all AP1 transcription factors [100]. TAM67 forms heterodimers with other AP1 transcription factors and these complexes bind to DNA, but the complexes are not able to activate transcription [100, 101]. Moreover, an early study, using a keratin promoter to drive expression, showed that TAM67 expression reduces TPA-stimulated invasion of mouse 308 cells through matrigel [65]. Further studies show that TAM67 inhibits invasion of human papillomavirus-immortalized human keratinocytes by suppressing AP1 transcription factor and NFκB signaling [102, 103]. These studies suggest that TAM67 is a useful construct for the study of cell function. Second, our use of the involucrin promoter permits targeting of TAM67 to the suprabasal epidermis [104–106] and alleviates problems that are observed with knockout mice where a specific AP1 transcription factor protein is lost from all layers. Third, a basal layer TAM67-targeted mouse model already existed [68, 70, 71, 107, 108] which permitted a direct comparison of the impact of basal versus suprabasal AP1 transcription factor inactivation. We will first discuss the impact of targeted expression of TAM67 in the epidermal basal layer.

5.1. TAM67 in the Basal Epidermis. In vivo studies in mouse epidermis show that TAM67-dependent inactivation of AP1 transcription factor function in the basal epidermal layer does not produce obvious changes in keratinocyte proliferation or epidermal or dermal appearance [68, 71, 107]. However, basal layer TAM67 expression does reduce susceptibility of SKH-1 hairless mice to UVB-dependent cancer progression [68, 71, 107]. Both tumor number and size are reduced and this is associated with reduced numbers of cyclin D1 positive cells in the tumors [107]. Expression of the E7 gene from human papillomavirus type 16 in mouse skin induces hyperplasia and enhances tumor promotion, and TAM67 protects mice from E7-enhanced tumorigenesis [70].

Some additional details are known regarding the mechanism of impact of AP1 transcription factor inaction in epidermal cancer cells. TPA treatment induces transformation of JB6/P+ cells. JB6/P+ cells are murine keratinocytes that undergo transformation following treatment with 12-O-tetradecanoylphorbol-13-acetate (TPA) [109]. Screening of microarrays from TPA-treated JB6/P+ cells, maintained in the presence or absence of TAM67 expression, revealed that high-mobility group A1 (HMGA1) protein is induced by TPA, and this induction is inhibited by TAM67. Further studies show that knockdown of HMGA1 with siRNA reduces JB6/P+ transformation, which is consistent with HMGA1 being an important AP1 transcription factor target [109]. A similar approach, also using JB6/P+ cells, identified sulfiredoxin as an additional gene that is required for TPA-induced transformation and is suppressed by TAM67 [110].

Sulfiredoxin is important for redox homeostasis and acts to reduce hyperoxidized peroxiredoxins. Cyclooxygenase-2, osteopontin, programmed cell death-4, and Wnt5a are additional proteins that may be important in transformation and have been identified [108, 111, 112]. It is possible that these proteins play a role in reducing tumor formation observed in mice where TAM67 is expressed in the basal layer.

5.2. TAM67 in the Suprabasal Epidermis. A recent study shows that targeted expression of TAM67 in the suprabasal epidermis results in extensive hyperplasia and hyperkeratosis [66]. This is associated with a substantial increase in proliferation of basal layer keratinocytes as measured by increased BrdU incorporation and increased appearance of Ki67-positive cells. This is not due to a direct effect of TAM67 on basal cells, as two different staining methods reveal that the TAM67-FLAG expression is confined to the suprabasal layers. Thus, inactivating suprabasal AP1 transcription factor function appears to feedback on the basal layer in a manner that stimulates basal layer cell division. In addition, differentiation appears to be delayed and incomplete. Consistent with delayed differentiation, keratins K5 and K14, which are normally exclusively expressed in the basal layer, are detected in all epidermal layers, and K6 is expressed in all epidermal layers. K6 is a keratin that is expressed under conditions of hyperproliferation but is not expressed in normal epidermis [66]. Thus, suprabasal TAM67 expression leads to increased basal layer proliferation and delayed differentiation and ultimately results in extensive hyperkeratosis. This is in marked contrast to the finding that targeting TAM67 to the epidermal basal layer using the keratin 14 promoter (K14-TAM67) produces no overt phenotype under resting conditions [71]. We propose that normal differentiation leads to accumulation of signals, generated by suprabasal cells, that suppress basal layer cell proliferation and that inhibiting differentiation opens this feedback loop leading to increased basal keratinocyte proliferation [66].

Because of the hyperproliferative phenotype, it was anticipated that mice expressing TAM67 in the suprabasal epidermis would be more susceptible to tumor formation. This was tested by treating control and suprabasal TAM67 mice with a DNA mutagenic agent, 7,12-dimethylbenz[α]anthracene (DMBA) to produce initiated cells, and then inducing TAM67 expression. Surprisingly, TAM67 expression, and the associated increase in cell proliferation, did not drive tumor formation in DMBA treated mice. This is interesting, because cell proliferation is thought to predispose tissue to enhanced tumor formation [113]. Treatment with carcinogen (7,12-dimethylbenz[α]anthracene, DMBA) followed by tumor promoter (12-O-tetradecanoylphorbol-13-acetate, TPA) is known to cause tumor formation [113]. However, in a protocol where mice were treated with DMBA, followed by treatment with TPA, TAM67 expression reduced tumor formation. The possibility that TAM67 may interfere with the proliferation promoting activity of TPA in the carcinogenesis protocol was considered; however, these experiments suggest that TAM67-expressing epidermis is fully competent to respond to TPA. Taken together, these findings show that inaction of AP1 transcription factor function in the suprabasal epidermis increases epidermal proliferation but reduces carcinogen/tumor promoter-induced cancer development. The underlying mechanism responsible for these surprising observations is under study.

Thus, although the basal and suprabasal targeted TAM67 mice produce very different epidermal phenotypes, these mice share features in common [66, 71]. First, TAM67 basal and suprabasal epidermal mice respond to stress agents (okadaic acid, TPA, etc.) with increased basal cell proliferation, and this response is not reduced when compared to control mice. Second, both strains display a reduced sensitivity to DMBA/TPA induced tumor formation. The fact that inactivating AP1 factor function in the basal or suprabasal epidermis reduces tumor formation, clearly suggest that, on balance, AP1 factors have an essential role in driving tumor formation.

6. Summary

A variety of genetic approaches have been used to study the *in vivo* role of AP1 transcription factors in epidermis. It is clear from these studies that AP1 transcription factors play a key role in controlling differentiation of epidermal keratinocytes and that perturbing this process results in a variety of disease phenotypes including psoriasis and cancer. It is also clear that some AP1 transcription factors function as procancer proteins (e.g., c-jun, c-fos), while others inhibit cancer development (e.g., JunB, ATF2). Additional studies suggest that a host of cytokines and chemokines is involved in generation of the disease and cancer phenotypes that develop when AP1 transcription factor function is perturbed, and these studies suggest that the epidermis can act as an endocrine organ to influence the function of other organs. It also appears that AP1 transcription factors have differing roles in basal and suprabasal epidermis, as inactivation of AP1 transcription factor function in these compartments produces no change (basal targeted TAM67 expression) or hyperproliferation (suprabasal targeted TAM67 expression).

References

[1] R. L. Eckert, G. Adhikary, S. Balasubramanian et al., "Biochemistry of epidermal stem cells," *Biochimica et Biophysica Acta*, vol. 1830, no. 2, pp. 2427–2434, 2013.

[2] C. Blanpain, V. Horsley, and E. Fuchs, "Epithelial stem cells: turning over new leaves," *Cell*, vol. 128, no. 3, pp. 445–458, 2007.

[3] G. Cotsarelis, "Epithelial stem cells: a folliculocentric view," *Journal of Investigative Dermatology*, vol. 126, no. 7, pp. 1459–1468, 2006.

[4] A. E. Kalinin, A. V. Kajava, and P. M. Steinert, "Epithelial barrier function: assembly and structural features of the cornified cell envelope," *BioEssays*, vol. 24, no. 9, pp. 789–800, 2002.

[5] P. M. Steinert, "A model for the hierarchical structure of the human epidermal cornified cell envelope," *Cell Death and Differentiation*, vol. 2, no. 1, pp. 33–40, 1995.

[6] R. L. Eckert, J. F. Crish, and N. A. Robinson, "The epidermal keratinocyte as a model for the study of gene regulation and

cell differentiation," *Physiological Reviews*, vol. 77, no. 2, pp. 397–424, 1997.

[7] R. L. Eckert, J. F. Crish, E. B. Banks, and J. F. Welter, "The epidermis: genes on—genes off," *Journal of Investigative Dermatology*, vol. 109, no. 4, pp. 501–509, 1997.

[8] J. F. Welter and R. L. Eckert, "Differential expression of the fos and jun family members c-fos, fosB, Fra-1, Fra-2, c-jun, junB and junD during human epidermal keratinocyte differentiation," *Oncogene*, vol. 11, no. 12, pp. 2680–2687, 1995.

[9] R. L. Eckert, T. Efimova, S. R. Dashti et al., "Keratinocyte survival, differentiation, and death: many roads lead to mitogen-activated protein kinase," *Journal of Investigative Dermatology Symposium Proceedings*, vol. 7, no. 1, pp. 36–40, 2002.

[10] R. L. Eckert, T. Efimova, S. Balasubramanian, J. F. Crish, F. Bone, and S. Dashti, "p38 mitogen-activated protein kinases on the body surface—a function for p38δ," *Journal of Investigative Dermatology*, vol. 120, no. 5, pp. 823–828, 2003.

[11] R. L. Eckert, J. F. Crish, T. Efimova et al., "Regulation of involucrin gene expression," *Journal of Investigative Dermatology*, vol. 123, no. 1, pp. 13–22, 2004.

[12] T. Efimova and R. L. Eckert, "Regulation of human involucrin promoter activity by novel protein kinase C isoforms," *Journal of Biological Chemistry*, vol. 275, no. 3, pp. 1601–1607, 2000.

[13] T. Efimova, P. LaCelle, J. F. Welter, and R. L. Eckert, "Regulation of human involucrin promoter activity by a protein kinase C, Ras, MEKK1, MEK3, p38/RK, AP1 signal transduction pathway," *Journal of Biological Chemistry*, vol. 273, no. 38, pp. 24387–24395, 1998.

[14] T. Efimova, A. Deucher, T. Kuroki, M. Ohba, and R. L. Eckert, "Novel protein kinase C isoforms regulate human keratinocyte differentiation by activating a p38δ mitogen-activated protein kinase cascade that targets CCAAT/enhancer-binding protein α," *Journal of Biological Chemistry*, vol. 277, no. 35, pp. 31753–31760, 2002.

[15] R. J. Davis, "Transcriptional regulation by MAP kinases," *Molecular Reproduction and Development*, vol. 42, no. 4, pp. 459–467, 1995.

[16] C. J. Caunt and S. M. Keyse, "Dual-specificity MAP kinase phosphatases (MKPs): shaping the outcome of MAP kinase signalling," *FEBS Journal*, vol. 280, no. 2, pp. 489–504, 2013.

[17] C. Q. Pan, M. Sudol, M. Sheetz, and B. C. Low, "Modularity and functional plasticity of scaffold proteins as p(l)acemakers in cell signaling," *Cellular Signalling*, vol. 24, no. 11, pp. 2143–2165, 2012.

[18] F. Zassadowski, C. Rochette-Egly, C. Chomienne, and B. Cassinat, "Regulation of the transcriptional activity of nuclear receptors by the MEK/ERK1/2 pathway," *Cellular Signalling*, vol. 24, no. 12, pp. 2369–2377, 2012.

[19] M. J. Robinson and M. H. Cobb, "Mitogen-activated protein kinase pathways," *Current Opinion in Cell Biology*, vol. 9, no. 2, pp. 180–186, 1997.

[20] Z. Chen, T. B. Gibson, F. Robinson et al., "MAP kinases," *Chemical Reviews*, vol. 101, no. 8, pp. 2449–2476, 2001.

[21] S. R. Kanade and R. L. Eckert, "Protein arginine methyltransferase 5 (PRMT5) signaling suppresses protein kinase Cdelta- and p38delta-dependent signaling and keratinocyte differentiation," *Journal of Biological Chemistry*, vol. 287, no. 10, pp. 7313–7323, 2012.

[22] T. Efimova, A. M. Broome, and R. L. Eckert, "A regulatory role for p38δ MAPK in keratinocyte differentiation: evidence for p38δ-ERK1/2 complex formation," *Journal of Biological Chemistry*, vol. 278, no. 36, pp. 34277–34285, 2003.

[23] T. Efimova, A. M. Broome, and R. L. Eckert, "Protein kinase Cδ regulates keratinocyte death and survival by regulating activity and subcellular localization of a p38δ-extracellular signal-regulated kinase 1/2 complex," *Molecular and Cellular Biology*, vol. 24, no. 18, pp. 8167–8183, 2004.

[24] C. A. Kraft, T. Efimova, and R. L. Eckert, "Activation of PKCδ and p38δ MAPK during okadaic acid dependent keratinocyte apoptosis," *Archives of Dermatological Research*, vol. 299, no. 2, pp. 71–83, 2007.

[25] P. Angel, A. Szabowski, and M. Schorpp-Kistner, "Function and regulation of AP-1 subunits in skin physiology and pathology," *Oncogene*, vol. 20, no. 19, pp. 2413–2423, 2001.

[26] M. Karin, Z. G. Liu, and E. Zandi, "AP-1 function and regulation," *Current Opinion in Cell Biology*, vol. 9, no. 2, pp. 240–246, 1997.

[27] E. Shaulian and M. Karin, "AP-1 as a regulator of cell life and death," *Nature Cell Biology*, vol. 4, no. 5, pp. E131–E136, 2002.

[28] E. Shaulian and M. Karin, "AP-1 in cell proliferation and survival," *Oncogene*, vol. 20, no. 19, pp. 2390–2400, 2001.

[29] H. Mizuno, Y. Y. Cho, W. Y. Ma, A. M. Bode, and Z. Dong, "Effects of MAP kinase inhibitors on epidermal growth factor-induced neoplastic transformation of human keratinocytes," *Molecular Carcinogenesis*, vol. 45, no. 1, pp. 1–9, 2006.

[30] B. Shi and R. R. Isseroff, "Epidermal growth factor (EGF)-mediated DNA-binding activity of AP-1 is attenuated in senescent human epidermal keratinocytes," *Experimental Dermatology*, vol. 14, no. 7, pp. 519–527, 2005.

[31] H. Takahashi, M. Ibe, S. Nakamura, A. Ishida-Yamamoto, Y. Hashimoto, and H. Iizuka, "Extracellular regulated kinase and c-Jun N-terminal kinase are activated in psoriatic involved epidermis," *Journal of Dermatological Science*, vol. 30, no. 2, pp. 94–99, 2002.

[32] G. Adhikary, J. Crish, J. Lass, and R. L. Eckert, "Regulation of involucrin expression in normal human corneal epithelial cells: a role for activator protein one," *Investigative Ophthalmology and Visual Science*, vol. 45, no. 4, pp. 1080–1087, 2004.

[33] D. Raj, D. E. Brash, and D. Grossman, "Keratinocyte apoptosis in epidermal development and disease," *Journal of Investigative Dermatology*, vol. 126, no. 2, pp. 243–257, 2006.

[34] E. Saez, S. E. Rutberg, E. Mueller et al., "c-fos is required for malignant progression of skin tumors," *Cell*, vol. 82, no. 5, pp. 721–732, 1995.

[35] C. R. Kahn, E. Young, Ihn Hwan Lee, and J. S. Rhim, "Human corneal epithelial primary cultures and cell lines with extended life span: in vitro model for ocular studies," *Investigative Ophthalmology and Visual Science*, vol. 34, no. 12, pp. 3429–3441, 1993.

[36] Q. B. She, N. Chen, A. M. Bode, R. A. Flavell, and Z. Dong, "Deficiency of c-Jun-NH2-terminal kinase-1 in mice enhances skin tumor development by 12-O-tetradecanoylphorbol-13-acetate," *Cancer Research*, vol. 62, no. 5, pp. 1343–1348, 2002.

[37] S. E. Rutberg, T. L. Adams, A. Glick, M. T. Bonovich, C. Vinson, and S. H. Yuspa, "Activator protein 1 transcription factors are fundamental to v-ras(Ha)-induced changes in gene expression in neoplastic keratinocytes," *Cancer Research*, vol. 60, no. 22, pp. 6332–6338, 2000.

[38] H. Iizuka, H. Takahashi, M. Honma, and A. Ishida-Yamamoto, "Unique keratinization process in psoriasis: late differentiation markers are abolished because of the premature cell death," *Journal of Dermatology*, vol. 31, no. 4, pp. 271–276, 2004.

[39] J. F. Welter, J. F. Crish, C. Agarwal, and R. L. Eckert, "Fos-related antigen (Fra-1), junB, and junD activate human involucrin promoter transcription by binding to proximal and distal AP1 sites to mediate phorbol ester effects on promoter activity," *Journal of Biological Chemistry*, vol. 270, no. 21, pp. 12614–12622, 1995.

[40] Y. Wu, X. Zhang, and Z. E. Zehner, "c-Jun and the dominant-negative mutant, TAM67, induce vimentin gene expression by interacting with the activator Sp1," *Oncogene*, vol. 22, no. 55, pp. 8891–8901, 2003.

[41] E. B. Banks, J. F. Crish, and R. L. Eckert, "Transcription factor Sp1 activates involucrin promoter activity in non-epithelial cell types," *Biochemical Journal*, vol. 337, part 3, pp. 507–512, 1999.

[42] E. B. Banks, J. F. Crish, J. F. Welter, and R. L. Eckert, "Characterization of human involucrin promoter distal regulatory region transcriptional activator elements—a role for Sp1 and AP1 binding sites," *Biochemical Journal*, vol. 331, part 1, pp. 61–68, 1998.

[43] C. Agarwal, T. Efimova, J. F. Welter, J. F. Crish, and R. L. Eckert, "CCAAT/enhancer-binding proteins. A role in regulation of human involucrin promoter response to phorbol ester," *Journal of Biological Chemistry*, vol. 274, no. 10, pp. 6190–6194, 1999.

[44] J. Schutte, J. D. Minna, and M. J. Birrer, "Deregulated expression of human c-jun transforms primary rat embryo cells in cooperation with an activated c-Ha-ras gene and transforms Rat-1a cells as a single gene," *Proceedings of the National Academy of Sciences of the United States of America*, vol. 86, no. 7, pp. 2257–2261, 1989.

[45] L. Bakiri, D. Lallemand, E. Bossy-Wetzel, and M. Yaniv, "Cell cycle-dependent variations in c-Jun and JunB phosphorylation: a role in the control of cyclin D1 expression," *EMBO Journal*, vol. 19, no. 9, pp. 2056–2068, 2000.

[46] E. Passegué and E. F. Wagner, "JunB suppresses cell proliferation by transcriptional activation of p16(INK4a) expression," *EMBO Journal*, vol. 19, no. 12, pp. 2969–2979, 2000.

[47] T. Deng and M. Karin, "JunB differs from c-Jun in its DNA-binding and dimerization domains, and respresses c-Jun by formation of inactive heterodimers," *Genes and Development*, vol. 7, no. 3, pp. 479–490, 1993.

[48] D. Mehic, L. Bakiri, M. Ghannadan, E. F. Wagner, and E. Tschachler, "Fos and Jun proteins are specifically expressed during differentiation of human keratinocytes," *Journal of Investigative Dermatology*, vol. 124, no. 1, pp. 212–220, 2005.

[49] M. Karin, "The regulation of AP-1 activity by mitogen-activated protein kinases," *Journal of Biological Chemistry*, vol. 270, no. 28, pp. 16483–16486, 1995.

[50] M. Karin, "Mitogen-activated protein kinase cascades as regulators of stress responses," *Annals of the New York Academy of Sciences*, vol. 851, pp. 139–146, 1998.

[51] L. Florin, J. Knebel, P. Zigrino et al., "Delayed wound healing and epidermal hyperproliferation in mice lacking JunB in the skin," *Journal of Investigative Dermatology*, vol. 126, no. 4, pp. 902–911, 2006.

[52] R. Zenz, R. Eferl, L. Kenner et al., "Psoriasis-like skin disease and arthritis caused by inducible epidermal deletion of Jun proteins," *Nature*, vol. 437, no. 7057, pp. 369–375, 2005.

[53] E. Passegué, W. Jochum, A. Behrens, R. Ricci, and E. F. Wagne, "JunB can substitute for Jun in mouse development and cell proliferation," *Nature Genetics*, vol. 30, no. 2, pp. 158–166, 2002.

[54] M. Schreiber, Z. Q. Wang, W. Jochum, I. Fetka, C. Elliott, and E. F. Wagner, "Placental vascularisation requires the AP-1 component Fra1," *Development*, vol. 127, no. 22, pp. 4937–4948, 2000.

[55] A. Fleischmann, F. Hafezi, C. Elliott, C. E. Remé, U. Rüther, and E. F. Wagner, "Fra-1 replaces c-Fos-dependent functions in mice," *Genes and Development*, vol. 14, no. 21, pp. 2695–2700, 2000.

[56] M. Schorpp-Kistner, Z. Q. Wang, P. Angel, and E. F. Wagner, "JunB is essential for mammalian placentation," *EMBO Journal*, vol. 18, no. 4, pp. 934–948, 1999.

[57] M. C. Gruda, J. van Amsterdam, C. A. Rizzo, S. K. Durham, S. Lira, and R. Bravo, "Expression of FosB during mouse development: normal development of FosB knockout mice," *Oncogene*, vol. 12, no. 10, pp. 2177–2185, 1996.

[58] Z. Q. Wang, C. Ovitt, A. E. Grigoriadis, U. Mohle-Steinlein, U. Ruther, and E. F. Wagner, "Bone and haematopoietic defects in mice lacking c-fos," *Nature*, vol. 360, no. 6406, pp. 741–745, 1992.

[59] R. S. Johnson, B. M. Spiegelman, and V. Papaioannou, "Pleiotropic effects of a null mutation in the c-fos proto-oncogene," *Cell*, vol. 71, no. 4, pp. 577–586, 1992.

[60] J. R. Brown, H. Ye, R. T. Bronson, P. Dikkes, and M. E. Greenberg, "A defect in nurturing in mice lacking the immediate early gene fosB," *Cell*, vol. 86, no. 2, pp. 297–309, 1996.

[61] R. S. Johnson, B. van Lingen, V. E. Papaioannou, and B. M. Spiegelman, "A null mutation at the c-jun locus causes embryonic lethality and retarded cell growth in culture," *Genes and Development*, vol. 7, no. 7B, pp. 1309–1317, 1993.

[62] F. Hilberg, A. Aguzzi, N. Howells, and E. F. Wagner, "c-Jun is essential for normal mouse development and hepatogenesis," *Nature*, vol. 365, no. 6442, pp. 179–181, 1993.

[63] R. Eferl, M. Sibilia, F. Hilberg et al., "Functions of c-Jun in liver and heart development," *Journal of Cell Biology*, vol. 145, no. 5, pp. 1049–1061, 1999.

[64] D. Thépot, J. B. Weitzman, J. Barra et al., "Targeted disruption of the murine junD gene results in multiple defects in male reproductive function," *Development*, vol. 127, no. 1, pp. 143–153, 2000.

[65] Z. Dong, H. C. Crawford, V. Lavrovsky et al., "A dominant negative mutant of jun blocking 12-O-tetradecanoylphorbol-13-acetate-induced invasion in mouse keratinocytes," *Molecular Carcinogenesis*, vol. 19, no. 3, pp. 204–212, 1997.

[66] E. A. Rorke, G. Adhikary, R. Jans, J. F. Crish, and R. L. Eckert, "AP1 factor inactivation in the suprabasal epidermis causes increased epidermal hyperproliferation and hyperkeratosis but reduced carcinogen-dependent tumor formation," *Oncogene*, vol. 29, no. 44, pp. 5873–5882, 2010.

[67] Q. Shen, Y. Zhang, I. P. Uray et al., "The AP-1 transcription factor regulates postnatal mammary gland development," *Developmental Biology*, vol. 295, no. 2, pp. 589–603, 2006.

[68] E. J. Thompson, J. MacGowan, M. R. Young, N. Colburn, and G. T. Bowden, "A dominant negative c-jun specifically blocks okadaic acid-induced skin tumor promotion," *Cancer Research*, vol. 62, no. 11, pp. 3044–3047, 2002.

[69] J. W. Tichelaar, Y. Yan, Q. Tan et al., "A dominant-negative c-jun mutant inhibits lung carcinogenesis in mice," *Cancer Prevention Research*, vol. 3, no. 9, pp. 1148–1156, 2010.

[70] M. R. Young, L. Farrell, P. Lambert, P. Awasthi, and N. H. Colburn, "Protection against human papillomavirus type 16-E7 oncogene-induced tumorigenesis by in vivo expression of dominant-negative c-jun," *Molecular Carcinogenesis*, vol. 34, no. 2, pp. 72–77, 2002.

[71] M. R. Young, J. J. Li, M. Rincón et al., "Transgenic mice demonstrate AP-1 (activator protein-1) transactivation is required for tumor promotion," *Proceedings of the National Academy of Sciences of the United States of America*, vol. 96, no. 17, pp. 9827–9832, 1999.

[72] R. Zenz, R. Eferl, C. Scheinecker et al., "Activator protein 1 (Fos/Jun) functions in inflammatory bone and skin disease," *Arthritis Research and Therapy*, vol. 10, no. 1, article 201, 2008.

[73] M. L. Carrozza, H. Jacobs, D. Acton, I. Verma, and A. Berns, "Overexpression of the FosB2 gene in thymocytes causes aberrant development of T cells and thymic epithelial cells," *Oncogene*, vol. 14, no. 9, pp. 1083–1091, 1997.

[74] A. E. Grigoriadis, K. Schellander, Z. Q. Wang, and E. F. Wagner, "Osteoblasts are target cells for transformation in c-fos transgenic mice," *Journal of Cell Biology*, vol. 122, no. 3, pp. 685–701, 1993.

[75] G. Sabatakos, N. A. Sims, J. Chen et al., "Overexpression of ΔFosB transcription factor(s) increases bone formation and inhibits adipogenesis," *Nature Medicine*, vol. 6, no. 9, pp. 985–990, 2000.

[76] M. Schorpp, R. Jäger, K. Schellander et al., "The human ubiquitin C promoter directs high ubiquitous expression of transgenes in mice," *Nucleic Acids Research*, vol. 24, no. 9, pp. 1787–1788, 1996.

[77] R. Zenz and E. F. Wagner, "Jun signalling in the epidermis: from developmental defects to psoriasis and skin tumors," *International Journal of Biochemistry and Cell Biology*, vol. 38, no. 7, pp. 1043–1049, 2006.

[78] R. Eferl and E. F. Wagner, "AP-1: a double-edged sword in tumorigenesis," *Nature Reviews Cancer*, vol. 3, no. 11, pp. 859–868, 2003.

[79] E. Passegué, W. Jochum, M. Schorpp-Kistner, U. Möhle-Steinlein, and E. F. Wagner, "Chronic myeloid leukemia with increased granulocyte progenitors in mice lacking JunB expression in the myeloid lineage," *Cell*, vol. 104, no. 1, pp. 21–32, 2001.

[80] J. B. Weitzman, L. Fiette, K. Matsuo, and M. Yaniv, "JunD protects cells from p53-dependent senescence and apoptosis," *Molecular Cell*, vol. 6, no. 5, pp. 1109–1119, 2000.

[81] O. Yazgan and C. M. Pfarr, "Differential binding of the menin tumor suppressor protein to JunD isoforms," *Cancer Research*, vol. 61, no. 3, pp. 916–920, 2001.

[82] C. M. Pfarr, F. Mechta, G. Spyrou, D. Lallemand, S. Carillo, and M. Yaniv, "Mouse JunD negatively regulates fibroblast growth and antagonizes transformation by ras," *Cell*, vol. 76, no. 4, pp. 747–760, 1994.

[83] D. Lu, S. Chen, X. Tan et al., "Fra-1 promotes breast cancer chemosensitivity by driving cancer stem cells from dormancy," *Cancer Research*, vol. 72, no. 14, pp. 3451–3456, 2012.

[84] M. Vaz, N. Machireddy, A. Irving et al., "Oxidant-induced cell death and Nrf2-dependent antioxidative response are controlled by Fra-1/AP-1," *Molecular and Cellular Biology*, vol. 32, no. 9, pp. 1694–1709, 2012.

[85] S. Yang, Y. Li, J. Gao et al., "MicroRNA-34 suppresses breast cancer invasion and metastasis by directly targeting Fra-1," *Oncogene*, 2012.

[86] R. Zenz, H. Scheuch, P. Martin et al., "c-Jun regulates eyelid closure and skin tumor development through EGFR signaling," *Developmental Cell*, vol. 4, no. 6, pp. 879–889, 2003.

[87] N. C. Luetteke, T. H. Qiu, R. L. Peiffer, P. Oliver, O. Smithies, and D. C. Lee, "TGFα deficiency results in hair follicle and eye abnormalities in targeted and waved-1 mice," *Cell*, vol. 73, no. 2, pp. 263–278, 1993.

[88] K. J. Fowler, F. Walker, W. Alexander et al., "A mutation in the epidermal growth factor receptor in waved-2 mice has a profound effect on receptor biochemistry that results in impaired lactation," *Proceedings of the National Academy of Sciences of the United States of America*, vol. 92, no. 5, pp. 1465–1469, 1995.

[89] P. J. Miettinen, J. E. Berger, J. Meneses et al., "Epithelial immaturity and multiorgan failure in mice lacking epidermal growth factor receptor," *Nature*, vol. 376, no. 6538, pp. 337–341, 1995.

[90] D. W. Threadgill, A. A. Dlugosz, L. A. Hansen et al., "Targeted disruption of mouse EGF receptor: effect of genetic background on mutant phenotype," *Science*, vol. 269, no. 5221, pp. 230–234, 1995.

[91] J. Y. Jin, H. Ke, R. P. Hall, and J. Y. Zhang, "C-Jun promotes whereas JunB inhibits epidermal neoplasia," *Journal of Investigative Dermatology*, vol. 131, no. 5, pp. 1149–1158, 2011.

[92] P. Pflegerl, P. Vesely, B. Hantusch et al., "Epidermal loss of JunB leads to a SLE phenotype due to hyper IL-6 signaling," *Proceedings of the National Academy of Sciences of the United States of America*, vol. 106, no. 48, pp. 20423–20428, 2009.

[93] A. Meixner, R. Zenz, H. B. Schonthaler et al., "Epidermal JunB represses G-CSF transcription and affects haematopoiesis and bone formation," *Nature Cell Biology*, vol. 10, no. 8, pp. 1003–1011, 2008.

[94] H. B. Schonthaler, R. Huggenberger, S. K. Wculek, M. Detmar, and E. F. Wagner, "Systemic anti-VEGF treatment strongly reduces skin inflammation in a mouse model of psoriasis," *Proceedings of the National Academy of Sciences of the United States of America*, vol. 106, no. 50, pp. 21264–21269, 2009.

[95] J. Guinea-Viniegra, R. Zenz, H. Scheuch et al., "TNFα shedding and epidermal inflammation are controlled by Jun proteins," *Genes and Development*, vol. 23, no. 22, pp. 2663–2674, 2009.

[96] J. Guinea-Viniegra, R. Zenz, H. Scheuch et al., "Differentiation-induced skin cancer suppression by FOS, p53, and TACE/ADAM17," *The Journal of Clinical Investigation*, vol. 122, no. 8, pp. 2898–2910, 2012.

[97] D. M. Benbrook and N. C. Jones, "Heterodimer formation between CREB and JUN proteins," *Oncogene*, vol. 5, no. 3, pp. 295–302, 1990.

[98] H. van Dam and M. Castellazzi, "Distinct roles of Jun:Fos and Jun:ATF dimers in oncogenesis," *Oncogene*, vol. 20, no. 19, pp. 2453–2464, 2001.

[99] A. Bhoumik, B. Fichtman, C. DeRossi et al., "Suppressor role of activating transcription factor 2 (ATF2) in skin cancer," *Proceedings of the National Academy of Sciences of the United States of America*, vol. 105, no. 5, pp. 1674–1679, 2008.

[100] P. H. Brown, T. K. Chen, and M. J. Birrer, "Mechanism of action of a dominant-negative mutant of c-Jun," *Oncogene*, vol. 9, no. 3, pp. 791–799, 1994.

[101] B. Han, E. A. Rorke, G. Adhikary et al., "Suppression of AP1 transcription factor function in keratinocyte suppresses differentiation," *PLoS One*, vol. 7, no. 5, Article ID e36941, 2012.

[102] J. J. Li, J. S. Rhim, R. Schlegel, K. H. Vousden, and N. H. Colburn, "Expression of dominant negative Jun inhibits elevated AP-1 and NF-κB transactivation and suppresses anchorage independent growth of HPV immortalized human keratinocytes," *Oncogene*, vol. 16, no. 21, pp. 2711–2721, 1998.

[103] J. J. Li, Y. Cao, M. R. Young, and N. H. Colburn, "Induced expression of dominant-negative c-jun downregulates NFkappaB and AP-1 target genes and suppresses tumor phenotype in

human keratinocytes," *Molecular Carcinogenesis*, vol. 29, no. 3, pp. 159–169, 2000.

[104] J. F. Crish, J. M. Howard, T. M. Zaim, S. Murthy, and R. L. Eckert, "Tissue-specific and differentiation-appropriate expression of the human involucrin gene in transgenic mice: an abnormal epidermal phenotype," *Differentiation*, vol. 53, no. 3, pp. 191–200, 1993.

[105] J. F. Crish, T. M. Zaim, and R. L. Eckert, "The distal regulatory region of the human involucrin promoter is required for expression in epidermis," *Journal of Biological Chemistry*, vol. 273, no. 46, pp. 30460–30465, 1998.

[106] J. F. Crish, F. Bone, S. Balasubramanian et al., "Suprabasal expression of the human papillomavirus type 16 oncoproteins in mouse epidermis alters expression of cell cycle regulatory proteins," *Carcinogenesis*, vol. 21, no. 5, pp. 1031–1037, 2000.

[107] S. J. Cooper, J. MacGowan, J. Ranger-Moore, M. R. Young, N. H. Colburn, and G. T. Bowden, "Expression of dominant negative c-jun inhibits ultraviolet B-induced squamous cell carcinoma number and size in an SKH-1 hairless mouse model," *Molecular Cancer Research*, vol. 1, no. 11, pp. 848–854, 2003.

[108] C. P. Matthews, A. M. Birkholz, A. R. Baker et al., "Dominant-negative activator protein 1 (TAM67) targets cyclooxygenase-2 and osteopontin under conditions in which it specifically inhibits tumorigenesis," *Cancer Research*, vol. 67, no. 6, pp. 2430–2438, 2007.

[109] A. Dhar, J. Hu, R. Reeves, L. M. S. Resar, and N. H. Colburn, "Dominant-negative c-Jun (TAM67) target genes: HMGA1 is required for tumor promoter-induced transformation," *Oncogene*, vol. 23, no. 25, pp. 4466–4476, 2004.

[110] Q. Wei, H. Jiang, C. P. Matthews, and N. H. Colburn, "Sulfiredoxin is an AP-1 target gene that is required for transformation and shows elevated expression in human skin malignancies," *Proceedings of the National Academy of Sciences of the United States of America*, vol. 105, no. 50, pp. 19738–19743, 2008.

[111] M. R. Young, H. S. Yang, and N. H. Colburn, "Promising molecular targets for cancer prevention: AP-1, NF-κB and Pdcd4," *Trends in Molecular Medicine*, vol. 9, no. 1, pp. 36–41, 2003.

[112] M. I. Kang, A. R. Baker, C. R. Dextras, S. M. Cabarcas, M. R. Young, and N. H. Colburn, "Targeting of noncanonical Wnt5a signaling by AP-1 blocker dominant-negative Jun when it inhibits skin carcinogenesis," *Genes & Cancer*, vol. 3, no. 1, pp. 37–50, 2012.

[113] T. J. Slaga, J. DiGiovanni, L. D. Winberg, and I. V. Budunova, "Skin carcinogenesis: characteristics, mechanisms, and prevention," *Progress in Clinical and Biological Research*, vol. 391, pp. 1–20, 1995.

11

Histopathological Study of Skin Adnexal Tumours—Institutional Study in South India

Ankit Sharma,[1] Deepak G. Paricharak,[2] Jitendra Singh Nigam,[1] Shivani Rewri,[1] Priyanka Bhatia Soni,[1] Anita Omhare,[1] and Preethi Sekar[1]

[1] *Department of Pathology, D.D.U. Hospital, Hari Nagar, New Delhi 110066, India*
[2] *Department of Pathology, Dr. D. Y. Patil Medical College, Kolhapur, Maharashtra 416006, India*

Correspondence should be addressed to Jitendra Singh Nigam; nigamjs@gmail.com

Academic Editor: Iris Zalaudek

Objective. The aim of this study was correlation of skin adnexal tumors with age, sex, and location and determining its incidence in the Department of Pathology at Dr. D. Y. Patil Medical College and Hospital, Kolhapur, Maharashtra. *Material and Methods.* 56 cases were included in this study from Jan 2004 to June 2010 with respect to incidence of adnexal tumors, age, and sex distribution. All slides were stained with haematoxylin and eosin and then findings were corroborated with special stains like PAS and reticulin wherever required. *Results.* 80.36% (45/56) were benign and 19.64% (11/56) were malignant adnexal tumors. The sweat gland tumors constituted the largest group (42.86% 24/56) cases followed by the hair follicle tumors (35.71%, 20/56) of cases and sebaceous gland tumors (21.43%, 12/56) cases. Overall male : female ratio was 1.07 : 1. The commonest age group was 51–60 years and the commonest affected body part was head and neck region (64.28%, 36/56) followed by trunk (14.28%, 8/56). Clear cell hidradenoma and pilomatricoma were commonest benign tumors and sebaceous carcinoma was the only malignant tumor seen. *Conclusion.* The incidence of benign skin adnexal tumors was more as compared to the malignant tumors. Malignant tumors were seen in older age group, usually over 50 years of age.

1. Introduction

Skin adnexal tumors (SATs) are those neoplasms that differentiate toward or arise from pilosebaceous unit, eccrine sweat glands or apocrine sweat glands, and these tumors are classified into four groups that exhibit histologic features analogous to hair follicles, sebaceous glands, and eccrine glands [1]. These tumors are derived from multipotential undifferentiated cells present within the epidermis or its appendageal structures and the histologic features of a tumor are related to the activation of molecular pathways responsible for forming the mature adnexal structure [1].

Most of the benign SATs present as asymptomatic papules or nodules and often difficult to diagnose clinically however anatomic location, number and distribution of lesions provide important clue, No change required [2]. They are however confirmed by histopathology, and immunohistochemistry may helps in confirmation of the diagnosis [3]. This study was therefore undertaken to analyze adnexal tumors of the skin for their morphological, clinical, and histological features and to group them using the International Classification of World Health Organization (2006).

2. Material and Methods

The present study includes the cases from Jan 2004 to June 2010. 56 cases were included in this study, which were reported by the Histopathology Sections of the Department of pathology at Dr. D. Y. Patil Medical College and Hospital, Kolhapur, Maharashtra. The clinicopathological data was taken from the record office for the given period. The histopathological examination was done on formalin fixed tissues and paraffin embedded blocks were made. Haematoxylin and Eosin stained sections were examined and few special stains like PAS and reticulin were performed wherever required. However in our laboratory setup, the facility for

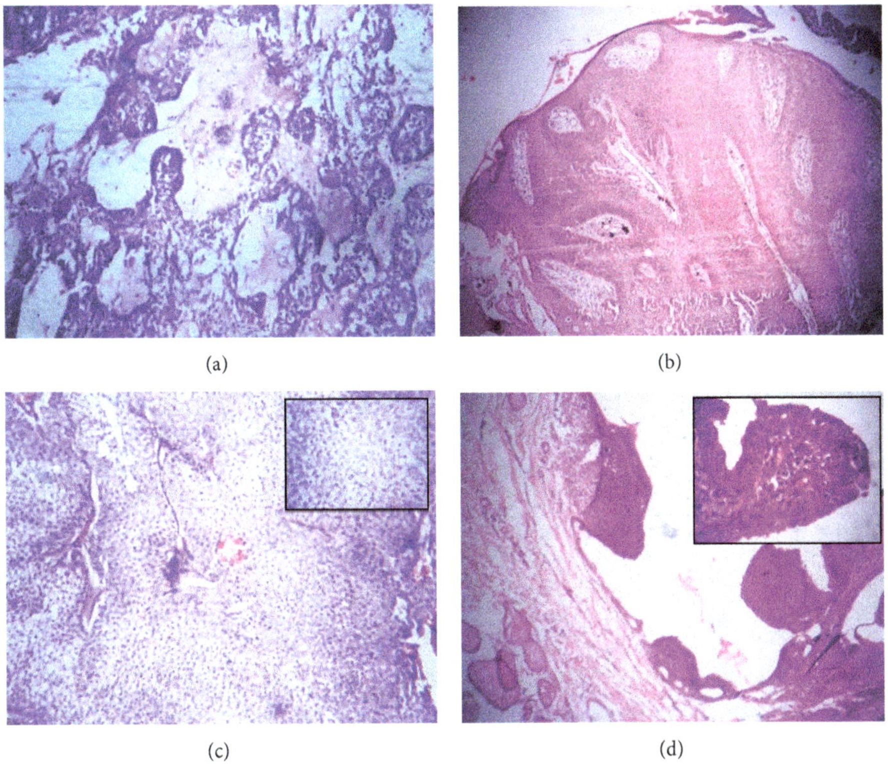

FIGURE 1: (a) Chondroid syringoma: tubular or ductular proliferation admixed with a chondroid stromal matrix. (H&E ×100). (b) Eccrine poroma: well-circumscribed tumor arising from lower portion of the epidermis extends downwards into dermis as cords and broad columns of uniform basaloid cells (H&E ×100). (c) Hidradenoma: Well-circumscribed nonencapsulated multilobulated tumor lobules with varying size and shape (H&E ×100), consisting of polyhedral cells with round nuclei with slightly basophilic cytoplasm and round cells with clear cytoplasm with small dark nuclei (Inset H&E ×400). (d) Syringocystadenoma papilliferum: epidermis with papillary projections extend into the lumina of the cystic invaginations. (H&E ×100) and the luminal row of high columnar cells with oval nuclei and faintly eosinophilic cytoplasm (Inset H&E ×400).

histochemical staining for enzymes like alkaline phosphatase, phosphorylase, succinic dehydrogenase, indoxyl esterase, and acid phosphatase was not available; they were not performed.

3. Results

In the present study, benign adnexal tumors constituted 80.36% (45/56) cases and malignant adnexal tumors constituted 19.64% (11/56) cases. The sweat gland tumors constituted the largest group involving 42.86% (24/56) cases followed by the hair follicle tumors 37.71% (20/56) cases followed by sebaceous gland tumors 21.43% (12/56) cases (Table 1). The male: female ratio was 1.07 : 1. Tumors were observed in all age groups ranging from 10 to 88 years. However, the highest incidence was observed in the age group of 51–60 years (26.78%, 15/56) followed by age groups of 31–40 (16.07%, 9/56) and 41–50 (14.28%, 8/56) years, respectively. The head and neck region was the most common site affected (64.28%, 36/56) followed by trunk (14.28%, 8/56) and then upper limb (12.5%, 7/56). In head and neck region 37.5% (21/56) cases were located on the face followed by scalp in 21.43% (12/56) cases. The neck region was least affected 5.36% (3/56) (Table 2).

TABLE 1: Adnexal tumors according to the direction of differentiation.

Sr. no.	Direction of differentiation	No. of cases	Percentage incidence (%)
1	Sweat gland tumors	24	42.86
2	Sebaceous gland tumors	12	21.43
3	Hair follicle tumors	20	35.71
	Total	56	100.00

The sweat glands tumors are comprised of chondroid syringoma, eccrine poroma, nodular clear cell hidradenoma, apocrine hidrocystoma, and syringocystadenoma papilliferum (Figure 1). Sebaceous glands tumors are comprised of sebaceous adenoma and sebaceous carcinoma. The hair follicle tumors are comprised of trichoepithelioma, trichofolliculoma (sebaceous), pilomatricoma, and proliferating trichilemmal cyst (Figure 2). Amongst the benign tumors; Clear cell hidradenoma and Pilomatricoma were the most common tumors representing 12 (21.43%) cases each, clear cell hidradenoma was observed in age ranging from 10 to 70 years. Most of the patients were above 40 years of age and female preponderance. pilomatricoma showed peak

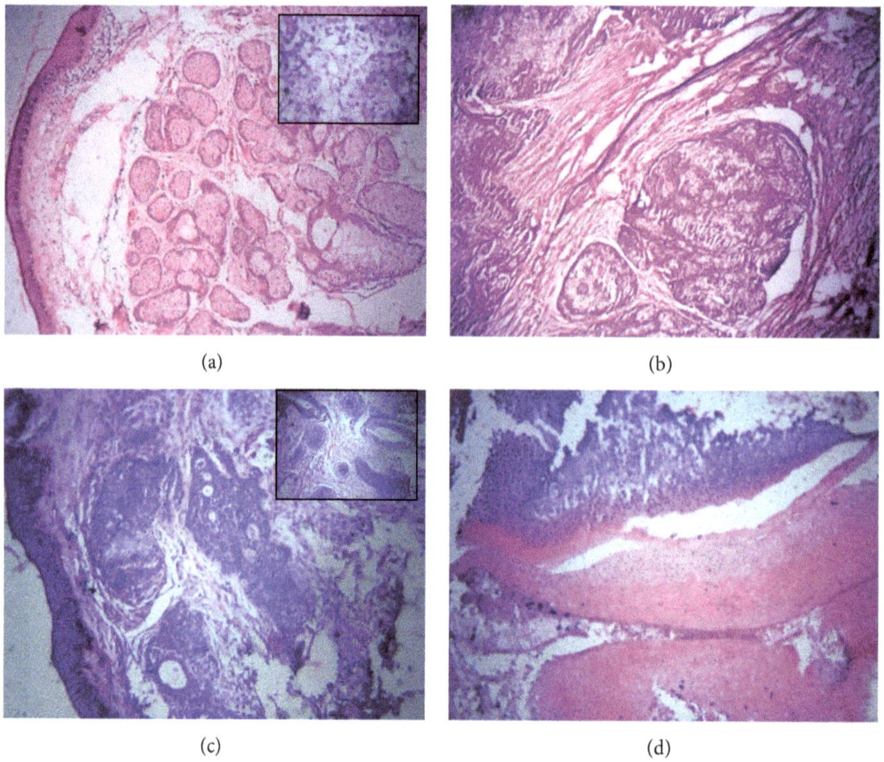

Figure 2: (a) Sebaceous adenoma: well-circumscribed tumor composed of sebaceous lobules of varying sizes and shapes (H&E ×100). Undifferentiated basaloid cells at the periphery while mature sebaceous cells were seen towards their center (Inset H&E ×400). (b) Sebaceous carcinoma: lobular arrangements of cells consist of small undifferentiated eosinophilic cells and large cells with clear to foamy cytoplasm. (H&E ×100). (c) Trichofolliculoma: dermis showing multiple cysts filled with keratin and lined by squamous epithelium (H&E ×100) and multiple cysts filled with keratin and lined by squamous epithelium. (Inset H&E ×100). (d) Pilomatricoma: Eosinophilic shadow cells predominantly and few basophilic cells with keratinization. (H&E ×100).

Table 2: The site and sex distribution of observed adnexal tumors.

Sr. no.	Site of tumor	Male	Female	Total	Percentage incidence (%)
	Head and neck				
1	Scalp	5	7	12	21.43
	Face	9	12	21	37.5
	Neck	2	1	3	5.36
2	Trunk	6	2	8	14.29
3	Upper limb	5	2	7	12.5
4	Lower limb	1	3	4	7.14
5	Not specified	1	—	1	1.78
	Total	29	27	56	100.00

incidence between 11 and 40 years of age and was more common in males. 6 (10.71%). cases of eccrine poroma were seen with age group ranged from 11 to 60 years and were more common in females. Chondroid syringoma came next, constituting 3 (5.36%) cases, out of which 2 (3.57%) were observed in patients above 30 years of age (Table 3). Amongst the malignant tumors sebaceous carcinoma was the only malignant tumor observed and constituted 19.64% (11/56). Most of them were meibomian gland carcinomas occurring in people above 50 years of age with maximum number of cases, that is, 4 observed in females above 70 years of age.

4. Discussion

Incidence of benign tumors is more as compared to malignant cases. In present study 80.36% (45/56) tumors were benign and 19.64% (11/56) tumors were malignant which was also seen in studies of Radhika et al. [4], Reddy et al. [5], and Samaila [6] who reported 77.14%, 69.41%, and 88.5% benign and 29.63%, 30.59%, and 11.5% malignant lesions, respectively. Nair [7] observed that sweat glands tumors are the commonest followed by hair follicle tumors and then sebaceous glands tumors. The present study also shows similar results. However, Radhika et al. [4] and Samalia [6] observed that sweat glands tumors are the commonest SATs followed by sebaceous glands tumors followed by tumors of hair follicle. Male : female ratio as observed by Nair [7] and Saha et al. [8] was 1 : 2.3 and 1 : 1.88, respectively. Radhika et al. also observed that majority of the patients are in the third decade and females outnumbered males [4]; however, present study showed male : female ratio as 1.07 : 1. Saha et al. [8] observed the mean age of onset of SATs was 24.15 ± 8.44. Nair [7] observed the commonest age group of presentation was 11–20 years; however, in the present study, commonest

TABLE 3: Age incidence of individual adnexal tumors observed in the present study.

Sr. no.	Tumors	Age groups (in years)							
		1–10	11–20	21–30	31–40	41–50	51–60	61–70	>70
				Sweat gland tumors					
1	Chondroid syringoma			1	1		1		
2	Eccrine poroma		1		1	2	2		
3	Nodular hidradenoma	2	2			4	3	1	
4	Apocrine hidrocystoma							1	
5	Syringocystadenoma papilliferum		1	1					
				sebaceous gland tumors					
6	Sebaceous adenoma						1		
7	Sebaceous carcinoma					1	4	2	4
				Hair follicle tumors					
8	Trichoepithelioma			1	1				
9	Trichofolliculoma (Sebaceous)			1	1				
10	Pilomatricoma	1	2	2	4	1	1	1	
11	Proliferating trichilemmal cyst				1		3		
	Total	3	6	6	9	8	15	5	4

age group was 51–60 years followed by 31–40 years. Samalia [6] observed that 46% of lesions were located in head and neck region which was also seen in our study. Song et al. observed that pilomatricoma was the most common benign tumor followed by dermoid cyst followed by steatocystoma multiplex, syringoma, and trichilemmal cyst [9]. Radhika et al. observed that the most common benign tumor is nodular hidradenoma followed by sebaceous naevus [4]. In present study, most common tumors were clear cell hidradenoma and pilomatricoma followed by eccrine poroma.

5. Conclusion

In Indian population, an overall incidence of skin adnexal tumors is very low. The incidence of benign skin adnexal tumors is more as compared to the malignant ones. Most of the malignant tumors occur in older age group usually over 50 years of age. However benign tumors show a wide age variation. Skin adnexal tumors can occur anywhere in the body; however head and neck region constitutes the most common site. Majority of the tumors can be classified into different subgroups on the basis of light microscopy alone. Skin adnexal tumors showing sweat gland differentiation are seen more frequently. In our institutional study, clear cell hidradenoma is the commonest tumor with sweat gland differentiation, while pilomatricoma is the most common type of hair follicle tumor. Amongst the tumors with sebaceous differentiation, sebaceous carcinoma (meibomian carcinoma) is commonest.

References

[1] T. S. S. Ahmed, J. D. Priore, and J. T. Seykora, "Tumors of epidermal appendages," in *Lever's Histopathology of the Skin*, D. E. Elder, R. Elenitsas, B. L. Johnson, and G. F. Murphy, Eds., pp. 867–868, Lippincott Williams & Wilkins, Philadelphia, Pa, USA, 9th edition, 2005.

[2] R. Stantaylor, J. B. Perone, S. Kaddu, and H. Kerl, "Appendage tumors and hamartomas of the skin," in *Fitzpatrick's Dermatology in General Medicine*, K. Wolff, L. Goldsmith, S. Katz, B. A. Gilchrest, A. S. Paller, and D. J. Leffell, Eds., pp. 1068–1087, McGraw Hill, New York, NY, USA, 7th edition, 2008.

[3] N. S. Penneys, "Immunohistochemistry of adnexal neoplasms," *Journal of Cutaneous Pathology*, vol. 11, no. 5, pp. 357–364, 1984.

[4] K. Radhika, B. V. Phaneendra, N. Rukmangadha, and M. K. Reddy, "A study of biopsy confirmed skin adnexal tumors: experience at a tertiary care teaching hospital," *Journal of Clinical and Scientific Research*, vol. 2, pp. 132–138, 2013.

[5] M. K. Reddy, A. J. Veliath, S. Nagarajan, and A. L. Aurora, "A clinicopathological study of adnexal tumours of skin," *Indian Journal of Medical Research*, vol. 75, no. 6, pp. 882–889, 1982.

[6] M. O. A. Samaila, "Adnexal skin tumors in Zaria, Nigeria," *Annals of African Medicine*, vol. 7, no. 1, pp. 6–10, 2008.

[7] P. S. Nair, "A clinico-histopathological study of skin appendageal tumors," *Indian Journal of Dermatology, Venereology and Leprology*, vol. 74, article 550, 2008.

[8] A. Saha, N. K. Das, R. C. Gharami, S. N. Chowdhury, and P. K. Datta, "A clinico-histopathological study of appendageal skin tumors, affecting head and neck region in patients attending the dermatology opd of a tertiary care centre in eastern india," *Indian Journal of Dermatology*, vol. 56, pp. 33–36, 2011.

[9] K. -Y. Song, D. -H. Yoon, E. -K. Ham, and Y. -S. Lee, "Clinicopathological study on the skin appendage tumors," *Korean Journal of Pathology*, vol. 23, pp. 111–121, 1989.

12

Gene Expression Differences Predict Treatment Outcome of Merkel Cell Carcinoma Patients

Loren Masterson,[1] Bryan J. Thibodeau,[2] Laura E. Fortier,[2] Timothy J. Geddes,[2] Barbara L. Pruetz,[2] Rajwant Malhotra,[3] Richard Keidan,[1] and George D. Wilson[2]

[1] *Department of General Surgery, Beaumont Health System, Royal Oak, MI 48073, USA*
[2] *Department of Beaumont BioBank, Beaumont Health System, 3811 West 13 Mile Road 105-RI, Royal Oak, MI 48073, USA*
[3] *Department of Anatomic Pathology, Beaumont Health System, Royal Oak, MI 48073, USA*

Correspondence should be addressed to Bryan J. Thibodeau; bryan.thibodeau@beaumont.edu

Academic Editor: Iris Zalaudek

Due to the rarity of Merkel cell carcinoma (MCC), prospective clinical trials have not been practical. This study aimed to identify biomarkers with prognostic significance. While sixty-two patients were identified who were treated for MCC at our institution, only seventeen patients had adequate formalin-fixed paraffin-embedded archival tissue and followup to be included in the study. Patients were stratified into good, moderate, or poor prognosis. Laser capture microdissection was used to isolate tumor cells for subsequent RNA isolation and gene expression analysis with Affymetrix GeneChip Human Exon 1.0 ST arrays. Among the 191 genes demonstrating significant differential expression between prognostic groups, keratin 20 and neurofilament protein have previously been identified in studies of MCC and were significantly upregulated in tumors from patients with a poor prognosis. Immunohistochemistry further established that keratin 20 was overexpressed in the poor prognosis tumors. In addition, novel genes of interest such as phospholipase A2 group X, kinesin family member 3A, tumor protein D52, mucin 1, and *KIT* were upregulated in specimens from patients with poor prognosis. Our pilot study identified several gene expression differences which could be used in the future as prognostic biomarkers in MCC patients.

1. Introduction

Merkel cell carcinoma (MCC) was first described in 1972 by Toker, which was initially thought to be derived from sweat glands [1]. In 1978, dense-core granules were found in these tumors consistent with neuroendocrine cells, and in particular Merkel cells [2]. MCC has gained recent attention not only due to its association with newly discovered Merkel polyomavirus but also due its increase in incidence [3]. In fact, the age-related incidence of MCC has nearly tripled from 1986 to 2001 [3]. Risk factors include advanced age, ultraviolet light exposure, and chronic immunosuppression. MCC are most commonly located in the head and neck, often accompanied by other primary cutaneous neoplasms, consistent with ultraviolet light exposure.

Prognosis of MCC is poor. Patients presenting with distant disease have two-year survival of only 32% [4]. Only 50% of patients have localized disease (Stage 1) at time of diagnosis. Staging is primarily based on tumor size and the extent of disease at the time of diagnosis [5]. Those patients diagnosed with disease and tumor size <2 cm without nodal involvement have a ten-year mortality between 29 and 39% [6]. This is more than four times the mortality rate for patients with melanoma diagnosis with the same disease stage [7]. Currently, prognosis is best determined by the extent of disease of initial diagnosis.

Due to rarity of MCC, prospective clinical trials have proven unfeasible [8]. More recently, several studies have focused on biomarker analysis in order to identify prognostic factors [9–11]. In this study, we performed global gene expression analysis of tumor specimens from patients with good, poor, and moderate outcomes to identify novel genes and pathways that might identify new prognostic markers or new treatment targets.

2. Materials and Methods

2.1. Patients and Specimens. We interrogated the Beaumont Hospital tumor registry for all patients treated for MCC within the last 10 years; 62 patients were identified. Patients were excluded who did not have tumor resection or tissue diagnosis at our institution due to lack of access to specimen. Patients were also excluded with inadequate followup or if their specimens failed to pass quality control measures for gene expression studies. All tissue paraffin block specimens were retrieved from anatomic pathology for validation and identification of disease by a single dermatopathologist (RM). After verification of tissue, MCC patients were stratified into one of three groups based upon status at 24 months following diagnosis. Poor prognosis patients either presented with or progressed to distant metastasis. Patients were considered to have a moderate prognosis if they presented with recurrent local disease or nodal disease at presentation but had no progression during followup of fewer than 24 months. Patients with favorable prognosis had local disease with no nodal disease at presentation and no progression during followup of at least 24 months [12]. Seventeen MCC patients satisfied all the inclusion criteria (6 poor prognosis, 3 moderate prognosis, and 8 good prognosis patients).

2.2. Laser Capture Microdissection (LCM). For LCM, 5 μm sections were cut from formalin-fixed paraffin-embedded (FFPE) tissue and mounted onto polyethylene naphthalate membrane glass slides (two sections per slide). Prior to deparaffinization, slides were placed into an oven at 60°C for 25 minutes then stained and dehydrated through a series of graded ethanol and xylene steps. Within 3 hours of sectioning, the pathologist-identified tumor areas were microdissected with both UV and IR lasers, where appropriate, using the Arcturus^{XT} Microdissection System (Molecular Devices) onto CapSure HS LCM Caps (Molecular Devices). Four caps were used per graded region from the dissection of 1–4 sections representing approximately 5,000 tumor cells (1-2 mm^2 area) captured per cap.

2.3. RNA Isolation. Total RNA was isolated from the LCM tissues using the PureLink FFPE RNA Isolation Kit (Invitrogen). The transfer film with the attached dissected material was separated from each CapSure HS LCM Cap and placed in deparaffinization melting buffer at 72°C for 10 min and then treated with Proteinase K at 60°C for 45 min. Following the manufacturer's protocol, total RNA was purified using spin cartridge technology, treated with DNase, quantified (Nanodrop 8000, Thermo Scientific), and stored at −80°C. RNA integrity was determined just prior to processing for expression microarray analysis. RNA integrity numbers ranged from 2.0 to 2.4, as determined by Bioanalyzer analysis (Agilent).

2.4. Whole Transcriptome (WT) Amplification, Purification, Fragmentation, and Hybridization. Total RNA was amplified and labeled using the WT-Ovation FFPE System V2, WT-Ovation Exon Module, and the Encore Biotin Module (NuGEN, Inc. San Carlos, CA, USA), which enables amplification and target preparation of the low quality RNA from FFPE, LCM samples. Amplifications were performed with 100 ng total RNA input following procedures described in the WT-Ovation FFPE System user guide. Target preparation for Affymetrix Human Exon 1.0 ST Arrays (Affymetrix, Santa Clara, CA, USA) was performed using 5 μg amplified cDNA and the Encore Biotin Module following the manufacturer's recommendations. Hybridization, washing and staining (with GeneChip Fluidics Station 450, Affymetrix), and scanning (with GeneChip Scanner 3000) were performed following manufacturer's protocols. Array scans from this process yielded signal intensities comparable to arrays prepared from high quality RNA from cell lines (data not shown). This method has also been independently reported recently to provide optimal RNA hybridization [13].

2.5. Gene Expression Analysis. The CEL files containing the raw intensity data from the Affymetrix GeneChip arrays were imported into Partek Genomics Suite (version 6.6 beta, build 6.11.1115) and normalized using the robust multichip average with a guanine-cytosine content background correction, quantile normalization, log2-transformation, and median polish probeset summarization. Exons were then summarized to genes using the average of the probesets. Differentially expressed genes were identified using ANOVA with two factors: prognosis and scan date (random variable). Unsupervised hierarchical clustering was carried out using Partek software (Partek Inc., St. Louis, MO, USA). Hierarchical clustering analysis was performed using Euclidean distance as similarity measure and average linkage for the agglomerative method. Gene set enrichment analysis (GSEA) and pathway analysis were performed using Pathway Studio 9.0 (Ariadne Genomics, Rockville, MD, USA). The data discussed in this publication have been deposited in NCBI's Gene Expression Omnibus [14] and are accessible through GEO Series accession number GSE36150.

2.6. Immunohistochemistry. Tissue sections from the corresponding FFPE tissue blocks were placed on slides, underwent high pH antigen retrieval, and were subsequently incubated with one of the following primary antibodies: mouse monoclonal anti-human keratin 20 (prediluted, Dako IS777), mouse monoclonal anti-human mucin 1 (1 : 100, Leica, NCL-HGM-45 mL), and rabbit polyclonal anti-human KIT (1 : 250, Dako A4502), rabbit polyclonal anti-human KIF3A (1 : 1200, Sigma K3513). The slides were then linked and visualized using the Dako Envision Flex system on a Dako Autostainer. Immunohistochemistry was scored based on intensity of staining with a 4-tier system (0 = absent, 1 = weak, 2 = intermediate, and 3 = intense). To address interobserver variability, scoring was performed by 2 independent investigators, and scores were averaged. Fisher's exact probability test was conducted comparing good and poor prognosis cohorts [15].

Table 1: Clinical characteristics of the 17 MCC patients utilized in study.

Feature	Good prognosis $n = 6$ (35%)	Moderate prognosis $n = 3$ (18%)	Poor prognosis $n = 8$ (47%)	Total $n = 17$
Gender				
Male	3 (50%)	2 (67%)	4 (50%)	9 (53%)
Female	3 (50%)	1 (33%)	4 (50%)	8 (47%)
Age, years: median, range	71.7 (54–82)	78.7 (71–84)	68.8 (44–83)	
Location				
Head and neck	3 (50%)	1 (33%)	2 (25%)	6 (35%)
Upper extremity	2 (33%)	1 (33%)	2 (25%)	5 (30%)
Lower extremity	1 (17%)	0 (0%)	3 (37.5%)	4 (23%)
Torso	0 (0%)	1 (33%)	1 (12.5%)	2 (12%)
AJCC stage at diagnosis				
(I)	2 (33%)	1 (33%)	0 (0%)	3 (18%)
(II)	3 (50%)	2 (67%)	5 (62.5%)	10 (59%)
(III)	1 (17%)	0 (0%)	3 (37.5%)	4 (23%)

3. Results

3.1. Identification and Isolation of Merkel Cell Samples. The patient demographics and lesion characteristics are outlined in Table 1. In this small cohort of patients, there was almost even number of male and females (53% versus 47%), and 53% (9 of 17 patients) of lesions were located on the extremities. While the majority (59%, 10 of 17) of patients were Stage II, 75% (3 of 4) of patients diagnosed with Stage III tumors had a poor prognosis.

Laser capture microdissection was used to isolate and remove as pure a population of tumor cells as possible based on morphological identification by a dermatopathologist. Figure 1 shows a typical lesion from a 49-year-old female with a Stage 2 lesion on a lower extremity; this lesion was from a poor prognosis patient that required surgery and salvage chemotherapy. The lesion showed a nodular arrangement of cells within the dermis with sparse cytoplasm with uniform, monotonous medium-sized nuclei (Figures 1(a) and 1(b)). The histological composition of the tumor clearly shows the importance of the laser capture microdissection approach taken in this study due to the presence of dermal and adnexal structures. Figures 1(c) and 1(d) show the selected outlined areas for dissection before and after laser capture microdissection.

3.2. Gene Expression Changes in MCC Related to Prognosis. The 17 samples of MCC were analyzed using the Human Exon 1.0 ST array from Affymetrix. Two arrays (one good prognosis and one poor prognosis) failed to pass array quality control metrics. In a comparison of the patients with poor prognosis ($n = 7$) versus those with good prognosis ($n = 5$), 191 genes were found to be differentially expressed ($P \leq 0.05$ and 1.5-fold cutoff, Table S1 in the Supplementary Material available online at http://dx.doi.org/10.1155/2014/596459). This includes 127 genes that are overexpressed in tumors from poor prognosis patients and 64 genes that are underexpressed. *NEFM* (neurofilament, medium polypeptide), *PLA2G10* (phospholipase A2, group X), and *KRT20* (keratin 20) are upregulated more than 3-fold in tumors with poor prognosis. *CYP2A6* (cytochrome P450, family 2, subfamily A, polypeptide 6), *MCART1* (mitochondrial carrier triple repeat 1), and *KRTAP19-5* (keratin associated protein 19-5) were downregulated at least 2.8-fold in poor prognosis samples.

Among the 191 differentially expressed genes, there is a subset of 45 genes that meet the stricter conditions of $P \leq 0.01$. Hierarchical clustering of the MCC samples was performed based upon these 45 differentially expressed genes. Clustering based upon the expression of these genes robustly delineated between the good and poor prognosis patients (Figure 2(a)). Inclusion of the 3 samples from patients with a moderate prognosis resulted in 2 patients clustering with the poor prognosis patients and 1 with the good prognosis patients (Figure 2(b)). The annotation for AJCC (American Joint Committee on Cancer) stage in these figures indicates that clustering based upon prognosis dependent gene expression is independent of stage.

3.3. Subnetwork Analysis. In order to better understand the biological context of the gene expression differences between MCC from good and poor prognosis patients, the expression microarray data was analyzed using Ariadne Pathway Studio's Subnetwork Enrichment Analysis tool [16, 17]. Pathway Studio utilizes MedScan, the literature mining program that searches publicly the available literature such as PubMed for relationships between entities [18]. A subnetwork consists of a single seed (i.e., disease or cell process) and genes associated to this seed by regulation of/by the seed [19]. The expression microarray dataset is interrogated with no prior significance filtering, and enrichment of the subnetwork is determined by both the level of regulation in the network and the size of the network. One type of network consists of genes associated with regulating diseases; that is, the "seed" of the subnetwork is a disease or disease condition. Interestingly, the top subnetwork identified is "genes associated with regulating neoplasm metastasis" (Figure 3). The visualized subnetwork was limited to include only those genes that were

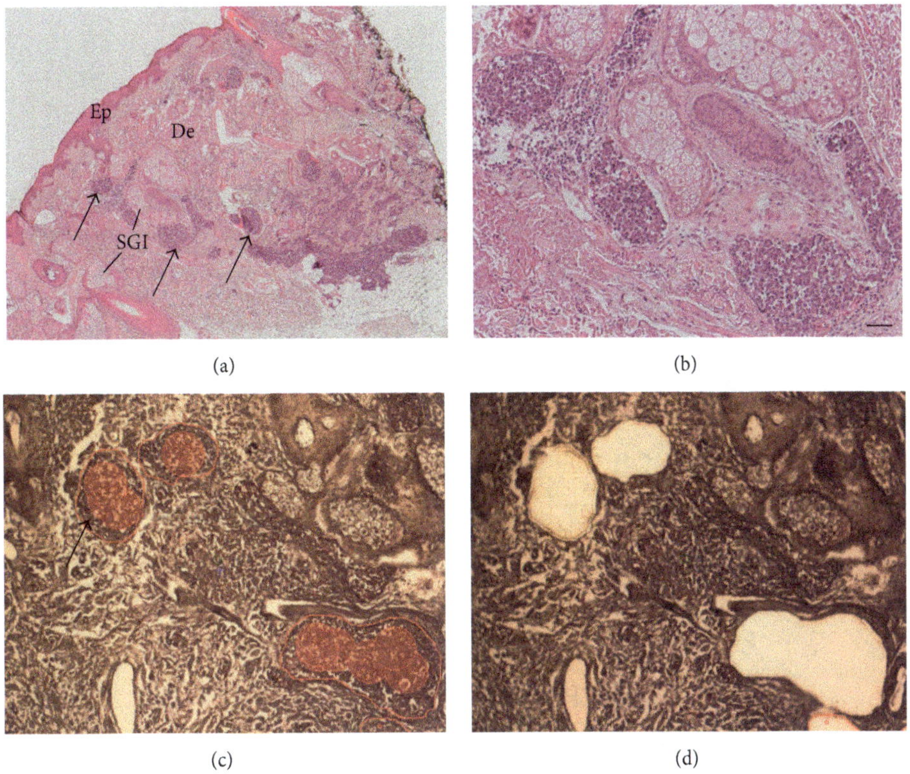

FIGURE 1: Representative example of histology of Merkel cell carcinoma from a tumor with poor prognosis. (a) Low power hematoxylin and eosin (H&E) stained photomicrograph. Arrows indicate regions of MCC to be microdissected. Dermis (De), epidermis (Ep), and sebaceous gland (SGI) are also indicated. (b) High power H&E image of same MCC. (c) Arcturus glass membrane hematoxylin counterstained serial section from same MCC. Areas to be laser capture microdissected are indicated by the arrow and red shading. The red punctate shading marks subsequent laser positioning. Using the Arcturus^{XT} Microdissection System (molecular devices), these regions were transferred onto CapSure HS LCM Caps (Molecular Devices). Four caps were used per patient sample from the dissection of 1-4 sections representing approximately 5,000 tumor cells (1-2 mm^2 area) captured per cap. (d) Image of the same membrane cut section after LCM. Magnification: (a) at 2X; (b), (c), and (d) at 10X. Scale bar = 50 μm.

differentially expressed at ANOVA $P \leq 0.10$ and a 1.5-fold cutoff. Less stringent conditions have previously been shown to be more appropriate for pathway analysis [20, 21].

Subnetwork enrichment analysis was then utilized to discover cell processes that are highly regulated by gene expression differences between tumors of good and poor prognosis patients (Table 2). Fourteen of the top twenty categories are related to growth, including regeneration, mitosis, invasive growth, and cell motility. In addition, two categories (neurite outgrowth and neurogenesis, Figure 3) suggest a connection to the neuroendocrine nature of MCC.

3.4. Immunohistochemistry. Several differentially expressed genes were further explored at the protein level. Immunohistochemistry was utilized to examine the protein products of MUC1, KIT, KIF3A, and KRT20 (Table 3). While the majority of all MCC samples (88%, 15 of 17) were positive for KRT20, the poor prognosis samples (Figure 4(a)) showed stronger staining than those from good prognosis patients (Figure 4(b)). Using Fisher's exact probability test comparing absent/weak staining to intermediate/intense staining, this result was significantly significant in this pilot study ($P \leq 0.03$). This agrees with the overexpression seen in the gene level analysis. KIF3A protein was detectable in 1 of 6 poor prognosis patient samples (Figure 4(c)), but no protein was evident in samples from the moderate or good prognosis patients (Figure 4(d)). MUC1 protein was undetectable in almost all samples with the exception of low level staining in the sample from one good prognosis patient. The protein levels of KIT did not corroborate the gene expression results. Despite 83% of good prognosis (5 of 6) and 75% of poor prognosis (6 of 8) samples being KIT positive, there was no pattern to the level of staining based upon prognosis ($P \leq 0.54$).

4. Discussion

Diagnosis of Merkel cell carcinoma can be difficult. Current treatment consists of surgical removal with very wide excision borders. Virtually, all patients receive radiation following wide surgical excision, while patients with positive lymph nodes or metastatic disease at time of diagnosis may be candidates for chemotherapy. No standard chemotherapy protocol has yet been established for the treatment of MCC. Because of the morphological and immunohistochemical similarity

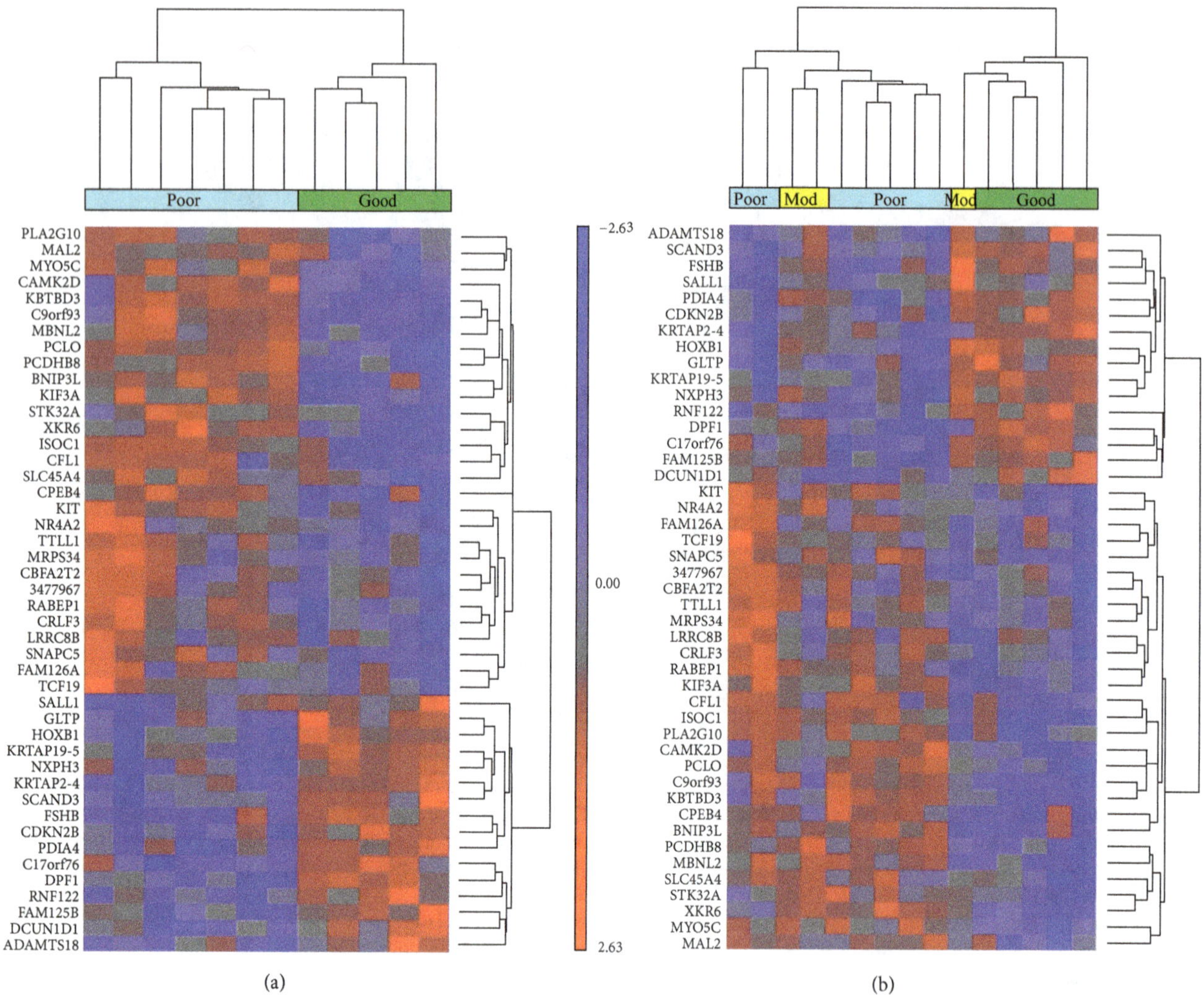

FIGURE 2: Hierarchical clustering of Merkel cell carcinoma samples. Samples were clustered based upon the expression pattern of 45 differentially expressed genes between tumors of poor and good prognosis patients ($P \leq 0.01$ and 1.5-fold cutoff). Individual samples are represented on the x-axis with poor prognosis patients in light blue ("poor"), good prognosis in green ("good"), and moderate prognosis in yellow ("mod"). Differentially expressed genes are shown on the y-axis. Clustering of (a) good and poor prognosis patients; (b) good, moderate, and poor prognosis patients. The scale of gene expression values are standardized such that genes are shifted to a mean of zero and scaled to a standard deviation of one.

of MCC to small cell lung carcinoma (SCLC), chemotherapy has been performed with protocols based largely on agents active in SCLC. A wide variety of chemotherapeutic agents have been discussed, including cytostatic drugs such as cyclophosphamide, doxorubicin, epirubicin, vincristine, etoposide, cisplatin, carboplatin, 5-fluorouracil, dacarbazine, mitoxantrone, bleomycin, and iphosphamide. Unfortunately, reports to date consist of only small studies and anecdotal evidence [22–24]. There is a need to move away from the largely empirical clinical management of MCC and find ways to understand and individualize treatment.

The ultimate goal of the study was to find markers that could identify poor prognosis patients at the time of diagnosis; these patients could benefit from increased or altered postsurgical therapy. In order to discover these novel biomarkers, expression microarray technology was utilized to examine global gene expression differences between patients that demonstrated a known prognosis (good prognosis or poor prognosis) based upon status 24 months following resection. This analysis resulted in a set of 191 genes being identified as differentially expressed. Hierarchical clustering of the patient samples based upon the expression of a subset of these genes (Figure 2(a)) demonstrated their utility in discriminating between the two prognoses. While definitive conclusions cannot be drawn due to the limited numbers in this pilot study, perhaps more interesting is the result of adding the patients with moderate prognosis to the clustering (Figure 2(b)). The good and poor prognosis patients remain segregated into two main clusters while one moderate patient cluster with the good prognosis patients and two with the poor prognosis patients. The patient that clustered with the good prognosis patients was a 71-year-old female whose

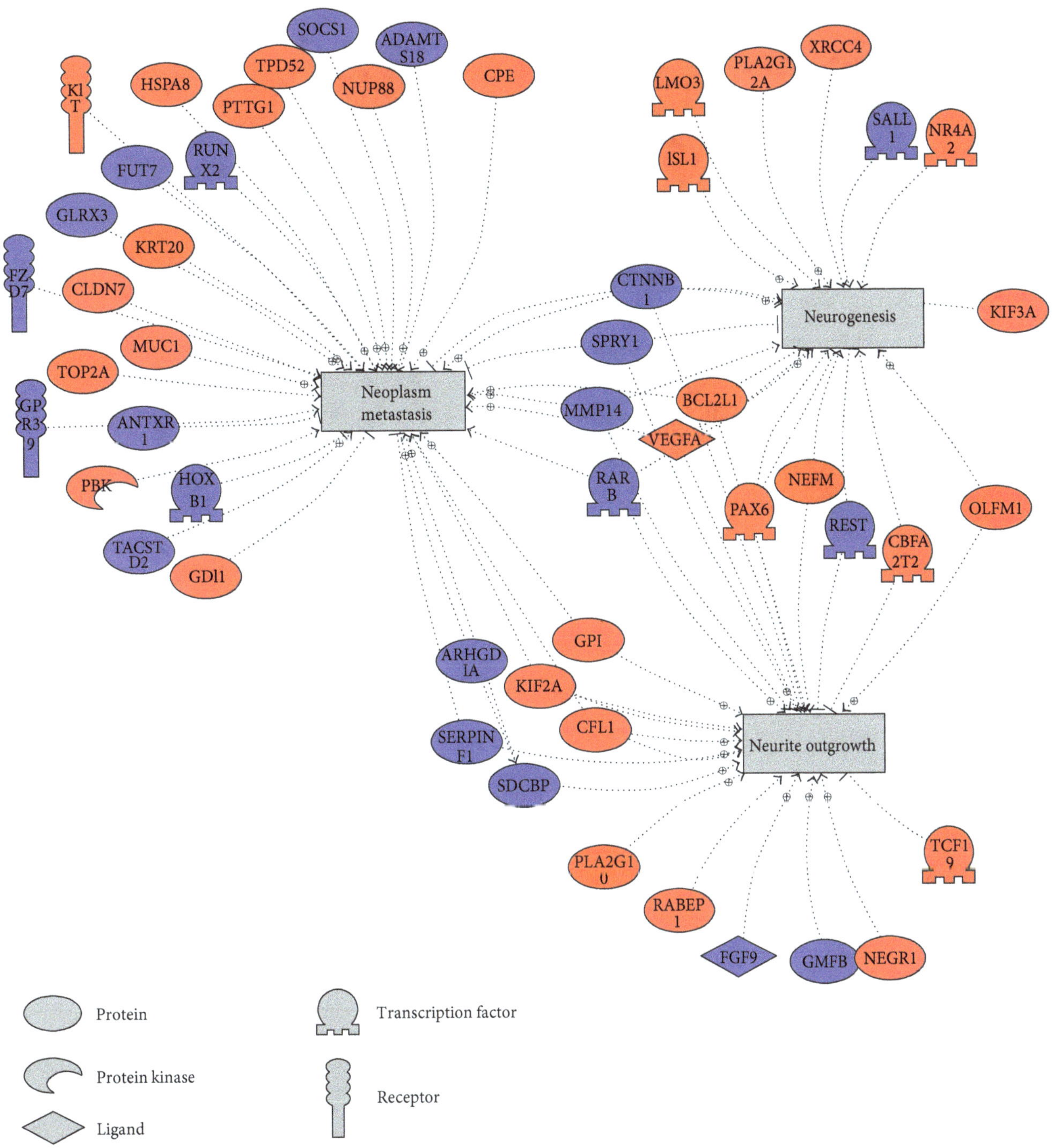

FIGURE 3: Subnetwork of genes involved in regulating neoplasm metastasis, neurite outgrowth, and neurogenesis. Genes in red are upregulated in poor prognosis; blue, downregulated.

primary was located on the breast. The patient samples that clustered with the poor prognosis patient samples were from an 84-year-old male with the primary located on the arm and an 81-year-old male with the primary on the lip. The moderate prognosis patients that group with the poor prognosis group represented the more "typical" MCC patient: male, older, and with the primary on a sun-exposed area. The moderate patient that clusters with the good prognosis patients had the primary at an atypical location and was female. In general, female MCC patients have been shown to have a better prognosis than male patients [6]. Longer term followup of these three patients could help to determine the accuracy of these projections to the good or poor prognosis groups based upon the expression of these 45 differentially expressed genes.

Further characterization of the expression microarray data using subnetwork enrichment analysis revealed that gene expression associated with neoplasm metastasis and neurite outgrowth was highly regulated between samples

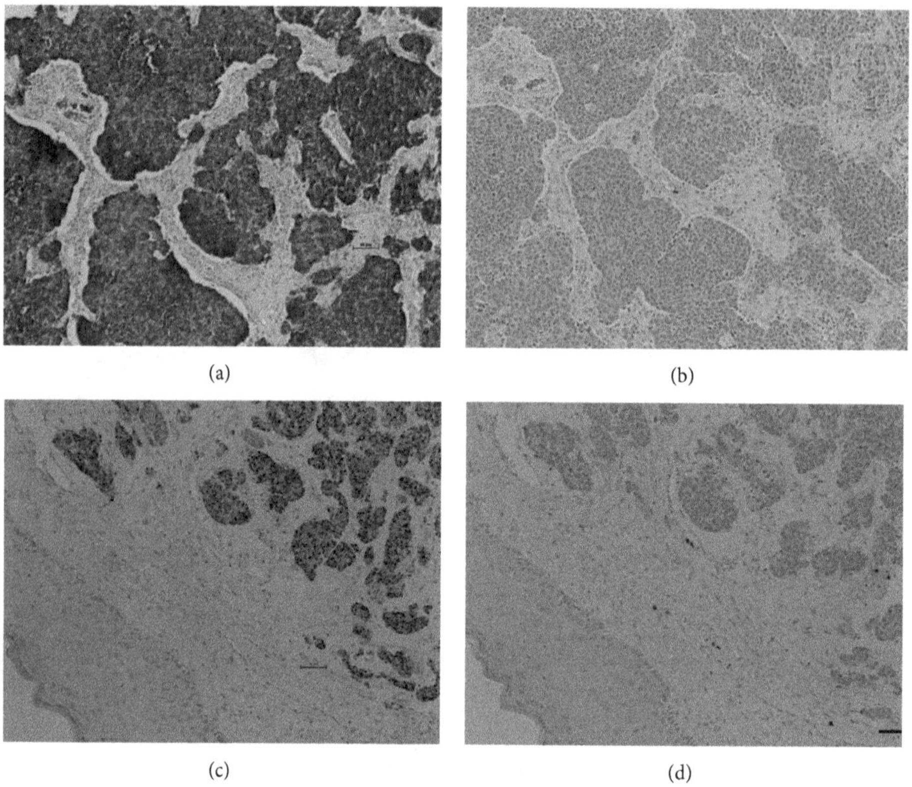

FIGURE 4: Immunohistochemistry in representative Merkel cell carcinoma tumors with good and poor prognoses. (a) intermediate KRT20 staining in poor prognosis tumor. (b) Weak KIF3A staining in poor prognosis tumor. (c) Weak punctate KRT20 staining in good prognosis tumor. (d) Negative (absent) KIF3A staining in good prognosis tumor. All images were taken at 10X magnification with Nikon digital DS-Fil high definition color camera on the Nikon Eclipse 90i. Scale bar = 50 μm.

TABLE 2: Subnetworks of genes involved in regulating cell processes that are highly regulated between patients with poor and good prognoses.

Gene set seed	P value
Neurite outgrowth	$3.36E-06$
Regeneration	$3.87E-05$
Kinetochore assembly	$8.02E-04$
Hair cell differentiation	$9.68E-04$
Olfactory bulb development	$9.79E-04$
Organogenesis	$9.96E-04$
Sertoli cell proliferation	$1.10E-03$
Spindle assembly	$1.72E-03$
Neural crest cell development	$2.18E-03$
Chondrogenesis	$2.41E-03$
Ureteric bud branching	$2.76E-03$
Protein polyubiquitination	$2.79E-03$
Ion channel clustering	$2.85E-03$
Chondrocyte differentiation	$2.86E-03$
Cytokinesis	$2.86E-03$

of patients with a good and poor prognoses. The neoplasm metastasis associated genes *KRT20*, tumor protein D52 (*TPD52*), *MUC1*, and *KIT* are upregulated in the poor prognosis tumors while homeobox B1 (*HOXB1*) is downregulated. *TPD52*, upregulated nearly 2-fold in tumors of poor prognosis patients, has been shown to be overexpressed in colorectal cancer [25] and ovarian cancer [26], and genomic amplification of *TPD52* has been seen in prostate cancer [27] and breast cancer [28]. *KIT* is also upregulated in the poor prognosis specimens. KIT is a transmembrane receptor for mast cell growth factor, also known as stem cell factor. Studies with MCC cell lines show that KIT is activated by paracrine or autocrine tumor cell-derived SCF which stimulates growth of MCC in vitro [29]. In one study looking at KIT expression in MCC tumors, Andea et al. showed dramatic survival differences between patients based upon KIT protein expression with high levels of KIT resulting in decreased 5-year survival [30]. *HOXB1*, which is downregulated in poor prognosis MCC, is a highly conserved transcription factor that plays an important role in morphogenesis and has been shown to be involved the metastatic potential of pancreatic cancer [31].

Genes associated with neurite outgrowth include the genes for *NEFM* and *PLA2G10*. Both of these genes are upregulated more than 3.5-fold in tumors of poor prognosis patients. NEFM encodes a type IV intermediate filament medium chain and is commonly used as a biomarker of neuronal damage. In one study, neuroendocrine cell lines expressed *NEFM* while nonneuroendocrine cell lines did not

TABLE 3: Immunohistochemistry results for KIF3A, KIT, KRT20, and MUC1. Results were grouped into absent/weak and intermediate/intense staining. Fisher's exact probability test compared good and poor prognosis results.

	Good prognosis	Moderate prognosis	Poor prognosis	P value
KIF3A				
Absent/weak	6	3	8	—
Intermediate/intense	0	0	0	
KIT				
Absent/weak	4	2	7	$P \leq 0.54$
Intermediate/intense	2	1	1	
KRT20				
Absent/weak	6	1	3	$P < 0.03$
Intermediate/intense	0	2	5	
MUC1				
Absent/weak	6	3	8	—
Intermediate/intense	0	0	0	

(—: P value not calculated due to $n = 0$ in intermediate/intense class).

[32]. Along with KRT20, NEFM was shown to be effective at discriminating MCC from small cell lung carcinoma with the majority of MCC being positive for both NEFM and KRT20 while NEFM and KRT20 were almost completely absent from small cell lung carcinoma [33].

In addition to these genes, there were other genes that were of interest and associated with cancer development or progression including dimethylarginine dimethylamino-hydrolase 1 (*DDAH1*), kinesin family member 3A (*KIF3A*), and *MUC1* which are all upregulated in the poor prognosis samples. The enzyme encoded by *DDAH1* is involved in nitric oxide generation through regulation of methylarginines. Nitric oxide metabolism has been implicated in carcinogenesis, tumor progression, angiogenesis, and response to therapy [34]; in particular, overexpression of *DDAH1* resulted in increased tumor growth and vascularization in a model of glioma tumorigenesis [35]. KIF3A activity is linked to Hedgehog signaling, which is upregulated in MCC [36]. KIF3A is required for the development of cilia which are present on most cells and are implicated in transducing Hedgehog signals during development [37]. The MUC1 protein is expressed on the apical surface of epithelial cells that line the mucosal surfaces of many different tissues. In a study by Kurzen et al., MUC1 was found to be expressed in Merkel cells and in about 82% of all MCC and 66% of metastases [38].

When examining the protein products of several of these differentially expressed genes by immunohistochemistry, the protein and gene expression results were in agreement for only 1 of 4 genes. KRT20 demonstrated increased mRNA and protein expression in the tumors of poor prognosis patients. KRT20 is an intermediate filament protein responsible for the structural integrity of epithelial cells. Our expression microarray analysis indicated 3.0-fold overexpression in poor prognosis tumors while the immunohistochemistry results confirmed an increase in the protein level. In earlier studies, 88–100% of MCC was positive for KRT20 [33, 39]. In particular, KRT20 was used as a marker for differentiating MCC from small cell carcinoma of the lung [33, 40]. Micrometastatic foci in sentinel lymph node biopsies stained strongly for KRT20 [41]. Unlike the positive results with KRT20, protein levels of KIF3A and MUC1 did not display a positive association with gene expression results. Despite the expression microarray evidence indicating robust gene expression in both prognoses groups, KIF3A and MUC1 proteins were each detected in only 1 sample. Similarly, the KIT protein levels did not correspond to prognosis group despite 67% (10 of 15) of MCC samples staining positive for KIT. This did, however, validate a previous study that found that 65% of MCC were KIT positive [42]. While there is limited agreement between the gene and protein expression data, there is substantial evidence in the literature to indicate that there is significant regulation of protein levels subsequent to mRNA transcription, thus allowing for differing results when comparing gene expression with protein expression [43].

The results of this study further develop a recently published gene expression analysis by Harms et al. [44]. While our comparison was among MCC patients based upon prognosis, they compared among MCC positive or negative for Merkel cell polyomavirus, squamous cell carcinoma (SCC), and normal skin. Intriguingly, the results comparing MCC with SCC and normal skin resulted in similar results reported here. Piccolo (*PCLO*), *KRT20*, and *KIT* were upregulated in MCC compared to SCC just as these 3 genes were upregulated in poor prognosis patient samples compared to good prognosis patient samples. In addition, functional classes found to be altered between MCC and SCC included categories such as nervous system development, neuron development, and neuron projection morphogenesis which is similar to those found in Table 2. In the comparison of MCC to normal skin, NEFM was found to be highly upregulated in MCC while our results showed that NEFM was upregulated more than 4-fold in poor prognosis patient samples.

5. Conclusions

In recent years, research has made rapid progress in identifying biological features of Merkel cell carcinoma; nevertheless, MCC represents a considerable challenge due to its relative rarity. While multiple studies have identified several biomarkers, prognostic value of these biomarkers has yet to be determined. This study is among the first to use LCM-captured MCC cells to investigate specific gene expression changes associated with prognosis of the tumor. Several of the gene expression changes presented here further implicate their role in MCC. Gene expression of *KRT20, KIT, MUC1,* and *NEFM* has been identified in earlier MCC studies. In addition, several new potential biomarkers were identified. Genes such as *TPD52, HOXB1,* and *KIF3A* have been implicated in other cancer types and are connected with MCC-associated signaling. Furthermore, KRT20 demonstrated elevated protein levels in poor prognosis patient samples. This complements results from Harms et al. showing elevated KRT20 protein in MCC compared with SCC. From these results, we conclude that genes such as *KIT, HOXB1,* and *KIF3A* may provide valuable insights into the biology of MCC and the possibility remains that novel therapeutic modalities may be discovered with continued understanding of these biomarkers. Additionally, protein expression levels of KRT20 will be of importance in evaluating the prognosis of MCC. Given the limited sample numbers in this pilot study, we aim to expand this study through collaborations with other institutions. Ongoing studies, including further analysis of data with longer patient followup and an assessment of the influence of polyomavirus in these patients, will be necessary in order to elucidate the ultimate potential of these new biomarkers.

Acknowledgments

The authors would like to thank the Department of Anatomical Pathology for their help with tumor pathology. This work was supported by the Beaumont Research Institute.

References

[1] C. Toker, "Trabecular carcinoma of the skin," *Archives of Dermatology*, vol. 105, no. 1, pp. 107–110, 1972.

[2] C. K. Tang and C. Toker, "Trabecular carcinoma of the skin. An ultrastructural study," *Cancer*, vol. 42, no. 5, pp. 2311–2321, 1978.

[3] S. K. Hussain, J. Sundquist, and K. Hemminki, "Incidence trends of squamous cell and rare skin cancers in the swedish national cancer registry point to calendar year and age-dependent increases," *Journal of Investigative Dermatology*, vol. 130, no. 5, pp. 1323–1328, 2010.

[4] B. D. Lemos, B. E. Storer, J. G. Iyer et al., "Pathologic nodal evaluation improves prognostic accuracy in Merkel cell carcinoma: analysis of 5823 cases as the basis of the first consensus staging system," *Journal of the American Academy of Dermatology*, vol. 63, no. 5, pp. 751–761, 2010.

[5] J. G. Iyer, S. Koba, and P. Nghiem, "Toward better management of Merkel cell carcinoma using a consensus staging system, new diagnostic codes and a recently discovered virus," *Actas Dermo-Sifiliograficas*, vol. 100, supplement 2, pp. 49–54, 2009.

[6] J. Albores-Saavedra, K. Batich, F. Chable-Montero, N. Sagy, A. M. Schwartz, and D. E. Henson, "Merkel cell carcinoma demographics, morphology, and survival based on 3870 cases: a population based study," *Journal of Cutaneous Pathology*, vol. 37, no. 1, pp. 20–27, 2010.

[7] C. M. Balch, J. E. Gershenwald, S. Soong et al., "Final version of 2009 AJCC melanoma staging and classification," *Journal of Clinical Oncology*, vol. 27, no. 36, pp. 6199–6206, 2009.

[8] T. Y. Eng, M. G. Boersma, C. D. Fuller et al., "A comprehensive review of the treatment of Merkel cell carcinoma," *The American Journal of Clinical Oncology*, vol. 30, no. 6, pp. 624–636, 2007.

[9] B. J. Hall, L. B. Pincus, S. S. Yu, D. H. Oh, A. R. Wilson, and T. H. McCalmont, "Immunohistochemical prognostication of Merkel cell carcinoma: p63 expression but not polyomavirus status correlates with outcome," *Journal of Cutaneous Pathology*, vol. 39, no. 10, pp. 911–917, 2012.

[10] S. Asioli, A. Righi, D. de Biase et al., "Expression of p63 is the sole independent marker of aggressiveness in localised (stage I-II) Merkel cell carcinomas," *Modern Pathology*, vol. 24, no. 11, pp. 1451–1461, 2011.

[11] A. Touzé, E. le Bidre, H. Laude et al., "High levels of antibodies against Merkel cell polyomavirus identify a subset of patients with Merkel cell carcinoma with better clinical outcome," *Journal of Clinical Oncology*, vol. 29, no. 12, pp. 1612–1619, 2011.

[12] K. G. Paulson, J. G. Iyer, A. R. Tegeder et al., "Transcriptome-wide studies of Merkel cell carcinoma and validation of intratumoral CD8+ lymphocyte invasion as an independent predictor of survival," *Journal of Clinical Oncology*, vol. 29, no. 12, pp. 1539–1546, 2011.

[13] M. Clément-Ziza, D. Gentien, S. Lyonnet, J. Thiery, C. Besmond, and C. Decraene, "Evaluation of methods for amplification of picogram amounts of total RNA for whole genome expression profiling," *BMC Genomics*, vol. 10, article 246, 2009.

[14] R. Edgar, M. Domrachev, and A. E. Lash, "Gene expression omnibus: NCBI gene expression and hybridization array data repository," *Nucleic Acids Research*, vol. 30, no. 1, pp. 207–210, 2002.

[15] K. J. Preacher and N. E. Briggs, "Calculation for Fisher's Exact Test: an interactive calculation tool for Fisher's exact probability test for 2 × 2 tables [Computer software]," 2001, http://quantpsy.org.

[16] A. Nikitin, S. Egorov, N. Daraselia, and I. Mazo, "Pathway studio—the analysis and navigation of molecular networks," *Bioinformatics*, vol. 19, no. 16, pp. 2155–2157, 2003.

[17] E. Kotelnikova, N. Ivanikova, A. Kalinin, A. Yuryev, and N. Daraselia, "Atlas of signaling for interpretation of microarray experiments," *PLoS ONE*, vol. 5, no. 2, Article ID e9256, 2010.

[18] S. Novichkova, S. Egorov, and N. Daraselia, "MedScan, a natural language processing engine for MEDLINE abstracts," *Bioinformatics*, vol. 19, no. 13, pp. 1699–1706, 2003.

[19] A. Yuryev, Z. Mulyukov, E. Kotelnikova et al., "Automatic pathway building in biological association networks," *BMC Bioinformatics*, vol. 7, article 171, 2006.

[20] F. M. Benes, D. Matzilevich, R. E. Burke, and J. Walsh, "The expression of proapoptosis genes is increased in bipolar disorder, but not in schizophrenia," *Molecular Psychiatry*, vol. 11, no. 3, pp. 241–251, 2006.

[21] M. V. Martin, B. Rollins, P. A. Sequeira et al., "Exon expression in lymphoblastoid cell lines from subjects with schizophrenia before and after glucose deprivation," *BMC Medical Genomics*, vol. 2, article 62, 2009.

[22] J. Jabbour, R. Cumming, R. A. Scolyer, G. Hruby, J. F. Thompson, and S. Lee, "Merkel cell carcinoma: assessing the effect of wide local excision, lymph node dissection, and radiotherapy on recurrence and survival in early-stage disease—results from a review of 82 consecutive cases diagnosed between 1992 and 2004," *Annals of Surgical Oncology*, vol. 14, no. 6, pp. 1943–1952, 2007.

[23] J. R. Clark, M. J. Veness, R. Gilbert, C. J. O'Brien, and P. J. Gullane, "Merkel cell carcinoma of the head and neck: is adjuvant radiotherapy necessary?" *Head and Neck*, vol. 29, no. 3, pp. 249–257, 2007.

[24] L. Desch and R. Kunstfeld, "Merkel cell carcinoma: chemotherapy and emerging new therapeutic options," *Journal of Skin Cancer*, vol. 2013, Article ID 327150, 9 pages, 2013.

[25] D. T. Petrova, A. R. Asif, V. W. Armstrong et al., "Expression of chloride intracellular channel protein 1 (CLIC1) and tumor protein D52 (TPD52) as potential biomarkers for colorectal cancer," *Clinical Biochemistry*, vol. 41, no. 14-15, pp. 1224–1236, 2008.

[26] J. A. Byrne, R. L. Balleine, M. S. Fejzo et al., "Tumor protein D52 (TPD52) is overexpressed and a gene amplification target in ovarian cancer," *International Journal of Cancer*, vol. 117, no. 6, pp. 1049–1054, 2005.

[27] M. A. Rubin, S. Varambally, R. Beroukhim et al., "Overexpression, amplification, and androgen regulation of TPD52 in prostate cancer," *Cancer Research*, vol. 64, no. 11, pp. 3814–3822, 2004.

[28] R. L. Balleine, M. S. Fejzo, P. Sathasivam, P. Basset, C. L. Clarke, and J. A. Byrne, "The hD52 (TPD52) gene is a candidate target gene for events resulting in increased 8q21 copy number in human breast carcinoma," *Genes, Chromosomes and Cancer*, vol. 29, no. 1, pp. 48–57, 2000.

[29] K. Krasagakis, I. Fragiadaki, M. Metaxari et al., "KIT receptor activation by autocrine and paracrine stem cell factor stimulates growth of Merkel cell carcinoma in vitro," *Journal of Cellular Physiology*, vol. 226, no. 4, pp. 1099–1109, 2011.

[30] A. A. Andea, R. Patel, S. Ponnazhagan et al., "Merkel cell carcinoma: correlation of KIT expression with survival and evaluation of KIT gene mutational status," *Human Pathology*, vol. 41, no. 10, pp. 1405–1412, 2010.

[31] F. U. Weiss, I. J. Marques, J. M. Woltering et al., "Retinoic acid receptor antagonists inhibit miR-10a expression and block metastatic behavior of pancreatic cancer," *Gastroenterology*, vol. 137, no. 6, pp. 2136.e7–2145.e7, 2009.

[32] E. Hofsli, T. E. Wheeler, M. Langaas, A. Lægreid, and L. Thommesen, "Identification of novel neuroendocrine-specific tumour genes," *The British Journal of Cancer*, vol. 99, no. 8, pp. 1330–1339, 2008.

[33] M. Bobos, P. Hytiroglou, I. Kostopoulos, G. Karkavelas, and C. S. Papadimitriou, "Immunohistochemical distinction between Merkel cell carcinoma and small cell carcinoma of the lung," *The American Journal of Dermatopathology*, vol. 28, no. 2, pp. 99–104, 2006.

[34] S. Singh and A. K. Gupta, "Nitric oxide: role in tumour biology and iNOS/NO-based anticancer therapies," *Cancer Chemotherapy and Pharmacology*, vol. 67, no. 6, pp. 1211–1224, 2011.

[35] J. K. R. Boult, S. Walker-Samuel, Y. Jamin, J. M. Leiper, G. S. J. Whitley, and S. P. Robinson, "Active site mutant dimethylarginine dimethylaminohydrolase 1 expression confers an intermediate tumour phenotype in C6 gliomas," *Journal of Pathology*, vol. 225, no. 3, pp. 344–352, 2011.

[36] M. Brunner, D. Thurnher, J. Pammer et al., "Expression of hedgehog signaling molecules in Merkel cell carcinoma," *Head and Neck*, vol. 32, no. 3, pp. 333–340, 2010.

[37] S. Y. Wong, A. D. Seol, P. So et al., "Primary cilia can both mediate and suppress Hedgehog pathway-dependent tumorigenesis," *Nature Medicine*, vol. 15, no. 9, pp. 1055–1061, 2009.

[38] H. Kurzen, S. Kaul, U. Egner, M. Deichmann, and W. Hartschuh, "Expression of MUC 1 and Ep-CAM in Merkel cell carcinomas: implications for immunotherapy," *Archives of Dermatological Research*, vol. 295, no. 4, pp. 146–154, 2003.

[39] M. Sidiropoulos, W. Hanna, S. J. Raphael, and Z. Ghorab, "Expression of TdT in Merkel cell carcinoma and small cell lung carcinoma," *The American Journal of Clinical Pathology*, vol. 135, no. 6, pp. 831–838, 2011.

[40] A. J. Hanly, G. W. Elgart, M. Jorda, J. Smith, and M. Nadji, "Analysis of thyroid transcription factor-1 and cytokeratin 20 separates Merkel cell carcinoma from small cell carcinoma of lung," *Journal of Cutaneous Pathology*, vol. 27, no. 3, pp. 118–120, 2000.

[41] L. D. Su, L. Lowe, C. R. Bradford, A. I. Yahanda, T. M. Johnson, and V. K. Sondak, "Immunostaining for cytokeratin 20 improves detection of micrometastatic Merkel cell carcinoma in sentinel lymph nodes," *Journal of the American Academy of Dermatology*, vol. 46, no. 5, pp. 661–666, 2002.

[42] B. L. Swick, R. Srikantha, and K. N. Messingham, "Specific analysis of KIT and PDGFR-alpha expression and mutational status in Merkel cell carcinoma," *Journal of Cutaneous Pathology*, vol. 40, no. 7, pp. 623–630, 2013.

[43] C. Vogel and E. M. Marcotte, "Insights into the regulation of protein abundance from proteomic and transcriptomic analyses," *Nature Reviews Genetics*, vol. 13, no. 4, pp. 227–232, 2012.

[44] P. W. Harms, R. M. Patel, M. E. Verhaegen et al., "Distinct gene expression profiles of viral- and nonviral-associated Merkel cell carcinoma revealed by transcriptome analysis," *Journal of Investigative Dermatology*, vol. 133, no. 4, pp. 936–945, 2013.

13

Dual S-100-AE1/3 Immunohistochemistry to Detect Perineural Invasion in Nonmelanoma Skin Cancers

Alma C. Berlingeri-Ramos,[1] Claire J. Detweiler,[2] Richard F. Wagner Jr.,[1] and Brent C. Kelly[1]

[1] *Department of Dermatology, University of Texas Medical Branch, 301 University Drive, Galveston, TX 77555-5302, USA*
[2] *Department of Pathology, Duke University Medical Center, Durham, NC 27710, USA*

Correspondence should be addressed to Alma C. Berlingeri-Ramos; alberlin@utmb.edu

Academic Editor: Silvia Moretti

Background. Perineural invasion (PNI) is an adverse prognostic histologic finding and increases the risk of local recurrence and metastasis. *Objective.* We aimed to determine if dual immunohistochemical (IHC) staining with S-100 and AE1/3 would increase the detection of PNI on nonmelanoma skin cancers (NMSCs). *Methods.* We collected 45 specimens of NMSCs in which there was clinical suspicion for PNI. Two dermatopathologists independently reviewed the tumors for the unequivocal presence of PNI. *Results.* Unequivocal PNI was present on 10 of the 45 tumors by H&E staining and on 15 of the 45 tumors by IHC staining. Large nerves (>0.1 mm) were involved in 3 of 10 H&E-stained cases and 3 of 15 IHC-stained cases, with 2 of the 4 cases demonstrating large nerve involvement with both staining methods. Of the 8 cases of PNI detected only on IHC, 7 were small nerves (≤0.1 mm). *Limitations.* All cases were selected because they were clinically suspicious for PNI, and this may be considered selection bias. *Conclusions.* PNI detection may be increased using dual S-100 and AE1/3 staining, but the majority of additional cases detected were small nerves. The clinical significance, given the small size of the involved nerves, is unclear.

1. Introduction

Perineural invasion (PNI) is growth of a tumor within the perineural space of a nerve or within the nerve fascicles [1–3]. PNI, particularly for cutaneous squamous cell carcinoma (cSCC), is considered an adverse prognostic histologic finding and increases the risk of local recurrence and metastasis [4, 5]. The current edition of the American Joint Committee on Cancer's Staging Manual includes PNI as a high risk feature for nonmelanoma skin cancers (NMSCs) because of its predictive value for aggressive behavior [6].

We aimed to determine if dual immunohistochemical (IHC) staining with both S-100 and AE1/3 would increase the detection of PNI on NMSCs on pathohistology.

2. Materials and Methods

Our electronic dermatopathology records were reviewed using an electronic SNOMED retrieval system for two types of NMSCs, basal cell carcinomas (BCCs) and squamous cell carcinomas (SCCs), in which the clinical information included the term "perineural" from June 2003 to June 2008. These records were evaluated and all cases (n = 45) of NMSC in which there was a clinical concern for PNI were included. The clinical information was reviewed and, in most cases, the clinician was concerned about PNI because of size of the tumor, pain, or suspicion based on Mohs frozen sections.

Tissue sections were cut at 3–5 microns and mounted on positively charged slides. Prior to treatment, all sections were dried in a slide oven at 60 degrees for 30 minutes to ensure that the sections adhered to the slides and were completely dry. Sections were deparaffinized in 4 changes of xylene for 5 minutes each and then rehydrated through a series of graded alcohols with a final rinse in distilled water. Endogenous peroxides were quenched by soaking sections in two changes of 3% methanol H_2O_2 for 5 minutes each.

Prior to IHC, sections were treated with antigen retrieval to facilitate antibody binding to antigen. Briefly, slides were

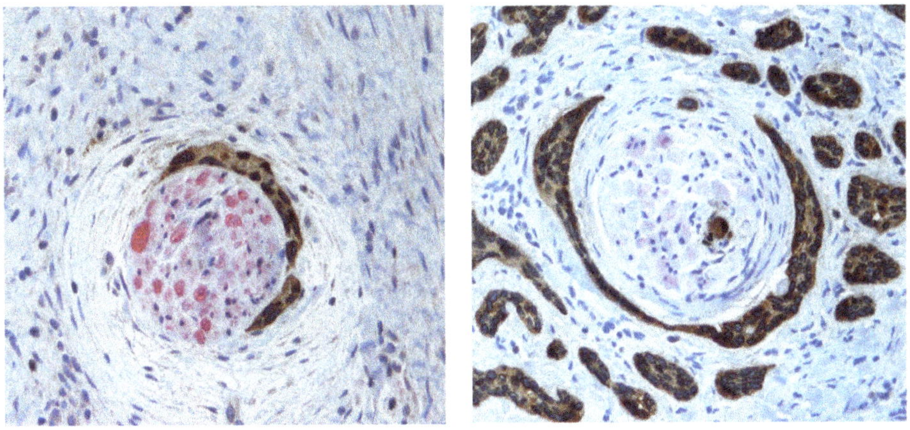

(a) (b)

Figure 1: Perineural invasion of squamous cell carcinoma (brown) inside the perineurium of the nerve (red). (a) IHC with dual staining for S-100 and AE1/3, original magnification ×200. Squamous cell carcinoma (brown) surrounding nerve, focally penetrating perineurium, and within fascicles. (b) IHC with dual staining for S-100 and AE1/3, original magnification ×200. IHC: immunohistochemistry.

incubated in the Black and Decker Vegetable Steamer for 20 minutes in Target Retrieval Solution (Dako Corporation, Carpinteria, CA; Cat. # S1699) preheated to 99°C. They were then taken out of the steamer and placed on an open counter to cool for 20 minutes in the solution. The slides were then rinsed in 3 changes of distilled water and placed into a container of tris-buffered saline (Signet Pathology Systems, Inc., Dedham, MA; Cat. # 2380) for 5 minutes to decrease the surface tension of the slides and facilitate coating by the following reagents.

Slides were loaded horizontally onto the Dako Autostainer where each of the following steps was automated. Tris-buffered saline was used to rinse the sections between each of the IHC steps. Both avidin and biotin from the Avidin Biotin Blocking Kit (Vector Laboratories, Burlingame, CA; Cat. # SP2001) were diluted in Antibody Diluent (Dako) at a ratio of 1 mL avidin or biotin to 5 mL diluent.

Diluted avidin was applied to sections and incubated for 7 minutes. AE1/3 (Signet number 464-01) at a concentration of 1 : 200 was incubated for 30 minutes. Sections were then incubated in LSAB2, universal secondary antibody (Dako) for 15 minutes, followed by LSAB2, label (Dako) for 15 minutes; then chromogen liquid DAB (Dako) was applied for 5 minutes. The slides were then run again in the autostainer using the primary antibody S-100 (Dako number Z0311) at a concentration of 1 : 4000 for 30 minutes. The tertiary reagent used here was a streptavidin-alkaline phosphatase conjugate (Millipore # 20841). Fast red was used as the chromogen. The slides were then taken off the autostainer and rinsed in distilled water, manually counterstained with Harris Hematoxylin (Fisher Scientific) for 1 minute, rinsed in distilled water followed by 0.25% ammonia water to blue and then a final rinse in distilled water. They were then dehydrated through graded series of alcohols and cleared in four changes of xylene and coverslipped with synthetic glass and Permount mounting media.

Dual IHC staining showed red chromogen staining of peripheral nerve nuclei and cytoplasm with S-100 and brown cytoplasmic staining of epithelial cells with AE1/3.

Two dermatopathologists independently reviewed the H&E sections and IHC sections for the unequivocal presence of PNI. PNI was defined as malignant appearing epithelial cells surrounding more than 50% of the nerve and tumor present within the perineurium or within the nerve fascicles [1–3]. Large nerves were defined as >0.1 mm, and small nerves were defined as ≤0.1 mm [1].

3. Results

Table 1 presents the findings for the 45 NMSCs (17 BCCs and 28 SCCs) studied. Examples of dual staining results are seen in Figure 1.

Overall, 18 cases (40%; 7 BCCs and 11 SCCs) had evidence of PNI on either routine examination or dual IHC staining. In the majority of cases (34 cases, 75.6%) the findings on H&E and dual IHC-stained tissue sections correlated with the presence or absence of PNI. This included 27 cases (60%) in which PNI was absent via both methods and 7 cases (15.6%) in which PNI was identified using both methods. In 8 cases (44.4%; 1 BCC and 7 SCCs) dual IHC was the only method by which PNI was demonstrated compared to 3 cases (16.7%; 1 BCC and 2 SCCs) in which H&E alone yielded positive findings (Figure 2).

Of these 3 cases identified via H&E alone, 1 corresponding IHC sample was inadequate due to loss of tissue. PNI on a second case was not found on dual IHC staining because IHC staining revealed that the tumor surrounded the nerve without invasion of perineurium.

Of the 8 cases in which PNI was found on dual IHC staining only, 7 cases (87.5%) involved small nerves (≤0.1 mm) (Figure 3). Seven of 8 (87.5%) were SCC cases, and 1 of 8 (12.5%) was a BCC case. Large nerves (>0.1 mm) were identified in 3 of 10 (30%) of H&E-stained cases and 3 of 15 (20%) of IHC-stained cases, with 2 of the 4 large nerve cases identified with both types of staining.

Out of the 7 cases in which PNI was identified via both methods there was 1 case in which H&E staining identified PNI in a large nerve, but IHC staining identified PNI in

TABLE 1: Detection of PNI on H&E and dual IHC staining.

Case number	Tumor type	PNI H&E	Nerve size (mm)	PNI dual IHC	Nerve size (mm)	Notes
1	BCC	−		−		
2	BCC	+	0.01	+	0.04	
3	BCC	−		−		
4	BCC	−		−		
5	BCC	+	0.06	−		
6	BCC	−		−		
7	BCC	−		−		
8	BCC	+	0.08	+	0.06	
9	BCC	+	0.11	+	0.08	
10	BCC	−		−		
11	BCC	−		−		
12	BCC	+	0.14	+	0.15	
13	BCC	−		−		
14	BCC	−		−		
15	BCC	+	0.07	+	0.07	
16	BCC	−		+	0.02	
17	BCC	−		−		
18	SCC	+	0.18	+	0.11	
19	SCC	−		+	0.03	
20	SCC	+	0.04	−		IHC staining more clearly demonstrated that tumor did not invade perineurium
21	SCC	−		−		
22	SCC	−		−		
23	SCC	−		−		
24	SCC	−		−		
25	SCC	−		−		
26	SCC	−		−		
27	SCC	−		−		
28	SCC	−		−		
29	SCC	−		−		
30	SCC	−		−		
31	SCC	−		−		
32	SCC	−		+	0.03	
33	SCC	−		+	0.03	
34	SCC	−		−		
35	SCC	+	0.06	−		Tissue block was cut through on sectioning for IHC
36	SCC	−		−		
37	SCC	−		+	0.06	
38	SCC	−		+	0.04	
39	SCC	+	0.05	+	0.02	
40	SCC	−		−		
41	SCC	−		−		
42	SCC	−		+	0.05	
43	SCC	−		+	0.12	
44	SCC	−		−		
45	SCC	−		−		

PNI: perineural invasion; H&E: hematoxylin and eosin; IHC: immunohistochemistry; BCC: basal cell carcinoma; SCC: squamous cell carcinoma.

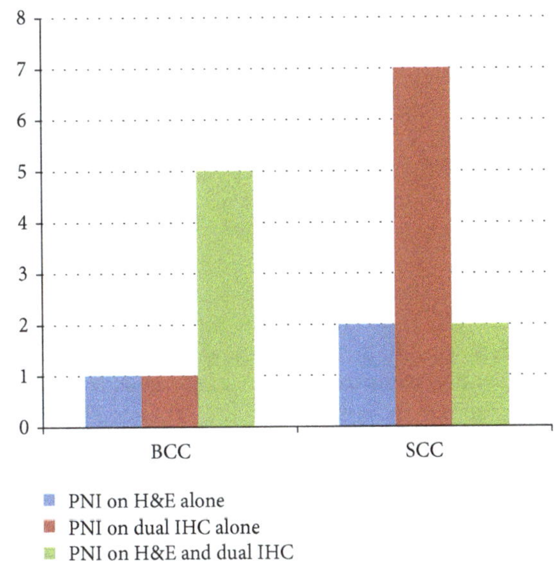

FIGURE 2: Comparative analysis between routine H&E examination and dual IHC using antibodies for S-100 and AE1/3 in the evaluation of PNI in cases of BCC and SCC. PNI: perineural invasion; H&E: hematoxylin and eosin; IHC: immunohistochemistry; BCC: basal cell carcinoma; SCC: squamous cell carcinoma.

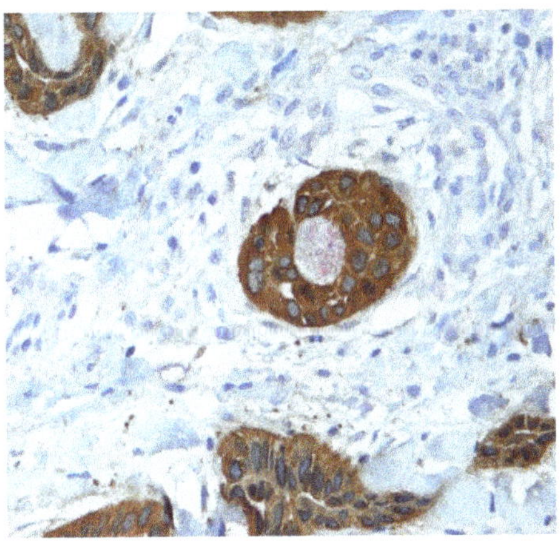

FIGURE 3: Perineural invasion. A small nerve branch (red) completely surrounded by squamous cell carcinoma (brown) in a case in which perineural invasion was not detected on H&E. IHC with dual staining for S-100 and AE1/3, original magnification ×200. H&E: hematoxylin and eosin; IHC: immunohistochemistry.

a small nerve. In the remaining 6 cases the diameter of the involved nerve found on H&E examination remained in the same nerve size category following IHC staining.

There were 0 cases in which the dermatopathologists differed in diagnosis of presence or absence of PNI.

4. Discussion

PNI in NMSC, particularly (cSCC), is considered to carry a more aggressive prognosis with increased rates of recurrence and metastasis [4, 5]. In a study by Rowe et al. [5] SCC of the skin, ear, and lip with histologic PNI had a local recurrence rate of 47.2% and a metastatic rate of 47.3%. In a study by Goepfert et al. [4] patients with cSCC with PNI had regional lymph node metastases (35% of patients) and distant metastases (15% of patients) significantly more frequently than in those without PNI.

Incidence of PNI varies greatly between studies depending on many potential variables, including number of histological sections examined, stains used, and diagnostic criteria. Leibovitch et al. [7, 8] found PNI in 283 of 10,035 basal cell carcinomas (BCCs) (2.74%) and in 70 of 1177 SCCs (5.95%) that were treated with Mohs surgery between 1993 and 2002. PNI is seen more commonly in SCCs than BCCs, and patients with SCC with PNI have a worse prognosis than those with BCC with PNI [7–9]. PNI is also more common in recurrent rather than previously untreated malignancies, and prognosis is worse for those with PNI in a recurrence [2, 4, 9]. Prognosis is also worse in patients with extensive rather than local PNI [9].

PNI is separated into clinical and incidental types. Clinical PNI describes patients with clinical symptoms or signs, such as cranial neuropathy and/or radiographic evidence of tumor involvement of a nerve [1, 10]. The most common symptom of PNI is paresthesias such as formication which can subsequently develop into feelings of pain, numbness, and/or weakness [10]. The trigeminal (CN V) and facial (CN VII) nerves are the most commonly involved [2, 4]. Imaging evidence of PNI is associated with a poorer prognosis [11]. Even with clinical symptoms of PNI, diagnosis can be delayed for more than 6 months to a year if suspicion is low [2]. Incidental PNI describes asymptomatic patients without radiographic evidence but with histopathologic evidence of PNI [1, 10]. Approximately 30% to 40% of patients with PNI have clinical evidence while for the majority of cases it is an incidental finding [2]. Patients with clinical PNI have a worse prognosis than those with incidental PNI [2, 10].

Detection of PNI is routinely performed histologically with H&E staining, but accurate identification of PNI can be difficult. Histological evidence of PNI is the presence of malignant cells within the perineural space of a nerve or within the nerve fascicles [1–3]. However, there is currently no standard definition of PNI, and some studies have included tumor near or abutting the outer perineurium [12]. Perineural inflammation and nerve fiber degeneration can be used as clues to nearby PNI [13]. Tumor cells can be hard to distinguish from normal perineurium and stroma [12]. Tumor cells in the perineural space may appear histologically different from the tumor from which they originate and may only show subtle signs of atypia [13]. There are at least four benign mimics of PNI that need to be considered and excluded when diagnosing PNI: peritumoral fibrosis, reexcision PNI, reparative PNI, and epithelial sheath neuroma [14]. Some studies say that perineural spread can have skip areas, where PNI is not visible on adjacent sections of tissue [12]. Other studies do not support the idea of skip areas. For example, Panizza et al. [15] did not find skip lesions in their study and suspected that skip areas are really a processing artifact. IHC staining for cSCC has been studied by Kelso et al. [16] who applied S-100 and $p75^{NGFR}$ IHC staining to cSCC cases and found increased detection of

PNI with the use of each. Standardized pathology protocols stringently defining PNI as tumor cells within the perineural space or between fascicles, staining of ambiguous cases, and documentation of the size of involved nerves could help increase the accuracy of PNI diagnosis and estimation of prognosis [1–3, 12].

Another factor to consider regarding PNI is the size of the nerve involved. It is currently unclear whether the size of the nerve involved plays a prognostic role in PNI. One variable contributing to this is the ambiguity of the words "large nerve" and "small nerve." Some studies define a large nerve as >0.1 mm, while others define it as ≥0.1 mm. There have been calls to officially define small nerves as ≤0.1 mm and large nerves as >0.1 mm, thus placing 0.1 mm nerves into the small nerve group [1]. Ross et al. [12] demonstrated that, in patients with SCC, PNI of large-caliber nerves (≥0.1 mm) had worse outcomes than PNI of small-caliber nerves (<0.1 mm). McCord et al. [17] also found a lower rate of local control with involvement of a named nerve pathway, though nerve diameter was not specifically defined. Carter et al. [18] demonstrated increased risk of nodal metastasis and death from disease with large nerve (≥0.1 mm) involvement. On the other hand, Lin et al. [9] demonstrated no difference in outcome in relation to the size of the involved nerve in patients with SCC or BCC when defining large nerves as >0.1 mm. Many studies have shown that large nerve PNI is associated with other risk factors such as recurrent tumor, larger tumor diameter, greater maximum depth of tumor, invasion beyond the subcutaneous fat, multiple nerve involvement, infiltrative growth, and lymphovascular invasion [12, 18]. It has been postulated that it is these associated risk factors rather than large nerve PNI that have resulted in poorer outcomes in patients [18]. Further studies are needed to truly determine significance, and universal guidelines for labeling of nerve sizes are needed for this area of research to progress.

There are no universal guidelines for the treatment of NMSC with PNI and current recommendations do not use PNI nerve size in the decision of treatment method [12]. Most are treated with radiotherapy with or without surgical excision via standard or Mohs micrographic surgery [1, 17, 19]. Mendenhall et al. [2] recommended treating NMSC with PNI with resection and postoperative radiotherapy if the cancer is resectable and treating with definitive radiotherapy for unresectable cases without consideration for PNI nerve size either way. Ross et al. [12] suggested adjuvant radiotherapy only when PNI involves large nerves greater than or equal to 0.1 mm. Currently, there are no clear evidence-based treatment guidelines, and physicians and patients are faced with choosing between surgery, radiotherapy, or both.

The 7th edition of the American Joint Committee on Cancer's Cancer Staging Manual (AJCC-7) for cSCC includes perineural invasion as a high risk feature, and the presence of two or more high risk features at any tumor size increases the stage from T1 to T2 [20]. Other high risk features include poorly differentiated or undifferentiated tumors, primary anatomical site on the ear or the nonhair bearing lip, thickness greater than 2 mm, and Clark level of at least IV [20]. There has been a proposal by Jambusaria-Pahlajani et al. [21] to classify the presence of one high risk factor as stage T2a, two to three high risk factors as stage T2b, and four high risk factors as stage T3. The results of their study showed worse outcomes (nodal metastases and death from cSCC) in T2b tumors compared to T2a tumors [21]. In a study by Schmitt et al. [22] it was shown that T2 tumors larger than 2 cm in the AJCC-7 criteria and T2b tumors in the alternative criteria by Jambusaria-Phlajani et al. have positive sentinel lymph node biopsy (SLNB) rates over 10% and thus warrant SLNB.

We simultaneously utilized the unique staining qualities of two different antibodies for the purpose of detection of PNI in NMSCs. In this pilot study, we did increase our detection of PNI compared to H&E alone. Dual IHC analysis using antibodies to S-100 and AE1/3 enhanced detection of suspicious foci by providing distinct staining patterns of peripheral nerves and malignant appearing epithelial cells, respectively. Dual IHC staining was particularly useful to resolve the diagnostic dilemma of perineurial proliferation and peritumoral fibrosis. The majority of these additional detections were in SCC cases (87.5%) and involved small nerves (87.5%). However, it is unclear if increased detection of small involved nerves would have clinical significance [9, 12]. All cases were selected because they were clinically suspicious for PNI, and this may be considered a form of selection bias and thus a pitfall of the study.

In cases with PNI, dual IHC did not significantly alter nerve diameter measurements. Dual IHC staining also increases the cost of diagnosis. Thus, additional dual IHC staining may not be warranted in cases in which PNI is clearly identified on initial H&E sections.

Dual IHC staining with S-100 and AE1/3 may be useful in cases where PNI is suspected but unclear on H&E analysis, especially in the case of peritumoral fibrosis and proliferation of perineurium.

Disclosure

The data in this paper was presented in poster form at the American Society for Dermatopathology annual meeting in 2010 and was published in abstract form in the Journal of Cutaneous Pathology 2011; 38(1):171.

References

[1] L. Buchanan, B. De'Ambrosis, K. Deambrosis et al., "Defining incidental perineural invasion: the need for a national registry," *Australasian Journal of Dermatology*, vol. 55, no. 2, pp. 107–110, 2014.

[2] W. M. Mendenhall, R. J. Amdur, L. S. Williams, A. A. Mancuso, S. P. Stringer, and N. P. Mendenhall, "Carcinoma of the skin of the head and neck with perineural invasion," *Head and Neck*, vol. 24, no. 1, pp. 78–83, 2002.

[3] D. Ratner, L. Lowe, T. M. Johnson, and D. J. Fader, "Perineural spread of basal cell carcinomas treated with Mohs micrographic surgery," *Cancer*, vol. 88, no. 7, pp. 1605–1613, 2000.

[4] H. Goepfert, W. J. Dichtel, and J. E. Medina, "Perineural invasion in squamous cell skin carcinoma of the head and neck," *The American Journal of Surgery*, vol. 148, no. 4, pp. 642–647, 1984.

[5] D. E. Rowe, R. J. Carroll, and C. L. Day Jr., "Prognostic factors for local recurrence, metastasis, and survival rates in squamous cell carcinoma of the skin, ear, and lip: implications for treatment modality selection," *Journal of the American Academy of Dermatology*, vol. 26, no. 6, pp. 976–990, 1992.

[6] T. Lardaro, S. M. Shea, W. Sharfman, N. Liégeois, and A. J. Sober, "Improvements in the staging of cutaneous squamous-cell carcinoma in the 7th edition of the AJCC *cancer staging manual*," *Annals of Surgical Oncology*, vol. 17, no. 8, pp. 1979–1980, 2010.

[7] I. Leibovitch, S. C. Huilgol, D. Selva, D. Hill, S. Richards, and R. Paver, "Cutaneous squamous cell carcinoma treated with Mohs micrographic surgery in Australia II. Perineural invasion," *Journal of the American Academy of Dermatology*, vol. 53, no. 2, pp. 261–266, 2005.

[8] I. Leibovitch, S. C. Huilgol, D. Selva, S. Richards, and R. Paver, "Basal cell carcinoma treated with Mohs surgery in Australia III. Perineural invasion," *Journal of the American Academy of Dermatology*, vol. 53, no. 3, pp. 458–463, 2005.

[9] C. Lin, L. Tripcony, J. Keller et al., "Perineural infiltration of cutaneous squamous cell carcinoma and basal cell carcinoma without clinical features," *International Journal of Radiation Oncology Biology Physics*, vol. 82, no. 1, pp. 334–340, 2012.

[10] C. J. Balamucki, A. A. Mancuso, R. J. Amdur et al., "Skin carcinoma of the head and neck with perineural invasion," *American Journal of Otolaryngology—Head and Neck Medicine and Surgery*, vol. 33, no. 4, pp. 447–454, 2012.

[11] L. S. Williams, A. A. Mancuso, and W. M. Mendenhall, "Perineural spread of cutaneous squamous and basal cell carcinoma: CT and MR detection and its impact on patient management and prognosis," *International Journal of Radiation Oncology Biology Physics*, vol. 49, no. 4, pp. 1061–1069, 2001.

[12] A. S. Ross, F. Miller Whalen, R. Elenitsas, X. Xu, A. B. Troxel, and C. D. Schmults, "Diameter of involved nerves predicts outcomes in cutaneous squamous cell carcinoma with perineural invasion: an investigator-blinded retrospective cohort study," *Dermatologic Surgery*, vol. 35, no. 12, pp. 1859–1866, 2009.

[13] A. M. Feasel, T. J. Brown, M. A. Bogle, J. A. Tschen, and B. R. Nelson, "Perineural invasion of cutaneous malignancies," *Dermatologic Surgery*, vol. 27, no. 6, pp. 531–542, 2001.

[14] M. Dunn, M. B. Morgan, T. W. Beer, K. T. K. Chen, and S. M. Acker, "Histologic mimics of perineural invasion," *Journal of Cutaneous Pathology*, vol. 36, no. 9, pp. 937–942, 2009.

[15] B. Panizza, T. A. Warren, C. A. Solares, G. M. Boyle, D. Lambie, and I. Brown, "Histopathological features of clinical perineural invasion of cutaneous squamous cell carcinoma of the head and neck and the potential implications for treatment," *Head and Neck*, vol. 36, no. 11, pp. 1611–1618, 2013.

[16] R. L. Kelso, M. I. Colome-Grimmer, T. Uchida, H. Q. Wang, and R. F. Wagner Jr., "p75^{NGFR} immunostaining for the detection of perineural invasion by cutaneous squamous cell carcinoma," *Dermatologic Surgery*, vol. 32, no. 2, pp. 177–183, 2006.

[17] M. W. McCord, W. M. Mendenhall, J. T. Parsons, and F. P. Flowers, "Skin cancer of the head and neck with incidental microscopic perineural invasion," *International Journal of Radiation Oncology Biology Physics*, vol. 43, no. 3, pp. 591–595, 1999.

[18] J. B. Carter, M. M. Johnson, T. L. Chua, P. S. Karia, and C. D. Schmults, "Outcomes of primary cutaneous squamous cell carcinoma with perineural invasion an 11-year cohort study," *JAMA Dermatology*, vol. 149, no. 1, pp. 35–42, 2013.

[19] A. Garcia-Serra, R. W. Hinerman, W. M. Mendenhall et al., "Carcinoma of the skin with perineural invasion," *Head & Neck*

carcinoma with perineural invasion an 11-year cohort study," *JAMA Dermatology*, vol. 149, no. 1, pp. 35–42, 2013.

[19] A. Garcia-Serra, R. W. Hinerman, W. M. Mendenhall et al., "Carcinoma of the skin with perineural invasion," *Head & Neck*

14

Delineating Molecular Mechanisms of Squamous Tissue Homeostasis and Neoplasia: Focus on p63

Kathryn E. King, Linan Ha, Tura Camilli, and Wendy C. Weinberg

Division of Monoclonal Antibodies, Office of Biotechnology Products, Center for Drug Evaluation and Research, US Food and Drug Administration, Bethesda, MD 20892, USA

Correspondence should be addressed to Kathryn E. King; kathryn.kingk@fda.hhs.gov

Academic Editor: Mitchell Denning

Mouse models have informed us that p63 is critical for normal epidermal development and homeostasis. The p53/p63/p73 family is expressed as multiple protein isoforms due to a combination of alternative promoter usage and C-terminal alternative splicing. These isoforms can mimic or interfere with one another, and their balance ultimately determines biological outcome in a context-dependent manner. While not frequently mutated, p63, and in particular the ΔNp63 subclass, is commonly overexpressed in human squamous cell cancers. *In vitro* keratinocytes and murine transgenic and transplantation models have been invaluable in elucidating the contribution of altered p63 levels to cancer development, and studies have identified the roles for ΔNp63 isoforms in keratinocyte survival and malignant progression, likely due in part to their transcriptional regulatory function. These findings can be extended to human cancers; for example, the novel recognition of NFκB/c-Rel as a downstream effector of p63 has identified a role for NFκB/c-Rel in human squamous cell cancers. These models will be critical in enhancing the understanding of the specific molecular mechanisms of cancer development and progression.

1. Introduction

p53 is a tumor suppressor that is upregulated and activated across organ systems as a tissue protective stress response mechanism [1]. *p63* is a member of the p53 gene family which also includes *p73*. In contrast to p53, both p63 and p73 exhibit cell-type-specific expression patterns and exert tissue-specific functions [2, 3]. Relevant to this review, p63 plays an essential role in the development and maintenance of normal stratified squamous epithelium. All *p53* family members encode multiple protein isoforms that act in overlapping or opposing manners both within and across family members. Given the complexity of the p53 family and the potential for the different family members to mimic or interfere with each other, the balance of p53 family isoforms in a given cellular context can impact the biological outcome. In this review, we highlight how information derived from mouse models has provided insight into molecular mechanisms of normal keratinocyte growth regulation and human cancer pathogenesis. In particular, we focus on the *p63* gene, the role of its gene products in normal epidermal development and homeostasis, and how dysregulation of p63 protein expression, which is tightly controlled under normal conditions, contributes to squamous carcinogenesis, not only of the skin, but also in other squamous epithelial cancers such as those of the head and neck.

2. Overview of p63 Structure/Function

Members of the p53 family were identified based on shared homology within their major functional domains: transactivation (TA), DNA binding (DBD), and oligomerization (OD); and exist as multiple protein isoforms due to a combination of alternate promoter usage and alternative splicing [4, 5]. Use of alternative promoters gives rise to isoforms of two classes: TA and ΔN. The TAp63 and TAp73 isoforms possess a transactivation domain with homology and function similar to that of p53, while the ΔNp63 and ΔNp73 isoforms lack this domain and can act to block TAp53-, TAp63-, and TAp73-mediated transcription [4] via the mechanisms discussed below. However, this does not imply that ΔNp63 isoforms lack transcriptional activation activity as alternate transactivation domains have been described both within the N-terminus of the ΔNp63 isoforms [6, 7] and in exons 11 and 12 of the C-terminus (transactivation domain 2 (TA2)) [8]. Further analysis has suggested that the second region is unlikely to be an independent activation domain [7]. Refined mapping studies indicate that this domain instead serves to modulate transcriptional activities associated with ΔNp63 isoforms [7]. Correspondingly, many positive transcriptional targets of ΔNp63 have been identified, which are discussed in this review.

All TA and ΔNp63 isoforms contain the DBD and OD domains but differ at the C-termini. This additional complexity is conferred on these proteins due to C-terminal alternative splicing, which in the case of p63 gives rise to TA and ΔN subclasses of p63α, β, γ, δ, and ε isoforms [4, 9] (Figure 1). Of these isoforms, α is the longest and contains a sterile alpha motif (SAM) protein-protein interaction domain [10] and a transcriptional inhibition domain (TID) [11]. The TID comprises 2 subdomains, one of which binds and masks the TA domain of TAp63α and the other, which is subject to sumoylation resulting in decreased intracellular p63α concentration and correspondingly to decreased activity [11–13]. Degradation of p63α is also promoted by the E3 ubiquitin ligase ITCH via ubiquitylation at the N-terminal border of the SAM domain of the p63α isoforms [14]. Regarding the other p63 C-terminal splice variants, exon 13 is spliced out of the β-isoform, which thus also lacks the SAM and TID domains. Both the α and β isoforms of p63 contain a phosphodegron motif utilized by Fbw7 E3 ubiquitin ligase in MDM2-mediated degradation [15]. The γ, δ, and ε isoforms all truncate shortly after the oligomerization domain, with each containing a unique C-terminal sequence [9]. Thus, all three isoforms lack the SAM and TID domains (Figure 1).

Like p53, the p63 and p73 proteins function as tetramers via their oligomerization domains. The oligomerization domains of p63 and p73, due to the presence of an additional α-helix, are more similar to one another than to that of p53 [16]. p63 and p73 were not observed to interact with p53 through their oligomerization domains but strongly interact with one another through this domain, with the p63/p73 heterotetramers exhibiting enhanced stability over homotetramers [16]. While p53 does not interact with p63/p73 through the oligomerization domain, WTp53 has been shown to target ΔNp63α for caspase-mediated degradation via interactions between the DNA binding domain of each protein [17], and mutated p53 has been shown to interact with the core DNA binding domains of p63 and p73, thereby impairing DNA binding and transactivation [18].

DNA binding is an area in which p53 family members can mimic or compete with each other. While p63 has been shown to bind to p53 responsive consensus sequences, distinct p63 responsive elements have also been identified [19–21]. It has been reported that the global DNA binding pattern of p73 does not differ from that of p63, but intensity of binding at given sites does vary depending on the cell type profiled [22]. This suggests that competition between the homo- and heterotetramers of different isoforms of p63 and p73, which are subject to cellular context, may define site occupancy. Beyond interactions with one another via their oligomerization domains or their DNA binding domains, and their competition at DNA response elements, p53 family members have been shown to be involved in feedback loops with one another that impact expression levels [23, 24]. Thus, at many levels dysregultion of any one family member may impact the fine balance that is involved in maintaining normal epidermal homeostasis.

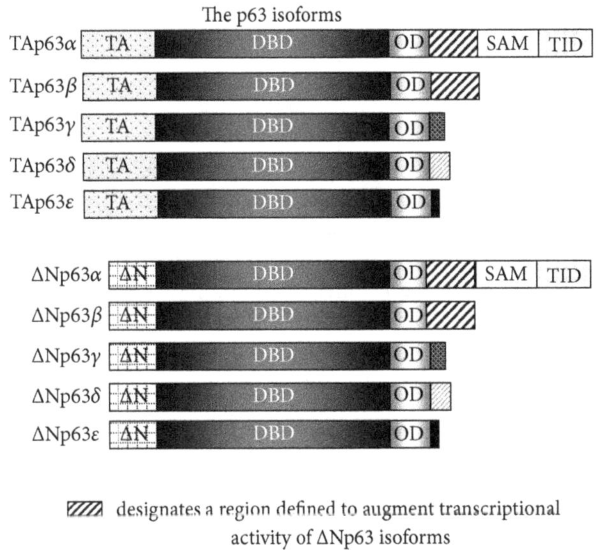

FIGURE 1: Use of alternative splicing gives rise to p63 isoforms of 2 subclasses: TAp63 and ΔNp63. Within each of these subclasses, C-terminal alternative splicing gives rise to α, β, γ, δ, and ε isoforms. The isoforms share homology in certain protein domains: TA (transactivation domain), ΔN, DBD (DNA binding domain), OD (oligomerization domain), SAM (sterile alpha motif domain), and TID (transactivation inhibition domain).

3. p63 and Normal Skin Biology

p63 is critical for normal epidermal morphogenesis [3, 25]. In the mature epidermis, the predominant p63 isoform expressed is ΔNp63α, and expression of this isoform is associated with the proliferative compartment [26]. Expression of this isoform is critical for the maintenance of the mature epidermis [27]. However, it is also the ΔNp63α isoform that is overexpressed in many squamous cell cancers [28]. As a starting point to understand how overexpression of a single isoform with ensuing disruption of the balance of p53 family members might contribute to squamous cancer pathogenesis, it is important to first understand the role of p63 both in normal epidermal morphogenesis and in homeostasis of the mature epidermis. Significant insight has been obtained through the use of mouse models outlined below.

3.1. Role of p63 in Mouse Models of Epidermal Morphogenesis and in Human Ectodermal Dysplasias

3.1.1. Mouse Models of Epidermal Morphogenesis. The criticality of p63 to normal epidermal development was highlighted by simultaneously published mouse models lacking functional *p63* [3, 25]. The mice were developed using distinct molecular strategies and upon gross phenotypic examination appeared similar; however, in-depth analysis of the epidermal phenotype gave rise to alternate hypotheses as to the role of p63 in epidermal development: epidermal progenitor cell maintenance versus commitment to stratification. In the mice developed by Yang et al., exons 6–8 corresponding to p63's DBD were replaced with the neomycin resistance gene [3]. In these mice, patches of disorganized epithelial cells positive for late markers of keratinocyte differentiation and negative for keratin 5 were evident, suggestive of a role for p63 in maintaining epidermal progenitor cells. Mice generated by Mills et al. were derived using an insertional gap repair mechanism [25]. Two strains generated by this approach, Brdml (truncating within exon 6) and Brdm2 (truncating after exon 10), appeared macroscopically identical, and thus, the strains were not distinguished in subsequent experiments in the seminal paper. Microscopic analysis of these mice revealed a layer of flattened cells expressing keratin 14 at low levels with no evidence of stratification or differentiation marker expression, suggestive of a failure to commit to a stratified epidermis. While no mRNA transcripts were detected from these mice by northern blotting, the transcript in the Brdm2 mouse model, which truncates after exon 10 [25], could in theory give rise to shortened ΔNp63 transcripts, similar to those described by Mangiulli et al. [9]. A recent recharacterization of a line of Brdm2 mice by Wolff et al. [29] revealed patches of keratinizing epidermis expressing truncated p63 at levels similar to wild type with stratification overlaying hair follicles. Based on further studies in embryos, the authors proposed these patches to be remnants of a more developed E15 epidermis 3–5 layers thick containing terminally differentiated epithelium that was transient in nature due to mechanical stress at birth, and suggested that the Brdm2 mice were equivalent to p63α/β knockout mice [29]. This observation and ensuing studies generated much controversy, as to whether the recharacterized mice were the same as those used by others or if perhaps a spontaneous genetic event might be at play [29–33], which to date remains unresolved.

Studies of the p63-deficient mouse lines provided strong evidence for the critical nature of the *p63* gene; however, interpretation of p63 function is confounded by the existence of multiple p63 protein isoforms. Therefore, single isoform knock-in mouse models have been developed on a *p63* null background to elucidate the role of specific p63 isoforms. These models have also generated controversy. Reconstitution of different p63 isoforms in the Brdm2 mice using tissue-specific inducible mouse models generated by separate groups gave rise to opposing conclusions as to the role of ΔNp63 in initiating stratification of simple epithelium [34, 35]. In one model, TAp63α, but not ΔNp63α, was found to drive stratification and keratin 5/keratin 14 expression of the simple lung epithelium [34], while in the other model, ΔNp63α or ΔNp63β caused stratification and keratin 5/keratin 14 expression in the simple lung epithelium [35]. With respect to the epidermis, differential results were also obtained by these two groups. In the first model, keratin 14-driven expression of TAp63α resulted in a severely hyperplastic epidermis exhibiting delayed differentiation [34], and based on their data the authors concluded that TAp63α is the initiating switch for epidermal stratification. In contrast, in the second model, expression of ΔNp63α or ΔNp63β under the control of the keratin 5 promoter did not result in complete restoration of epithelial integrity, but it did result in several areas of stratified epidermis, which expressed differentiation markers, indicating that the ΔNp63α and ΔNp63β can act to initiate stratification [35]. Further support for ΔNp63α as an initiator of stratification comes from other genetic complementation studies in which ΔNp63α or TAp63α, both under the keratin 5 promoter, was introduced into the *p63(−/−)* mice from Yang et al. [3, 36]. In these studies, ΔNp63α was able to partially restore the epidermal basal layer, but not differentiation marker expression, whereas TAp63α reconstitution resulted in a phenotype similar to *p63(−/−)* mice [36]. Reconstitution of a combination of ΔNp63α and TAp63α resulted in a more complete epidermis formation containing patches with a more organized structure that expressed markers of differentiation [36]. It is possible that differences with respect to the differentiation status of the epidermis generated by reconstitution of ΔNp63α in the later two studies could be due to the mouse model used, but in contrast to the first model discussed, partial epidermal restoration by ΔNp63α is a common feature of both.

Finally, subclass-specific knockout mice have been developed as a means of exploring functions attributable to the TAp63 or ΔNp63 subclasses in the presence of wild-type expression levels of the opposing subclass. Germline ablation of TAp63 did not impact normal epidermal morphogenesis in the presence of ΔNp63 isoforms [37]. In contrast, mice in which ΔN exon was replaced with GFP appeared phenotypically similar to *p63(−/−)* mice, and, like the *p63(−/−)* mice generated by Yang et al. [3], retained only disorganized patches of keratinocytes expressing terminal markers of differentiation [38]. However, in contrast to the mice generated by Yang et al. [3], these mice coexpressed keratin 5 along with the markers of terminal differentiation. Furthermore, expression of the basal transcription factor AP-2α indicated that in the absence of ΔNp63, basal patches can form, but these were observed to have decreased Ki67 staining. Taken together, this is suggestive of a role for ΔNp63 during epidermal morphogenesis in both progenitor cell maintenance and in epidermal commitment, closing the gap between the original interpretations of the pan-p63 mouse models [38].

3.1.2. p63 and Human Genetic Syndromes. In humans, heterozygous mutations in *p63* are linked to genetic syndromes that include ectodermal dysplasia as part of the disease phenotype [39]. Distinct phenotypes are associated with mutations in specific p63 domains, providing clues to structure/function relationships. For example, ankyloblepharon-ectodermal defects-cleft lip/palate (AEC) syndrome is associated with mutations in the SAM domain [40], while ectodermal dysplasia and cleft/lip palate (EEC) syndrome is associated with mutations within the DBD [41, 42]. Not all of the syndromes include skin involvement. Of the syndromes, skin involvement is most pronounced and severe in AEC, which is linked to missense mutations in the SAM domain [40, 43] and therefore implicates the α isoforms.

Unlike normal skin where ΔNp63 expression is associated with the basal proliferative compartment, in AEC patient skin samples, nuclear p63 expression extends beyond the basal layer to the terminally differentiating cells and is accompanied by coexpression of differentiation markers [40]. *In vitro* studies have shown that SAM domain mutations, as seen in AEC, block interaction between p63α and mRNA splicing/processing proteins critical to direct splicing of FGFR-2 to the isoform required for normal epithelial differentiation [44]. Characterization of the AEC L514F ΔNp63α mutant in stable cell lines revealed that activation of a cryptic splice site due to loss of these interactions resulted in production of a C-terminally truncated form of ΔNp63α exclusively located in the nucleus and resistant to proteosome degradation [45]. Mouse models have helped to further define the contribution of this genetic alteration to the phenotype of this syndrome. A knock-in mouse model developed for the L514F mutation recapitulates the expected AEC phenotype including hypoplastic and fragile skin with a transient reduction in proliferation during embryonic development [46]. Skin fragility in these mice, and in humans with AEC syndrome, was associated with altered desmosome gene expression mediated by mutant p63 [47]. To gain insight into further pathways impacted, intact and eroded AEC syndrome skin and normal skin were compared by microarray analysis. The findings revealed changes in expression of genes associated with epidermal adhesion, skin barrier formation, and hair follicle biology, all consistent with the clinical presentation [48]. Thus, SAM domain mutations highlight the importance of p63 and in particular ΔNp63α to normal epidermal morphogenesis/homeostasis.

3.2. p63 in Normal Epidermal Homeostasis. Maintenance of normal epidermal homeostasis involves mediation of processes including proliferation, differentiation, stem cell maintenance, senescence, viability, and cell adhesion. Evidence suggests that each of these is impacted by p63 protein expression (Figure 2). *In vivo*, in the adult human epidermis, p63 is highly expressed in the basal cells with proliferative potential [26] and is downregulated in the suprabasal layers [4]. *In vitro* depletion of p63 in human regenerating organotypic cultures resulted in hypoproliferation and a lack of stratification and differentiation [49]. These effects were found to be mainly due to the ΔNp63α isoform. In a mouse model, specific knockdown of ΔNp63α in the mature epidermis resulted in severe skin fragility with erosion [27]. A multitude of studies, primarily *in vitro*, focused on the downstream targets mediated by ΔNp63α have shed light on the network of target genes implicated in these ΔNp63α-mediated biological processes. While an extensive cataloguing of all of these studies is beyond the scope of this review, some of these studies, with a focus on those performed in keratinocytes, are discussed here to highlight the potential impact of dysregulated ΔNp63α on signaling pathways that may be assessed using mouse models of the skin.

3.2.1. Cell Cycle Regulation. Numerous examples serve to illustrate how perturbation of ΔNp63 expression could result in altered biological outcome. *In vitro*, in developmentally mature murine keratinocytes, we and others demonstrated that ΔNp63α is associated with maintenance of proliferative capacity [49–53]. Mimicking overexpression of ΔNp63α seen in squamous cell carcinomas blocks the normal growth arrest and induction of the cyclin-dependent kinase inhibitor $p21^{WAF1}$ in response to elevated Ca^{2+} conditions [50, 51] and correspondingly suppresses the differentiation markers keratin 10 and filaggrin, but not keratin 1. The α-tail of ΔNp63 is required for its suppressive effect on differentiation but not for the aberrant growth arrest response [51], which may be mediated at least in part by transcriptional repression of $p21^{WAF1}$ by binding of ΔNp63α to its promoter [52]. Regulation of $p21^{WAF1}$ is further impacted by crosstalk between p63 and Notch 1, whereby Notch 1 is negatively regulated by ΔNp63α in cells of high renewal potential but synergizes with ΔNp63α during early differentiation to induce keratin 1. Subsequently, Notch 1 downregulates ΔNp63α to permit the expression of the late differentiation marker involucrin [54]. This context-dependent crosstalk is implicated in maintaining the balance between keratinocyte growth arrest and differentiation.

In addition to the factors regulating $p21^{WAF1}$ described above, a balance exists between ΔNp63α and many other target genes involved in proliferation and differentiation that are critical for maintenance of or for the switch between the states. For example, the cell cycle inhibitor PTEN is negatively regulated by ΔNp63α. Depletion of either ΔNp63α or PTEN alone had opposite effects on colony growth in colony forming assays, but depletion of both ΔNp63α and PTEN at the same time had no impact, implying the balance between the two is critical to biological outcome [55]. Another example focuses on the epidermis of mice with mutant IRF6, which is hyperproliferative and fails to undergo differentiation [56]. This has been attributed to a failure of a feedback loop with ΔNp63α that controls ΔNp63α expression, thereby regulating the switch between proliferation and differentiation. In this feedback loop, IRF6 is a direct transcriptional target of ΔNp63α, which when upregulated induced proteasome-mediated degradation of ΔNp63α allowing for keratinocytes to exit the cell cycle [57]. In addition to regulation of levels of ΔNp63α impacting biological outcome as exemplified by the previous two examples, Runx1, a transcription factor involved both in keratinocyte proliferation and differentiation, is directly differentially regulated by ΔNp63α in proliferating versus differentiating keratinocytes by binding to distinct DNA binding sites on the Runx1 promoter. This represents

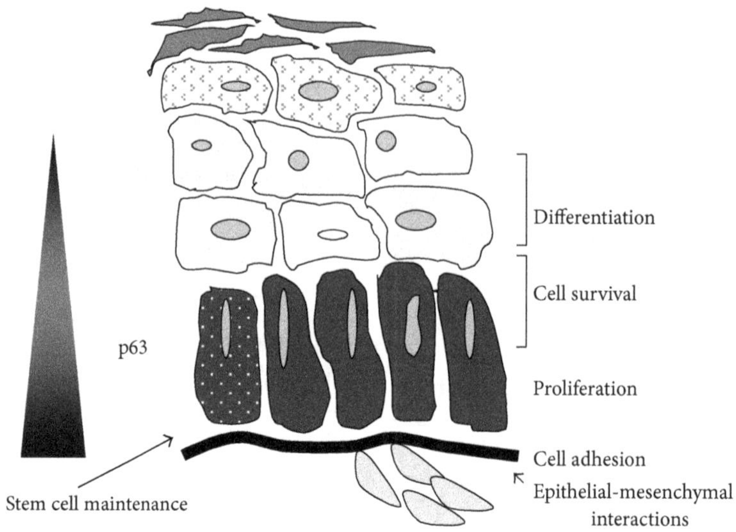

FIGURE 2: p63 impacts multiple biological endpoints involved in normal epidermal homeostasis. Overexpression of ΔNp63*α* impacts pathways that can contribute to cancer development.

a different mechanism of regulation [58], however, one that also could be perturbed by altered expression of ΔNp63*α*.

3.2.2. Differentiation. The mouse models described in Section 3.1.1 support a role for ΔNp63*α* not only in the maintenance of epidermal progenitor cells, but also, in the commitment to stratification. At a molecular level, ΔNp63*α* synergizes with Notch 1 to induce keratin 1 expression during differentiation, and the ΔNp63*α* target gene *IKKα* is necessary for epidermal differentiation [54, 59–63]. However, overexpression of ΔNp63*α* in primary murine keratinocyte cultures blocks expression of keratin 10 and filaggrin, but not keratin 1 [50] implying that a fine balance in levels of ΔNp63*α* is required for complete differentiation. Some examples of transcription factors which based on *in vitro* studies are thought to interplay with ΔNp63*α* during differentiation follow.

Basally expressed keratin 14 is a known direct transcriptional target of ΔNp63*α* [64]. The transcription factor Sknla (Octl1) blocks ΔNp63*α* induction of the keratin 14 promoter and promotes keratin 10 upregulation [65]. There is also evidence for ΔNp63*α* both blocking and inducing transcription factors that promote differentiation in a cell-context-dependent manner. For instance, ΔNp63*α* directly represses high-mobility group box protein 1 (HBP1), a transcription factor necessary for stratification of organotypic cultures [66]. In contrast, in differentiating keratinocytes ΔNp63*α* induces ZNF750, a transcription factor that is required for terminal epidermal differentiation [67]. Interestingly, ZNF750 is bound by ΔNp63*α* in both proliferating and differentiating keratinocytes, but expression is only induced in differentiating cells, suggesting that additional cofactors are involved for distinct biological endpoints. The contribution of cofactors is further exemplified by the case of Alox12, a granular layer protein important for epidermal barrier formation, which is induced by ΔNp63*α* only in differentiating keratinocytes [68].

ΔNp63*α* expression can be regulated at the transcriptional level as well as by altered protein stability, as noted above. Another means of controlling levels of ΔNp63*α* is by microRNAs, short RNA molecules that act as posttranscriptional regulators. They recognize seed sequences in the 3′UTR and serve to block protein translation or decrease RNA stability. Such an interaction was identified as part of a feedback loop between p63 and iASPP, an inhibitory member of the apoptosis stimulating protein of p53 family, critical for epidermal homeostasis [69]. In this loop, iASPP is a direct transcriptional target of p63 that positively regulates ΔNp63 via the repression of miRs 754-3p and 720 to allow for proliferation. Blocking iASPP expression allows for differentiation via upregulation of miRs 754-3p and 720, which downregulate ΔNp63*α*. Other examples include miR203, which directly targets p63 through its 3′UTR for degradation and promotes differentiation by restricting proliferative potential and promoting cell cycle exit [70]. miRs are also regulated by ΔNp63*α*. miR-34a and miR-34c, associated with cell cycle withdrawal, are negatively regulated by ΔNp63*α* [71]. In contrast, miR17, miR20b, miR30a, miR106a, miR143, and miR 455-3p are positively regulated by p63 and critical for the onset of keratinocyte differentiation via modulation of the MAPKs [72].

3.2.3. Epidermal-Dermal Interface and Adhesiveness and Viability. Adhesiveness and cell viability are two additional properties positively impacted by ΔNp63*α*. Epidermal-specific knockdown of ΔNp63 in mature keratinocytes in mice resulted in impaired differentiation and compromised basement membranes [63]. In an *in vitro* model, *Frasl*, which encodes for an extracellular matrix protein, was identified as a ΔNp63*α* regulated gene important for maintaining the epidermal-dermal interface integrity [63]. To maintain this interface, p63 prevents nonepidermal gene expression in keratinocytes via positive regulation of bone morphogenetic protein- (BMP-) 7 [73]. The importance of ΔNp63 in maintaining epithelial-mesenchymal crosstalk was highlighted by the discovery of *interleukin-1 α (Il-1α)* as a p63 target gene. IL-1α induces growth factors in fibroblasts that can bind to receptors on the basal keratinocytes to promote proliferation [74]. Cell-cell adhesiveness was found to be mediated by p63 via Perp, which is a critical desmosomal component for cell-cell adhesion in normal development and in wound healing [75, 76]. With respect to apoptosis, the proapoptotic protein, IGFBP3, is directly repressed by ΔNp63 in both normal and SCC cells [77]. Similarly, downregulation of p63 in primary human foreskin keratinocytes was found to induce apoptosis and to reduce both $\beta 1$ and $\beta 4$ integrin expression [78], linking adhesiveness with viability.

Taken together, the data presented in Sections 3.2.1–3.2.3 demonstrate that the network of genes regulated by ΔNp63α is large and perturbation of the balance between ΔNp63α and members of this network could have adverse biological consequences.

3.3. Stem Cell Maintenance and Senescence. The proliferative lifespan of cells is limited by replicative senescence during which the cells permanently withdraw from the cell cycle, yet remain viable [79, 80]. This phenomenon is associated with the normal ageing process of renewable tissues such as the epidermis. p63 has been proposed as a marker of human epidermal keratinocyte stem cells that is downregulated when keratinocytes become transient amplifying cells [81]. Consistent with these data and the hypothesis that epidermal progenitor cell exhaustion occurs in *p63(−/−)* mice, depletion of p63 in immature human epidermal keratinocytes resulted in reduced clonal growth [82]. Regulation of replicative senescence in human epidermal keratinocytes involves miRs-138, 181a, 181b, and 130b which promote senescence by targeting ΔNp63α and Sirt1 for degradation. However, in a feedback loop, these miRs are themselves targets of negative regulation by ΔNp63α [83]; thus, overexpression of ΔNp63α could also perturb senescence.

Mouse models provide support for a role for p63 in the maintenance of stem cell proliferative capacity. Characteristics of accelerating ageing were noted in *p63(+/−)* mice observed for extended periods generated by two groups using the mice developed by both Yang et al. and Mills et al. [3, 25, 84, 85]. Germline or somatic *p63* depletion under control of the keratin 5 promoter gave rise to enhanced senescence marker expression [84], suggesting a role for p63 in the negative regulation of senescence. Indeed, overexpression of ΔNp63α in primary mouse keratinocytes overcame replicative senescence in association with delayed and diminished induction of INK4/p16 and Arf/p19 [86]. Consistent with these findings, crossing of *p63(−/−)* mice developed by Yang et al. [3] with *INK4/p16(−/−)* or *Arf/p19(−/−)* mice was able to partially rescue the proliferation and differentiation defects observed in *p63(−/−)* mice [87], reinforcing a role for p63 in blocking senescence. While these mice display reepithelialization, skin from *p63(−/−)* mice crossed with *Ink4a/p16(−/−)* or *Arf/p19(−/−)* mice is fragile and easily detachable, suggestive of defective adhesion, which also can be attributed to p63.

In the mouse models described above, all p63 isoforms were knocked down. A TAp63-specific knockdown mouse model that supports a role for TAp63 in adult stem cell maintenance was generated by crossing TAp63 floxed mice with germline-specific promoter cre or keratin 14-cre mice [37]. *TAp63(−/−)* mice exhibited signs of premature ageing. Interestingly, overexpression of ΔNp63α under control of the keratin 14 promoter resulted in a phenotype similar to that reported in mice lacking TAp63 [88]. Skin-derived precursor (SKP) cells are multipotent precursor cells derived from the dermis that can differentiate into mesodermal and neural cells [89]. In the *TAp63(−/−)* mice, SKP cells proliferate more rapidly than wild-type SKP cells, and thus, undergo senescence more rapidly. As adult stem cell populations are not immortal, this enhanced proliferation in *TAp63(−/−)* cells would be expected to lead to stem cell exhaustion, which is associated with accelerated ageing.

4. p63 and Neoplasia

4.1. Observational Studies of Human Tumors. The *p53* tumor suppressor gene is commonly mutated in human cancer [1]. Due to the similarity of the TAp63 isoforms with p53, it was hypothesized that mutation of *p63* could provide a mechanistic explanation for tumors in which *p53* was not mutated. It was found, instead, that mutation of *p63* is a rare event in human cancer cell lines [90], but that p63 overexpression is seen in human squamous cell cancers including esophageal squamous cell carcinoma [91, 92], nasopharyngeal carcinoma [93], and squamous cell carcinoma of the skin [94, 95]. Overexpression of the ΔNp63 protein in primary squamous cell carcinomas (SCCs) of the head, neck, and lung correlates with amplification of the p63 gene locus, which occurs frequently in these cancers [28, 96]. While there is agreement that ΔNp63α is overexpressed in lung SCCs, conflicting results have been published as to whether this correlates with prognosis [96, 97].

In squamous cell carcinomas of the skin, a significant increase in p63 expression, both in terms of intensity and distribution, is seen relative to normal skin, as the proliferative fraction is expanded in tumors [26, 95]. Examination of skin lesions ranging from keratoacanthoma to a grade IV spindle cell carcinoma revealed very strong p63 immunoreactivity in grade 3 SCC with decrease in a single grade IV spindle SCC. In these tumors, carcinoma *in situ* was characterized by p63 immunoreactivity in all layers [94]. While ΔNp63α was shown to be the most overexpressed isoform in squamous cell tumors, careful characterization of the TA and ΔN isoforms from different tissue and tumor types revealed that individual isoforms are differentially expressed in the neoplastic transformation of different tissue types [98], implying specific contributions of the isoform expressed in a context-dependent manner. While ΔNp63α is overexpressed in primary skin tumors, expression of TAp63 is not a common event but has been reported to be downregulated relative to normal skin using PCR-based methods [99]. It is clear that ΔNp63α is overexpressed in skin SCCs, however, whether it actively plays a role in tumor formation or is a bystander has been unclear. Further insight into this question has been gained by *in vitro* and *in vivo* studies, as discussed below.

4.2. In Vitro/Molecular Studies with Human Cancer Cell Lines and Primary Keratinocytes

4.2.1. Impact on Signaling Pathways. In particular, *in vitro* studies in SCC cells have provided insight into the potential signaling pathways impacted by p63 dysregulation in squamous cell carcinoma. As discussed previously, IRF6 is involved in a negative feedback loop with ΔNp63α that is necessary for the downregulation of ΔNp63α seen with differentiation [57], and an appropriate balance between these factors is required for the switch between proliferation and differentiation in the normal epidermis [100]. Correspondingly, expression of IRF6 was found to be strongly downregulated in human SCC [101]. Reexpression of IRF-6 in the context of primary human keratinocytes expressing both ΔNp63α and a mutant v-ras 12 oncogene was found to abolish the ability of ΔNp63α to promote colony growth and restore oncogene induced senescence [101], supporting a role for IRF6 in regulating ΔNp63α as part of its tumor suppressor function. In other studies, ΔNp63α has been shown to upregulate Hsp70, a protein colocalized with ΔNp63 in primary SCCs of the head and neck (HNSCCs) that is associated with proliferation and viability of HNSCC [102]. Likewise, accumulation of β-catenin in the nucleus and activation of downstream signaling pathways common to many cancers are induced by ΔNp63α in HNSCC cells [103].

Consistent with a role in promoting adhesion, ΔNp63 is negatively regulated by the epithelial-to-mesenchymal transition (EMT) promoting transcription factors snail and slug, and this association is observed in primary human cervical, head and neck, and esophageal SCCs. This decrease in ΔNp63α is associated with increased migration in SCC cell lines [104]. ΔNp63α also physically sequesters YB-1, a positive translational mediator of snail, thereby preventing both enhanced snail activity and YB1's function in actin cytoskeleton reorganization, both of which lead to cancer cell migration and invasion [105]. Another direct transcriptional target of ΔNp63α is the vitamin D receptor (VDR) [106], which is induced by multiple p63 isoforms. Downregulation of VDR expression results in increased cell migration of A431 epidermoid carcinoma cells, which can be rescued by ΔNp63α or VDR [107]. A role for ΔNp63α in preventing metastasis is further supported by the finding that antagonism of ΔNp63α by mutant-p53/Smad complex allows TGF-β to convert from a tumor suppressor role to a role in promoting metastases [108]. In line with this, knockdown of p63 in squamous cancer cell lines, in which the predominant isoform expressed was ΔNp63, led to an increase of mesenchymal and neural markers and upregulation of genes associated with invasion and motility [109].

Based on the data, it is enticing to contemplate that ΔNp63α plays a role in cancer development by promoting proliferation and viability at earlier stages, while it may need to be downregulated during progression to allow for the necessary enhanced motility, invasiveness, and EMT [110] that allow metastases to form.

4.2.2. Altered Responsiveness to Genotoxic Stress. ΔNp63α can impact cellular response to genotoxic stress. A mouse model in which ΔNp63 was overexpressed under control of the loricrin promoter showed that downregulation of ΔNp63 is required for UVB-induced apoptosis of the epidermis [111]. Mechanistically, degradation of ΔNp63α in keratinocytes exposed to apoptotic doses of UV was shown to be mediated by p38 MAPK, which phosphorylates ΔNp63α. This led to its detachment from p53-dependent promoters and results in apoptosis induction [112]. Consistent with this report, occupancy of binding sites involved in cell cycle arrest and apoptosis switched following adriamycin or UV treatment of human epidermal keratinocytes from ΔNp63α to p53 occupancy, which would be expected to result in increased apoptosis or cell cycle arrest [113].

Many therapeutic agents used in cancer treatment promote genotoxic stress as a means to reduce or control tumor growth. Expression of high levels of ΔNp63α predicts responsiveness of primary HNSCC to platinum-based therapies [114]. Upon exposure to cisplatin, ΔNp63α is proteosomally degraded via stratifin-mediated nuclear export and Rackl targeting [114, 115]. An interaction between the p63 proteins and the NF-κB pathway also plays a role in responsiveness to chemotherapeutics. In JHU-022 oral cavity SCC cells, IKKβ, a known activator of RelA, promotes ΔNp63α degradation in response to cisplatin [116]. In this cell line, cisplatin treatment resulted in a physical interaction between RelA and ΔNp63α that abrogates ΔNp63α mediated $p21^{WAF1}$ promoter repression and targets ΔNp63α for proteosomal degradation [117]. The presence of c-Abl, which has been implicated as an oncogene, in HNSCC cells treated with cisplatin stabilizes ΔNp63α expression. This stabilization of ΔNp63α leads to enhanced cell viability [118], which could be anticipated to result in clinical consequences.

Survival of HNSCC cells that overexpress ΔNp63α is dependent on the presence of ΔNp63α, which functions by blocking TAp73-driven apoptosis both via promoter binding and physical interaction with p73 in a p53-independent manner [119]. TAp73 and ΔNp63α are engaged in a feedback loop involving miR-193a-5p, which is repressed by ΔNp63α and activated by TAp73 and targets the p73 UTR. Cisplatin treatment results in ΔNp63α degradation and TAp73-mediated activation of miR-193a-5p, limiting TAp73's pro-apoptotic effects and chemosensitivity [23]. Reimplantation in the presence or absence of a miR-193a-5p antagomir of disaggregated cells from primary mouse SCCs generated by a chemical carcinogenesis protocol revealed that knockdown of this miR resulted in reduced tumor formation and enhanced chemosensitivity [23], indicating that a strategy targeting both ΔNp63α and miR-193a-5p might be more effective in this scenario. HNSCC cells can circumvent the requirement for ΔNp63α expression for survival by the overexpression of Bcl2 [119]. In addition to blocking p73 to promote survival of

HNSCC, ΔNp63α associates with histone deacetylase 1 and 2 forming an apoptotic transcriptional repressor complex. This complex is sensitive to breakdown by cisplatin and HDAC inhibitors, in the presence of low, but not high, levels of endogenous Bcl-2 indicating once again that the context of the tumor impacts the success of chemotherapy [120]. Unlike the case of TAp73 described above, in HaCaT cells in response to chemotherapy, ΔNp63α is involved in an antiapoptotic feedback loop in which it, as well as mutant p53, induces ΔNp63α [24]. Thus, response to genotoxic stress is another biological endpoint that can be impacted by dysregulated ΔNp63α.

4.3. Modeling Human Cancers in Mouse to Assess the Contribution of p63 to Neoplasia. Cancer arises as a multistep process that can be reiterated in well-established mouse models in a controlled fashion [121]. Results of the studies presented above suggest that TAp63 would harbor tumor suppressor properties and overexpressed ΔNp63 would harbor oncogenic properties. In this section, we highlight the use of mouse models to dissect out how altered p63 levels contribute biologically to prevention or development of cancer, either alone or in altered balance with other family members or other oncogenic pathways. Approaches discussed utilize mice with a heterozygous null mutation in *p63* on a background of wild type, *p53(+/−)* and/or *p73(+/−)*; TA-isoform-specific knockout mice; and mouse models where the elevated levels of ΔNp63α observed in human SCC are mimicked in cultured keratinocytes and transplanted to nude mice.

4.3.1. TAp63 as a Tumor Suppressor. The potential role for physiological levels of p63 acting as a tumor suppressor with respect to spontaneous tumor development was explored by two groups in the context of alteration of other p53 family members [85, 122]. In a mouse model in which the *p63* genotype was contributed by mice developed by Yang et al. [3], mice heterozygous for a null mutation in both *p63* and *p73* displayed a higher incidence of spontaneous tumor formation relative to wild-type mice. Furthermore, mice heterozygous for *p53*, *p63*, and *p73* developed a higher incidence and formed more aggressive tumors than mice heterozygous for the *p53* null mutation alone. These findings suggest that p63 and p73 share a tumor suppressor role as has been long established for p53 [1, 85]. In the absence of additional genetic mutations, these *p63(+/−)* mice developed squamous cell carcinomas (10%), adenomas (15%), and histiocytic sarcomas (20%) at 10%, 15%, and 20% greater rates, respectively, than wild type. In contrast, in a study using mice with a p63 genotype contributed by the mice developed by Mills et al. [25], *p63(+/−)/p53(+/−)* mice were found to be less prone to spontaneous tumors than p53 +/− mice alone. Additionally, these *p63(+/−)* mice were shown to have decreased susceptibility to chemically induced carcinogenesis, suggesting that p63 does not contribute a tumor suppressor activity in cancer. To date, this controversy remains unresolved.

In the mouse models described above, all p63 isoforms were targeted. TAp63-subclass-specific knockdown mice allow distinction between the TA and ΔN subclass properties. Following observation for 2.5 years, an enhanced incidence of carcinoma, including SCC of the skin and sarcoma development, was observed in *TAp63(+/−)* and *TAp63(−/−)* mice relative to wild-type mice [123], again supporting a tumor suppressive role for TAp63. It was noted that tumors from the *TAp63(+/−)* and *TAp63(−/−)* mice were highly metastatic, and at a mechanistic level TAp63 was found to positively regulate Dicer, a protein critical for miR processing, and miR 130b. Reexpression of both Dicer and miR130b in *TAp63(−/−)* MEFs decreased invasiveness of these cells, suggesting that TAp63's tumor suppressor role could be mediated at least in part through Dicer and miR130b [123]. As mentioned previously, miR130b targets ΔNp63α for degradation [83].

4.3.2. Overexpressed ΔNp63α Facilitates Tumor Progression. The mouse models described above focused on the TAp63 isoforms and were performed at wild-type or decreased levels of endogenous p63. However, overexpression of ΔNp63α is a common event in squamous cancers. Two independent studies have used similar approaches to mimic this overexpression with the goal of examining the *in vivo* functional consequences of ΔNp63α overexpression in the epidermis. Results from both lab groups support a contributory role for ΔNp63α in the cancer phenotype with mechanistic distinctions. In studies performed in our laboratory, wild-type primary murine keratinocytes were transduced with retrovirus encoding a v-rasHA oncogene in combination with a lentivirus encoding either a control GFP construct or ΔNp63α and grafted onto the dorsum of nude mice in combination with primary dermal fibroblasts [86]. This model allows growth of normal keratinocytes as well as benign and malignant tumor phenotypes in the graft site. Mice were observed up to a month following cell grafting for tumor formation. No lesions were observed in graft sites following transplantation of keratinocytes expressing only GFP or ΔNp63α alone. Grafting of keratinocytes expressing v-Ras^{HA} + GFP resulted, as expected, in the formation of well differentiated papillomas, while grafting of keratinocytes expressing v-Ras^{HA} + ΔNp63α resulted in 100% malignant conversion to carcinoma [86]. Although elevated levels of ΔNp63α alone are insufficient to confer a tumor phenotype *in vivo*, we found that ΔNp63α blocks oncogene-induced senescence by inhibiting p16^{ink4a}/p19^{arf} pathways and cooperates with oncogenic v-Ras^{HA} to enhance malignant conversion *in vivo*. This study supports a contributory role for ΔNp63α in cancer pathogenesis and a mechanistic link to cell survival by overriding oncogene-induced senescence through inhibition of p16^{ink4a} and p19^{arf}, key mediators of cellular senescence.

Using a similar approach, Keyes et al. [124] demonstrated that overexpressing ΔNp63α in keratinocytes in the presence of oncogenic ras resulted in growth of malignant carcinomas following subcutaneous injection. In this study also, the malignant phenotype was associated with a bypass of oncogene-induced senescence. Overexpression of ΔNp63α was further shown to enhance stem-like proliferation of keratinocytes and maintain survival of the keratin 15-positive stem cell population. Furthermore, chromatin-remodeling protein Lsh was identified as a new target of ΔNp63α and as an essential mediator of senescence bypass. Although p19^{arf} was not detectable in the tumors derived from ras/ΔNp63α keratinocytes in this study, an *in vitro* component of the study indicated that p16^{ink4a} and p19^{arf} were not reduced during the initial stages of senescence bypass. Therefore, contrary to our study, it was proposed that the initiating events through which ΔNp63α inhibits senescence do not occur via p16^{ink4a}/p19^{arf} pathways. Although the difference in p16^{ink4a}/p19^{arf} between these two studies may be due to the different time courses used, it further indicates the complexity of the pathways interacting with p63 family members and underscores the need for additional studies to understand the role of p63 and its downstream effectors in tumorigenesis and senescence.

An oncogenic role for ΔNp63 is further supported by studies in a mouse model containing a dominant negative 14-3-3σ mutation (*Er/+*). 14-3-3σ, a protein associated with keratinocyte differentiation, is a direct target for ΔNp63α repression in undifferentiated human epidermal keratinocytes [52]. Treatment of *Er/+* mice on a *p63(+/+)* background with a two-stage carcinogenesis protocol resulted in the formation of tumors in which ΔNp63α was strongly expressed, while loss of function of an endogenous allele of p63 in this context, which generated (*Er/+/p63+/−*) mice, resulted in reduced sensitivity to this protocol, suggestive of cooperation of ΔNp63α in Ras/14-3-3σ-induced tumorigenesis [125].

A Role for NF-κB/c-Rel in ΔNp63α-Mediated Carcinogenesis. In a transcription factor profiling exercise, we identified activation of NF-κB in keratinocytes following the overexpression of ΔNp63α. The NF-κB family comprises 5 members functioning as hetero- and homodimers [126]. Only NF-κB/c-Rel was found to be modulated by ΔNp63α under these conditions, with nuclear accumulation of phosphorylated c-Rel but none of the other NFκB subunits enhanced in the presence of overexpressed ΔNp63α. NF-κB is associated with multiple human diseases, including cancer, for which therapeutics targeting its constitutive NF-κB activation are under development [127, 128]. Of the five family members, RelA, p50, and c-Rel subunits have been implicated in the maintenance of normal epidermal homeostasis [129, 130], and in SCC, the RelA/p50 heterodimer has been shown to promote or repress malignancy in a context-dependent manner [131, 132]. Nuclear c-Rel expression is associated with both solid breast tumors and hematopoietic malignancies [133]; however, it had not previously been investigated in SCC of the skin. The increase in nuclear c-Rel accumulation seen with elevated ΔNp63α levels was found to be critical to the ability of ΔNp63α overexpressing keratinocytes to proliferate under conditions that normally induce growth arrest [134]. Mechanistically, this is correlated with a physical interaction between ΔNp63α and c-Rel on the promoter of the p21^{WAF1} gene in these cells, both *in vitro* and *in vivo*, which represses p21^{WAF1} expression. These findings extended to primary human HNSCC, in which we found that ΔNp63α and c-Rel colocalized in the nuclei throughout the tumor sections, as opposed to a more restricted expression in normal tissue.

In an extension of these studies, Lu et al. characterized a dynamic mechanism whereby c-Rel, ΔNp63α, and TAp73, which are coexpressed in the nuclei of a subset of HNSCC cell lines, control expression on binding sites including p21^{WAF1}, Noxa, and Puma [135]. Exposure of HNSCC cell line cultures to TNF-α to mimic inflammation in the tumor environment was found to induce nuclear accumulation of c-Rel. In the absence of this stimulus, ΔNp63α was found to physically interact with TAp73. Similar to our results in untreated primary keratinocytes upon overexpression of ΔNp63α, a physical interaction between endogenous ΔNp63α and c-Rel was observed following TNF-α treatment in these HNSCC cell lines. Interestingly, under conditions of c-Rel overexpression, the interaction between ΔNp63α and TAp73 was blocked and TAp73 was translocated to the cytoplasm. This suggests that c-Rel displaces TAp73. ChIP assays indicated that this regulation occurred on the promoters of genes involved in growth arrest and apoptosis, resulting in their downregulation [135].

5. Summary/Future Directions: Challenging *In Vitro* Findings in *In Vivo Models*

Primary murine cell cultures and *in vivo* murine models have been instrumental in elucidating the multistep nature of carcinogenesis [121] and in challenging the role of specific genetic alterations, such as those observed in *p63*, in cancer pathogenesis [86, 124]. The mouse models described in this review have provided us with a clear picture of the importance of p63 to normal epidermal development and homeostasis and have highlighted the roles for specific p63 isoforms in neoplasia. However, given the complexity of the p63 family members, their interactions, and the context-specific manner in which they can exert their effects, much remains to be defined.

Mouse models with molecular alterations that allow targeting of specific gene products will be indispensible in deepening our understanding of and resolving controversy related to the role of *p63* both in normal tissue and in disease. Once a pathway has been implicated, primary cultures from mouse epidermis can be readily manipulated to express or eliminate a particular protein presumed active upstream or downstream to assess the impact. Applied in combination with keratinocytes from genetically altered mice, both *in vitro* and *in vivo* findings can be challenged further for the consequences of the alterations. However, it is important to remember that all models have limitations, and a deeper understanding of the role of p63 in normal epidermal homeostasis and neoplasia will ultimately be derived from an iterative process involving *in vitro* observations in primary cells, cell lines and primary tumors, *in vivo* queries of these findings, and reexamination of the outcomes in the context of human tumors. Mouse models comprise a critical component of this process.

As an example, the observation in primary mouse keratinocytes that c-Rel acts downstream of ΔNp63α in modulating keratinocyte growth regulation led to a further novel observation that c-Rel levels are enhanced in primary

HNSCC of humans and links this protein accumulation to altered NFκB/c-Rel activity in human head and neck squamous cell cancer cells [134]. The requirement for c-Rel in these cancers can be tested by modulating c-Rel and ΔNp63α independently using lentiviral gene transduction followed by grafting. Long-term overexpression of ΔNp63α has been shown to support sustained high levels of nuclear c-Rel expression, and c-Rel shRNA lentiviruses are capable of depleting c-Rel in keratinocytes for extended time (unpublished observations). Assessing the impact of these modulations *in vivo* will clarify the interplay between these alterations and their relevance to cancer development and progression.

References

[1] B. Vogelstein, D. Lane, and A. J. Levine, "Surfing the p53 network," *Nature*, vol. 408, no. 6810, pp. 307–310, 2000.

[2] A. Yang, N. Walker, R. Bronson et al., "p73-Deficient mice have neurological, pheromonal and inflammatory defects but lack spontaneous tumours," *Nature*, vol. 404, no. 6773, pp. 99–103, 2000.

[3] A. Yang, R. Schweitzer, D. Sun et al., "p63 is essential for regenerative proliferation in limb, craniofacial and epithelial development," *Nature*, vol. 398, no. 6729, pp. 714–718, 1999.

[4] A. Yang, M. Kaghad, Y. Wang et al., "p63, a p53 homolog at 3q27-29, encodes multiple products with transactivating, death-inducing, and dominant-negative activities," *Molecular Cell*, vol. 2, no. 3, pp. 305–316, 1998.

[5] M. Kaghad, H. Bonnet, A. Yang et al., "Monoallelically expressed gene related to p53 at 1p36, a region frequently deleted in neuroblastoma and other human cancers," *Cell*, vol. 90, no. 4, pp. 809–819, 1997.

[6] M. Dohn, S. Zhang, and X. Chen, "p63α and ΔNp63α can induce cell cycle arrest and apoptosis and differentially regulate p53 target genes," *Oncogene*, vol. 20, no. 25, pp. 3193–3205, 2001.

[7] E. S. Helton, J. Zhu, and X. Chen, "The unique NH2-terminally deleted (ΔN) residues, the PXXP motif, and the PPXY motif are required for the transcriptional activity of the ΔN variant of p63," *Journal of Biological Chemistry*, vol. 281, no. 5, pp. 2533–2542, 2006.

[8] P. Ghioni, F. Bolognese, P. H. G. Duijf, H. Van Bokhoven, R. Mantovani, and L. Guerrini, "Complex transcriptional effects of p63 isoforms: identification of novel activation and repression domains," *Molecular and Cellular Biology*, vol. 22, no. 24, pp. 8659–8668, 2002.

[9] M. Mangiulli, A. Valletti, M. F. Caratozzolo et al., "Identification and functional characterization of two new transcriptional variants of the human p63 gene," *Nucleic Acids Research*, vol. 37, no. 18, pp. 6092–6104, 2009.

[10] C. D. Thanos and J. U. Bowie, "p53 Family members p63 and p73 are SAM domain-containing proteins," *Protein Science*, vol. 8, no. 8, pp. 1708–1710, 1999.

[11] Z. Serber, H. C. Lai, A. Yang et al., "A C-terminal inhibitory domain controls the activity of p63 by an intramolecular mechanism," *Molecular and Cellular Biology*, vol. 22, no. 24, pp. 8601–8611, 2002.

[12] W. E. Straub, T. A. Weber, B. Schäfer et al., "The C-terminus of p63 contains multiple regulatory elements with different functions," *Cell Death and Disease*, vol. 1, no. 1, article e5, 2010.

[13] P. Ghioni, Y. D'Alessandra, G. Mansueto et al., "The protein stability and transcriptional activity of p63α are regulated by SUMO-1 conjugation," *Cell Cycle*, vol. 4, no. 1, pp. 183–190, 2005.

[14] M. Rossi, R. I. Aqeilan, M. Neale et al., "The E3 ubiquitin ligase Itch controls the protein stability of p63," *Proceedings of the National Academy of Sciences of the United States of America*, vol. 103, no. 34, pp. 12753–12758, 2006.

[15] F. Galli, M. Rossi, Y. D'Alessandra et al., "MDM2 and Fbw7 cooperate to induce p63 protein degradation following DNA damage and cell differentiation," *Journal of Cell Science*, vol. 123, no. 14, pp. 2423–2433, 2010.

[16] D. Coutandin, F. Löhr, F. H. Niesen et al., "Conformational stability and activity of p73 require a second helix in the tetramerization domain," *Cell Death and Differentiation*, vol. 16, no. 12, pp. 1582–1589, 2009.

[17] E. A. Ratovitski, M. Patturajan, K. Hibi, B. Trink, K. Yamaguchi, and D. Sidransky, "p53 associates with and targets ΔNp63 into a protein degradation pathway," *Proceedings of the National Academy of Sciences of the United States of America*, vol. 98, no. 4, pp. 1817–1822, 2001.

[18] S. Strano, G. Fontemaggi, A. Costanzo et al., "Physical interaction with human tumor-derived p53 mutants inhibits p63 activities," *Journal of Biological Chemistry*, vol. 277, no. 21, pp. 18817–18826, 2002.

[19] M. Osada, H. L. Park, Y. Nagakawa et al., "Differential recognition of response elements determines target gene specificity for p53 and p63," *Molecular and Cellular Biology*, vol. 25, no. 14, pp. 6077–6089, 2005.

[20] C. A. Perez, J. Ott, D. J. Mays, and J. A. Pietenpol, "p63 consensus DNA-binding site: identification, analysis and application into a p63MH algorithm," *Oncogene*, vol. 26, no. 52, pp. 7363–7370, 2007.

[21] K. Ortt and S. Sinha, "Derivation of the consensus DNA-binding sequence for p63 reveals unique requirements that are distinct from p53," *FEBS Letters*, vol. 580, no. 18, pp. 4544–4550, 2006.

[22] A. Yang, Z. Zhu, A. Kettenbach et al., "Genome-wide mapping indicates that p73 and p63 Co-occupy target sites and have similar DNA-binding profiles *in vivo*," *PLoS ONE*, vol. 5, no. 7, Article ID e11572, 2010.

[23] B. Ory, M. R. Ramsey, C. Wilson et al., "A microRNA-dependent program controls p53-independent survival and chemosensitivity in human and murine squamous cell carcinoma," *Journal of Clinical Investigation*, vol. 121, no. 2, pp. 809–820, 2011.

[24] M. Lanza, B. Marinari, M. Papoutsaki et al., "Cross-talks in the p53 family: ΔNp63 is an anti-apoptotic target for ΔNp73α and p53 gain-of-function mutants," *Cell Cycle*, vol. 5, no. 17, pp. 1996–2004, 2006.

[25] A. A. Mills, B. Zheng, X. J. Wang, H. Vogel, D. R. Roop, and A. Bradley, "p63 is a p53 homologue required for limb and epidermal morphogenesis," *Nature*, vol. 398, no. 6729, pp. 708–713, 1999.

[26] R. Parsa, A. Yang, F. McKeon, and H. Green, "Association of p63 with proliferative potential in normal and neoplastic human keratinocytes," *Journal of Investigative Dermatology*, vol. 113, no. 6, pp. 1099–1105, 1999.

[27] M. I. Koster, B. Marinari, A. S. Payne, P. N. Kantaputra, A. Costanzo, and D. R. Roop, "ΔNp63 knockdown mice: a mouse model for AEC syndrome," *American Journal of Medical Genetics A*, vol. 149, no. 9, pp. 1942–1947, 2009.

[28] K. Hibi, B. Trink, M. Patturajan et al., "AIS is an oncogene amplified in squamous cell carcinoma," *Proceedings of the*

National Academy of Sciences of the United States of America, vol. 97, no. 10, pp. 5462–5467, 2000.

[29] S. Wolff, F. Talos, G. Palacios, U. Beyer, M. Dobbelstein, and U. M. Moll, "The α/β carboxy-terminal domains of p63 are required for skin and limb development. New insights from the Brdm2 mouse which is not a complete p63 knockout but expresses p63 γ-like proteins," *Cell Death and Differentiation*, vol. 16, no. 8, pp. 1108–1117, 2009.

[30] M. L. Mikkola, A. Costanzo, I. Thesleff, D. R. Roop, and M. I. Koster, "Treasure or artifact: a decade of p63 research speaks for itself," *Cell Death and Differentiation*, vol. 17, no. 1, pp. 180–183, 2010.

[31] F. Talos, S. Wolff, U. Beyer, M. Dobbelstein, and U. M. Moll, "Brdm2-an aberrant hypomorphic p63 allele," *Cell Death and Differentiation*, vol. 17, no. 1, pp. 184–186, 2010.

[32] R. Shalom-Feuerstein, A. M. Lena, H. Zhou et al., "Δnp63 is an ectodermal gatekeeper of epidermal morphogenesis," *Cell Death and Differentiation*, vol. 18, no. 5, pp. 887–896, 2011.

[33] D. Aberdam and R. Mantovani, "A new p63-deficient mouse model or a fresh look at an old one?" *Cell Death and Differentiation*, vol. 16, no. 8, pp. 1073–1074, 2009.

[34] M. I. Koster, S. Kim, A. A. Mills, F. J. DeMayo, and D. R. Roop, "p63 is the molecular switch for initiation of an epithelial stratification program," *Genes and Development*, vol. 18, no. 2, pp. 126–131, 2004.

[35] R. A. Romano, K. Ortt, B. Birkaya, K. Smalley, and S. Sinha, "An active role of the ΔN isoform of p63 in regulating basal keratin genes K5 and K14 and directing epidermal cell fate," *PLoS ONE*, vol. 4, no. 5, Article ID e5623, 2009.

[36] E. Candi, A. Rufini, A. Terrinoni et al., "Differential roles of p63 isoforms in epidermal development: selective genetic complementation in p63 null mice," *Cell Death and Differentiation*, vol. 13, no. 6, pp. 1037–1047, 2006.

[37] X. Su, M. Paris, Y. J. Gi et al., "TAp63 prevents premature aging by promoting adult stem cell maintenance," *Cell Stem Cell*, vol. 5, no. 1, pp. 64–75, 2009.

[38] R. A. Romano, K. Smalley, C. Magraw et al., "DeltaNp63 knockout mice reveal its indispensable role as a master regulator of epithelial development and differentiation," *Development*, vol. 139, pp. 772–782, 2012.

[39] T. Rinne, H. G. Brunner, and H. Van Bokhoven, "p63-associated disorders," *Cell Cycle*, vol. 6, no. 3, pp. 262–268, 2007.

[40] J. A. McGrath, P. H. G. Duijf, V. Doetsch et al., "Hay-Wells syndrome is caused by heterozygous missense mutations in the SAM domain of p63," *Human Molecular Genetics*, vol. 10, no. 3, pp. 221–229, 2001.

[41] J. Celli, P. Duijf, B. C. J. Hamel et al., "Heterozygous germline mutations in the p53 homolog p63 are the cause of EEC syndrome," *Cell*, vol. 99, no. 2, pp. 143–153, 1999.

[42] H. Van Bokhoven, B. C. J. Hamel, M. Bamshad et al., "p63 gene mutations in EEC syndrome, limb-mammary syndrome, and isolated split hand-split foot malformation suggest a genotype-phenotype correlation," *American Journal of Human Genetics*, vol. 69, no. 3, pp. 481–492, 2001.

[43] H. G. Brunner, B. C. J. Hamel, and H. Van Bokhoven, "The p63 gene in EEC and other syndromes," *Journal of Medical Genetics*, vol. 39, no. 6, pp. 377–381, 2002.

[44] A. Fomenkov, Y. P. Huang, O. Topaloglu et al., "p63α mutations lead to aberrant splicing of keratinocyte growth factor receptor in the Hay-Wells syndrome," *Journal of Biological Chemistry*, vol. 278, no. 26, pp. 23906–23914, 2003.

[45] Y. P. Huang, Y. Kim, Z. Li, T. Fomenkov, A. Fomenkov, and E. A. Ratovitski, "AEC-associated p63 mutations lead to alternative splicing/protein stabilization of p63 and modulation of notch signaling," *Cell Cycle*, vol. 4, no. 10, pp. 1440–1447, 2005.

[46] G. Ferone, H. A. Thomason, D. Antonini et al., "Mutant p63 causes defective expansion of ectodermal progenitor cells and impaired FGF signalling in AEC syndrome," *EMBO Molecular Medicine*, vol. 4, pp. 192–205, 2012.

[47] G. Ferone, M. R. Mollo, H. A. Thomason et al., "p63 control of desmosome gene expression and adhesion is compromised in AEC syndrome," *Human Molecular Genetics*, vol. 22, pp. 531–543, 2012.

[48] S. E. Clements, T. Techanukul, J. E. Lai-Cheong et al., "Mutations in AEC syndrome skin reveal a role for p63 in basement membrane adhesion, skin barrier integrity and hair follicle biology," *British Journal of Dermatology*, vol. 167, pp. 134–144, 2012.

[49] A. B. Truong, M. Kretz, T. W. Ridky, R. Kimmel, and P. A. Khavari, "p63 regulates proliferation and differentiation of developmentally mature keratinocytes," *Genes and Development*, vol. 20, no. 22, pp. 3185–3197, 2006.

[50] K. E. King, R. M. Ponnamperuma, T. Yamashita et al., "ΔNp63α functions as both a positive and a negative transcriptional regulator and blocks *in vitro* differentiation of murine keratinocytes," *Oncogene*, vol. 22, no. 23, pp. 3635–3644, 2003.

[51] K. E. King, R. M. Ponnamperuma, M. J. Gerdes et al., "Unique domain functions of p63 isotypes that differentially regulate distinct aspects of epidermal homeostasis," *Carcinogenesis*, vol. 27, no. 1, pp. 53–63, 2006.

[52] M. D. Westfall, D. J. Mays, J. C. Sniezek, and J. A. Pietenpol, "The ΔNp63α phosphoprotein binds the p21 and 14-3-3σ promoters *in vivo* and has transcriptional repressor activity that is reduced by Hay-Wells syndrome-derived mutations," *Molecular and Cellular Biology*, vol. 23, no. 7, pp. 2264–2276, 2003.

[53] M. P. DeYoung, C. M. Johannessen, C. O. Leong, W. Faquin, J. W. Rocco, and L. W. Ellisen, "Tumor-specific p73 up-regulation mediates p63 dependence in squamous cell carcinoma," *Cancer Research*, vol. 66, no. 19, pp. 9362–9368, 2006.

[54] B. C. Nguyen, K. Lefort, A. Mandinova et al., "Cross-regulation between Notch and p63 in keratinocyte commitment to differentiation," *Genes and Development*, vol. 20, no. 8, pp. 1028–1042, 2006.

[55] M. K. Leonard, R. Kommagani, V. Payal, L. D. Mayo, H. N. Shamma, and M. P. Kadakia, "DeltaNp63alpha regulates keratinocyte proliferation by controlling PTEN expression and localization," *Cell Death & Differentiation*, vol. 18, pp. 1924–1933, 2011.

[56] R. J. Richardson, J. Dixon, S. Malhotra et al., "Irf6 is a key determinant of the keratinocyte proliferation-differentiation switch," *Nature Genetics*, vol. 38, no. 11, pp. 1329–1334, 2006.

[57] F. Moretti, B. Marinari, N. L. Iacono et al., "A regulatory feedback loop involving p63 and IRF6 links the pathogenesis of 2 genetically different human ectodermal dysplasias," *Journal of Clinical Investigation*, vol. 120, no. 5, pp. 1570–1577, 2010.

[58] I. Masse, L. Barbollat-Boutrand, M. Molina et al., "Functional interplay between p63 and p53 controls RUNX1 function in the transition from proliferation to differentiation in human keratinocytes," *Cell Death & Disease*, vol. 3, article e318, 2012.

[59] Y. Xin, Q. Lu, and Q. Li, "IKK1 control of epidermal differentiation is modulated by Notch signaling," *American Journal of Pathology*, vol. 178, no. 4, pp. 1568–1577, 2011.

[60] S. Liu, Z. Chen, F. Zhu, and Y. Hu, "IkappaB kinase alpha and cancer," *Journal of Interferon & Cytokine Research*, vol. 32, pp. 152–158, 2012.

[61] Q. Li, Q. Lu, J. Y. Hwang et al., "IKK1-deficient mice exhibit abnormal development of skin and skeleton," *Genes and Development*, vol. 13, no. 10, pp. 1322–1328, 1999.

[62] E. Candi, A. Terrinoni, A. Rufini et al., "p63 is upstream of IKKα in epidermal development," *Journal of Cell Science*, vol. 119, no. 22, pp. 4617–4622, 2006.

[63] M. I. Koster, D. Dai, B. Marinari et al., "p63 induces key target genes required for epidermal morphogenesis," *Proceedings of the National Academy of Sciences of the United States of America*, vol. 104, no. 9, pp. 3255–3260, 2007.

[64] R. A. Romano, B. Birkaya, and S. Sinha, "A functional enhancer of keratin14 is a direct transcriptional target of ΔNp63," *Journal of Investigative Dermatology*, vol. 127, no. 5, pp. 1175–1186, 2007.

[65] A. M. Lena, R. Cipollone, I. Amelio et al., "Skn-1a/Oct-11 and ΔNp63α exert antagonizing effects on human keratin expression," *Biochemical and Biophysical Research Communications*, vol. 401, no. 4, pp. 568–573, 2010.

[66] S. Borrelli, E. Candi, B. Hu et al., "The p63 target HBP1 is required for skin differentiation and stratification," *Cell Death and Differentiation*, vol. 17, no. 12, pp. 1896–1907, 2010.

[67] G. L. Sen, L. D. Boxer, D. E. Webster et al., "ZNF750 is a p63 target gene that induces KLF4 to drive terminal epidermal differentiation," *Developmental Cell*, vol. 22, pp. 669–677, 2012.

[68] S. Kim, I. F. Choi, J. R. Quante, L. Zhang, D. R. Roop, and M. I. Koster, "P63 directly induces expression of Alox12, a regulator of epidermal barrier formation," *Experimental Dermatology*, vol. 18, no. 12, pp. 1016–1021, 2009.

[69] A. Chikh, R. N. Matin, V. Senatore, M. Hufbauer, D. Lavery et al., "iASPP/p63 autoregulatory feedback loop is required for the homeostasis of stratified epithelia," *The EMBO Journal*, vol. 30, pp. 4261–4273, 2011.

[70] R. Yi, M. N. Poy, M. Stoffel, and E. Fuchs, "A skin microRNA promotes differentiation by repressing 'stemness'," *Nature*, vol. 452, no. 7184, pp. 225–229, 2008.

[71] D. Antonini, M. T. Russo, L. De Rosa, M. Gorrese, L. Del Vecchio, and C. Missero, "Transcriptional repression of miR-34 family contributes to p63-mediated cell cycle progression in epidermal cells," *Journal of Investigative Dermatology*, vol. 130, no. 5, pp. 1249–1257, 2010.

[72] N. Wu, E. Sulpice, P. Obeid et al., "The miR-17 family links p63 protein to MAPK signaling to promote the onset of human keratinocyte differentiation," *PLoS One*, vol. 7, Article ID e45761, 2012.

[73] L. De Rosa, D. Antonini, G. Ferone et al., "P63 suppresses non-epidermal lineage markers in a bone morphogenetic protein-dependent manner via repression of Smad7," *Journal of Biological Chemistry*, vol. 284, no. 44, pp. 30574–30582, 2009.

[74] C. E. Barton, K. N. Johnson, D. M. Mays et al., "Novel p63 target genes involved in paracrine signaling and keratinocyte differentiation," *Cell Death and Disease*, vol. 1, no. 9, article e74, 2010.

[75] R. A. Ihrie, M. R. Marques, B. T. Nguyen et al., "Perp is a p63-regulated gene essential for epithelial integrity," *Cell*, vol. 120, no. 6, pp. 843–856, 2005.

[76] V. G. Beaudry, R. A. Ihrie, S. B. Jacobs et al., "Loss of the desmosomal component perp impairs wound healing *in vivo*," *Dermatology Research and Practice*, vol. 2010, Article ID 759731, 11 pages, 2010.

[77] C. E. Barbieri, C. A. Perez, K. N. Johnson, K. A. Ely, D. Billheimer, and J. A. Pietenpol, "IGFBP-3 is a direct target of transcriptional regulation by ΔNp63α in squamous epithelium," *Cancer Research*, vol. 65, no. 6, pp. 2314–2320, 2005.

[78] D. K. Carroll, J. S. Carroll, C. O. Leong et al., "p63 regulates an adhesion programme and cell survival in epithelial cells," *Nature Cell Biology*, vol. 8, no. 6, pp. 551–561, 2006.

[79] L. Hayflick and P. S. Moorhead, "The serial cultivation of human diploid cell strains," *Experimental Cell Research*, vol. 25, no. 3, pp. 585–621, 1961.

[80] L. Hayflick, "The limited *in vitro* lifetime of human diploid cell strains," *Experimental Cell Research*, vol. 37, no. 3, pp. 614–636, 1965.

[81] G. Pellegrini, E. Dellambra, O. Golisano et al., "p63 identifies keratinocyte stem cells," *Proceedings of the National Academy of Sciences of the United States of America*, vol. 98, no. 6, pp. 3156–3161, 2001.

[82] M. Senoo, F. Pinto, C. P. Crum, and F. McKeon, "p63 is essential for the proliferative potential of stem cells in stratified epithelia," *Cell*, vol. 129, no. 3, pp. 523–536, 2007.

[83] V. Rivetti d, A. M. Lena, M. Nicoloso et al., "p63-microRNA feedback in keratinocyte senescence," *Proceedings of the National Academy of Sciences of the United States of America*, vol. 109, pp. 1133–1138, 2012.

[84] W. M. Keyes, Y. Wu, H. Vogel, X. Guo, S. W. Lowe, and A. A. Mills, "p63 deficiency activates a program of cellular senescence and leads to accelerated aging," *Genes and Development*, vol. 19, no. 17, pp. 1986–1999, 2005.

[85] E. R. Flores, S. Sengupta, J. B. Miller et al., "Tumor predisposition in mice mutant for p63 and p73: evidence for broader tumor suppressor functions for the p53 family," *Cancer Cell*, vol. 7, no. 4, pp. 363–373, 2005.

[86] L. Ha, R. M. Ponnamperuma, S. Jay, M. S. Ricci, and W. C. Weinberg, "Dysregulated δNp63α inhibits expression of ink4a/arf, blocks senescence, and promotes malignant conversion of keratinocytes," *PLoS ONE*, vol. 6, no. 7, Article ID e21877, 2011.

[87] X. Su, M. S. Cho, Y. J. Gi, B. A. Ayanga, C. J. Sherr, and E. R. Flores, "Rescue of key features of the p63-null epithelial phenotype by inactivation of Ink4a and Arf," *The EMBO Journal*, vol. 28, no. 13, pp. 1904–1915, 2009.

[88] M. Sommer, N. Poliak, S. Upadhyay et al., "ΔNp63α overexpression induces downregulation of Sirt1 and an accelerated aging phenotype in the mouse," *Cell Cycle*, vol. 5, no. 17, pp. 2005–2011, 2006.

[89] J. G. Toma, I. A. McKenzie, D. Bagli, and F. D. Miller, "Isolation and characterization of multipotent skin-derived precursors from human skin," *Stem Cells*, vol. 23, no. 6, pp. 727–737, 2005.

[90] K. Hagiwara, M. G. McMenamin, K. Miura, and C. C. Harris, "Mutational analysis of the p63/p73L/p51/p40/CUSP/KET gene in human cancer cell lines using intronic primers," *Cancer Research*, vol. 59, no. 17, pp. 4165–4169, 1999.

[91] J. N. Glickman, A. Yang, A. Shahsafaei, F. McKeon, and R. D. Odze, "Expression of p53-related protein p63 in the gastrointestinal tract and in esophageal metaplastic and neoplastic disorders," *Human Pathology*, vol. 32, no. 11, pp. 1157–1165, 2001.

[92] H. Hu, S. H. Xia, A. D. Li et al., "Elevated expression of p63 protein in human esophageal squamous cell carcinomas," *International Journal of Cancer*, vol. 102, no. 6, pp. 580–583, 2002.

[93] T. Crook, J. M. Nicholls, L. Brooks, J. O'Nions, and M. J. Allday, "High level expression of ΔN-p63: a mechanism for the inactivation of p53 in undifferentiated nasopharyngeal carcinoma (NPC)?" *Oncogene*, vol. 19, no. 30, pp. 3439–3444, 2000.

[94] J. S. Reis-Filho, B. Torio, A. Albergaria, and F. C. Schmitt, "p63 expression in normal skin and usual cutaneous carcinomas," *Journal of Cutaneous Pathology*, vol. 29, no. 9, pp. 517–523, 2002.

[95] D. A. Wrone, S. Yoo, L. K. Chipps, and R. L. Moy, "The expression of p63 in actinic keratosis, seborrheic keratosis, and cutaneous squamous cell carcinomas," *Dermatologic Surgery*, vol. 30, no. 10, pp. 1299–1302, 2004.

[96] P. P. Massion, P. M. Taflan, S. M. J. Rahman et al., "Significance of p63 amplification and overexpression in lung cancer development and prognosis," *Cancer Research*, vol. 63, no. 21, pp. 7113–7121, 2003.

[97] G. Pelosi, F. Pasini, C. O. Stenholm et al., "p63 immunoreactivity in lung cancer: yet another player in the development of squamous cell carcinomas?" *Journal of Pathology*, vol. 198, no. 1, pp. 100–109, 2002.

[98] K. Nylander, P. J. Coates, and P. A. Hall, "Characterization of the expression pattern of p63 alpha and delta Np63 alpha in benign and malignant oral epithelial lesions," *International Journal of Cancer*, vol. 87, pp. 368–372, 2000.

[99] M. Senoo, I. Tsuchiya, Y. Matsumura et al., "Transcriptional dysregulation of the p73L/p63/p51/p40/KET gene in human squamous cell carcinomas: expression of δNp73L, a novel dominant-negative isoform, and loss of expression of the potential tumour suppressor p51," *British Journal of Cancer*, vol. 84, no. 9, pp. 1235–1241, 2001.

[100] R. J. Richardson, J. Dixon, S. Malhotra et al., "Irf6 is a key determinant of the keratinocyte proliferation-differentiation switch," *Nature Genetics*, vol. 38, no. 11, pp. 1329–1334, 2006.

[101] E. Botti, G. Spallone, F. Moretti et al., "Developmental factor IRF6 exhibits tumor suppressor activity in squamous cell carcinomas," *Proceedings of the National Academy of Sciences of the United States of America*, vol. 108, pp. 13710–13715, 2011.

[102] G. Wu, M. Osada, Z. Guo et al., "ΔNp63α up-regulates the Hsp70 gene in human cancer," *Cancer Research*, vol. 65, no. 3, pp. 758–766, 2005.

[103] M. Patturajan, S. Nomoto, M. Sommer et al., "ΔNp63 induces β-catenin nuclear accumulation and signaling," *Cancer Cell*, vol. 1, no. 4, pp. 369–379, 2002.

[104] M. Herfs, P. Hubert, M. Suarez-Carmona et al., "Regulation of p63 isoforms by snail and slug transcription factors in human squamous cell carcinoma," *American Journal of Pathology*, vol. 176, no. 4, pp. 1941–1949, 2010.

[105] C. A. Di, A. Troiano, M. O. Di et al., "The p63 protein isoform DeltaNp63alpha modulates Y-box binding protein 1 in its subcellular distribution and regulation of cell survival and motility genes," *The Journal of Biological Chemistry*, vol. 287, pp. 30170–30180, 2012.

[106] R. Kommagani, T. M. Caserta, and M. P. Kadakia, "Identification of vitamin D receptor as a target of p63," *Oncogene*, vol. 25, no. 26, pp. 3745–3751, 2006.

[107] R. Kommagani, M. K. Leonard, S. Lewis, R. A. Romano, S. Sinha, and M. P. Kadakia, "Regulation of VDR by ΔNp63α is associated with inhibition of cell invasion," *Journal of Cell Science*, vol. 122, no. 16, pp. 2828–2835, 2009.

[108] M. Adorno, M. Cordenonsi, M. Montagner et al., "A mutant-p53/Smad complex opposes p63 to empower TGFβ-induced metastasis," *Cell*, vol. 137, no. 1, pp. 87–98, 2009.

[109] C. E. Barbieri, L. J. Tang, K. A. Brown, and J. A. Pietenpol, "Loss of p63 leads to increased cell migration and up-regulation of genes involved in invasion and metastasis," *Cancer Research*, vol. 66, no. 15, pp. 7589–7597, 2006.

[110] R. Kalluri and R. A. Weinberg, "The basics of epithelial-mesenchymal transition," *Journal of Clinical Investigation*, vol. 119, no. 6, pp. 1420–1428, 2009.

[111] K. M. Liefer, M. I. Koster, X. J. Wang, A. Yang, F. McKeon, and D. R. Roop, "Down-regulation of p63 is required for epidermal UV-B-induced apoptosis," *Cancer Research*, vol. 60, no. 15, pp. 4016–4020, 2000.

[112] M. Papoutsaki, F. Moretti, M. Lanza et al., "A p38-dependent pathway regulates ΔNp63 DNA binding to p53-dependent promoters in UV-induced apoptosis of keratinocytes," *Oncogene*, vol. 24, no. 46, pp. 6970–6975, 2005.

[113] K. L. Schavolt and J. A. Pietenpol, "p53 and Δnp63α differentially bind and regulate target genes involved in cell cycle arrest, DNA repair and apoptosis," *Oncogene*, vol. 26, no. 42, pp. 6125–6132, 2007.

[114] R. Zangen, E. Ratovitski, and D. Sidransky, "ΔNp63α levels correlate with clinical tumor response to cisplatin," *Cell Cycle*, vol. 4, no. 10, pp. 1313–1315, 2005.

[115] A. Fomenkov, R. Zangen, Y. P. Huang et al., "RACK1 and stratifin target ΔNp63α for a proteasome degradation in head and neck squamous cell carcinoma cells upon DNA damage," *Cell Cycle*, vol. 3, no. 10, pp. 1285–1295, 2004.

[116] A. Chatterjee, X. Chang, T. Sen, R. Ravi, A. Bedi, and D. Sidransky, "Regulation of p53 family member isoform ΔNp63α by the nuclear factor-κB targeting kinase IκB kinase β," *Cancer Research*, vol. 70, no. 4, pp. 1419–1429, 2010.

[117] T. Sen, X. Chang, D. Sidransky, and A. Chatterjee, "Regulation of ΔNp63α by NFκB," *Cell Cycle*, vol. 9, no. 24, pp. 4841–4847, 2010.

[118] M. Yuan, P. Luong, C. Hudson, K. Gudmundsdottir, and S. Basu, "C-Abl phosphorylation of Δnp63α is critical for cell viability," *Cell Death and Disease*, vol. 1, no. 1, article e16, 2010.

[119] J. W. Rocco, C. O. Leong, N. Kuperwasser, M. P. DeYoung, and L. W. Ellisen, "p63 mediates survival in squamous cell carcinoma by suppression of p73-dependent apoptosis," *Cancer Cell*, vol. 9, no. 1, pp. 45–56, 2006.

[120] M. R. Ramsey, L. He, N. Forster, B. Ory, and L. W. Ellisen, "Physical association of HDAC1 and HDAC2 with p63 mediates transcriptional repression and tumor maintenance in squamous cell carcinoma," *Cancer Research*, vol. 71, no. 13, pp. 4373–4379, 2011.

[121] S. Frame, R. Crombie, J. Liddell et al., "Epithelial carcinogenesis in the mouse: correlating the genetics and the biology," *Philosophical Transactions of the Royal Society B*, vol. 353, no. 1370, pp. 839–845, 1998.

[122] W. M. Keyes, H. Vogel, M. I. Koster et al., "p63 heterozygous mutant mice are not prone to spontaneous or chemically induced tumors," *Proceedings of the National Academy of Sciences of the United States of America*, vol. 103, no. 22, pp. 8435–8440, 2006.

[123] X. Su, D. Chakravarti, M. S. Cho et al., "TAp63 suppresses metastasis through coordinate regulation of Dicer and miRNAs," *Nature*, vol. 467, no. 7318, pp. 986–990, 2010.

[124] W. M. Keyes, M. Pecoraro, V. Aranda et al., "Δnp63α is an oncogene that targets chromatin remodeler Lsh to drive skin stem cell proliferation and tumorigenesis," *Cell Stem Cell*, vol. 8, no. 2, pp. 164–176, 2011.

[125] Q. Li, S. A. Sambandam, H. J. Lu, A. Thomson, S. H. Kim et al., "14-3-3sigma and p63 play opposing roles in epidermal tumorigenesis," *Carcinogenesis*, vol. 32, pp. 1782–1788, 2011.

[126] T. D. Gilmore, "Introduction to NF-κB: players, pathways, perspectives," *Oncogene*, vol. 25, no. 51, pp. 6680–6684, 2006.

[127] G. Courtois and T. D. Gilmore, "Mutations in the NF-κB signaling pathway: implications for human disease," *Oncogene*, vol. 25, no. 51, pp. 6831–6843, 2006.

[128] C. Van Waes, "Nuclear factor-κB in development, prevention, and therapy of cancer," *Clinical Cancer Research*, vol. 13, no. 4, pp. 1076–1082, 2007.

[129] C. S. Seitz, Q. Lin, H. Deng, and P. A. Khavari, "Alterations in NF-κB function in transgenic epithelial tissue demonstrate a growth inhibitory role for NF-κB," *Proceedings of the National Academy of Sciences of the United States of America*, vol. 95, no. 5, pp. 2307–2312, 1998.

[130] R. Gugasyan, A. Voss, G. Varigos et al., "The transcription factors c-rel and RelA control epidermal development and homeostasis in embryonic and adult skin via distinct mechanisms," *Molecular and Cellular Biology*, vol. 24, no. 13, pp. 5733–5745, 2004.

[131] A. Loercher, T. L. Lee, J. L. Ricker et al., "Nuclear factor-kappaB is an important modulator of the altered gene expression profile and malignant phenotype in squamous cell carcinoma," *Cancer Research*, vol. 64, pp. 6511–6523, 2004.

[132] M. Dajee, M. Lazarov, J. Y. Zhang et al., "NF-κB blockade and oncogenic Ras trigger invasive human epidermal neoplasia," *Nature*, vol. 421, no. 6923, pp. 639–643, 2003.

[133] M. A. Sovak, R. E. Bellas, D. W. Kim et al., "Aberrant nuclear factor-κb/Rel expression and the pathogenesis of breast cancer," *Journal of Clinical Investigation*, vol. 100, no. 12, pp. 2952–2960, 1997.

[134] K. E. King, R. M. Ponnamperuma, C. Allen et al., "The p53 homologue ΔNp63α interacts with the nuclear factor-κB pathway to modulate epithelial cell growth," *Cancer Research*, vol. 68, no. 13, pp. 5122–5131, 2008.

[135] H. Lu, X. Yang, P. Duggal et al., "TNF-alpha promotes c-REL/DeltaNp63alpha interaction and TAp73 dissociation from key genes that mediate growth arrest and apoptosis in head and neck cancer," *Cancer Research*, vol. 71, pp. 6867–6877, 2011.

15

Squamous Cell Carcinomas of the Skin Explore Angiogenesis-Independent Mechanisms of Tumour Vascularization

Ievgenia Pastushenko,[1] Tamara Gracia-Cazaña,[1] Sandra Vicente-Arregui,[2] Gert G. Van den Eynden,[3] Mariano Ara,[1] Peter B. Vermeulen,[3] Francisco José Carapeto,[4] and Steven J. Van Laere[2,5]

[1] *Department of Dermatology, University Hospital "Clinico Lozano Blesa," Calle San Juan Bosco 15, 50009 Zaragoza, Spain*
[2] *Department of Pathology, University Hospital "Miguel Servet," Paseo Isabel la Católica 1-3, 50009 Zaragoza, Spain*
[3] *Translational Cancer Research Unit Antwerp, Oncology Centre, General Hospital Sint-Augustinus, Oosterveldlaan 24, 2610 Wilrijk, Belgium*
[4] *Department of Medicine, Psychiatry and Dermatology, School of Medicine, University of Zaragoza, Calle Domingo Miral s/n, 50009 Zaragoza, Spain*
[5] *Department of Oncology, KU of Leuven, Herestraat 49, 3000 Leuven, Belgium*

Correspondence should be addressed to Ievgenia Pastushenko; jane.pastushenko@gmail.com

Academic Editor: Giuseppe Argenziano

Aims. To evaluate the vascularization in basal cell carcinomas (BCCs) and squamous cell carcinomas (SCCs) of the skin. *Methods.* We performed CD31 (i.e., panendothelial marker) and CD105 (i.e., proliferating endothelium marker) immunostaining on samples of 70 SCCs and 70 BCCs of the skin. We evaluated the relative blood vessel area using the Chalkley counting method in each histologic subtype of these tumours. We calculated the degree of proliferation of blood vessel endothelium dividing CD105-Chalkley score by CD31-Chalkley score. *Results.* We found significantly higher peritumoral and intratumoral blood vessel area in SCC when compared to BCC (both with CD31 and CD105). Chalkley counts differed significantly between groups with different BCC histologic subtypes and SCC with different grade of differentiation. Surprisingly, the degree of proliferation of blood vessel endothelium was higher in BCC when compared to SCC. *Conclusions.* While SCC exhibited significantly higher intratumoral and peritumoral blood vessel areas compared to BCC, the relatively low rate of proliferating endothelium in this tumour type suggests the existence of endothelial-sprouting-independent mechanisms of vascularization in SCC.

1. Introduction

Basal cell carcinoma (BCC) and squamous cell carcinoma (SCC) of the skin are the most common human solid malignant tumours. One of the key biological processes that appear to be relevant to the establishment and prognosis of most forms of cancer, including skin cancer, is angiogenesis [1]. Using the mouse model Eichten et al. demonstrated that during squamous skin carcinogenesis blood vessels undergo increase in endothelial cell proliferation, vessel diameter, vessel density and leakage [2]. Although several studies evaluated the role of microvessel density in the progression of epithelial skin cancer, the proliferation of vascular endothelium or blood vessel area (BVA) has not yet been investigated.

For many years, the process of tumour vascularization was thought to proceed mainly through the sprouting of new blood vessels from the preexisting vasculature. However, in recent years, additional endothelial-sprouting-independent mechanisms have been described, such as vascular cooption, intussusceptive angiogenesis, mosaic vessels, vasculogenesis, and/or vasculogenic mimicry [3].

The quantification of angiogenesis is complicated by the fact this is dynamic process. Two international consensus on quantification of angiogenesis in solid tumours were published [4, 5], considering the Chalkley counting technique as a more reproducible and clinically applicable technique. Chalkley counting score reflects the relative vessel area, gibing an estimate of the total perfusion of the tumor. It is important to note that two categories of endothelial cell specific antibodies are currently available for immunohistochemistry: the panendothelial cell markers, characterized by equal intensity of staining for small and large blood vessels, and antibodies that bind selectively to proliferating endothelium [6]. In order to evaluate the degree of proliferating blood vessels we used the proliferating-endothelium marker CD105 and we compared the results with those obtained with CD31 immunostain.

2. Materials and Methods

2.1. Patients and Tissue Samples. A total of 70 formalin-fixed, paraffin-embedded surgical specimens of patients presenting with SCCs and 70 with BCCs at the University Hospital "Clínico Lozano Blesa" (Zaragoza, Spain) between 2008 and 2010 were included in our study. The following clinicopathologic variables were recorded: sex, date of birth, date of diagnosis, anatomic site of the tumor, BCC histologic subtype (superficial, nodular, and aggressive), SCC histological grading (well-, moderately, and poorly differentiated), lymphovascular invasion, and perineural invasion. In the "aggressive" BCC group, we included infiltrative, morpheaform, and micronodular histotypes.

2.2. Immunohistochemistry. Immunohistochemical stainings were performed using DAKO autostainer system and commercially available endothelial markers CD31 (monoclonal mouse anti-human platelet endothelial cell adhesion molecule- (PECAM-) 1 antibody, Clone JC70A, DAKO, Glostrup, Denmark; dilution: 1 : 50 for 1 hour) and CD105 (monoclonal mouse anti-human endoglin antibody, Clone SN6h, DAKO, Glostrup, Denmark; dilution: 1 : 100 for 1 hour). As positive control, a sample of breast cancer with a known high MVD was used.

2.3. Evaluation of Relative Blood Vessel Area and Proliferating Endothelium. The relative blood vessel area was determined both in intratumoral (IT) and peritumoral (PT) areas using Chalkley counting technique. PT vessels were defined as CD34 positive vessels located at the interface of tumour and adjacent dermis (Chalkley method is based on the use of an eyepiece graticule containing 25 randomly positioned dots, which is rotated so that the maximum number of points is on or within the vessels). Thus, the Chalkley count is the number of points that hit stained vessels. The average of three highest values for each tumor section was used for the analysis.

2.4. Statistical Analysis. All analyses were performed using the statistical package SPSS ver. 19.0 for Mac. Associations between different categorical variables were assessed by Pearson's χ^2 test. The unpaired Student's t-test was used variables following normal distribution. The CD31 and CD105 Chalkley counts did not follow the normal distribution (Kolmogorov-Smirnov = 0.12, $P < 0.0001$, and Kolmogorov-Smirnov = 0.10, $P = 0.002$, resp.); therefore, the Mann-Whitney test, Wilcoxon signed-rank test, or Spearman's rank correlation was used as appropriate. The intraobserver and interobserver agreement for classifying the tumours as Chalkley count high or low (using as a cut-off point the mean Chalkley count value) were evaluated by kappa statistic.

3. Results

The median age of included patients was 77.6 years (range 60.2–88.3) in SCC group and 75.5 years (range 53.5–88.9) in BCC group at the time of surgery ($P < 0.05$). The main clinical and pathologic characteristics of patients included in the study are compiled in Table 1.

In all histological slides CD31 or CD105 positive staining could be detected. The costaining of inflammatory cells has been observed in slides immunostained with CD31, but these could be distinguished from endothelial cells on the basis of morphological differences. No clear hot spots were observed in SCC or in BCC. Median peritumoural- (PT-) CD31-Chalkley count was 8.33 (SD = 1.98) points for SCC and 5.81 (SD = 1.05) for BCC ($P < 0.001$) (Figure 1(a)), while median PT-CD105-Chalkley count was 7.84 (SD = 1.76) points for SCC and 5.19 (SD = 1.19) for BCC ($P < 0.001$) (Figure 1(b)). Median intratumoral- (IT-) CD31-Chalkley count was 4.67 (SD = 1.23) for SCC and 0.00 (SD = 1.67) for BCC ($P < 0.001$), while median IT-CD105-Chalkley count was 2.33 (SD = 1.71) and median IT-CD105-Chalkley count was 0.00 (SD = 0.67) ($P > 0.001$). Moreover, both PT and IT-rBVA differed between superficial, nodular, and aggressive BCC ($P_{CD31} < 0.001$, $P_{CD105} < 0.001$) and between well-, moderately, and poorly differentiated SCC ($P_{CD31} = 0.007$, $P_{CD105} = 0.03$) (Table 2). Figure 2 shows samples of CD31 and CD105 immunostaining in BCC and SCC. There was a strong correlation between CD31 and CD105 Chalkley score (Pearson's $R = 0.8$; $P < 0.001$). We next proceeded to evaluate the degree of proliferating endothelium by dividing the CD105-Chalkley score by the CD31-Chalkley score. The mean CD105/CD31 quotient was 0.96 for BCC (SD = 0.16) and 0.79 for SCC (SD = 0.16) ($P = 0.024$).

In a subset of cases ($n = 30$; 15 SCCs and 15 BCCs), the intraobserver and the interobserver agreement were evaluated by kappa statistic (both for CD31 and CD105). These slides were examined by IP two times and one time by TGC. The intraobserver agreement between the two examinations by IP for classifying the tumors as high or low Chalkley counting values (taking the mean value for each antibody as a cut-point) was $k = 0.65$ for CD31 and $k = 0.80$ for CD105, whereas the interobserver agreement between IP and TGC was $k = 0.54$ for CD34 and $k = 0.67$ for CD105 (k-values between 0.41 and 0.60 indicate moderate strength of agreement and k-values between 0.61 and 0.80 substantial strength of agreement).

TABLE 1: Summary of the main clinical and histological characteristics of patients included in the study.

Category	BCC	SCC
Number of patients		
Male	53	49
Female	17	21
Total	**70**	**70**
Age of diagnosis	73.3 (53.5–88.9)	76.2 (60.2–88.3)
Anatomic site		
Head and neck	51 (72.8%)	53 (75.7%)
Extremities	6 (8.6%)	15 (21.4%)
Trunk	13 (18.6%)	2 (2.9%)
Histologic subtype	Superficial BCC: 23 (32.9%) Nodular BCC: 42 (60.0%) Aggressive* BCC: 5 (7.1%)	Well-differentiated SCC: 30 (42.8%) Moderately differentiated SCC: 37 (52.9%) Poorly differentiated SCC: 3 (4.3%)
Presence of LVI	0 (0%)	3 (4.3%)
Presence of PNI	0 (0%)	1 (1.4%)

BCC: basal cell carcinoma; SCC: squamous cell carcinoma; LVI: lymphovascular invasion; PNI: perineural invasion.
*Aggressive BCC group includes infiltrative, morpheaform, and micronodular subtypes.

TABLE 2: Chalkley score according to histotype in basal and squamous cell carcinomas.

CD31			K-W	CD105			K-W
Basal cell carcinoma							
Superficial ($n = 23$)	Nodular ($n = 42$)	Aggressive ($n = 5$)	$P < 0.001$	Superficial ($n = 23$)	Nodular ($n = 42$)	Aggressive ($n = 5$)	$P < 0.001$
5.2 (SD = 0.64)	6.0 (SD = 0.94)	7.2 (SD = 1.17)		4.2 (SD = 0.73)	5.4 (SD = 0.86)	7.7 (SD = 0.69)	
Squamous cell carcinoma							
Well-diff. ($n = 30$)	Moderately diff. ($n = 37$)	Poorly diff. ($n = 3$)	$P = 0.07$	Well-diff. ($n = 30$)	Moderately diff. ($n = 37$)	Poorly diff. ($n = 3$)	$P = 0.03$
7.7 (SD = 1.43)	8.7 (SD = 1.91)	12.1 (SD = 2.14)		7.3 (SD = 1.53)	8.2 (SD = 1.54)	11.4 (SD = 1.2)	

The CD31 and CD105 Chalkley counts did not follow the normal distribution (Kolmogorov-Smirnov = 0.12, $P < 0.0001$, and Kolmogorov-Smirnov = 0.10, $P = 0.002$, resp.). Therefore, K-W (=Kruskal-Wallis) test has been applied.

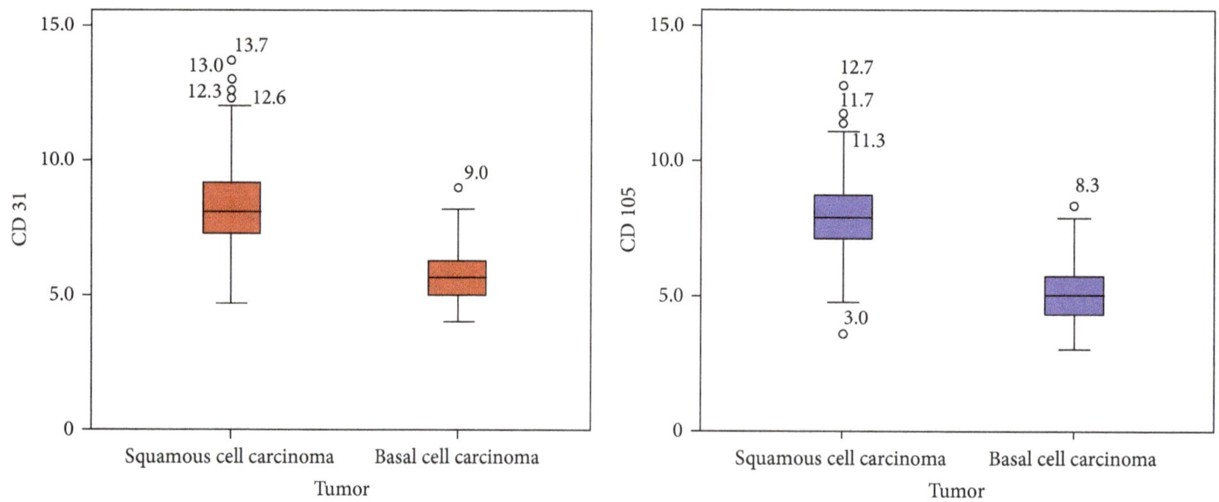

(a) CD31 Chalkley score

(b) CD105 Chalkley score

FIGURE 1: CD31 and CD105 Chalkley counts in basal and squamous cell carcinomas. Box plots for the Chalkley score for CD31 (a) and CD105 (b).

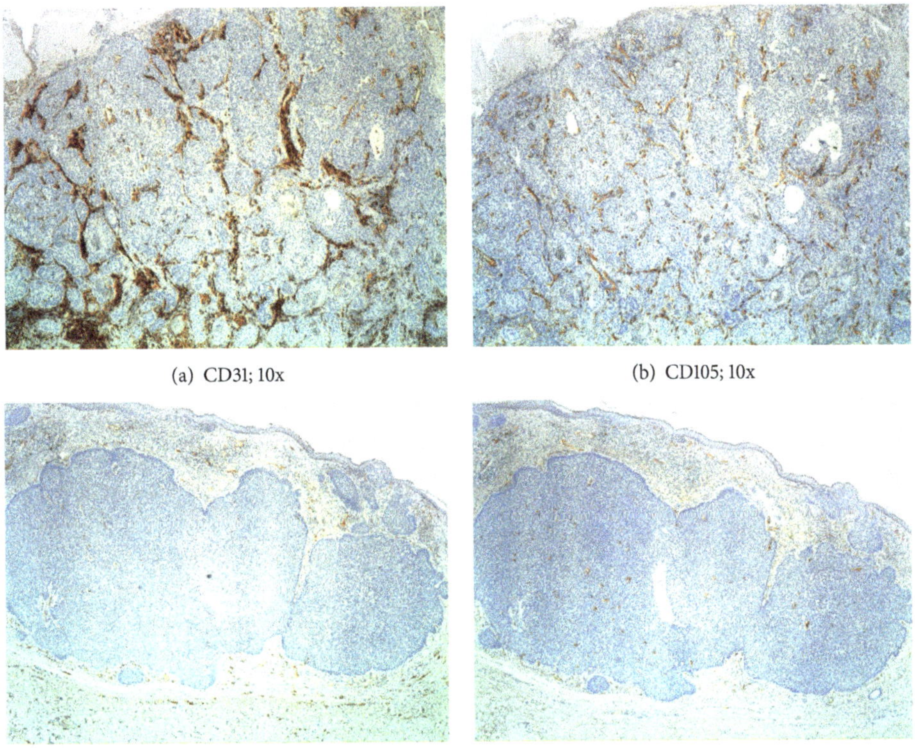

(a) CD31; 10x (b) CD105; 10x (c) CD31; 10x (d) CD105; 10x

FIGURE 2: Blood vessels in basal cell carcinoma and squamous cell carcinomas. Sections of squamous cell carcinoma ((a) and (b)) showing a notably higher vessel density than basal cell carcinoma, both for CD31 (c) and CD105 (d).

4. Discussion

In our present study, we found statistically greater relative PT and IT blood vessel areas in SCC compared to BCC, both with CD31 and CD105 antibodies. These findings seem to be logical, since high degree of vascularization provides oxygen and nutrients for tumour growth, explaining, at least in part, the differences in clinical behavior between BCC and SCC. While most studies evaluating the role of angiogenesis in cancer, including epithelial skin tumours, used the technique described by Weidner et al., based on the number of microvessels quantification, we evaluated the blood vessel area, reflecting the global tumour perfusion. Loggini et al. investigated the angiogenesis pattern in BCC and SCC of the skin, demonstrating that the majority of samples with high vascularization belonged to the squamous histotype, while the majority of BCC showed a significantly lower number of microvessels [7]. Chin et al. evaluated vascular patterns in SCCs, BCCs, and trichoepitheliomas (TEs) using CD31 mAb. The SCC blood vessel counts were significantly higher if compared to BCCs or TEs [8]. Differences between the neovascularization in BCC with benign course and BCC with aggressive behavior have been found [9, 10]. From the clinical perspective, the phase II clinical trial based on 31 patients with advanced cutaneous SCC treated with Cetuximab showed a disease control rate in 69% and response rate in 28% of included patients [11].

However and surprisingly, BCC exhibited significantly higher proportion of proliferating endothelium than SCC, apparently contradicting the abovementioned results. There is at least one explanation for these findings, based on angiogenesis-independent mechanisms of tumour vascularization. Intussusceptive angiogenesis occurs by the insertion of the interstitial tissue column into the lumen of preexisting vessels inducing partition of the vessel lumen [3]. This type of angiogenesis is faster and more economical than sprouting, occurs within hours of even minutes, and does not primarily depend on EC proliferation. The ability for growing by coopting the massive vascular plexus present in the peritumoural connective tissue was described in aggressive tumours localized in highly vascularized tissues. Thus, our results suggest that SCC, characterized by more rapid growth and aggressive clinical behaviour, explores other mechanisms of tumour vascularization which allow faster oxygen and nutrient transport, while BCC growth mainly depends on proliferation of vascular endothelium. Importantly, angiogenesis-independent mechanisms of tumour vascularization were described to be more resistant to antiangiogenic therapy.

Angiogenesis is a dynamic process, making its quantification inherently difficult. Since no decisions have to be made on whether adjacent stained structures are the reflection of one single microvessel or two separate microvessels, Chalkley counting is considered a more objective approach than Weidner technique [5]. We evaluated the reproducibility of this technique, showing both inter- and intraobserver moderate to substantial strength of agreement. Slightly lower agreement in CD31-immunostained slides could be explained by the presence of costaining of inflammatory cells, which could result in the erroneous incorporation of inflammatory cell count into the final score.

In conclusion, our results suggest that the existence of angiogenesis-independent mechanisms of tumour vascularization may be considered as a hallmark of epithelial tumors with more aggressive clinical behaviour.

Acknowledgment

This research was supported by grants from the University of Zaragoza.

References

[1] I. Pastushenko, P. B. Vermeulen, F. J. Carapeto et al., "Blood microvessel density, lymphatic microvessel density and lymphatic invasion in predicting melanoma metastases: systematic review and meta-analysis," *British Journal of Dermatology*, vol. 170, no. 1, pp. 66–77, 2013.

[2] A. Eichten, W. C. Hyun, and L. M. Coussens, "Distinctive features of angiogenesis and lymphangiogenesis determine their functionality during de novo tumor development," *Cancer Research*, vol. 67, no. 11, pp. 5211–5220, 2007.

[3] I. Pastushenko, P. B. Vermeulen, G. G. van den Eynden et al., "Mechanisms of tumour vascularisation in cutaneous malignant melanoma: clinical implications," *British Journal of Dermatology*, 2014.

[4] P. E. Vermeulen, G. Gasparini, S. B. Fox et al., "Quantification of angiogenesis in solid human tumours: an international consensus on the methodology and criteria of evaluation," *European Journal of Cancer Part A*, vol. 32, no. 14, pp. 2474–2484, 1996.

[5] P. B. Vermeulen, G. Gasparini, S. B. Fox et al., "Second international consensus on the methodology and criteria of evaluation of angiogenesis quantification in solid human tumours," *European Journal of Cancer*, vol. 38, no. 12, pp. 1564–1579, 2002.

[6] J. Hasan, R. Byers, and G. C. Jayson, "Intra-tumoural microvessel density in human solid tumours," *British Journal of Cancer*, vol. 86, no. 10, pp. 1566–1577, 2002.

[7] B. Loggini, L. Boldrini, S. Gisfredi et al., "CD34 microvessel density and VEGF expression in basal and squamous cell carcinoma," *Pathology Research and Practice*, vol. 199, no. 11, pp. 705–712, 2003.

[8] C. W. S. Chin, A. J. E. Foss, A. Stevens, and J. Lowe, "Differences in the vascular patterns of basal and squamous cell skin carcinomas explain their differences in clinical behaviour," *Journal of Pathology*, vol. 200, no. 3, pp. 308–313, 2003.

[9] A. Carbone, P. Viola, S. Varrati, D. Angelucci, A. Tulli, and P. Amerio, "Microvessel density and VEGF expression seems to correlate with invasiveness of basal cell carcinoma," *European Journal of Dermatology*, vol. 21, no. 4, pp. 608–609, 2011.

[10] S. Staibano, A. Boscaino, G. Salvatore, P. Orabona, L. Palombini, and G. de Rosa, "The prognostic significance of tumor angiogenesis in nonaggressive and aggressive basal cell carcinoma of the human skin," *Human Pathology*, vol. 27, no. 7, pp. 695–700, 1996.

[11] E. Maubec, P. Petrow, I. Scheer-Senyarich et al., "Phase II study of cetuximab as first-line single-drug therapy in patients with unresectable squamous cell carcinoma of the skin," *Journal of Clinical Oncology*, vol. 29, no. 25, pp. 3419–3426, 2011.

16

Role of Stat3 in Skin Carcinogenesis: Insights Gained from Relevant Mouse Models

Everardo Macias,[1] Dharanija Rao,[1] and John DiGiovanni[1,2,3]

[1] *Division of Pharmacology and Toxicology, College of Pharmacy, The University of Texas at Austin, Austin, TX 78723, USA*
[2] *Department of Nutritional Sciences, College of Natural Sciences, The University of Texas at Austin, Austin, TX 78723, USA*
[3] *Dell Pediatric Research Institute, The University of Texas at Austin, 1400 Barbara Jordan Boulevard, Austin, TX 78723, USA*

Correspondence should be addressed to John DiGiovanni; john.digiovanni@austin.utexas.edu

Academic Editor: Ajit K. Verma

Signal transducer and activator of transcription 3 (Stat3) is a cytoplasmic protein that is activated in response to cytokines and growth factors and acts as a transcription factor. Stat3 plays critical roles in various biological activities including cell proliferation, migration, and survival. Studies using keratinocyte-specific Stat3-deficient mice have revealed that Stat3 plays an important role in skin homeostasis including keratinocyte migration, wound healing, and hair follicle growth. Use of both constitutive and inducible keratinocyte-specific Stat3-deficient mouse models has demonstrated that Stat3 is required for both the initiation and promotion stages of multistage skin carcinogenesis. Further studies using a transgenic mouse model with a gain of function mutant of Stat3 (Stat3C) expressed in the basal layer of the epidermis revealed a novel role for Stat3 in skin tumor progression. Studies using similar Stat3-deficient and gain-of-function mouse models have indicated its similar roles in ultraviolet B (UVB) radiation-mediated skin carcinogenesis. This paper summarizes the use of these various mouse models for studying the role and underlying mechanisms for the function of Stat3 in skin carcinogenesis. Given its significant role throughout the skin carcinogenesis process, Stat3 is an attractive target for skin cancer prevention and treatment.

1. Introduction

Signal transducers and activators of transcription (Stats) are proteins that are activated by extracellular signaling proteins, such as growth factors, cytokines and various peptides [1]. Stats can also be activated via nonreceptor tyrosine kinases (e.g., src and abl) [1]. Cell-surface-mediated receptor activation causes the phosphorylation of tyrosine kinases, such as Janus-associated-kinase (Jak), which provides docking sites for the src homology (SH2) domain, enabling the binding and subsequent phosphorylation of Stats. The reciprocal interaction between the SH2 domains of two phosphorylated Stat monomers results in the formation of a functional Stat dimer. By this process, the Stat proteins are recruited to Jaks and are phosphorylated at their critical tyrosine residues. The phosphorylated Stats dimerize, translocate to the nucleus, and drive transcription of their target genes (Figure 1) [2].

While activation of Stats downstream of ligand-induced receptor activation is linked to differentiation and growth regulation functions, constitutive activation of Stats is often associated with deregulated cell growth [1]. There are seven different Stat proteins, Stat1 through Stat6, including two isoforms of Stat5 (Stat5a and Stat5b). Stat1, Stat3, Stat4, Stat5a, and Stat5b all form homodimers. In addition, Stat1, Stat2, and Stat3 can form heterodimers. Phenotypic analysis of genetically targeted mouse models for individual Stat genes has aided in delineating their biological roles. Interestingly, of all the Stat proteins only deletion of Stat3 leads to embryonic lethality [3]. Stat3 was originally identified as an IL-6-dependent transcription factor that promotes acute phase gene expression [4, 5]. However, subsequent studies have shown Stat3 activation by various cytokines, growth factors, and hormones [1]. In addition to its role in numerous cellular functions, there is strong evidence correlating Stat3

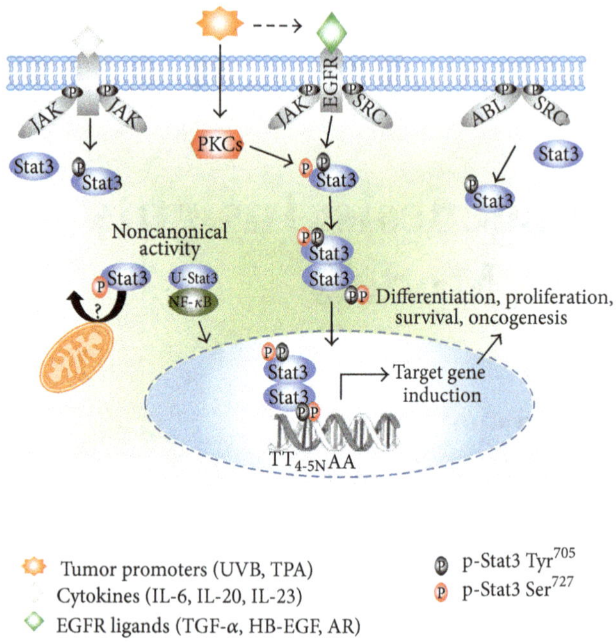

FIGURE 1: Pathways associated with Stat3 activation. Stat3 is activated downstream of receptor tyrosine kinases (e.g., EGFR), cytokine receptors via associated Janus family kinases (JAKs) (e.g., IL-6 receptor), and nonreceptor-associated tyrosine kinases (e.g., c-src). Tumor promoters such as TPA and UVB activate Stat3 in keratinocytes primarily via the EGFR. Activation of PKCs by tumor promoters leads to the processing of membrane-bound proforms of EGFR ligands such as heparin-binding EGF (HB-EGF) by matrix metalloproteinases (MMPs). In addition, PKCs associate with and phosphorylate Stat3 at Ser^{727}, which is necessary for maximal Stat3 transcriptional activity. Furthermore, transcriptional induction of cytokines and EGF ligands can lead to autocrine stimulation and sustained Stat3 phosphorylation. After phosphorylation, STAT3 dimerizes and translocates to the nucleus, where Stat3 dimers directly regulate gene expression of transcriptional targets including Bcl-x_L, cyclin D1, c-myc, Twist and Survivin. STAT3-mediated regulation of target gene expression is involved in various cellular functions including cell differentiation, proliferation, survival, and oncogenesis. Stat3 can also act through noncanonical signaling pathways. In this regard, unphosphorylated Stat3 (U-Stat3) can drive gene expression of a subset of genes that are different from p-Stat3 dimers in an NF-κB-dependent and independent manner. In addition, p-Stat3 Ser^{727} can translocate into the mitochondria and influence mitochondrial respiratory chain activity. These noncanonical Stat3 signaling pathways have protumorigenic roles in certain cell/tissue types; however their role in epithelial carcinogenesis has not been evaluated.

activation and cancer. Stat3 is found constitutively activated in cells transformed by the oncogenes v-Src and v-Abl, as well as in various human cancers, including hematologic, pancreas, breast, head and neck, and prostate cancer [6, 7]. Although there is substantial data in the literature on the protumorigenic effects of Stat3, there have been reports that activation of Stat3 can have an opposite, tumor-suppressive role (e.g., PTEN wt versus null gliomas) [8] and that activated Stat3 is associated with better prognosis in leiomyosarcoma and human papillary thyroid carcinoma [9, 10].

The mouse skin model of multistage carcinogenesis has been used for over 60 years and is one of the most well-established *in vivo* models for studying the stepwise and chronological development of epithelial tumors [11, 12]. Multistage chemical carcinogenesis in this model can be subdivided into three stages: initiation, promotion, and progression. The initiation step involves application of a subcarcinogenic dose of a carcinogen such as 7,12-dimethylbenz[a]anthracene (DMBA), which induces mutations in gene(s) through metabolism to reactive diol-epoxide metabolites and their subsequent covalent binding to DNA forming DNA adducts. The Ha-ras gene is a primary target of DMBA in this model and is routinely found mutated at codon 61 (A to T mutation) in tumors generated by initiation with polycyclic aromatic hydrocarbon [11]. Subsequently, the process of tumor promotion is accomplished by the repeated application of a tumor-promoting agent, most commonly the phorbol ester, 12-*O*-tetradecanoylphorbol-13-acetate (TPA). TPA treatment induces epidermal proliferation and clonal expansion of initiated cells. Lastly, the tumor progression stage occurs stochastically and leads to the conversion of skin papillomas to squamous cell carcinomas (SCCs) [11–14]. In this model of skin carcinogenesis, Stat3 is activated very early in the epidermis following treatment with different classes of tumor promoters, including TPA, okadaic acid, and chrysarobin [15]. In addition, Stat3 is upregulated and constitutively activated in skin papillomas and SCCs generated by the two-stage protocol. The primary mechanism for activation of Stat3 in mouse keratinocytes exposed to tumor promoters is through activation of epidermal growth factor receptor (EGFR) (Figure 1) [15], although other pathways may also contribute to its activation during tumor promotion. Given the unique embryonic lethal phenotype of Stat3 targeting, tissue-specific knockout and inducible knockout strategies using the Cre-*loxP* system have been used to elucidate the role(s) of Stat3 in skin biology and skin carcinogenesis [16]. Loss-of-function studies have been complimented by a Stat3 mouse model expressing a constitutively activated Stat3 protein (Stat3C) under the control of the keratin 5 promoter (K5.Stat3C transgenic mice). Studies from this comprehensive set of skin-specific knockout and transgenic Stat3 mouse models have shown that Stat3 plays a major role in skin carcinogenesis. Herein, we review the use of these mouse models and the insights gained regarding the role of Stat3 in skin carcinogenesis.

2. Skin-Specific Deletion of Stat3 Reveals Roles in Wound Healing and Hair Cycle

Due to the embryonic lethality of $Stat3^{-/-}$ mice, mice with conditional deletion of Stat3 in the skin were generated by crossing $Stat3^{flox/-}$ mice with a transgenic line expressing Cre recombinase under the control of the human keratin 5 promoter (K5.*Cre*) [17, 18]. The K5 promoter drives gene expression in the basal cell layer of the epidermis and follicular keratinocytes [19]. Thus, expression of Cre recombinase under control of K5 allowed for deletion of the Stat3 gene throughout the epidermis and the outer root sheath of hair follicles [18, 19]. Unlike Stat3$^{-/-}$ mice, K5.*Cre* × Stat3$^{flox/-}$ mice were viable, developed normally, and exhibited normal skin at a young age. However, Stat3 disruption in these mice impaired keratinocyte migration during the wound healing process both *in vivo* and *in vitro*. In addition, Stat3 loss compromised mainly the second anagen phase of the hair cycle [17]. Thus, older mice developed a sparse hair coat and also developed spontaneous skin ulcers due to impaired wound healing. From these studies it was concluded that Stat3 was not involved in skin morphogenesis but that it plays a significant role in skin remodeling through its effects on wound healing and the hair cycle [17, 20].

3. Skin-Specific Deletion of Stat3 Reveals Roles in both the Initiation and Promotion Stages of Two-Stage Chemical Carcinogenesis

Various forms of skin wounding are known to promote skin tumors in mice [11]. As mentioned above, studies using mice with a keratinocyte-specific deletion of Stat3 revealed a significant role for Stat3 in skin wound healing. Therefore, further studies were conducted to examine the possible role of Stat3 in skin carcinogenesis. For these studies, mice containing both floxed Stat3 alleles (i.e., Stat3$^{flox/flox}$ mice) were used to reduce the severity of the wounding defect seen in mice harboring one floxed allele and one null allele (i.e., Stat3$^{flox/-}$ mice) in the original studies [17]. Stat3$^{flox/flox}$ mice were crossed with K5.Cre mice to produce an epidermis-specific deficiency Stat3 [21]. Thus, use of this skin-specific Stat3-deficient mouse model demonstrated that Stat3 was absolutely required for development of skin tumors using the two-stage DMBA-TPA protocol. In this regard, loss of Stat3 completely suppressed the development of skin papillomas. Further studies using these mice revealed that Stat3 deficiency sensitized keratinocytes to DMBA-induced apoptosis both *in vivo* and *in vitro* [21]. Interestingly, Stat3-deficient keratinocytes that underwent apoptosis after DMBA treatment *in vivo* were localized in the bulge region adjacent to label-retaining cells (LRCs) [21]. The proximity of DMBA-sensitive cells to LRCs raised the possibility that the loss of Stat3 induced a loss of initiated keratinocyte stems cells in this model (discussed in more detail below). These data suggested that Stat3 played a role during the initiation stage of skin carcinogenesis through its ability to regulate genes involved in keratinocyte survival during the process of tumor initiation.

The repeated treatment with TPA after initiation is used to induce epidermal proliferation and clonal expansion of initiated cells that harbor Ha-ras mutations, which ultimately leads to development of premalignant papillomas [11, 12]. Loss of Stat3 in K5.Cre × Stat3$^{flox/flox}$ mice resulted in a significant reduction of epidermal hyperproliferation (assessed by bromodeoxyuridine (BrdU) labeling index) compared to control littermates following TPA treatment [15, 21]. Mechanistic studies showed that recovery of cell cycle regulatory proteins cyclin D1 and cyclin E was delayed and c-myc expression was persistently downregulated in the epidermis of K5.Cre × Stat3$^{flox/flox}$ mice after topical treatment with TPA in comparison to control mice. Thus, constitutive deletion of Stat3 in the basal layer of epidermis inhibited TPA-induced epidermal hyperproliferation during tumor promotion. Additional studies investigating the role of Stat3 in clonal expansion of initiated cells during promotion were conducted using the TG.AC mouse model. TG.AC transgenic mice express a fusion protein of the activated v-Ha-Ras oncogene and the mouse zeta-globin gene [29]. In this model expression of activated v-Ha-Ras replaces the initiation step (DMBA treatment) of the two-stage chemical carcinogenesis protocol. Promotion in TG.AC mice with TPA results in development of multiple papillomas that progress to SCCs [29]. Inhibition of Stat3 using an oligonucleotide decoy targeting Stat3 inhibited TPA-induced papilloma formation in TG.AC mice, confirming that Stat3 is required for the clonal expansion of initiated cells during the promotion phase of two-stage skin carcinogenesis [21]. Moreover, intratumoral injection of Stat3 decoy caused regression in preexisting skin papillomas [21]. Collectively, these studies using K5.Cre × Stat3$^{flox/flox}$ mice indicated that Stat3 is required for survival of keratinocytes that have accumulated DNA damage during initiation with DMBA and that initiated keratinocytes harboring Ha-ras mutations require Stat3 for proliferation and clonal expansion during tumor promotion with TPA.

4. Inducible Stat3 Deficiency Using K5.CreER^{T2} × Stat3$^{flox/flox}$ Mice Directly Confirms a Role for Stat3 in Both the Initiation and Promotion Stages of Skin Carcinogenesis

While the studies using K5.Cre × Stat3$^{flox/flox}$ mice provided strong evidence that Stat3 was involved in both the initiation and promotion stages of skin carcinogenesis, more direct evidence was obtained using an inducible system where Stat3 could be deleted in a temporal manner. Thus, intercross of Stat3$^{flox/flox}$ mice with a transgenic mouse expressing a tamoxifen inducible *Cre* (i.e., Cre-ER^{T2}) gene under the control of the K5 promoter (K5.CreER^{T2} mice) provided a temporally controlled and inducible epidermis-specific Stat3-deficient mouse model [24, 30]. Using this mouse model, temporal disruption of Stat3 at the time of initiation resulted in an increased number of apoptotic cells following DMBA treatment [24]. In a two-stage carcinogenesis experiment, tamoxifen treatment prior to DMBA treatment of inducible Stat3-deficient mice significantly delayed tumor onset and reduced the number of papillomas per mouse [24]. Similarly, inducible deletion of Stat3 prior to each TPA treatment during the tumor promotion stage delayed tumor onset and tumor multiplicity. Mechanistic studies confirmed that deletion of Stat3 using this inducible system led to reduced levels of survival proteins such as Bcl-x$_L$ and S-phase proteins such as cyclin D1, cyclin E, and c-myc supporting the earlier observations using K5.Cre × Stat3$^{flox/flox}$ mice.

The availability of an inducible Stat3 knockout model also allowed deletion of Stat3 in skin papillomas generated by the DMBA-TPA protocol. In this regard, deletion of Stat3 in skin papillomas by i.p. injection of tamoxifen inhibited subsequent growth of these tumors. Collectively, these studies using an inducible Stat3 knockout system provided direct evidence for a role of Stat3 in both the initiation and promotion stages of skin carcinogenesis. Furthermore, these studies showed that deletion of Stat3 reduced the levels of both survival proteins and cell cycle proteins involved in G1 to S-phase transition. Finally, the use of these models demonstrated the requirement for Stat3 activation for continued growth of skin papillomas.

5. Stat3C Transgenic Mice Reveal a Novel Role for Stat3 in Skin Tumor Progression

Constitutive activation of Stat3 is observed in a variety of human tumors [6, 7] as noted above. This persistent activation can be recapitulated experimentally by substituting residues A661 and N663 for cysteine residues, allowing for cysteine-cysteine sulfhydryl bonds between Stat3 monomers and the formation of Stat3 homodimers without the phosphorylation of Tyr^{705} [31]. This form of Stat3, referred to as Stat3C, was initially shown to transform mouse and rat fibroblasts as demonstrated by anchorage-independent growth in soft agar and formation of tumors when these cells were injected into nude mice [31]. Further study of the role of Stat3 in skin carcinogenesis was facilitated by the generation of mice that express this constitutively active/dimerized form of Stat3 targeted to the proliferative compartment of epidermis using the bovine K5 promoter (i.e., K5.Stat3C transgenic mice) [27]. K5.Stat3C transgenic mice did not develop spontaneous tumors but did exhibit a mild hyperproliferative epidermis and developed spontaneous psoriatic skin lesions with age [28]. In addition, K5.Stat3C mice showed an increased BrdU labeling index after TPA treatment compared to nontransgenic littermates. Expression of Stat3C in the basal compartment of the epidermis significantly protected keratinocytes from DMBA-induced apoptosis [27]. In a DMBA-TPA skin carcinogenesis protocol, K5.Stat3C mice developed skin tumors in greater number and with a shortened latency compared to nontransgenic littermates. Notably, 100% of skin tumors that developed in K5.Stat3C transgenic mice bypassed the premalignant (papilloma) stage and initially developed as carcinoma *in situ*. Histological and immunohistochemical analyses revealed that these tumors were highly vascularized and poorly differentiated, and invasion into surrounding dermal/mesenchymal tissue was observed at a very early stage. Expression of K10, filaggrin, and E-cadherin was completely lost in skin tumors from K5.Stat3C transgenic mice by 20 weeks [27]. Thus, expression of a constitutively active form of Stat3 significantly increased the rate of tumor progression in this model system. This effect of Stat3 was associated with increased expression of Twist, a transcription factor known to regulate genes involved in epithelial-mesenchymal transition (EMT) [27, 32]. Thus, use of this unique mouse model led to the discovery that Stat3 plays an important role not only in the initiation and promotion stages of skin carcinogenesis but also during the progression stage.

6. Deletion of Stat3 in Bulge Region Keratinocyte Stem Cells

Keratinocyte stem cells (KSCs) located in the bulge region of hair follicles are self-renewing cells that provide transit-amplifying cells necessary for hair regrowth and skin homeostasis [33]. In addition, KSCs in the bulge region are believed to be target cells for tumor development in two-stage chemical carcinogenesis of mouse skin [34, 35]. The K15 promoter has been reported to be specifically active in the bulge region of the murine hair follicle and has been used to characterize KSCs in the bulge region. For loss-of-function studies of bulge region KSCs, Morris [35] generated K15.CrePR1 transgenic mice. Cre-PR1 is a fusion protein that consists of Cre recombinase and a truncated form of the progesterone receptor that binds to the progesterone antagonist RU486 but not to endogenous progesterone [35, 36]. To further investigate the role of Stat3 in bulge region keratinocytes during multistage skin carcinogenesis, Dae et al. [25] utilized the K15.CrePR1 transgenic mouse model in combination with $Stat3^{flox/flox}$ mice. Using this inducible model, Stat3 deletion at the time of initiation in bulge region keratinocytes led to a significant reduction in tumor incidence and multiplicity (~80% reduction in papilloma formation). The K15.CrePR1 inducible system is not 100% efficient and the small number of papillomas obtained from these knockout mice stained positive for Stat3. This data indicated that Stat3 is absolutely necessary for tumor development, since the remaining Stat3-positive KSCs were selected during tumor promotion. In addition, DMBA treatment led to a significant increase in the number of apoptotic keratinocytes in the bulge region of the knockout mice. FACS analysis showed that there was a reduction in the percentage of bulge region KSCs that were positive for CD34 and α6-integrin in the knockout mice compared to the control mice 24 hours after DMBA treatment. Furthermore, the α6+CD34+ population from K15.CrePR1 × $Stat3^{flox/flox}$ mice showed a reduction of the signature Ha-ras codon 61 A^{182} to T mutation induced by topical application of DMBA [25]. Hence, Stat3 status influenced survival of DNA-damaged KSCs, since the absence of Stat3 led to increased apoptosis of bulge region KSCs following treatment with DMBA ultimately leading to reduced number of mutated cells available for clonal expansion during tumor promotion [25]. These data suggested that Stat3 plays an important role in the behavior of bulge region KSCs during the initiation step of skin tumor development by the two-stage chemical carcinogenesis protocol.

7. Stat3 in UVB-Induced Skin Carcinogenesis

The availability of both loss-of-function and gain-of-function mouse models for Stat3 in skin keratinocytes facilitated further study of this important molecule in skin carcinogenesis mediated by ultraviolet B (UVB) exposure. UV radiation, and in particular UVB exposure, is the major risk factor for nonmelanoma skin cancer in humans [37]. Following exposure to UVB, the level of phosphorylated Stat3 (p-Stat3) is initially decreased, followed by a significant increase at later time points in the mouse epidermis. The levels of Stat3 target genes, such as cyclin D1, Bcl-x_L, and c-Myc, followed the changes in activated Stat3 in response to UVB irradiation [38]. Epidermis-specific Stat3-deficient mice were found to be very sensitive to UVB radiation as revealed by a higher number of sunburned and apoptotic cells following irradiation with UVB [22]. On the other hand, the epidermis of K5.Stat3C mice was significantly resistant to UVB-induced apoptosis [23]. Furthermore, additional studies showed that protection against UVB-induced apoptosis in Stat3C transgenic mice was not due to impaired DNA damage response. Instead, the status of Stat3 influenced the survival of cells containing UVB-induced DNA photoproducts, including those cells located in the bulge region of the hair follicles through regulation of antiapoptotic genes such as Bcl-x_L [23, 26]. In line with these observations, overexpression of Stat3C in K5.Stat3C mice enhanced UVB-induced skin carcinogenesis (both incidence and tumor multiplicity) compared to the wild-type controls [23]. In contrast, Stat3-deficient mice were resistant to UVB skin carcinogenesis compared to wild-type controls [23]. Thus, based on these studies Stat3 appears to play a strikingly similar role in both chemical and UVB-mediated skin carcinogenesis.

8. Studies Using Other Mouse Models Support an Important Role of Stat3 in Skin Carcinogenesis

As noted above Bcl-x_L is one of several antiapoptotic proteins regulated by Stat3 [39]. Deletion of Stat3 in keratinocytes leads to a concomitant and dramatic reduction in levels of Bcl-x_L [24]. To study the functional role of Bcl-x_L in skin carcinogenesis, skin-specific Bc-x_L-deficient mice were generated. In this model, Bcl-x_L expression is disrupted in the basal compartment of mouse epidermis using the bovine K5 promoter to drive expression of Cre recombinase (i.e., K5.Cre × Bcl-$x_L^{flox/flox}$ mice). A significant increase in apoptosis induced by either UVB irradiation or DMBA treatment was observed in the epidermis of Bcl-x_L-deficient mice. Furthermore, an increase in apoptotic cells was noted in hair follicle keratinocytes, including those located in the bulge region. Cell proliferation was not affected by Bcl-x_L deficiency following exposure to either UVB or TPA. Bcl-x_L-deficient mice were more resistant than wild-type controls to skin tumor development with delayed onset and reduced number of tumors using either UVB complete carcinogenesis or the DMBA/TPA two-stage regimen. Moreover, Bcl-2, Mcl-1, and survivin protein levels were increased in the epidermis of Bcl-x_L-deficient mice in the absence of stimuli. Furthermore, levels of these antiapoptotic proteins were also high in skin tumors from Bcl-x_L-deficient mice that developed in response to either UVB or two-stage carcinogenesis protocols. Collectively, these studies demonstrated that Bcl-x_L plays a role early in skin carcinogenesis through its antiapoptotic functions to enhance survival of keratinocytes, including bulge region KSCs, following DNA damage. These data also demonstrated that one of the antiapoptotic genes known to be regulated by Stat3 was likely mediating at least some of its action during the initiation stage of multistage skin carcinogenesis. However, deletion of Bcl-x_L did not fully recapitulate the actions of Stat3 deletion during initiation indicating that other Stat3-regulated genes are also likely involved in the action of Stat3.

It is also noteworthy that Stat3 function appears to be necessary for epidermal hyperplasia and susceptibility to skin tumor formation in other transgenic mouse models. In this regard, Stat3 has been implicated in proteins kinase c epsilon (PKCε) mediated UV skin carcinogenesis. Stat3 Tyr^{705} and Ser^{727} phosphorylation is increased in K5. PKCε transgenic epidermis after UV irradiation compared to controls. Like Stat3C, overexpression of PKCε in mouse skin (K5.PKCε) inhibited apoptosis, promoted cell survival, and induced development of SCCs in UVB skin carcinogenesis experiments [40–42]. These studies show an interaction between PKCε and Stat3 that leads to Stat3 activation by phosphorylation at Ser^{727}. Phosphorylation at Ser^{727} is necessary for full transcriptional activity of Stat3 *in vivo* and may aid in the development of SCCs in K5.PKCε transgenic mice [43]. Collectively, these studies demonstrate that Stat3 plays a critical role in the development of UVB-induced skin tumors through its effects on both survival and proliferation of keratinocytes [23].

In other studies, overexpression of human papillomavirus 8 (HPV8) in mouse skin using the K14 promoter (i.e., K14.HPV8 transgenic mice) leads to epidermal hyperplasia and the development of spontaneous SCCs [44]. These tumors exhibited an increased level of p-Stat3 Tyr^{705} [44]. In a two-stage carcinogenesis bioassay, loss of a single Stat3 allele reduced HPV8-mediated epidermal hyperplasia and skin tumorigenesis [44]. Loss of Stat3 also produced similar effects in a mouse model of basal cell carcinoma [45]. In this model, SmoM2 expression in the basal epidermal layer was also driven by the K14 promoter (i.e., K14.SmoM2 transgenic mice). Epidermal-specific knockout of Stat3 in the K14.SmoM2 transgenic mice significantly reduced SmoM2-mediated epidermal hyperplasia and tumor development [45]. These studies further demonstrate the importance of Stat3 in skin carcinogenesis.

9. Stat3 and Human Skin Cancer

Activation of Stat3 appears to play an important role in the development of human nonmelanoma skin cancer. Stat3 is found constitutively activated in UVB-induced SCCs from both mouse and human skin [22]. Increased p-Stat3 expression in human SCCs and basal cell carcinomas (BCCs) in comparison to normal skin has been observed in various retrospective studies [46–49]. This increased expression of p-Stat3 is inversely associated with cellular differentiation, with expression in poorly differentiated SCCs being significantly higher than in well-differentiated SCCs [46, 47]. A positive correlation between p-Stat3 expression and depth of tumor invasion, but not tumor size, was also observed [46, 47].

Furthermore, like SCCs derived from K5.Stat3C transgenic mice, human SCCs display a negative correlation between the expression of p-Stat3 and E-cadherin [27, 46]. Stat3-mediated downregulation of E-cadherin, in conjunction with Stat3-mediated induction of twist as observed in K5.Stat3C-derived SCCs, may promote EMT and contribute to the metastatic potential of SCCs. These data suggest that Stat3 plays an important role in the development and progression of human SCCs.

Head and neck cancers are a group of biologically similar cancers that stem from the lip, oral cavity, nasal cavity, paranasal sinuses, pharynx, and larynx. In this group of cancers, it is estimated that 90% are SCCs or head and neck squamous cell carcinoma (HNSCC), which originate from the mucosal lining (epithelium) in these tissues [50]. HNSCCs are very similar histologically to SCCs of the skin and both share a number of similar molecular alterations. In particular, as observed in cutaneous SCCs, preclinical and clinical studies have implicated Stat3 in the development and progression of HNSCCs [51–54]. In head and neck tumor tissue, Stat3 is found upregulated and constitutively activated (phosphorylated) and has a positive correlation with poor prognosis [51, 54]. Preclinical studies have shown that HNSCC cell lines stably transfected with a constitutively active STAT3 construct expressed elevated levels of STAT3 target genes, including Bcl-x_L and cyclin D1, leading to increased proliferation *in vitro* and more rapid tumor growth rates *in vivo* [55]. In addition, targeting Stat3 increases tumor cell apoptosis and decreased Bcl-x_L expression in a head and neck xenograft model [53]. In addition, reducing Stat3 activity by targeting upstream proteins has shown promise in HNSCC preclinical and clinical studies. In this regard, inhibiting EGFR-Stat3 pathway in 4-nitroquinoline-1-oxide (4-NQO-) induced murine model of oral carcinogenesis by erlotinib, a small molecule inhibitor of EGFR, inhibited development of preneoplastic lesions and oral tumors by approximately 70% with a concomitant decrease of Stat3 levels in erlotinib-treated mice [56]. Similarly, primary human oral cavity squamous cell cancers showed reduced levels of both EGFR and p-Stat3 after treatment with erlotinib compared to pretreated paired tissue [57]. Moreover, combined molecular targeting of Stat3 sensitizes cells to radiotherapy and small molecule chemotherapeutic agents *in vitro* [58, 59]. Together, these data have provided the basis for targeting Stat3 in HNSCC in a clinical setting (discussed below).

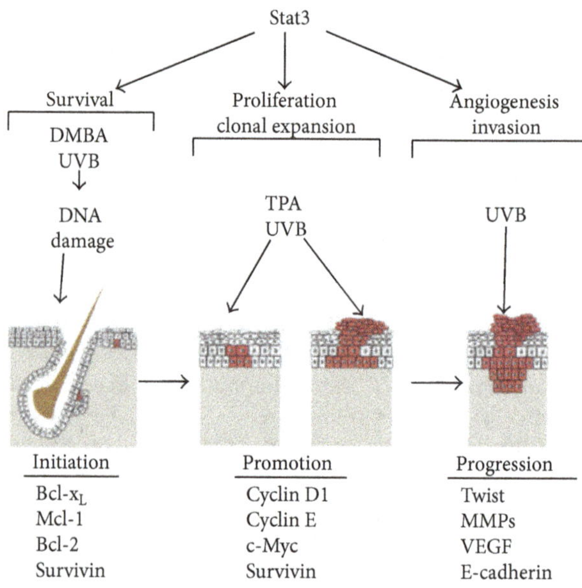

FIGURE 2: From studies in loss-of-function and gain-of-function mouse models, Stat3 has been shown to have a critical role in all three stages of skin carcinogenesis whether induced by chemicals (using the standard DMBA-TPA protocol) or by complete carcinogenesis with UVB. During the initiation stage, Stat3 aids in the survival of DNA-damaged keratinocyte stem cells (bulge region and possibly those in the interfollicular epidermis) induced by DMBA or UVB-irradiation by upregulation of prosurvival proteins such as bcl-x_L, bcl-2, mcl-1, and survivin. Clonal expansion of initiated cells (promotion) is carried out through repeated treatment with TPA or UVB. In this stage, Stat3-mediated induction of cell cycle regulatory proteins (e.g., cyclin D1, cyclin E, c-myc, and survivin) is necessary for keratinocyte proliferation, epidermal hyperplasia, and development of papillomas/premalignant lesions. Progression or conversion of papillomas to SCCs is denoted as a downward invading lesion that traverses into the dermal compartment. Stat3 plays a role in the progression stage by regulating genes involved in angiogenesis and invasion (e.g., VEGF, MMPs, twist, E-cadherin).

10. Perspectives and Future Directions

Collectively, the comprehensive set of skin-specific gain- and loss-of-function mouse models described above have revealed that Stat3 plays a critical role in all three stages of skin carcinogenesis induced by either chemical exposure or UVB irradiation (see Table 1 for a listing of these mouse models). Stat3 is required for survival of DNA-damaged KSCs and the proliferation necessary for clonal expansion of initiated cells during tumor promotion. In addition, Stat3 also appears to have a role in driving malignant conversion of skin tumors. Although UVB is a complete carcinogen, it possesses both initiating and promoting activity that can be distinguished experimentally. From the available data, Stat3 appears to play a very similar mechanistic role during UVB-mediated skin carcinogenesis. Figure 2 summarizes our current state of knowledge regarding Stat3 function in skin carcinogenesis.

The current data also suggest that targeting Stat3 activation may provide an effective strategy for both the prevention and treatment of skin cancer. However, targeting Stat3 directly has proven to be difficult and this molecule has largely seemed "undruggable" [60]. Many approaches have been taken to target Stat3 activity, including inhibition of upstream proteins such as receptor and nonreceptor tyrosine kinases, targeting of Stat3 SH2 domains to prevent phosphorylation/dimerization, inhibition of Stat3 DNA-binding activity, and inhibition of nuclear import [61]. Until recently, inhibition of upstream regulatory proteins has made the most progress in clinical trials [62]. Phase 0 (University of Pittsburgh, Pittsburgh, PA) and phase 1 clinical trials (MD Anderson Cancer Center, Houston, TX, USA and Otsuka Pharmaceuticals, Princeton, NJ, USA) evaluating

TABLE 1: Mouse models for evaluating Stat3 function in skin carcinogenesis.

Mouse model	Skin phenotype	Susceptibility to skin carcinogenesis	References
K5.Cre × $Stat3^{flox/-}$	(i) Defective wound healing (ii) Defective hair cycle from 2nd anagen onward	Not tested	[17]
K5.Cre × $Stat3^{flox/flox}$	No visible phenotype	Reduced susceptibility to both DMBA-TPA and UVB carcinogenesis	[21–23]
K5.$CreER^{T2}$× $Stat3^{flox/flox}$	No visible phenotype	Reduced susceptibility to both tumor initiation with DMBA and tumor promotion with TPA; UVB not tested	[24]
K15.CrePR1 × $Stat3^{flox/flox}$	No visible phenotype	Reduced susceptibility to tumor initiation by DMBA; UVB not tested	[25]
K5.Cre × Bcl-$x_L^{flox/flox}$	No visible phenotype	Reduced susceptibility to both DMBA-TPA and UVB carcinogenesis	[26]
K5.Stat3C	(i) Enlarged blood vessels in skin at birth (ii) Sparse hair coat (iii) Increased skin vascularization in adult mice (iv) Hypervascularization in response to mild wounding (e.g., tape stripping) (v) Develop scaly, hyperkeratotic lesions on tail (psoriasis) (vi) No spontaneous skin tumors	Enhanced susceptibility to DMBA-TPA and UVB skin carcinogenesis Enhanced progression of skin tumors to SCCs	[22, 23, 27, 28]

Stat3 inhibitors have recently been completed. In addition, a phase 1 (Isis Pharmaceuticals, San Diego, CA, USA) and an observational clinical trial (New York University, New York, NY, USA) are in the recruiting stages. The completed phase 0 clinical trial evaluated the safety of an oligonucleotide decoy targeting Stat3 by intratumoral injection in patients with HNSCC [63]. Interestingly, a single intratumoral injection with a Stat3 decoy showed decreased Stat3 target gene expression of cyclin D1 and Bcl-x_L in HNSCC biopsies [63]. Moreover, by circularizing the 15-base pair oligonucleotide with two hexaethylene glycol linkages, Sen and colleagues were able to inhibit tumor growth in preclinical mouse xenografts via systemic administration [63]. These studies offer promise for expanded phase 1 clinical trials in HNSCC patients and a wide range of malignancies that are dependent on Stat3 activation, including nonmelanoma skin cancers.

Recent evidence suggests a novel role for Stat3 in mitochondrial respiration, presumably via its interaction with electron transport chain components [64] and see again Figure 1. Mitochondrial localized Stat3 (referred to as mitoStat3) is necessary for Ha-ras-mediated transformation of mouse embryonic fibroblasts independent of Stat3 nuclear activity or tyrosine phosphorylation [65]. In addition, unphosphorylated Stat3 (U-Stat3), which was previously thought to be an inactive protein, has recently been shown to regulate gene transcription through a mechanism distinct from that of tyrosine-phosphorylated Stat3 dimers [66–68]. U-Stat3 has been shown to interact with nuclear factor-κB (NF-κB) (Figure 1) and regulate genes with κB elements, but it can also induce a cohort of genes through an NF κB independent mechanism [67]. Expression of U-Stat3 enhances hepatocellular carcinoma (HCC) formation in Ras-transformed $p19^{ARF-/-}$ hepatocytes [67, 69]. Whether mitoStat3 or U-Stat3 plays a role in epithelial carcinogenesis is unclear at the present time. Future studies should also evaluate these potential mechanisms and will likely require the development of additional mouse models. In addition, targeting or exploiting these noncanonical activities associated with Stat3 for both prevention and treatment strategies may also be warranted.

Acknowledgments

The authors thank Linda Beltran and Lauren Pascale for their assistance in the preparation of this paper. Original research was supported by NIH Grant CA76520 (to J. DiGiovanni).

References

[1] J. Bromberg and J. E. Darnell Jr., "The role of STATs in transcriptional control and their impact on cellular function," *Oncogene*, vol. 19, no. 21, pp. 2468–2473, 2000.

[2] D. E. Levy and J. E. Darnell Jr., "Stats: transcriptional control and biological impact," *Nature Reviews Molecular Cell Biology*, vol. 3, no. 9, pp. 651–662, 2002.

[3] T. Kisseleva, S. Bhattacharya, J. Braunstein, and C. W. Schindler, "Signaling through the JAK/STAT pathway, recent advances and future challenges," *Gene*, vol. 285, no. 1-2, pp. 1–24, 2002.

[4] Z. Zhong, Z. Wen, and J. E. Darnell Jr., "Stat3: a STAT family member activated by tyrosine phosphorylation in response to epidermal growth factor and interleukin-6," *Science*, vol. 264, no. 5155, pp. 95–98, 1994.

[5] J. E. Darnell Jr., I. M. Kerr, and G. R. Stark, "Jak-STAT pathways and transcriptional activation in response to IFNs and other extracellular signaling proteins," *Science*, vol. 264, no. 5164, pp. 1415–1421, 1994.

[6] T. Bowman, R. Garcia, J. Turkson, and R. Jove, "STATs in oncogenesis," *Oncogene*, vol. 19, no. 21, pp. 2474–2488, 2000.

[7] J. Turkson and R. Jove, "STAT proteins: novel molecular targets for cancer drug discovery," *Oncogene*, vol. 19, no. 56, pp. 6613–6626, 2000.

[8] N. de la Iglesia, G. Konopka, S. V. Puram et al., "Identification of a PTEN-regulated STAT3 brain tumor suppressor pathway," *Genes and Development*, vol. 22, no. 4, pp. 449–462, 2008.

[9] J. P. Couto, L. Daly, A. Almeida et al., "STAT3 negatively regulates thyroid tumorigenesis," *Proceedings of the National Academy of Sciences of the United States of America*, vol. 109, no. 35, pp. E2361–E2370, 2012.

[10] N. Setsu, K. Kohashi, M. Endo et al., "Phosphorylation of signal transducer and activator of transcription 3 in soft tissue leiomyosarcoma is associated with a better prognosis," *International Journal of Cancer*, vol. 132, no. 1, pp. 109–115, 2013.

[11] J. DiGiovanni, "Multistage carcinogenesis in mouse skin," *Pharmacology and Therapeutics*, vol. 54, no. 1, pp. 63–128, 1992.

[12] E. L. Abel, J. M. Angel, K. Kiguchi, and J. DiGiovanni, "Multistage chemical carcinogenesis in mouse skin: fundamentals and applications," *Nature Protocols*, vol. 4, no. 9, pp. 1350–1362, 2009.

[13] T. J. Slaga, S. M. Fischer, C. E. Weeks, and A. J. Klein-Szanto, "Multistage chemical carcinogenesis in mouse skin," *Current Problems in Dermatology*, vol. 10, pp. 193–218, 1980.

[14] T. J. Slaga, "Multistage skin carcinogenesis: a useful model for the study of the chemoprevention of cancer," *Acta Pharmacologica et Toxicologica*, vol. 55, supplement 2, pp. 107–124, 1984.

[15] K. S. Chan, S. Carbajal, K. Kiguchi, J. Clifford, S. Sano, and J. DiGiovanni, "Epidermal growth factor receptor-mediated activation of Stat3 during multistage skin carcinogenesis," *Cancer Research*, vol. 64, no. 7, pp. 2382–2389, 2004.

[16] K. Takeda, K. Noguchi, W. Shi et al., "Targeted disruption of the mouse Stat3 gene leads to early embryonic lethality," *Proceedings of the National Academy of Sciences of the United States of America*, vol. 94, no. 8, pp. 3801–3804, 1997.

[17] S. Sano, S. Itami, K. Takeda et al., "Keratinocyte-specific ablation of Stat3 exhibits impaired skin remodeling, but does not affect skin morphogenesis," *The EMBO Journal*, vol. 18, no. 17, pp. 4657–4668, 1999.

[18] M. Tarutani, S. Itami, M. Okabe et al., "Tissue-specific knockout of the mouse Pig-a gene reveals important roles for GPI-anchored proteins in skin development," *Proceedings of the National Academy of Sciences of the United States of America*, vol. 94, no. 14, pp. 7400–7405, 1997.

[19] C. Byrne and E. Fuchs, "Probing keratinocyte and differentiation specificity of the human K5 promoter in vitro and in transgenic mice," *Molecular and Cellular Biology*, vol. 13, no. 6, pp. 3176–3190, 1993.

[20] S. Sano, K. S. Chan, and J. DiGiovanni, "Impact of Stat3 activation upon skin biology: a dichotomy of its role between homeostasis and diseases," *Journal of Dermatological Science*, vol. 50, no. 1, pp. 1–14, 2008.

[21] K. S. Chan, S. Sano, K. Kiguchi et al., "Disruption of Stat3 reveals a critical role in both the initiation and the promotion stages of epithelial carcinogenesis," *Journal of Clinical Investigation*, vol. 114, no. 5, pp. 720–728, 2004.

[22] S. Sano, K. S. Chan, M. Kira et al., "Signal transducer and activator of transcription 3 is a key regulator of keratinocyte survival and proliferation following UV irradiation," *Cancer Research*, vol. 65, no. 13, pp. 5720–5729, 2005.

[23] D. J. Kim, J. M. Angel, S. Sano, and J. DiGiovanni, "Constitutive activation and targeted disruption of signal transducer and activator of transcription 3 (Stat3) in mouse epidermis reveal its critical role in UVB-induced skin carcinogenesis," *Oncogene*, vol. 28, no. 7, pp. 950–960, 2009.

[24] K. Kataoka, D. J. Kim, S. Carbajal, J. L. Clifford, and J. DiGiovanni, "Stage-specific disruption of Stat3 demonstrates a direct requirement during both the initiation and promotion stages of mouse skin tumorigenesis," *Carcinogenesis*, vol. 29, no. 6, pp. 1108–1114, 2008.

[25] J. K. Dae, K. Kataoka, D. Rao, K. Kiguchi, G. Cotsarelis, and J. DiGiovanni, "Targeted disruption of Stat3 reveals a major role for follicular stem cells in skin tumor initiation," *Cancer Research*, vol. 69, no. 19, pp. 7587–7594, 2009.

[26] J. K. Dae, K. Kataoka, S. Sano, K. Connolly, K. Kiguchi, and J. DiGiovanni, "Targeted disruption of Bcl-xL in mouse keratinocytes inhibits both UVB- and chemically induced skin carcinogenesis," *Molecular Carcinogenesis*, vol. 48, no. 10, pp. 873–885, 2009.

[27] K. S. Chan, S. Sano, K. Kataoka et al., "Forced expression of a constitutively active form of Stat3 in mouse epidermis enhances malignant progression of skin tumors induced by two-stage carcinogenesis," *Oncogene*, vol. 27, no. 8, pp. 1087–1094, 2008.

[28] S. Sano, K. S. Chan, S. Carbajal et al., "Stat3 links activated keratinocytes and immunocytes required for development of psoriasis in a novel transgenic mouse model," *Nature Medicine*, vol. 11, no. 1, pp. 43–49, 2005.

[29] A. Leder, A. Kuo, R. D. Cardiff, E. Sinn, and P. Leder, "v-Ha-ras transgene abrogates the initiation step in mouse skin tumorigenesis: effects of phorbol esters and retinoic acid," *Proceedings of the National Academy of Sciences of the United States of America*, vol. 87, no. 23, pp. 9178–9182, 1990.

[30] A. K. Indra, X. Warot, J. Brocard et al., "Temporally-controlled site-specific mutagenesis in the basal layer of the epidermis: comparison of the recombinase activity of the tamoxifen-inducible Cre-ER(T) and Cre-ER(T2) recombinases," *Nucleic Acids Research*, vol. 27, no. 22, pp. 4324–4327, 1999.

[31] J. F. Bromberg, M. H. Wrzeszczynska, G. Devgan et al., "Stat3 as an oncogene," *Cell*, vol. 98, no. 3, pp. 295–303, 1999.

[32] J. Yang, S. A. Mani, and R. A. Weinberg, "Exploring a new twist on tumor metastasis," *Cancer Research*, vol. 66, no. 9, pp. 4549–4552, 2006.

[33] R. Ghadially, "25 years of epidermal stem cell research," *Journal of Investigative Dermatology*, vol. 132, no. 3, part 2, pp. 797–810, 2012.

[34] R. J. Morris, "Keratinocyte stem cells: targets for cutaneous carcinogens," *Journal of Clinical Investigation*, vol. 106, no. 1, pp. 3–8, 2000.

[35] R. J. Morris, "A perspective on keratinocyte stem cells as targets for skin carcinogenesis," *Differentiation*, vol. 72, no. 8, pp. 381–386, 2004.

[36] R. J. Morris, Y. Liu, L. Marles et al., "Capturing and profiling adult hair follicle stem cells," *Nature Biotechnology*, vol. 22, no. 4, pp. 411–417, 2004.

[37] D. S. Preston and R. S. Stern, "Nonmelanoma cancers of the skin," *The New England Journal of Medicine*, vol. 327, no. 23, pp. 1649–1662, 1992.

[38] D. J. Kim, M. L. Tremblay, and J. DiGiovanni, "Protein tyrosine phosphatases, TC-PTP, SHP1, and SHP2, cooperate in rapid dephosphorylation of Stat3 in keratinocytes following UVB irradiation," *PLoS ONE*, vol. 5, no. 4, Article ID e10290, 2010.

[39] J. M. Grad, X. R. Zeng, and L. H. Boise, "Regulation of Bcl-xL: a little bit of this and a little bit of STAT," *Current Opinion in Oncology*, vol. 12, no. 6, pp. 543–549, 2000.

[40] M. H. Aziz, H. T. Manoharan, and A. K. Verma, "Protein kinase Cε, which sensitizes skin to sun's UV radiation-induced cutaneous damage and development of squamous cell carcinomas, associates with Stat3," *Cancer Research*, vol. 67, no. 3, pp. 1385–1394, 2007.

[41] M. H. Aziz, H. T. Manoharan, J. M. Sand, and A. K. Verma, "Protein kinase Cε interacts with Stat3 and regulates its activation that is essential for the development of skin cancer," *Molecular Carcinogenesis*, vol. 46, no. 8, pp. 646–653, 2007.

[42] J. M. Sand, M. H. Aziz, N. E. Dreckschmidt et al., "PKCε overexpression, irrespective of genetic background, sensitizes skin to uvr-induced development of squamous-cell carcinomas," *Journal of Investigative Dermatology*, vol. 130, no. 1, pp. 270–277, 2010.

[43] Y. Shen, K. Schlessinger, X. Zhu et al., "Essential role of STAT3 in postnatal survival and growth revealed by mice lacking STAT3 serine 727 phosphorylation," *Molecular and Cellular Biology*, vol. 24, no. 1, pp. 407–419, 2004.

[44] M. de Andrea, M. Ritta, M. M. Landini et al., "Keratinocyte-specific stat3 heterozygosity impairs development of skin tumors in human papillomavirus 8 transgenic mice," *Cancer Research*, vol. 70, no. 20, pp. 7938–7948, 2010.

[45] D. Gu, Q. Fan, X. Zhang, and J. Xie, "A role for transcription factor STAT3 signaling in oncogene smoothened-driven carcinogenesis," *The Journal of Biological Chemistry*, vol. 287, no. 45, pp. 38356–38366, 2012.

[46] C. Suiqing, Z. Min, and C. Lirong, "Overexpression of phosphorylated-STAT3 correlated with the invasion and metastasis of cutaneous squamous cell carcinoma," *Journal of Dermatology*, vol. 32, no. 5, pp. 354–360, 2005.

[47] S. Q. Cai, L. R. Chen, H. J. Wang, L. F. Yao, and M. Zheng, "Effect of STAT3 phosphorylation and p53 expression on human epidermal non melanoma cutaneous tumors," *Zhejiang Da Xue Xue Bao Yi Xue Ban* , vol. 33, no. 4, pp. 331–334, 2004.

[48] S. Y. Chen, S. Takeuchi, Y. Moroi et al., "Overexpression of phosphorylated-ATF2 and STAT3 in cutaneous squamous cell carcinoma, Bowen's disease and basal cell carcinoma," *Journal of Dermatological Science*, vol. 51, no. 3, pp. 210–215, 2008.

[49] Z. L. Liu, Y. Li, Q. Y. Kong et al., "Immunohistochemical profiling of Wnt, NF-κB, Stat3 and Notch signaling in human epidermal tumors," *Journal of Dermatological Science*, vol. 52, no. 2, pp. 133–136, 2008.

[50] D. G. Pfister, K. K. Ang, D. M. Brizel et al., "Head and neck cancers," *Journal of the National Comprehensive Cancer Network*, vol. 9, no. 6, pp. 596–650, 2011.

[51] M. Masuda, M. Suzui, R. Yasumatu et al., "Constitutive activation of signal transducers and activators of transcription 3 correlates with cyclin D1 overexpression and may provide a novel prognostic marker in head and neck squamous cell carcinoma," *Cancer Research*, vol. 62, no. 12, pp. 3351–3355, 2002.

[52] J. I. Song and J. R. Grandis, "STAT signaling in head and neck cancer," *Oncogene*, vol. 19, no. 21, pp. 2489–2495, 2000.

[53] J. R. Grandis, S. D. Drenning, Q. Zeng et al., "Constitutive activation of Stat3 signaling abrogates apoptosis in squamous cell carcinogenesis in vivo," *Proceedings of the National Academy of Sciences of the United States of America*, vol. 97, no. 8, pp. 4227–4232, 2000.

[54] J. K. Nagpal, R. Mishra, and B. R. Das, "Activation of Stat-3 as one of the early events in tobacco chewing-mediated oral carcinogenesis," *Cancer*, vol. 94, no. 9, pp. 2393–2400, 2002.

[55] T. Kijima, H. Niwa, R. A. Steinman et al., "STAT3 activation abrogates growth factor dependence and contributes to head and neck squamous cell carcinoma tumor growth in vivo," *Cell Growth and Differentiation*, vol. 13, no. 8, pp. 355–362, 2002.

[56] R. J. Leeman-Neill, R. R. Seethala, S. V. Singh et al., "Inhibition of EGFR-STAT3 signaling with erlotinib prevents carcinogenesis in a chemically-induced mouse model of oral squamous cell carcinoma," *Cancer Prevention Research*, vol. 4, no. 2, pp. 230–237, 2011.

[57] C. I. Tsien, M. K. Nyati, A. Ahsan et al., "Effect of erlotinib on epidermal growth factor receptor and downstream signaling in oral cavity squamous cell carcinoma," *Head & Neck*, 2012.

[58] J. A. Bonner, E. S. Yang, H. Q. Trummell, S. Nowsheen, C. D. Willey, and K. P. Raisch, "Inhibition of STAT-3 results in greater cetuximab sensitivity in head and neck squamous cell carcinoma," *Radiotherapy and Oncology*, vol. 99, no. 3, pp. 339–343, 2011.

[59] J. A. Bonner, H. Q. Trummell, C. D. Willey, B. A. Plants, and K. P. Raisch, "Inhibition of STAT-3 results in radiosensitization of human squamous cell carcinoma," *Radiotherapy and Oncology*, vol. 92, no. 3, pp. 339–344, 2009.

[60] P. Koppikar and J. Bromberg, "STATe of the art approach: using oligonucleotide decoys to target the, 'undruggable'," *Cancer Discovery*, vol. 2, no. 8, pp. 670–672, 2012.

[61] S. Haftchenary, M. Avadisian, and P. T. Gunning, "Inhibiting aberrant Stat3 function with molecular therapeutics: a progress report," *Anti-Cancer Drugs*, vol. 22, no. 2, pp. 115–127, 2011.

[62] P. Sansone and J. Bromberg, "Targeting the interleukin-6/Jak/stat pathway in human malignancies," *Journal of Clinical Oncology*, vol. 30, no. 9, pp. 1005–1014, 2012.

[63] M. Sen, S. M. Thomas, S. Kim et al., "First-in-human trial of a STAT3 decoy oligonucleotide in head and neck tumors: implications for cancer therapy," *Cancer Discovery*, vol. 2, no. 8, pp. 694–705, 2012.

[64] J. Wegrzyn, R. Potla, Y. J. Chwae et al., "Function of mitochondrial Stat3 in cellular respiration," *Science*, vol. 323, no. 5915, pp. 793–797, 2009.

[65] D. J. Gough, A. Corlett, K. Schlessinger, J. Wegrzyn, A. C. Larner, and D. E. Levy, "Mitochondrial STAT3 supports Ras-dependent oncogenic transformation," *Science*, vol. 324, no. 5935, pp. 1713–1716, 2009.

[66] J. Yang, M. Chatterjee-Kishore, S. M. Staugaitis et al., "Novel roles of unphosphorylated STAT3 in oncogenesis and transcriptional regulation," *Cancer Research*, vol. 65, no. 3, pp. 939–947, 2005.

[67] J. Yang, X. Liao, M. K. Agarwal, L. Barnes, P. E. Auron, and G. R. Stark, "Unphosphorylated STAT3 accumulates in response to

IL-6 and activates transcription by binding to NFκB," *Genes and Development*, vol. 21, no. 11, pp. 1396–1408, 2007.

[68] G. Peña, B. Cai, J. Liu et al., "Unphosphorylated STAT3 modulates alpha7 nicotinic receptor signaling and cytokine production in sepsis," *European Journal of Immunology*, vol. 40, no. 9, pp. 2580–2589, 2010.

[69] D. Schneller, G. Machat, A. Sousek et al., "p19^{ARF}/p14^{ARF} controls oncogenic functions of signal transducer and activator of transcription 3 in hepatocellular carcinoma," *Hepatology*, vol. 54, no. 1, pp. 164–172, 2011.

17

The Pink Rim Sign: Location of Pink as an Indicator of Melanoma in Dermoscopic Images

Ryan K. Rader,[1] Katie S. Payne,[1] Uday Guntupalli,[2] Harold S. Rabinovitz,[3] Maggie C. Oliviero,[3] Rhett J. Drugge,[4] Joseph J. Malters,[5] and William V. Stoecker[1]

[1] *Stoecker & Associates, LLC, 10101 Stoltz Drive, Rolla, MO 65401-7714, USA*
[2] *Missouri University of Science & Technology, G20 Emerson Electric Co. Hall, Rolla, MO 65409 0040, USA*
[3] *Skin and Cancer Associates, 201 NW 82nd Avenue, Bennett Medical Plaza, Suite 501, Plantation, FL 33324, USA*
[4] *Sheard & Drugge PC, 50 Glenbrook Road, Unit 1C, Stamford, CT 06902, USA*
[5] *The Dermatology Center, LLC, 10101 Stoltz Drive, Rolla, MO 65401, USA*

Correspondence should be addressed to William V. Stoecker; wvs@mst.edu

Academic Editor: Mohammed Kashani-Sabet

Background. In dermoscopic images, multiple shades of pink have been described in melanoma without specifying location of these areas within the lesion. *Objective.* The purpose of this study was to determine the statistics for the presence of centrally and peripherally located pink melanoma and benign melanocytic lesions. *Methods.* Three observers, untrained in dermoscopy, each retrospectively analyzed 1290 dermoscopic images (296 melanomas (170 *in situ* and 126 invasive), 994 benign melanocytic nevi) and assessed the presence of any shade of pink in the center and periphery of the lesion. *Results.* Pink was located in the peripheral region in 14.5% of melanomas and 6.3% of benign melanocytic lesions, yielding an odds ratio of 2.51 (95% CI: 1.7 3.8, $P < 0.0001$). Central pink was located in 12.8% of melanomas and 21.8% of benign lesions, yielding an odds ratio of 0.462 (95% CI: 0.67, $P = 0.204$). Pink in melanoma *in situ* tended to be present throughout the lesion (68% of pink lesions). Pink in invasive melanoma was present in 17% of cases, often presenting as a pink rim. *Conclusions.* The presence of pink in the periphery or rim of a dermoscopic melanocytic lesion image provides an indication of malignancy. We offer the "pink rim sign" as a clue to the dermoscopic diagnosis of invasive melanoma.

1. Introduction

Any pink color within a melanocytic lesion can be regarded as a marker for inflammation and has long been recognized as a clinical clue to melanoma [1, 2]. In melanomas without significant pigmentation, either amelanotic or hypomelanotic, a subset of these dermoscopically visible areas has been called "milky-red areas" [3–5]. Johr published a series of cases that characterized amelanotic melanoma with pink regions [2]. Menzies et al. listed more than one shade of pink being a statistically significant positive indicator of melanoma (odds ratio = 2.3, sensitivity = 32.4%, and specificity = 82.9%) versus all nonmelanomas [5].

Our goal in this study was to see if the presence of pink can be detected, even by those unskilled in dermoscopy, with the goal of earlier identification of melanoma. In this research, the term "pink" is not defined other than the color pink as understood by dermoscopically naïve observers. We sought additionally to determine whether location of pink in the lesion is important. Preliminary analysis determined that pink located in the periphery of dermoscopic lesions could assist in early detection of melanoma.

2. Methods

The image set used in this study consists of 1290 digital, contact nonpolarized dermoscopic images of melanocytic lesions, acquired during the National Institutes of Health-funded study SBIR R44 CA-101639-02A2. These contact images were obtained with gel interface and minimal pressure. This image set included 296 invasive malignant melanomas and melanomas *in situ* and 994 benign

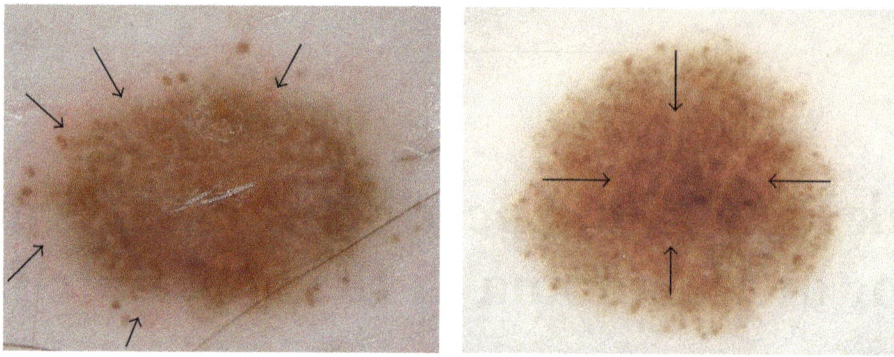

(a) (b)

FIGURE 1: (a) *In situ* melanoma arising within a congenital lesion, 4 mm, abdomen, 34-year-old male. Peripheral pink with some eccentric pink centrally: *in situ* melanoma, 4 mm wide, right abdomen, arising within a superficial compound congenital nevus; pink rim sign is present (arrows) just external to irregular network lacking pink. Note negative network and peripheral globules that are fairly uniform and symmetric. (b) Pink throughout lesion: benign nevus, not biopsied, 5 mm nevus on upper arm in 35-year-old female; pink is present at rim but is most prominent centrally (arrows). Pink rim sign is absent. Note similar architecture and symmetrically arranged globules in both lesions.

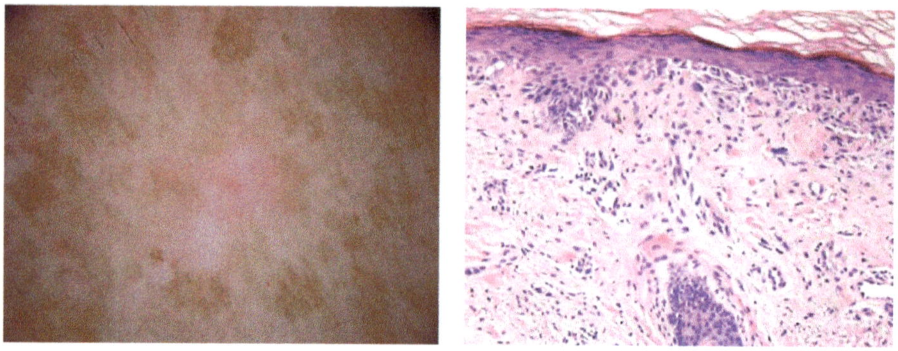

(a) (b)

FIGURE 2: (a) Noncircumferential peripheral and central pink: completely amelanotic invasive melanoma, on right upper arm, 42-year-old female, depth 0.55 mm, 5 mm wide; patient had not noticed the lesion. Pink is present; pink rim sign is absent. (b) Histopathology for melanoma.

melanocytic lesions including 461 dysplastic nevi with mild atypia, 70 dysplastic nevi with moderate atypia, 271 nevocellular nevi without atypia, and 192 congenital nevi. Images were acquired at four clinics: Skin and Cancer Associates (Plantation, FL), the Dermatology Center (Rolla, MO), Columbia Dermatology (Columbia, MO), and Sheard and Drugge PC (Stamford, CT). The images had a resolution of 1024 × 768 pixels. The Phelps County Regional Medical Center Institutional Review Board (Rolla, Missouri) approved this research and each subject or subject's parent or guardian signed a consent form for this research. All melanomas were biopsied and examined by a dermatopathologist and all benign lesions were either biopsied or followed and determined to have no change. The high *in situ* to invasive melanoma ratio (1.35) reflects the detection of melanomas at an early stage in four dermatology private practices in the USA [6]. Lesions were included if they were biopsied or if either patient or physician suspected the possibility of melanoma. The NIH study lesions comprised a convenience sample of all lesions seen in these four clinics. All melanocytic lesions in this NIH study were included in the current study except the following classes: Spitz-Reed nevi, nevi with known previous treatment (nevus recurrens), lesions with multiple diagnoses/collision tumors, and lesions with high-grade atypia, blue nevi, and metastatic melanomas.

Each image was analyzed without knowledge of diagnosis by three untrained observers: two premedical students with eight months' clinical research experience finding borders for lesions in dermoscopic images (RKR, KSP) and an engineering graduate student (UG) with no clinical experience and six months of image processing experience. The three observers independently determined if any peripherally located or centrally located pink areas were present. Consensus agreement was obtained after individual assessments were completed. The study was supervised by a dermatologist with 18 years of experience in dermoscopy (WVS).

Pink coloration can be present in various shades. We offer several examples of pink, including light pink (Figures 1 and 2), dark pink (Figure 4(a)), and pink-orange (Figure 5(a)). We did not demand any particular shade or any medical diagnosis, such as erythema, but rather sought to include all lesions for which the untrained observers agreed that there

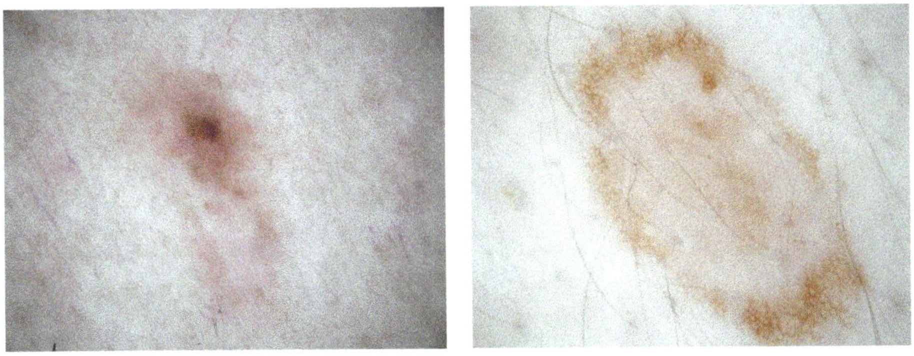

(a) (b)

FIGURE 3: (a) Invasive melanoma, 8 mm wide, back, 62-year-old female, depth 0.55 mm. Nearly circumferential peripheral and central pink. (b) Clark compound nevus, 9 mm wide, 17-year-old male, biopsy confirmed. Central-only pink. Pink rim sign is absent in both (a) and (b).

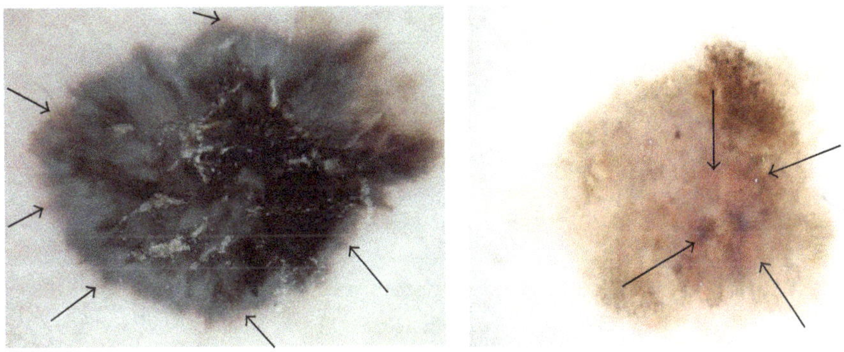

(a) (b)

FIGURE 4: (a) Invasive melanoma, 10 mm wide, chest, 50-year-old male, 0.80 mm thick, peripheral-only pink, with circumferential pink rim sign (most prominent at arrows). (b) Clark compound nevus with moderate atypia, 5.5 mm wide, on shoulder, 25-year-old female. Note architectural disorder, irregularly distributed globules, atypical pigment net, and pink and blue color. Pink is most prominent at center (arrows), negative pink rim sign.

was some shade of pink present. For people with fair skin, with an identifiably pink background, pink must be increased from the background, as in Figures 1(a) and 1(b). The lesion was not considered pink if there was no change in pink from the background skin color.

For peripheral pink, the pink color was present at the lesion rim in a large enough area to be easily detected (area diameter > 1 mm on 10 mm wide dermoscopic images) but need not be present circumferentially. Similarly, central pink was considered present if pink was present somewhere inside the lesion rim, occupying the same minimal area. Any discrepancies between the two observers were resolved by consensus on presence or absence of pink area. These findings were reviewed by a dermatologist (WVS). Figures 1–6 show dermoscopic views of malignant and benign lesions that had central pink, peripheral pink, or pink throughout the lesion. Histopathological imaging for Figures 3(a), 4(a), and 5(a) are seen in Figures 7, 8, and 9, respectively.

Sensitivity, specificity, and odds ratios were computed for the peripheral pink feature. The P values were computed from the chi-square distribution using the Wald chi-square value (Pearson uncorrected). Standard sensitivity and specificity were calculated as sensitivity: (true positive/(true positive + false negative)) and specificity: (true negative/(false positive + true negative)). Odds ratios were calculated as the odds of melanoma with peripheral pink present divided by the odds of melanoma without the feature: ((true positive × true negative)/(false negative × false positive)).

3. Results

Of the entire pigmented lesion set, 1154/1290 (89%) had some pink in the lesion. Of the 296 malignant melanomas overall, 93% had pink color present in the lesion. The majority 899/1290 (70%) of lesions had pink color present somewhere in the lesion periphery. The invasive melanomas had a slightly higher percentage of peripheral-only pink (21/126 = 16.7%) compared to the *in situ* melanomas (22/170 = 12.9%). Of the 994 benign nevi, 64 (6.4%) had peripheral-only pink. The odds ratio for the presence of peripheral-only pink for all malignant melanomas is 2.51 (95% CI: 1.7–3.8, $P < 0.0001$) while the odds ratio for central-only pink is 0.462 (95% CI: 0.32–0.67, $P = 0.204$).

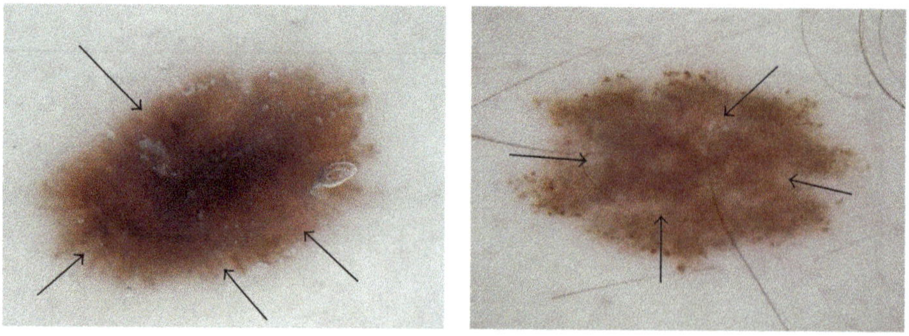

(a) (b)

FIGURE 5: (a) Invasive melanoma, 5 mm wide, lateral abdomen, 32-year-old male, 0.44 mm thick, peripheral pink, with pink rim sign (arrows). (b) Enlarging melanocytic lesion with congenital features, 8 mm wide, abdomen, 21-year-old male. Pink is more prominent centrally than peripherally, negative pink rim sign.

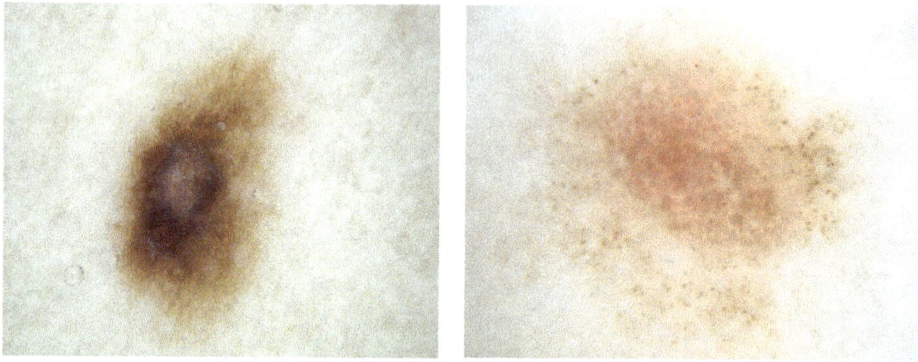

(a) (b)

FIGURE 6: (a) Benign nevus. Central pink only. (b) Congenital nevus, no biopsy, central-only pink. In this nevus, pink extends nearly to the periphery but diminished at the far rim. Neither lesion was biopsied.

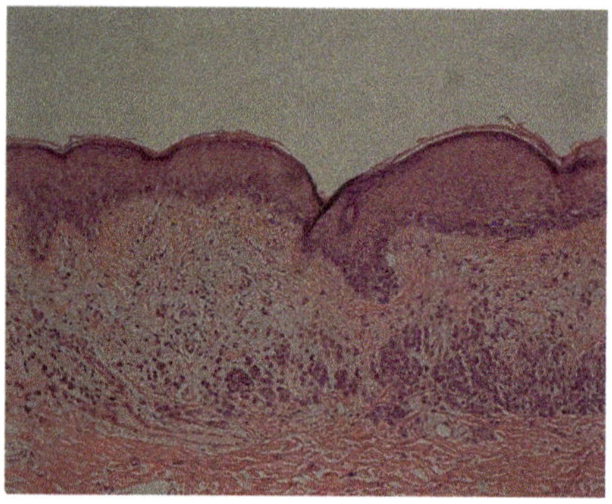

FIGURE 7: Histopathology for Figure 3(a), melanoma 0.55 mm depth.

Pink color was present confined to the center of the lesion in 38/296 (12.8%) of melanomas and in 217/994 (21.8%) of benign lesions. Percentages of lesion types are shown in Table 1. A rim of pink at the outside of a pigmented lesion, in some cases even resembling the sun visible around the darker lunar object in a lunar eclipse or a rim of sun at sunset, can be termed the "pink rim sign." The pink rim sign is present in the melanoma *in situ* in Figure 1(a) and the two invasive melanomas in Figures 4(a) and 5(a).

4. Discussion

The differentiation in the clinic of early malignant melanoma from benign pigmented lesions, even with dermoscopy, remains a difficult challenge. At the earliest stages, especially in melanomas lacking significant pigmentation, few dermoscopic clues may be present to aid in this differentiation. Irregular pigment network, negative network, atypical vascular patterns, and blue-gray granular peppering are helpful features if they are present [3, 7–11]. Yet these structures have specific patterns which can be challenging for those still learning dermoscopy. Pink color observed without magnification is a clinical clue for presence of malignancy, including primarily nonmelanocytic lesions, such as basal cell and squamous cell carcinoma [2]. Data presented here supports the hypothesis that any pink coloration observed dermoscopically confined to the periphery of a lesion increases the likelihood of melanoma (odds ratio 2.5), whereas pink observed only in the central, nonperipheral portion of the lesion decreases the likelihood of melanoma (odds ratio 0.46). We must indicate that any pink coloration includes a generous definition of pink. For example, pink-orange, light pink, and dark pink were all counted as pink. Menzies et al. noted that milky-red pink areas conferred an odds ratio of 2.5 for the diagnosis of melanoma among a group of

TABLE 1: Number of lesion types by location of pink coloration.

Lesion type	Peripheral-only pink (lesion type total)	Central-only pink	Pink throughout entire lesion
Invasive melanoma*	21 (126); 16.7%**	15 (126); 11.9%	80 (126); 63.5%
Melanoma *in situ*	22 (170); 12.9%	23 (170); 13.5%	115 (170); 67.7%
Nevus without atypia	18 (271); 6.6%	54 (271); 19.9%	181 (271); 19.9%
Dysplastic nevus, mild atypia	26 (461); 5.6%	103 (461); 22.3%	268 (461); 58.1%
Dysplastic nevus, moderate atypia	2 (70); 2.86%	13 (70); 18.6%	48 (70); 68.6%
Congenital nevus	18 (192); 9.4%	47 (192); 24.5%	101 (192); 52.6%

*Median Breslow depth: 0.41 mm. **Differences in lesion totals represent lesions with no pink.

amelanotic lesions and an odds ratio of 2.3 for the finding of more than one shade of pink [5]. Thus, our findings extend the findings of the Menzies group to most nevocellular lesions, with a similar odds ratio for peripheral pink. As our study demonstrates with dermoscopically naive observers, training in dermoscopy is not required for the detection of pink. In cases where other structures are absent, such as for hypomelanotic melanoma (Figure 3(a)) or symmetric lesions with few other features of melanoma (Figure 1(a)), the finding of pink color in the periphery can help lead to earlier excision.

The type of dermoscopy can affect results. Dermoscopic features related to vascularity, including pink color, can be altered by excess pressure caused by direct skin contact with the dermatoscope. However, our image set shows pink coloration preserved in the majority of contact dermoscopy images, demonstrating that contact dermoscopy can be a reliable detection method for pink coloration. In addition, Benvenuto-Andrade et al., in a study comparing dermoscopy techniques, showed greater preservation of pink veil by polarized dermoscopy [12]. However, our image set shows that with proper minimal-pressure technique using a gel interface, pink coloration is preserved in the majority of these contact dermoscopy images. Images in the Benvenuto-Andrade study show that pink coloration becomes redder in some non contact polarized dermoscopy images and appears in some benign images, creating a false-positive pink rim sign, such as what was seen in a dysplastic nevus and a blue nevus in that study [12]. We conclude that contact non polarized dermoscopy using proper technique, with gel and minimal pressure, gives the best color balance to allow reliable detection of the pink rim sign.

We may apply this clinical observation to analytic techniques to increase the accuracy of both computer-based diagnostic systems and human detection of melanoma. In computer-based systems, it is anticipated that combined color and location analysis can provide diagnostic assistance to practitioners. The pink rim sign might serve as an adjunct feature for such systems by applying the ratio of pink in the periphery to pink in the center of the lesion. For practitioners, in cases where it is difficult to determine whether structural features of melanoma are present, the finding of a pink rim sign can increase the index of suspicion for melanoma and may lead to earlier excision. Additionally, the presence of pink may be determined on clinical examination, without dermoscopy. Therefore pink serves as not only a dermoscopy warning sign but also an aid to localization of significant lesions.

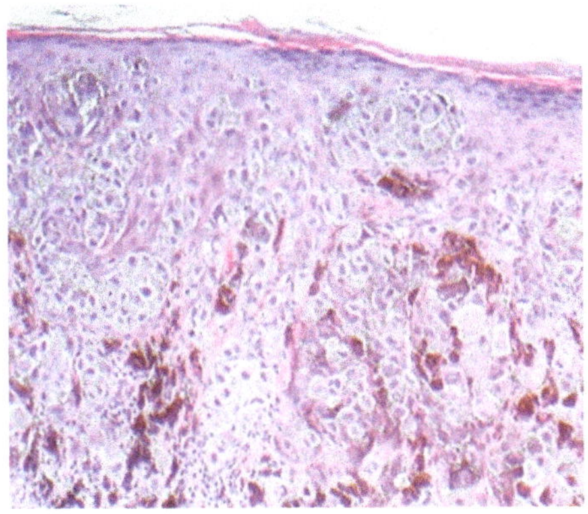

FIGURE 8: Histopathology for Figure 4(a), invasive melanoma 0.80 mm depth.

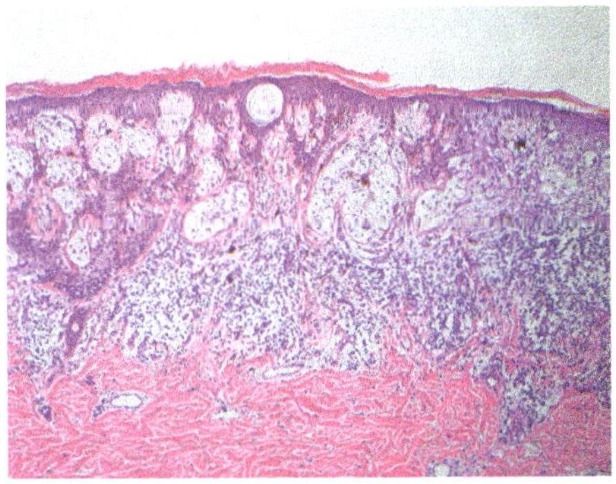

FIGURE 9: Histopathology for Figure 5(a), invasive melanoma 0.44 mm thick.

At least two specific pink structures in dermoscopy have already been described. These include milky-red areas or globules [4] and pink veil [12]. Milky-red areas are vascular structures seen in hypomelanotic or amelanotic melanoma. Pink veil may be seen in benign lesions, including dermatofibroma, as well as basal cell carcinoma and melanoma [12]. Our findings for pink reflect those of Pizzichetta et al. for milky-red areas, who found for a group of benign and malignant amelanotic and hypomelanotic lesions that milky-red areas are present more frequently in melanomas (93% in thick melanomas; 31% in thin melanomas) versus 17% in benign lesions [4].

Our study avoids anyterminology specific to dermoscopy in defining "pink." The three observers were not given any specific structural definition that they needed to learn but rather were instructed to just decide whether pink color was present at the lesion rim or center. Our definition of pink is more inclusive than "milky-red areas," and more lesions will be described as pink. In our experience, nevi in people with fair skin (Fitzpatrick 1 and 2 skin types) generally contain pink color. The frequency of pink color observed in lesions will vary among populations. Thus the high frequency of pink color observed in our series cannot be generalized to all populations. We found that, in our thicker melanomas, for example, the 0.8 mm melanoma in Figure 4, pink is confined to the rim of the lesion because of more advanced central pigmentation, whereas in earlier melanomas pink was found throughout the lesion, as in the melanoma *in situ* in Figure 1 and the 0.55 mm melanomas in Figures 2 and 3. There is experimental support for the hypothesis that pink color in the periphery can indicate malignancy. Terushkin et al. showed that the blood volume visible by transillumination techniques exceeds the area of pigmented lesions seen on dermoscopy [13]. They also showed a correlation between the degree of atypia and the blood volume. On the spectrum from mild to moderate to severe atypia to malignant melanoma, blood volume was found to have been increased.

The finding of increased blood volume could help explain the reason that pink in the periphery is correlated with malignancy in pigmented lesions. We also found an increase in the presence of peripheral pink with more advanced diagnosis. Peripheral pink was present in 6.6% of nevocellular nevi, 12.9% of *in situ* melanomas, and 16.7% of invasive melanomas. This correlation did not extend to degree of atypia in benign lesions, however, as more nevi with mild atypia (5.64% had peripheral pink than those with moderate atypia (2.86%)). Otherwise, the progressive increase in blood volume with increasing atypia observed in the Terushkin study correlates overall with our observed increase in peripheral pink percentages as well as the progression of milky-red areas in the Pizzichetta study (93% in thick melanomas; 31% in thin melanomas) versus 17% in benign lesions [4]. The findings of the Terushkin transillumination study provide a physiologic reason why pink in the periphery may have more discriminatory power for any skin cancer than pink in other areas.

Although pink is correlated with erythema, vascularity, and blood volume, there is no 1 : 1 correlation. Pink is a more inclusive and less specific criterion. The advantage to pink as a sign for melanoma is that it can be detected by naive observers.

Our study is limited by the nonconsecutive acquisition of a convenience sample of lesions in the four clinics above, with clinical and dermoscopic digital photographs obtained between 2007 and 2011. These lesions comprise the majority of melanomas found in these clinics during this interval. For this study, we eliminated two of the most difficult diagnostic categories of lesions—collision tumors and melanocytic lesions with high-grade dysplasia. The first category, collision tumors, those difficult lesions that can show features of both benign and malignant lesions, must be analyzed piecewise, requiring advanced dermoscopy skills. For the second category, high-grade dysplastic lesions, the analysis can be complicated by disagreement among dermatopathologists. Another limitation present in our study is that we employed only student observers, neither of whom was formally trained in dermoscopy. These nonphysician observers may nonetheless model the skills of physicians beginning training in dermoscopy, and, as dermoscopy is more widely employed by nonspecialists, the pink rim sign could be used by these physicians.

Another limitation is the possibility of unconscious introduction of bias, using a different technique such as applying less central pressure when acquiring melanoma images, resulting in more apparent erythema in the periphery. Nevi have less erythema and when capturing the image the photographer would not likely have paid attention to the amount of pressure being applied resulting in the vasculature being blanched. As this is a pilot study, future studies are needed to confirm this observation. Future studies could be done with noncontact dermoscopy, and lesions could be evaluated by those with experience in dermoscopy to further explore these findings.

5. Conclusion

A pink rim in a melanocytic lesion is a clue to the diagnosis of melanoma. An odds ratio of 2.5 was calculated for any shade of pink confined to the periphery of dermoscopic images of melanocytic lesions. We did not restrict the shade of pink. Pink-orange and dark pink were considered pink. These pink areas can be detected by people without formal dermoscopic training. This pink color likely corresponds to increased blood volume. When pink color is observed in the periphery of a dermoscopic image of a melanocytic lesion, this feature suggests consideration of melanoma within the differential diagnosis.

Disclaimer

The contents of this paper are solely the responsibility of the authors and do not necessarily represent the official views of NIH, the sponsor. The sponsor had no role in the design and conduct of the study; in the collection, analysis, and interpretation of data; or in the preparation, review, or approval of the paper.

Authors' Contribution

Ryan K. Rader, Katie S. Payne, and William V. Stoecker had full access to all the data in the study and take responsibility for the integrity of the data and the accuracy of the data analysis. William V. Stoecker was responsible for study concept and design. Ryan K. Rader, Katie S. Payne, William V. Stoecker, Harold S. Rabinovitz, Maggie C. Oliviero, Joseph J. Malters, and Rhett J. Drugge contributed to acquisition of data.William V. Stoecker, Ryan K. Rader, Katie S. Payne, Harold S. Rabinovitz, Uday Guntupalli, Maggie C. Oliviero, Rhett J. Drugge, and Joseph J. Malters contributed to analysis and interpretation of data. Ryan K. Rader, William V. Stoecker were involved with drafting of the paper. Ryan K. Rader, Katie S. Payne, William V. Stoecker, Harold S. Rabinovitz, Maggie C. Oliviero, Rhett J. Drugge, and Joseph J. Malters contributed to critical revision of the paper for important intellectual content. Ryan K. Rader, Katie S. Payne, William V. Stoecker contributed to statistical analysis.

Acknowledgments

The authors wish to thank Jason Hagerty, who served as system administrator, and Dr. Elizabeth Drugge for data procurement. This paper was made possible by Grant no. SBIR R44 CA-101639-02A2 of the National Institutes of Health (NIH).

References

[1] R. J. Friedman, D. S. Rigel, and A. W. Kopf, "Early detection of malignant melanoma: the role of physician examination and self-examination of the skin," *Ca-A Cancer Journal for Clinicians*, vol. 35, no. 3, pp. 130–151, 1985.

[2] R. H. Johr, "Pink lesions," *Clinics in Dermatology*, vol. 20, no. 3, pp. 289–296, 2002.

[3] G. Argenziano, I. Zalaudek, R. Corona et al., "Vascular structures in skin tumors: a dermoscopy study," *Archives of Dermatology*, vol. 140, no. 12, pp. 1485–1489, 2004.

[4] M. A. Pizzichetta, R. Talamini, I. Stanganelli et al., "Amelanotic/hypomelanotic melanoma: clinical and dermoscopic features," *British Journal of Dermatology*, vol. 150, no. 6, pp. 1117–1124, 2004.

[5] S. W. Menzies, J. Kreusch, K. Byth et al., "Dermoscopic evaluation of amelanotic and hypomelanotic melanoma," *Archives of Dermatology*, vol. 144, no. 9, pp. 1120–1127, 2008.

[6] S. M. Stricklin, W. V. Stoecker, J. M. Malters et al., "Melanoma in situ in a private practice setting 2005 through 2009: location, lesion size, lack of concern," *Journal of the American Academy of Dermatology*, vol. 67, no. 3, pp. e105–e109, 2012.

[7] G. Argenziano, C. Catricalà, M. Ardigo et al., "Seven-point checklist of dermoscopy revisited," *British Journal of Dermatology*, vol. 164, no. 4, pp. 785–790, 2011.

[8] M. A. Pizzichetta, R. Talamini, A. A. Marghoob et al., "Negative pigment network: an additional dermoscopic feature for the diagnosis of melanoma," *Journal of the American Academy of Dermatology*, vol. 68, no. 4, pp. 552–559, 2013.

[9] R. P. Braun, O. Gaide, M. Oliviero et al., "The significance of multiple blue-grey dots (granularity) for the dermoscopic diagnosis of melanoma," *British Journal of Dermatology*, vol. 157, no. 5, pp. 907–913, 2007.

[10] W. Stolz, O. Braun-Falco, P. Bilek, M. Landthaler, W. H. C. Burgdorf, and A. Cognetta, *Color Atlas of Dermatoscopy*, Blackwell Science, Berlin, Germany, 2nd edition, 2002.

[11] H. P. Soyer, G. Argenziano, R. Hofmann-Wellenhof, and R. Johr, Eds., *Color Atlas of Melanocytic Lesions of the Skin*, Springer, Berlin, Germany, 2007.

[12] C. Benvenuto-Andrade, S. W. Dusza, A. L. C. Agero et al., "Differences between polarized light dermoscopy and immersion contact dermoscopy for the evaluation of skin lesions," *Archives of Dermatology*, vol. 143, no. 3, pp. 329–338, 2007.

[13] V. Terushkin, S. W. Dusza, N. A. Mullani et al., "Transillumination as a means to differentiate melanocytic lesions based on their vascularity," *Archives of Dermatology*, vol. 145, no. 9, pp. 1060–1062, 2009.

18

Latest Approved Therapies for Metastatic Melanoma: What Comes Next?

Farid Menaa

Department of Oncology, Stem Cells and Nanomedicine, Fluorotronics, Inc., 2453 Cades Way, Building C, San Diego, CA 92081, USA

Correspondence should be addressed to Farid Menaa; dr.fmenaa@gmail.com

Academic Editor: M. Lebwohl

Nowadays, oncogene-directed therapy and immunotherapy represent the two most promising avenues for patients with metastatic melanoma. The recent oncogene-directed therapeutic, vemurafenib, usually produces high level of tumor shrinkage and survival benefits in many patients with *B-RAF*^{V600E} mutant melanomas, although the fast and high degrees of responses are likely short-lived. Conversely, the newly-approved immunotherapeutic, ipilimumab, produces durable responses in patients presenting CTLA-4 T-cell surface protein. Nevertheless, the possible synergy in combining these two therapeutic strategies primarily rely on the rational design of medical protocols (e.g., sequence and timing of agent administration; drug selectivity; compatibility of combined therapies i.e., adoptive T cell or agents, i.e., MEK inhibitor trametinib, PD-1 and PDL-1 blockers). Improved therapeutic protocols shall overcome therapeutic limitations such as the (i) tolerability and safety (i.e., minimal toxic side-effects); (ii) progression free survival (e.g., reduced relapse disease frequency); (iii) duration response (i.e., decreased drug resistance). Eventually, multidisciplinary approaches are still requested (e.g., genomics for personalized medicine, nanomedicine to overcome low free-drug bioavailability and targeting, systematic search of "melanoma stem cells" to enhance the prognosis and develop more valuable theranostics). In this paper, I will mainly present and discuss the latest and promising treatments for advanced cutaneous melanomas.

1. Introduction

Melanoma (from Greek—melas: "dark") is a tumor originated from malignant transformation of melanocytes (i.e., melanin pigment-producing cells) that can be found in the skin, bowel, and eye [1].

According to the estimations provided by the American Cancer Society (ACS) in 2010, 68.130 new cases of melanomas were diagnosed and approximately 8.700 people died from this cancer [2]. The incidence of melanoma in the US has increased of about three folds between the last three decades (i.e., from 7.89 per 100.000 in 1975 to 22.52 per 100.000 in 2008) [3]. Clinical and epidemiological data suggest that several risk factors can contribute to the increased incidence: (i) extensive or repeated exposure to sunlight [4]; (ii) individuals with family history of melanoma (5–12% of all reported cases) [5]; (iii) high nevi count and dysplastic nevus [6], thereby suggesting the need to perform a biopsy of the suspicious lesion. The biopsy permits to establish not only an accurate diagnosis but also to define the optimal staging and proceed earlier with the appropriate therapy (e.g., surgery, chemotherapy, and/or radiotherapy).

Metastatic melanoma (i.e., advanced malignant melanoma) is the most aggressive form of skin cancer with a median overall survival (OS) of only few months (8 to 18 months) [2]. This fact could be mainly explained by the modest results obtained with dacarbazine (DITC) and high-dose interleukin 2 (HD IL-2), the two unique FDA-approved therapies for metastatic melanoma until 2011 [7–9]. Indeed, DITC is limited by a low response rate (RR of 5% to 15%) and an insufficient OS (about 8 months) [7]. Besides, HD IL-2 is also limited by a low RR (6% to 10%), a short duration of responses in most patients as well as a severe toxicity [8, 9]. Since 2011, 3 new agents have been approved for the treatment of advanced melanoma by the Food and Drug Administration (FDA) [10–12]: (i) vemurafenib, a mutant

B-RAF^{V600E} inhibitor, recommended for unresectable or metastatic melanoma [10]; (ii) ipilimumab, an anti-CTLA-4 monoclonal antibody, also preconized for the treatment of unresectable or metastatic melanoma [11]; (iii) pegylated interferon alpha-2b (PEG-IFN), a covalent conjugate of the polyethylene glycol (PEG) with the recombinant α-2b interferon (IFN), long-time used to treat chronic hepatitis patients infected with hepatitis c virus [12], and currently recommended as adjuvant treatment for stage III melanoma [13].

Vemurafenib has emerged as a highly selective mutant *B-RAF*^{V600E} inhibitor with little effect on wild type *B-RAF*, thereby demonstrating significant tumor regression (>40%) while minimizing side effects in a large number of patients with metastatic melanoma [14–16]. Nevertheless, the single use of this oncogene-targeted agent presents the following main disadvantages: (i) short median duration of response (MDR) and progression-free survival (PFS) (i.e., about 6 months only) [16]; (ii) low RR in patients who harbor mutations other than $V_{600}E$. The proportion of these patients ranges between 10% and 30% (e.g., $V_{600}K$ is present in 5% to 20% of patients with melanoma) [17, 18].

Ipilimumab was designed and developed to block the cytotoxic T-lymphocyte-associated antigen 4 (CTLA-4), thereby increasing the T-cell activity and promoting antitumor activity in patients with cancers [19]. Thereby, in patients with unresectable or metastatic melanoma, ipilimumab plus DITC versus DITC alone significantly improved the OS (about 11 months versus 9 months, resp.) and RR (about 15% versus 10%, resp.) [20, 21].

PEG-IFN, similarly to high-dose interferon (HDI or Intron A) [1, 22], has been approved for the adjuvant treatment (after surgical resection) of stage III melanoma patients. This approval was mainly based on final results of a recent randomized phase III trial organized by the European Organization for Research and Treatment of Cancer (EORTC) 18991 that showed greater relapse-free survival (RFS of 45.6%) in comparison to observation (38.9%), although no significant effect on OS was noticed [12, 23]. Previously, in an open-label phase 2 study, the efficacy and safety of PEG-IFN in combination with temozolomide were investigated in patients with metastatic melanoma without brain metastases [24]. The RR of this combination reached 31% of the patients, the median OS was 12 months, and no patient developed brain metastases while receiving study treatment, which was besides well tolerated. Up to date, and in the best of my knowledge, it remains unknown whether PEG-IFN can provide better efficacy and safety results than the biochemotherapy combining cisplatin, vinblastine, DTIC plus IL-2 (Proleukin), and interferon. Indeed, a recent phase 3 trial (SWOG S0008) only assessed the efficacy and safety of this biochemotherapy versus HDI in patients with high-risk melanoma [25]. The results showed major improvement in the median RFS in favor of biochemotherapy (4.3 years versus 1.9 years with HDI). OS, however, was exactly the same (56% at 5 years), and acute grade 4 toxicity was more frequent with biochemotherapy. All together, the biochemotherapy can be considered as a better adjuvant treatment than HDI. Currently, both HDI and PEG-IFN are considered as category 2B due to their limited benefits, and so will not be further detailed in this paper.

Eventually, in one hand, these new exciting chemotherapies represent a great hope for the physicians and patients with advanced melanoma. In the other hand, their respective limitations clearly emphasize the importance of developing novel treatment strategies (e.g., cell-based therapies, advanced and rational combinatorial therapeutic approaches, nanodrug formulations). These alternative therapeutic options might help to improve OS, PFS, RFS, RR, and MDR while minimizing toxic adverse events, thereby contributing *in fine* to the quality of the patient's life.

In this paper, most recent FDA-approved treatments against advanced cutaneous melanoma (stage III and IV) are highlighted, and possible enhanced therapeutic strategies to overcome their respective associated limitations are discussed.

2. Latest FDA-Approved Drugs for Advanced/Metastatic Melanoma

Most patients with unresectable stage III or stage IV disease require systemic treatment rather than metastasectomy.

2.1. Oncogene-Directed Therapy: Mutant B-RAF Inhibitors. Melanoma is a molecularly heterogeneous disease with approximately half (40%–60%) of the cutaneous melanoma cells harboring an activating mutation in the *B-RAF* gene, which encodes a serine/threonine kinase protein kinase, and most of the mutations (>70%) are $V_{600}E$ (i.e., substitution of valine for glutamate at amino acid position 600) [17, 26–28]. Because mutated *B-RAF* leads to constitutive activation of the mitogen-activated protein kinase pathway (MAPK) that, in turn, increases the cellular proliferation and drives the oncogenic activity [29, 30], intensive research has consisted to selectively inhibit mutated *B-RAF* in patients with melanoma (e.g., studies with sorafenib, a multitargeted kinase inhibitor), but the results were globally disappointing due to off-target side effects mainly induced through inhibition of wild type *B-RAF* [14, 31–35].

Among highly selective *B-RAF* inhibitors, only the recent FDA-approved vemurafenib (formerly PLX4032, currently marketed as Zelboraf and initially developed by Genentech Roche) is capable of silencing mutant *B-RAF*^{V600E} without interfering with wild type *B-RAF*. Indeed, in a phase 2 clinical trial involving patients with metastatic melanoma harboring *B-RAF*^{V600E} mutation (n = 132), vemurafenib demonstrated substantial tumor regression in 81% of the cases, a RR of 52%, and a MDR of 6.8 months [14–16]. Further, in a phase 3 clinical trial (BRIM3) involving previously untreated patients (n = 675), vemurafenib was much better than DITC in terms of RR (48% versus 5%, resp.), PFS (5.3 months versus 1.6 months, resp.), and percent of patients alive at six months (OS of 84% versus 64%, resp.) [10]. Also, in a recent open-label pilot study, it was stated that vemurafenib could be beneficial for previously treated metastatic melanoma patients with brain metastases [36]. Besides, common adverse events associated with vemurafenib included accelerated growth of cutaneous squamous cell carcinomas (SCCs) and keratoacanthomas [10, 37–40], most probably through paradoxical activation of MAPK signaling (about 20–25% of the patients with advanced melanoma) [37–40].

Eventually, vemurafenib represents an excellent model for successful targeted anticancer therapy (i.e., high RR and low toxicity) in patients with *B-RAF*^{V600E} mutations [41]. Nevertheless, these clinical benefits are counterbalanced by the relatively short MDR, high selectivity for the *B-RAF*^{V600E} mutation, and related toxicities of the drug. Owing to consideration that 10% to 30% of patients have a non-*BRAF*^{V600E} mutation (e.g., *B-RAF*^{V600k} mutation is present in 5% to 20% of melanoma patients) [17, 18], further studies are required to examine the efficacy of vemurafenib, alone or in combination, in patients with a non-*BRAF*^{V600E} mutation. These studies are important to avoid useless administration of vemurafenib in a subset of patients, who might otherwise become resistant to the drug. Alternatively, rational combination of vemurafenib with other agents (e.g., ipilimumab) might circumvent an eventual drug resistance and/or further improve the clinical outcome of the patients (e.g., MDR, OS).

2.2. Immunotherapy: CTLA-4 Inhibitors. Melanoma is one of the most immunogenic tumors due to the presence of tumor infiltrating lymphocytes (TIL) in resected melanoma, clinical responses to immune stimulation, and occasional spontaneous regressions. CTLA-4 expression is necessary for activation of self-regulation of T cells, and so CTLA-4 inhibitors could represent serious therapeutic options to generate T-cell hyperresponsiveness and overcome tumor immune escape [19].

Up to date, ipilimumab (formerly MDX-010, MDX-101, or MDX-CTLA-4, currently marketed as Yervoy and initially developed by Bristol-Myers Squibb) is a fully human IgG1 monoclonal antibody that blocks CTLA-4, subsequently increasing the T-cell activity and promoting an antitumor activity and represents the only approved immunotherapeutic agent for systemic treatment [20]. In the first phase 3 randomized trial involving patients with previously treated unresectable stage III or IV melanoma (n = 676), ipilimumab compared to the glycoprotein 100 peptide (gp100) vaccine demonstrated an improved median OS (10.1 months versus 6.4 months, resp.) and a much better RR (10.9% versus 1.5%, resp.), *albeit* the occurrence of toxicities with ipilimumab, including grade 3 or 4 immune-related adverse events (e.g., enterocolitis, hepatitis, and dermatitis) and deaths, was higher than with gp100 (10–15% versus 3%, resp.) [11]. Ipilimumab plus gp100, compared to gp100, did not improve the OS observed with ipilimumab alone (10.0 months versus 10.1 months, resp.) [11]. In the second phase 3 randomized trial involving previously untreated patients with metastatic melanoma (n = 502), ipilimumab combined with DITC demonstrated a modest but statistically significant improvement in OS compared to DITC plus placebo (11.2 months versus 9.1 months, resp.) as well a better overall RR (15.2% versus 10.3%, resp.) [20, 21]. Interestingly, survival rates over the years were always significantly higher in the ipilimumab-DITC group than in the group treated with the single agent DITC (at 1 year: 47.3% versus 36.3%; at 2 years: 28.5% versus 17.9%; at 3 years: 20.8% versus 12.2%, resp.), clearly demonstrating that ipilimumab is able to confer a durable response (MDR of 19.3 months versus 8.1 months, resp.). Nevertheless, median PFS was barely improved (2.8 months versus 2.6 months, resp.). Also, grade 3 or 4 adverse events (e.g., hepatitis) occurred more frequently in patients treated with ipilimumab plus DITC than in patients treated with DITC (plus placebo) (56.3% versus 27.5%, resp.), although low rates of gastrointestinal events and no drug-related deaths occurred in the ipilimumab-DITC group [20, 21].

Eventually, although the OS and MDR noticed with ipilimumab are higher than that one observed with vemurafenib, the most important limitation of this drug tested alone or in combination remains the modest RR. This strongly suggests a need for rational combination between ipilimumab and other commercially available free- or nanoencapsulated drugs (e.g., vemurafenib and bevacizumab, resp.) that might provide complementary clinical benefits.

3. Therapeutic Perspectives for Improving the Effects of FDA-Approved Drugs

3.1. Promising Molecular Targets to Overcome the Resistance Associated with B-RAF Inhibitors. Since approximately 50% of patients with melanoma harbor *B-RAF* mutations and might be then eligible for treatment with the novel *B-RAF* inhibitors, this means that another half of the patients with advanced melanoma might not fully benefit from vemurafenib (i.e., specific *B-RAF*^{V600E} targeting drug). Therefore, it appears reasonable to develop drugs that specifically target gene mutations other than $V_{600}E$ (e.g., *B-RAF*^{V600k} targeting agents). Also, at a larger extent, targeting any molecular alterations that occur (frequently or rarely) in specific melanoma related pathways (including those which are involved in "melanoma stem cells") shall provide additive or synergistic clinical benefits. For instance, molecules involved in the mitogen-activated protein kinase (MAPK) signaling could represent interesting targets to overcome the melanoma resistance. Indeed, it has been previously shown that MAPK activation by mutants *B-RAF* drives melanoma tumor proliferation, and that the resistance to *B-RAF* inhibitors—responsible for their short-duration response—can be (or not) associated with reactivation of the MAPK pathway ("escape route") [41–43]. Recent studies demonstrated that MAPK-dependent acquired resistance to *B-RAF* inhibition in melanomas can involve (i) upregulation of receptor tyrosine kinases (RTKs) and N-RAS [44]; (ii) elevated expression of COT kinase through MAPK pathway reactivation [45]; (iii) activation of MAPK kinase (MEK *aka* MAPK/ERK) [46, 47]; (iv) elevation of C-RAF [48]. Besides, MAPK-independent molecules involved in the melanoma resistance mechanism include (i) upregulation of IGF-1R [49]; (ii) PI3K/AKT signaling through the activation of c-KIT (a RTK also known as CD117) [50]; (iii) loss of PTEN through the suppression of BIM expression [51].

Recent promising results from clinical trials mainly implicate MEK-1 and c-KIT inhibitors. Indeed, a recent phase III trial (METRIC study) involving patients with advanced or metastatic melanoma harboring *B-RAF*$^{V600E/k}$ mutant and without prior brain metastases (n = 332) reported the great efficacy of a reversible and highly selective allosteric inhibitor of MEK1/2 activity, trametinib (formerly GSK 1120212), when compared with "chemotherapy" (DITC or paclitaxel, but not vemurafenib) [52]. Thereby, significant improvements have been observed in favor of trametinib, mainly at the median PFS (4.8 months versus 1.4 months with chemotherapy) and the overall RR (24% versus 7% with chemotherapy). In spite of crossovers, at 6 months, OS was also significantly improved in favor of trametinib (74% versus 56% with "chemotherapy"). Globally, trametinib was well tolerated and safe (e.g., most side effects included skin rash and hypertension), validating that targeting the MEK pathway is a viable strategy. Besides, ongoing trials are evaluating the safety and efficacy of c-KIT inhibitors (i.e., imatinib, nilotinib, and dasatinib) [53–55], and their combinations with *B-RAF* inhibitors are underway. Indeed, *c-KIT* is mutated in approximately 20% of sun-damaged skin [56] and, once its corresponding protein is activated by its ligand called SCF (Stem Cell Factor), mediates cell growth and cell survival signals through signaling pathways such as P13K-AKT-mTOR and RAS-RAF-MEK-ERK. Thereby, *c-KIT* has been implicated in the pathogenesis of several cancers including metastatic melanoma [57, 58], and previous clinical trials demonstrated a durable overall RR (16–24%) as well as a median OS ranging from 11 to 14 months [50, 53, 59].

Eventually, rational combination of *B-RAF* inhibitors (e.g., vemurafenib, dabrafenib) with drugs that specifically target one of the above-mentioned molecules (e.g., MEK, c KIT, or CTLA-4) would further improve the clinical outcome of the patients with advanced/metastatic melanoma. A current nonrandomized open-label phase 1/2 trial (NCT01400451 study) that aims to evaluate the efficacy and safety of vemurafenib with ipilimumab in adult subjects with *B-RAF*^{V600} mutation-positive metastatic melanoma is ongoing but is not recruiting participants, yet [60]. The results of this challenging study are expected for August 2015 [60]. Interestingly, the selective *B-RAF* inhibitor, dabrafenib (formerly GSK2118436), previously showed similar efficacy to vemurafenib [35], and several clinical trials in patients with *B-RAF*^{V600} mutant melanoma showed promising results with dabrafenib as a single agent [61–63] or in combo with trametinib [64–66]. Thereby, a recent multicentre, open-label phase 1/2 trial (BREAK-MB study), investigated the efficacy and safety of oral dabrafenib in adult patients with *B-RAF*$^{V600E/k}$ mutant melanoma metastatic to the brain (n = 172) [61, 62]. 29 of 74 (39.2%) patients with *B-RAF*^{V600E} mutant melanoma and only 1 of 15 (6.7%) patients with *B-RAF*^{V600k} mutant melanoma in cohort A (n = 89 patients who had not received previous local treatment for brain metastases) achieved an overall intracranial response with dabrafenib. Comparatively, 20 of 65 (30.8%) patients with *B-RAF*^{V600k} mutant melanoma and 4 of 18 (22%) with *B-RAF*^{V600k} mutant melanoma in cohort B (n = 83 patients who had progressive brain metastases after previous local treatments) achieved an overall intracranial response with dabrafenib. Further, the treatment-related adverse events of grade 3 or worse occurred in 38 (22%) patients from the cohort A and in 51 (30%) patients from the cohort B. The three most frequent serious events were pyrexia (6%), intracranial hemorrhage (6%), and SCC (6%). To sum up, these impressive results were mainly obtained in patients with *B-RAF*^{V600E} mutant melanoma and brain metastases, irrespective of whether they were previously treated or untreated, clearly showing that dabrafenib is safe (e.g., lack of skin toxicity) and can confer robust activity in intracranial disease, suggesting possible elimination of whole brain radiotherapy in similar subsets of patients. Further, in a randomized open-label multicenter phase 3 trial (BREAK-3 study) involving previously untreated patients with *B-RAF*^{V600E} mutant melanoma (n = 250) [63], dabrafenib compared to DITC led to (i) a significant improvement of the median PFS (5.1 months versus 2.7 months, resp.); (ii) a greater RR (53% versus 19%, resp.). The OS data were immature at the time of the study analysis. Further, hyperkeratosis (37%), pyrexia (28%), and skin papillomas (24%) were among the most frequent adverse events observed in patients treated with dabrafenib, and interestingly, only few cases of SCC (7%) and keratoacanthomas (3%) were noticed [63]. Other recent results, obtained from an open-label study involving patients with metastatic melanoma and *B-RAF*^{V600} mutations (n = 247), showed that dabrafenib and trametinib can be safely combined at full monotherapy doses (150 mg and 2 mg, resp.) [64–66]. Indeed, for the combo therapy group of patients, compared to the monotherapy group (dabrafenib only), the following end points were observed (i) the rate of pyrexia was increased (71% versus 26%, resp.); (ii) the rate of proliferative skin lesions (i.e., the incidence of cutaneous SCC) was not significantly reduced (7% versus 19%, resp.); according to me, this observation might be explained by the presence of MEK-independent subsets of mutant RAS, since MEK-dependent and -independent subsets of mutant RAS have been identified in tumor cell lines [67, 68]; (iii) PFS was significantly improved (9.4 months versus 5.8 months, resp.); (iv) RR was significantly improved (76% versus 54%, resp.); (v) the duration of response was also much better (10.5 months versus 5.6 months, resp.). However, OS could not be compared because of the relatively short-term followup. These overall exciting experimental results will need to be confirmed in ongoing phase 3 larger studies before combo therapy likely replaces monotherapy (i.e., *B-RAF* inhibitor as a single agent). Indeed, larger studies might demonstrate whether *B-RAF*/MEK combo therapy can (i) both delay and prevent onset of resistance to therapy; (ii) significantly reduce the incidence of SCC formation fevers, chills, and MEK inhibitor-induced dermatitis; (iii) extend overall survival or if ipilimumab shall be implemented to confer a survival benefit in case of treatment failures (e.g., disease progression, unacceptable adverse events); (iv) recover patients that initially failed with monotherapy or provide potential benefit to initial monotherapy in order to further improve PFS.

3.2. Promising Molecular Targets to Overcome Low-Response Rate Associated with Immunotherapeutic Agents. Although ipilimumab can induce long-term responses in a subset of patients, the relatively low RR (10%–15%) observed with this immunotherapeutic agent limits its use. Possible ways to overcome this limitation would be (i) increase of the dose (e.g., 3 to 10 mg/kg); (ii) selection/stratification of the patients (i.e., personalized medicine); (iii) rationale combination with other treatment modalities (e.g., molecularly targeted therapy, radiation therapy, adoptive T-cell therapy, melanoma initiating/propagating cells).

The low response rate of ipilimumab is thought to be caused by melanoma immune escape, a mechanism that involves the expression of programmed death ligand 1 (PD-L1), which once bound to its ligand PD-1 (programmed death-1) of activated lymphocytes, would cause apoptosis of the activated lymphocytes and subsequent immune tolerance [69–71]. Interestingly, a phase 1 study led on specific human anti-PD-1 antibody (formerly MDX-1106 *aka* BMS-936558), a fully recombinant human immunoglobulin G4 [72], offered clinical benefits in a variety of previously treated refractory solid tumors including melanoma, without generating significant toxicities [72]. Thereby, a dose-escalation study of the combination of MDX-1106 with ipilimumab has been started [53], and phase 1 trials of anti-PD-L1 are also underway. Recently, the clinical activity and safety of MDX-1106 intravenously administrated in escalating doses every two weeks in patients with advanced melanoma ($n = 94$), have been reported [73]. The overall RR was 28%, and 6% of patients achieved stable disease after 24 weeks. Most side effects were immune related, though three treatment-related deaths occurred on study, including two due to pneumonitis. Interestingly, a subanalysis of the data hinted that the PD-L1 protein might serve as a biomarker of response. Indeed, more than one-third of patients expressing PD-L1 responded to immunotherapy, whereas responses were not observed among patients lacking PD-L1 expression. Eventually, these preliminary data strongly suggest that blockage of the PD-1 pathway may represent a new immune therapy.

Besides, pertinent clinical studies are assessing the combinatorial effects of ipilimumab with promising antiangiogenic drugs (e.g., bevacizumab, an antivascular endothelial growth factor A (VEGF-A)), immunostimulators (e.g., sargramostim, a recombinant human granulocyte macrophage colony-stimulating factor (GM-CSF)), and/or anticancer agents (e.g., fotemustine, a nitrosourea alkylating agent, or the *B-RAF* inhibitor vemurafenib) based on previous studies [74–76]. Indeed, a recent randomized phase 2 trial (BEAM study) involving patients with previously untreated advanced melanoma ($n = 214$) has evaluated the activity of the FDA-approved drug bevacizumab (Avastin) combined with carboplatin plus paclitaxel (BCP) versus placebo carboplatin plus paclitaxel (CP) [74]. Although the results were not as good as expected (median PFS: 5.6 months with BCP versus 4.2 months with CP; overall RR: 25.5% with BCP versus 16.4% with CP; median OS: 12.3 months with BCP versus 8.6 months with CP), the trial might be considered as positive. Further, no new safety signals were observed. Interestingly, the hazard rate (0.79) for improvement in OS at the last time point was the same seen with BCP that led the US FDA to approve bevacizumab for lung cancer [75]. Therefore, a trial of chemotherapy combining bevacizumab with the first-line therapeutic agents for metastatic melanoma (e.g., ipilimumab, vemurafenib) might be beneficial. In this regard, the first combination study, a recent nonrandomized open-label phase 1 trial, did investigate potential synergies of ipilimumab and bevacizumab in a limited number of evaluable adult patients with unresectable stage III or stage IV melanoma ($n = 21$) [76]. This preliminary and promising study showed that ipilimumab plus bevacizumab could (i) display synergistic effects and provide clinical benefit in a large number of patients as shown in 14/21 of the enrolled patients; (ii) be safely administered with management of noted toxicities, which were mostly immune related (e.g., grade 3-4 hepatitis, grade 2 colitis, arteritis, hypophysitis, thyroiditis, bilateral uveitis,). Further, studies with the immunostimulator sargramostim (Leukine/Prokine) show that this drug may help the immune system recover from the side effects of treatment in patients with metastatic melanoma and so could be tested as a combinatory agent with ipilimumab. Indeed, a previous investigation (NCCTG study) has consisted to perform a dose-escalation clinical trial with aerosolized sargramostim in HLA-A2 patients with metastatic melanoma to the lung ($n = 40$). The data showed that the toxicity was acceptable for all tested doses and the greatest increase in antitumor T-cell immune responses was achieved at the highest doses [77]. Then, a hypothesis-generating study was conducted to evaluate the safety and efficacy of prolonged administration of sargramostim as surgical adjuvant therapy in patients with melanoma at high risk of recurrence ($n = 98$) [78]. The prolonged administration of the drug was well tolerated among patients, and the 5-year melanoma-specific survival rate was 60%, providing preliminary evidence that sargramostim can be administered as adjuvant therapy for patients with melanoma at high risk of recurrence. Interestingly, an ongoing recent randomized open-label phase 2 longitudinal trial (NCT01134614) is studying how well giving ipilimumab with (arm I) or without (arm II) sargramostim works in treating adult patients with stage III or stage IV melanoma without brain metastases (estimated enrollment $n = 220$) [79]. However, the effects (e.g., OS, PFS, RR, MDR, safety) of ipilimumab plus sargramostim versus ipilimumab alone, in treating patients with advanced melanoma, remain unknown. Eventually, fotemustine (Muphoran), a non-FDA-approved drug available in Europe, is known to rapidly cross the blood-brain barrier and to display encouraging activity in patients with brain metastases [80]. Also, in a phase 3 trial involving patients with metastatic melanoma ($n = 229$) [81], fotemustine compared to DITC was associated with (i) an improved overall RR (15.5% versus 6.8%, resp.); (ii) a trend toward improved OS (7.3 versus 5.6 months, resp.); (iii) a longer median time to development of brain metastases (22.7 months versus 7.2 months, resp.) in patients without brain metastases at inclusion; (iv) a similar MDR (5.8 months versus 6.9 months); (v) a similar time to progression (1.8 months versus 1.9 months); (vi) a similar quality of life; (vii) more adverse events such as myelosuppression (i.e., grade 3 to 4 neutropenia 51% versus 5%, resp. and thrombocytopenia 43%

versus 6%, resp.) and alopecia. Interestingly, a recent open-label, single-arm phase 2 trial (NIBIT-M1 study) is investigating the efficacy and safety of ipilimumab plus fotemustine in adult patients ($n = 86$) with metastatic melanoma and with or without asymptomatic brain metastases [82]. As primarily results, this medicinal combination achieved disease control in 40 patients (46.5%) with metastatic melanoma, including those with brain metastases. Nevertheless, the treatment-related adverse effects (e.g., grade 3 or 4 myelotoxicity and hepatotoxicity) were present in 47 patients (55%).

Eventually, the use of nanomaterials to formulate nanodrugs (e.g., drug nanocarriers such as solid lipid nanoparticles (SLN) or nanostructured lipid carriers (NLC)) might be useful to possibly enhance efficacy (e.g., systemic bioavailability, targeting), tolerability, and safety of free drugs presenting clinical benefit for patients with metastatic melanoma (e.g., ipilimumab, vemurafenib). In general, it is well accepted that administration of appropriate nanodrug formulations can contribute to enhance the duration response, the response rate, the OS, and PFS in patients with a given type of cancer [83, 84]. In this regard and based on a recent study announcing the preparation of nanoliposomes-encapsulated bevacizumab with beneficial effects in prolonging the residency of bevacizumab in the vitreous [85], it might be interesting to test ipilimumab plus nanoencapsulated bevacizumab in patients with unresectable stage III or stage IV melanoma. Besides, "adoptive T-cell therapy" (ACT), which presents several conceptual similarities with hematopoietic stem-cell transplantations (HSCTs) in terms of advantages and disadvantages can constitute another therapeutic option to overcome the low response associated with immunotherapeutic agents (e.g., ipilimumab). Indeed, successful isolation-expansion-infusion of TIL has shown clinical benefits for the treatment of patients with metastatic melanoma [86–91]. For instance, the RR (72%) was higher when using nonmyeloablative lymphodepletion with cytotoxic chemotherapy and with or without total body irradiation (TBI) than when ipilimumab was combined with IL-2 [86–91]. Interestingly, preclinical work suggested that selective *B-RAF*^{V600E} inhibition enhances T-cell recognition of melanoma without affecting lymphocyte function, providing a rational for the combination of *B-RAF* inhibitors (e.g., vemurafenib or dabrafenib) with stimulatory immune agents (e.g., ipilimumab or PD-1/PD-L1) [92].

4. Conclusions

The incidence of metastastic melanoma is increasing worldwide. Vemurafenib and ipilimumab, based on their respective success rates, are bringing hopes to physicians and patients. Vemurafenib has emerged as a highly selective *B-RAF*^{V600E} mutant melanoma inhibitor and could display good response rates in patients with unresectable or metastatic melanoma. Nevertheless, its main disadvantage remains the short median duration response as well as its limited use to patients who harbor mutations other than *B-RAF*^{V600E} (e.g., *B-RAF*^{V600k}). Besides, ipilimumab was developed to block the cytotoxic T-lymphocyte-associated antigen 4 (CTLA-4) in patients with unresectable or metastatic melanoma. Interestingly, ipilimumab presents the opposite main advantage and disadvantage than vemurafenib. Several clinical trials are underway to address the question of rational combination of those two approved drugs, together and/or separately with other potential therapeutic targets (PD-1, PD-L1, c-KIT, MEK1, VEGF-A...). Cell therapy such as adoptive T cell is encouraging. Nanoencapsulation of the recent FDA-approved free drugs (e.g., vemurafenib, ipilimumab), using proper nanocarriers, or rational combination of these free drugs with available adjuvant nanotherapeutics might be beneficial as they might enhance the overall pharmacological features (e.g., bioavailability and targeting). The importance of direct targeting of potential melanoma initiating/propagating cells within a given patient was not detailed in this paper but might be important in order to avoid immune resistance, immune escape, and disease relapse. Owing to consideration that the incidence of advanced/metastatic melanoma in the younger population is increasing, clinical trials in pediatric patients appear necessary. Eventually, the rational molecular or cellular combo therapy is a key strategy, as it shall beneficiate a larger number of patients. The recent results reported in this paper are quite exciting and, undeniably, constitute a new hope for patients and healthcare professionals.

Abbreviations

ACT: Adoptive T-cell therapy
ACS: American cancer society
BCP: Bevacizumab/carboplatin/paclitaxel
CTL A4: Cytotoxic T-lymphocyte-associated antigen 4
DITC: Dacarbazine
FDA: Food and drug administration
HDI: High-dose interferon
HSCT: Hematopoietic stem cell transplantation
IL-2: Interleukin-2
PD-1: Programmed death-1
PEG-IFN: Pegylated interferon alpha-2b
MAPK: Mitogen-activated protein kinase
MDR: Median duration response
MEK: MAPK/extracellular signal-regulated kinase (ERK)
MEKi: MEK inhibitor
OS: Overall survival
PEG: Polyethylene glycol
PFS: Progression-free survival
RAF: Ras-activating factor
RFS: Relapse/recurrence free survival
RR: Response rate
SCC: Squamous cell carcinoma
TBI: Total body irradiation
TIL: Tumor infiltrating lymphocytes.

Acknowledgments

The author would like to thank Dr. Abder Menaa, M. D. for his pertinent suggestions and critical review of this paper.

References

[1] V. T. DeVita, T. S. Lawrence, and S. A. Rosenberg, *DeVita, Hellman, and Rosenberg's Cancer: Principles & Practice of Oncology*, Wolters Kluwer/Lippincott Williams & Wilkins, Philadelphia, Pa, USA, 8th edition, 2008.

[2] A. Jemal, R. Siegel, J. Xu, and E. Ward, "Cancer statistics, 2010," *CA: Cancer Journal for Clinicians*, vol. 60, no. 5, pp. 277–300, 2010.

[3] N. Howlader, L. A. G. Ries, A. B. Mariotto, M. E. Reichman, J. Ruhl, and K. A. Cronin, "Improved estimates of cancer-specific survival rates from population-based data," *Journal of the National Cancer Institute*, vol. 102, no. 20, pp. 1584–1598, 2010.

[4] R. Bestak and G. M. Halliday, "Chronic low-dose UVA irradiation induces local suppression of contact hypersensitivity, Langerhans cell depletion and suppressor cell activation in C3H/HeJ mice," *Photochemistry and Photobiology*, vol. 64, no. 6, pp. 969–974, 1996.

[5] F. G. Haluska and F. S. Hodi, "Molecular genetics of familial cutaneous melanoma," *Journal of Clinical Oncology*, vol. 16, no. 2, pp. 670–682, 1998.

[6] K. H. Kraemer, M. M. Lee, A. D. Andrews, and W. C. Lambert, "The role of sunlight and DNA repair in melanoma and nonmelanoma skin cancer: the xeroderma pigmentosum paradigm," *Archives of Dermatology*, vol. 130, no. 8, pp. 1018–1021, 1994.

[7] G. J. Hill, E. T. Krementz, and H. Z. Hill, "Dimethyl triazeno imidazole carboxamide and combination therapy for melanoma. IV. Late results after complete response to chemotherapy (Central Oncology Group Protocols 7130, 7131, and 7131A)," *Cancer*, vol. 53, no. 6, pp. 1299–1305, 1984.

[8] M. B. Atkins, M. T. Lotze, J. P. Dutcher et al., "High-dose recombinant interleukin 2 therapy for patients with metastatic melanoma: analysis of 270 patients treated between 1985 and 1993," *Journal of Clinical Oncology*, vol. 17, no. 7, pp. 2105–2116, 1999.

[9] G. Q. Phan, P. Attia, S. M. Steinberg, D. E. White, and S. A. Rosenberg, "Factors associated with response to high-dose interleukin-2 in patients with metastatic melanoma," *Journal of Clinical Oncology*, vol. 19, no. 15, pp. 3477–3482, 2001.

[10] P. B. Chapman, A. Hauschild, C. Robert et al., "Improved survival with vemurafenib in melanoma with BRAF V600E mutation," *The The New England Journal of Medicine*, vol. 364, no. 26, pp. 2507–2516, 2011.

[11] F. S. Hodi, S. J. O'Day, D. F. McDermott et al., "Improved survival with ipilimumab in patients with metastatic melanoma," *The New England Journal of Medicine*, vol. 363, no. 8, pp. 711–723, 2010.

[12] F. Carrat, F. Bani-Sadr, S. Pol et al., "Pegylated interferon alfa-2b versus standard interferon alfa-2b, plus ribavirin, for chronic hepatitis C in HIV-infected patients: a randomized controlled trial," *The Journal of the American Medical Association*, vol. 292, no. 23, pp. 2839–2848, 2004.

[13] A. M. Eggermont, S. Suciu, M. Santinami et al., "Adjuvant therapy with pegylated interferon alfa-2b versus observation alone in resected stage III melanoma: final results of EORTC 18991, a randomised phase III trial," *The Lancet*, vol. 372, no. 9633, pp. 117–126, 2008.

[14] K. T. Flaherty, I. Puzanov, K. B. Kim et al., "Inhibition of mutated, activated BRAF in metastatic melanoma," *The New England Journal of Medicine*, vol. 363, no. 9, pp. 809–819, 2010.

[15] K. S. M. Smalley and V. K. Sondak, "Melanoma—an unlikely poster child for personalized cancer therapy," *The New England Journal of Medicine*, vol. 363, no. 9, pp. 876–878, 2010.

[16] A. Ribas, K. Kim, L. Schuchter, R. Gonzalez et al., "BRIM-2: an open label, multicenter phase II study of vemurafenib in previously treated patients with BRAF V600E mutation-positive metastatic melanoma," *Journal of Clinical Oncology*, vol. 29, abstract no. 8509, 2011.

[17] L. Si, Y. Kong, X. Xu et al., "Prevalence of BRAF V600E mutation in Chinese melanoma patients: large scale analysis of BRAF and NRAS mutations in a 432-case cohort," *European Journal of Cancer*, vol. 48, no. 1, pp. 94–100, 2012.

[18] A. M. Menzies, L. Visintin, M. D. Chatfield et al., "Long. BRAF mutation by age-decade and body mass index in metastatic melanoma," *Journal of Clinical Oncology*, vol. 29, abstract no. 8507, 2011.

[19] I. Melero, S. Hervas-Stubbs, M. Glennie, D. M. Pardoll, and L. Chen, "Immunostimulatory monoclonal antibodies for cancer therapy," *Nature Reviews Cancer*, vol. 7, no. 2, pp. 95–106, 2007.

[20] C. Robert, L. Thomas, I. Bondarenko et al., "Ipilimumab plus dacarbazine for previously untreated metastatic melanoma," *The New England Journal of Medicine*, vol. 364, no. 26, pp. 2517–2526, 2011.

[21] J. D. Wolchok, L. Thomas, I. N. Bondarenko et al., "Phase III randomized study of ipilimumab (IPI) plus dacarbazine (DTIC) versus DTIC alone as first-line treatment in patients with unresectable stage III or IV melanoma," *Journal of Clinical Oncology*, vol. 29, abstract no. LBA5, 2011.

[22] B. F. Cole, R. D. Gelber, J. M. Kirkwood, A. Goldhirsch, E. Barylak, and E. Borden, "Quality-of-life-adjusted survival analysis of interferon alfa-2b adjuvant treatment of high-risk resected cutaneous melanoma: an Eastern cooperative oncology group study," *Journal of Clinical Oncology*, vol. 14, no. 10, pp. 2666–2673, 1996.

[23] A. M. Eggermont, S. Suciu, M. Santinami et al., "EORTC, 18991 phase III trial: long-term adjuvant pegylated interferon-α2b (PEG-IFN) versus observation in resected stage III melanoma: long-term results at 7. 6-years follow-up," *Journal of Clinical Oncology*, vol. 29, no. 15, abstract no. 8506b, 2011.

[24] W. J. Hwu, K. S. Panageas, J. H. Menell et al., "Phase II study of temozolomide plus pegylated interferon-α-2b for metastatic melanoma," *Cancer*, vol. 106, no. 11, pp. 2445–2451, 2006.

[25] L. E. Flaherty, J. Moon, M. B. Atkins et al., "Phase III trial of high-dose interferon α-2b versus cisplatin, vinblastine, DTIC plus IL-2 and interferon in patients with high-risk melanoma (SWOG S0008): an Intergroup study of CALGB, COC, ECOG and SWOG," *Journal of Clinical Oncology*, vol. 30, abstract no. 8504, 2012.

[26] H. Davies, G. R. Bignell, C. Cox et al., "Mutations of the BRAF gene in human cancer," *Nature*, vol. 417, no. 6892, pp. 949–954, 2002.

[27] J. A. Curtin, J. Fridlyand, T. Kageshita et al., "Distinct sets of genetic alterations in melanoma," *The New England Journal of Medicine*, vol. 353, no. 20, pp. 2135–2147, 2005.

[28] J. A. Jakob, R. L. Bassett, C. S. Ng et al., "Clinical characteristics and outcomes associated with BRAF and NRAS mutations in

metastatic melanoma," *Cancer*, vol. 118, no. 16, pp. 4014–4023, 2011.

[29] N. Dhomen and R. Marais, "BRAF signaling and targeted therapies in melanoma," *Hematology/Oncology Clinics of North America*, vol. 23, no. 3, pp. 529–545, 2009.

[30] G. S. Inamdar, S. V. Madhunapantula, and G. P. Robertson, "Targeting the MAPK pathway in melanoma: why some approaches succeed and other fail," *Biochemical Pharmacology*, vol. 80, no. 5, pp. 624–637, 2010.

[31] S. M. Wilhelm, C. Carter, L. Tang et al., "BAY 43-9006 exhibits broad spectrum oral antitumor activity and targets the RAF/MEK/ERK pathway and receptor tyrosine kinases involved in tumor progression and angiogenesis," *Cancer Research*, vol. 64, no. 19, pp. 7099–7109, 2004.

[32] T. Eisen, T. Ahmad, K. T. Flaherty et al., "Sorafenib in advanced melanoma: a phase II randomised discontinuation trial analysis," *British Journal of Cancer*, vol. 95, no. 5, pp. 581–586, 2006.

[33] D. F. McDermott, J. A. Sosman, R. Gonzalez et al., "Double-blind randomized phase II study of the combination of sorafenib and dacarbazine in patients with advanced melanoma: a report from the 11715 study group," *Journal of Clinical Oncology*, vol. 26, no. 13, pp. 2178–2185, 2008.

[34] A. Hauschild, S. S. Agarwala, U. Trefzer et al., "Results of a phase III, randomized, placebo-controlled study of sorafenib in combination with carboplatin and paclitaxel as second-line treatment in patients with unresectable stage III or stage IV melanoma," *Journal of Clinical Oncology*, vol. 27, no. 17, pp. 2823–2830, 2009.

[35] R. Kefford, H. Arkenau, M. Brown, M. Millward et al., "Phase I/II study of GSK2118436, a selective inhibitor of oncogenic mutant BRAF kinase, in patients with metastatic melanoma and other solid tumors," *Journal of Clinical Oncology*, vol. 28, abstract no. 8503, 2010.

[36] R. Dummer, J. Rinderknecht, S. M. Goldinger et al., "An open-label pilot study of vemurafenib in previously treated metastatic melanoma patients with brain metastases," *Journal of Clinical Oncology*, vol. 29, abstract no. 8548, 2011.

[37] F. Su, A. Viros, C. Milagre et al., "RAS mutations in cutaneous squamous-cell carcinomas in patients treated with BRAF inhibitors," *The New England Journal of Medicine*, vol. 366, no. 3, pp. 207–215, 2012.

[38] E. Y. Chu, K. A. Wanat, C. J. Miller et al., "Diverse cutaneous side effects associated with BRAF inhibitor therapy: a clinicopathologic study," *Journal of the American Academy of Dermatology*, vol. 67, no. 6, pp. 1265–1272, 2012.

[39] P. A. Oberholzer, D. Kee, P. Dziunycz et al., "RAS mutations are associated with the development of cutaneous squamous cell tumors in patients treated with RAF inhibitors," *Journal of Clinical Oncology*, vol. 30, no. 3, pp. 316–321, 2012.

[40] M. E. Lacouture, K. O'Reilly, N. Rosen, and D. B. Solit, "Induction of cutaneous squamous cell carcinomas by RAF inhibitors: cause for concern?" *Journal of Clinical Oncology*, vol. 30, no. 3, pp. 329–330, 2012.

[41] N. Wagle, C. Emery, M. F. Berger et al., "Dissecting therapeutic resistance to RAF inhibition in melanoma by tumor genomic profiling," *Journal of Clinical Oncology*, vol. 29, no. 22, pp. 3085–3096, 2011.

[42] M. E. Gorre, M. Mohammed, K. Ellwood et al., "Clinical resistance to STI-571 cancer therapy caused by BCR-ABL gene mutation or amplification," *Science*, vol. 293, no. 5531, pp. 876–880, 2001.

[43] L. M. Ellis and D. J. Hicklin, "Resistance to targeted therapies: refining anticancer therapy in the era of molecular oncology," *Clinical Cancer Research*, vol. 15, no. 24, pp. 7471–7478, 2009.

[44] R. Nazarian, H. Shi, Q. Wang et al., "Melanomas acquire resistance to B-RAF(V600E) inhibition by RTK or N-RAS upregulation," *Nature*, vol. 468, no. 7326, pp. 973–977, 2010.

[45] C. M. Johannessen, J. S. Boehm, S. Y. Kim et al., "COT drives resistance to RAF inhibition through MAP kinase pathway reactivation," *Nature*, vol. 468, no. 7326, pp. 968–972, 2010.

[46] J. Villanueva, A. Vultur, J. T. Lee et al., "Acquired resistance to BRAF inhibitors mediated by a RAF kinase switch in melanoma can be overcome by cotargeting MEK and IGF-1R/PI3K," *Cancer Cell*, vol. 18, no. 6, pp. 683–695, 2010.

[47] C. M. Emery, K. G. Vijayendran, M. C. Zipser et al., "MEK1 mutations confer resistance to MEK and B-RAF inhibition," *Proceedings of the National Academy of Sciences of the United States of America*, vol. 106, no. 48, pp. 20411–20416, 2009.

[48] C. Montagut, S. V. Sharma, T. Shioda et al., "Elevated CRAF as a potential mechanism of acquired resistance to BRAF inhibition in melanoma," *Cancer Research*, vol. 68, no. 12, pp. 4853–4861, 2008.

[49] M. Guix, A. C. Faber, S. E. Wang et al., "Acquired resistance to EGFR tyrosine kinase inhibitors in cancer cells is mediated by loss of IGF-binding proteins," *Journal of Clinical Investigation*, vol. 118, no. 7, pp. 2609–2619, 2008.

[50] R. D. Carvajal, C. R. Antonescu, J. D. Wolchok et al., "KIT as a therapeutic target in metastatic melanoma," *The Journal of the American Medical Association*, vol. 305, no. 22, pp. 2327–2334, 2011.

[51] K. H. T. Paraiso, Y. Xiang, V. W. Rebecca et al., "PTEN loss confers BRAF inhibitor resistance to melanoma cells through the suppression of BIM expression," *Cancer Research*, vol. 71, no. 7, pp. 2750–2760, 2011.

[52] C. Robert, K. T. Flaherty, P. Hersey et al., "METRIC phase III study: efficacy of trametinib (T), a potent and selective MEK inhibitor (MEKi), in progression-free survival (PFS) and overall survival (OS), compared with chemotherapy (C) in patients (pts) with BRAFV600E/K mutant advanced or metastatic melanoma (MM)," *Journal of Clinical Oncology*, vol. 30, no. 18, absrtact no. LBA8509, 2012.

[53] Clinical trials investigating c-KIT inhibitors for advanced melanoma http://www.clinicaltrials.gov/ct2/results?term=cKIT+inhibitors&cond=%22Melanoma%22.

[54] H. M. Kluger, A. Z. Dudek, C. McCann et al., "A phase 2 trial of dasatinib in advanced melanoma," *Cancer*, vol. 117, no. 10, pp. 2202–2208, 2011.

[55] S. E. Woodman, J. C. Trent, K. Stemke-Hale et al., "Activity of dasatinib against L576P KIT mutant melanoma: molecular, cellular, and clinical correlates," *Molecular Cancer Therapeutics*, vol. 8, no. 8, pp. 2079–2085, 2009.

[56] J. A. Curtin, K. Busam, D. Pinkel, and B. C. Bastian, "Somatic activation of KIT in distinct subtypes of melanoma," *Journal of Clinical Oncology*, vol. 24, no. 26, pp. 4340–4346, 2006.

[57] H. Kitayama, Y. Kanakura, T. Furitsu et al., "Constitutively activating mutations of c-kit receptor tyrosine kinase confer factor-independent growth and tumorigenicity of factor-dependent hematopoietic cell lines," *Blood*, vol. 85, no. 3, pp. 790–798, 1995.

[58] K. B. Kim, O. Eton, D. W. Davis et al., "Phase II trial of imatinib mesylate in patients with metastatic melanoma," *British Journal of Cancer*, vol. 99, no. 5, pp. 734–740, 2008.

[59] J. Guo, L. Si, Y. Kong et al., "Phase II, open-label, single-arm trial of imatinib mesylate in patients with metastatic melanoma harboring c-Kit mutation or amplification," *Journal of Clinical Oncology*, vol. 29, no. 21, pp. 2904–2909, 2011.

[60] "Clinical trials investigating vemurafenib plus ipilimumab for advanced melanoma," http://www.clinicaltrials.gov/ct2/show/NCT01400451?term=vemurafenib&cond=%22Melanoma%22&rank=21.

[61] G. V. Long, U. Trefzer, M. A. Davies et al., "Dabrafenib in patients with Val600Glu or Val600Lys BRAF-mutant melanoma metastatic to the brain (BREAK-MB): a multicentre, open-label, phase 2 trial," *The Lancet Oncology*, vol. 13, no. 11, pp. 1087–1095, 2012.

[62] J. M. Kirkwood, G. V. Long, U. Trefzer et al., "BREAK-MB: a phase II study assessing overall intracranial response rate to dabrafenib (GSK2118436) in patients with BRAF V600E/k mutation-positive melanoma with brain metastases," *Journal of Clinical Oncology*, vol. 30, abstract no. 8501, 2012.

[63] A. Hauschild, J. J. Grob, L. V. Demidov et al., "Phase III, randomized, open-label, multicenter trial (BREAK-3) comparing the BRAF kinase inhibitor dabrafenib (GSK2118436) with dacarbazine (DTIC) in patients with BRAFV600E-mutated melanoma," *Journal of Clinical Oncology*, vol. 30, abstract no. LBA8500, 2012.

[64] J. R. Infante, G. S. Falchook, D. P. Lawrence, J. S. Weber et al., "Phase I/II study to assess safety, pharmacokinetics, and efficacy of the oral MEK 1/2 inhibitor GSK1120212 dosed in combination with oral BRAF inhibitor," *Journal of Clinical Oncology*, vol. 29, abstract no. CRA8503, 2011.

[65] J. S. Weber, K. T. Flaherty, J. R. Infante et al., "Updated safety and efficacy results from a phase I/II study of the oral BRAF inhibitor dabrafenib (GSK2118436) combined with the oral MEK 1/2 inhibitor trametinib (GSK1120212) in patients with BRAFi-naive metastatic melanoma," *Journal of Clinical Oncology*, vol. 30, abstract no. 8510, 2012.

[66] K. T. Flaherty, J. R. Infante, A. Daud et al., "Combined BRAF and MEK inhibition in melanoma with BRAF V600 mutations," *The New England Journal of Medicine*, vol. 367, no. 18, pp. 1694–1703, 2012.

[67] S. Wee, Z. Jagani, K. X. Xiang et al., "PI3K pathway activation mediates resistance to MEK inhibitors in KRAS mutant cancers," *Cancer Research*, vol. 69, no. 10, pp. 4286–4293, 2009.

[68] E. Halilovic, Q. B. She, Q. Ye et al., "PIK3CA mutation uncouples tumor growth and cyclin D1 regulation from MEK/ERK and mutant KRAS signaling," *Cancer Research*, vol. 70, no. 17, pp. 6804–6814, 2010.

[69] M. E. Keir, M. J. Butte, G. J. Freeman, and A. H. Sharpe, "PD-1 and its ligands in tolerance and immunity," *Annual Review of Immunology*, vol. 26, pp. 677–704, 2008.

[70] J. L. Riley, "PD-1 signaling in primary T cells," *Immunological Reviews*, vol. 229, no. 1, pp. 114–125, 2009.

[71] T. Okazaki and T. Honjo, "The PD-1-PD-L pathway in immunological tolerance," *Trends in Immunology*, vol. 27, no. 4, pp. 195–201, 2006.

[72] J. R. Brahmer, C. G. Drake, I. Wollner et al., "Phase I study of single-agent anti-programmed death-1 (MDX-1106) in refractory solid tumors: safety, clinical activity, pharmacodynamics, and immunologic correlates," *Journal of Clinical Oncology*, vol. 28, no. 19, pp. 3167–3175, 2010.

[73] F. S. Hodi, M. Sznol, D. F. McDermott et al., "Clinical activity and safety of anti-PD-1 (BMS-936558, MDX-1106) in patients with advanced melanoma," *Journal of Clinical Oncology*, vol. 20, abstract no. 8507, 2012.

[74] K. B. Kim, J. A. Sosman, J. P. Fruehauf et al., "BEAM: a randomized phase II study evaluating the activity of bevacizumab in combination with carboplatin plus paclitaxel in patients with previously untreated advanced melanoma," *Journal of Clinical Oncology*, vol. 30, no. 1, pp. 34–41, 2012.

[75] A. Sandler, R. Gray, M. C. Perry et al., "Paclitaxel-carboplatin alone or with bevacizumab for non-small-cell lung cancer," *The New England Journal of Medicine*, vol. 355, no. 24, pp. 2542–2550, 2006.

[76] F. S. Hodi, P. A. Friedlander, M. B. Atkins et al., "A phase I trial of ipilimumab plus bevacizumab in patients with unresectable stage III or stage IV melanoma," *Journal of Clinical Oncology*, vol. 29, abstract no. 8511, 2011.

[77] S. N. Markovic, V. J. Suman, W. K. Nevala et al., "A dose-escalation study of aerosolized sargramostim in the treatment of metastatic melanoma: an NCCTG study," *American Journal of Clinical Oncology*, vol. 31, no. 6, pp. 573–579, 2008.

[78] L. E. Spitler, R. W. Weber, R. E. Allen et al., "Recombinant human granulocyte-macrophage colony-stimulating factor (GM-CSF, sargramostim) administered for 3 years as adjuvant therapy of stages II(T4), III, and IV melanoma," *Journal of Immunotherapy*, vol. 32, no. 6, pp. 632–637, 2009.

[79] "Ipilimumab with or without sargramostim in treating patients with stage III or stage IV melanoma that cannot be removed by surgery," http://clinicaltrials.gov/show/NCT01134614.

[80] D. Khayat, B. Giroux, J. Berille et al., "Fotemustine in the treatment of brain primary tumors and metastases," *Cancer Investigation*, vol. 12, no. 4, pp. 414–420, 1994.

[81] M. F. Avril, S. Aamdal, J. J. Grob et al., "Fotemustine compared with dacarbazine in patients with disseminated malignant melanoma: a phase III study," *Journal of Clinical Oncology*, vol. 22, no. 6, pp. 1118–1125, 2004.

[82] A. M. Di Giacomo, P. A. Ascierto, L. Pilla et al., "Ipilimumab and fotemustine in patients with advanced melanoma (NIBIT-M1): an open-label, single-arm phase 2 trial," *The Lancet Oncology*, vol. 13, no. 9, pp. 879–886, 2012.

[83] F. Menaa and B. Menaa, "Development of mitotane lipid nanocarriers and enantiomers: two-in-one solution to efficiently treat adreno-cortical carcinoma," *Current Medicinal Chemistry*, vol. 19, no. 34, pp. 5854–5862, 2012.

[84] H. L. McArthur, H. Rugo, B. Nulsen et al., "A feasibility study of bevacizumab plus dose-dense doxorubicin-cyclophosphamide (AC) followed by nanoparticle albumin-bound paclitaxel in early-stage breast cancer," *Clinical Cancer Research*, vol. 17, no. 10, pp. 3398–3407, 2011.

[85] M. Abrishami, S. Zarei-Ghanavati, D. Soroush, M. Rouhbakhsh, M. R. Jaafari, and B. Malaekeh-Nikouei, "Preparation, characterization, and in vivo evaluation of nanoliposomes-encapsulated bevacizumab (avastin) for intravitreal administration," *Retina*, vol. 29, no. 5, pp. 699–703, 2009.

[86] S. A. Rosenberg, B. S. Packard, P. M. Aebersold et al., "Use of tumor-infiltrating lymphocyts and interleukin-2 in the immunotherapy of patients with metastatic melanoma. A preliminary report," *The New England Journal of Medicine*, vol. 319, no. 25, pp. 1676–1680, 1988.

[87] S. A. Rosenberg, J. R. Yannelli, J. C. Yang et al., "Treatment of patients with metastatic melanoma with autologous tumor-infiltrating lymphocytes and interleukin 2," *Journal of the National Cancer Institute*, vol. 86, no. 15, pp. 1159–1166, 1994.

[88] S. A. Rosenberg and M. E. Dudley, "Cancer regression in patients with metastatic melanoma after the transfer of autologous antitumor lymphocytes," *Proceedings of the National Academy of Sciences of the United States of America*, vol. 101, no. 2, pp. 14639–14645, 2004.

[89] M. E. Dudley, J. R. Wunderlich, J. C. Yang et al., "Adoptive cell transfer therapy following non-myeloablative but lymphodepleting chemotherapy for the treatment of patients with refractory metastatic melanoma," *Journal of Clinical Oncology*, vol. 23, no. 10, pp. 2346–2357, 2005.

[90] S. A. Rosenberg, J. C. Yang, R. M. Sherry et al., "Durable complete responses in heavily pretreated patients with metastatic melanoma using T-cell transfer immunotherapy," *Clinical Cancer Research*, vol. 17, no. 13, pp. 4550–4557, 2011.

[91] M. E. Dudley, "Adoptive cell therapy for patients with melanoma," *Journal of Cancer*, vol. 2, pp. 360–362, 2011.

[92] A. Boni, A. P. Cogdill, P. Dang et al., "Selective BRAFV600E inhibition enhances T-cell recognition of melanoma without affecting lymphocyte function," *Cancer Research*, vol. 70, no. 13, pp. 5213–5219, 2010.

19

Simulators of Squamous Cell Carcinoma of the Skin: Diagnostic Challenges on Small Biopsies and Clinicopathological Correlation

Kong-Bing Tan,[1] Sze-Hwa Tan,[1] Derrick Chen-Wee Aw,[2] Huma Jaffar,[2] Thiam-Chye Lim,[3] Shu-Jin Lee,[4] and Yoke-Sun Lee[1]

[1] *Department of Pathology, Yong Loo Lin School of Medicine, National University Health System, National University of Singapore, Lower Kent Ridge Road, Singapore 119074*
[2] *University Medicine Cluster, National University Health System, Singapore 119074*
[3] *University Surgical Cluster, National University Health System, Singapore 119074*
[4] *Departments of Otorhinolaryngology and Hand and Reconstructive Microsurgery, National University Health System, Singapore 119074*

Correspondence should be addressed to Kong-Bing Tan; kong_bing_tan@nuhs.edu.sg

Academic Editor: Giuseppe Argenziano

Squamous cell carcinoma (SCC) is a common and important primary cutaneous malignancy. On skin biopsies, SCC is characterized by significant squamous cell atypia, abnormal keratinization, and invasive features. Diagnostic challenges may occasionally arise, especially in the setting of small punch biopsies or superficial shave biopsies, where only part of the lesion may be assessable by the pathologist. Benign mimics of SCC include pseudoepitheliomatous hyperplasia, eccrine squamous syringometaplasia, inverted follicular keratosis, and keratoacanthoma, while malignant mimics of SCC include basal cell carcinoma, melanoma, and metastatic carcinoma. The careful application of time-honored diagnostic criteria, close clinicopathological correlation and a selective request for a further, deeper, or wider biopsy remain the most useful strategies to clinch the correct diagnosis. This review aims to present the key differential diagnoses of SCC, to discuss common diagnostic pitfalls, and to recommend ways to deal with diagnostically challenging cases.

1. Introduction

Squamous cell carcinoma (SCC) is amongst the top 3 common skin cancers, ranking behind basal cell carcinoma (BCC) and ahead of melanoma [1]. It is a tumor that is locally invasive and which has the capacity to metastasize. Prognostically, it also occupies an intermediate position between BCC and melanoma, with BCC being locally invasive but typically nonmetastasizing, while melanoma having the well-known capability to metastasize. Histopathologically, most cases of SCC are readily diagnosable. However, diagnostic challenges are occasionally encountered and contributed mainly by the myriad of histopathologic mimics of SCC and small biopsies that sample only part of the lesion [2].

For the simulators of SCC, on the one hand, there are benign squamous lesions that appear to be infiltrative histopathologically. On the other hand, there are other malignant skin tumors that may display squamous differentiation or which elicit squamous proliferation that mimic SCC. Misdiagnosis of benign lesions as SCC would result in unnecessarily extensive surgery, while delayed diagnosis of SCC could lead to local tissue destruction by tumor, sometimes metastatic disease, and even death. Some malignant differential diagnostic entities, for example, melanoma and Merkel cell carcinoma (MCC), have worse prognosis or require different surgical strategies and differ in the need for adjuvant treatment [3, 4]. This review will present all the salient benign and malignant differential diagnoses of

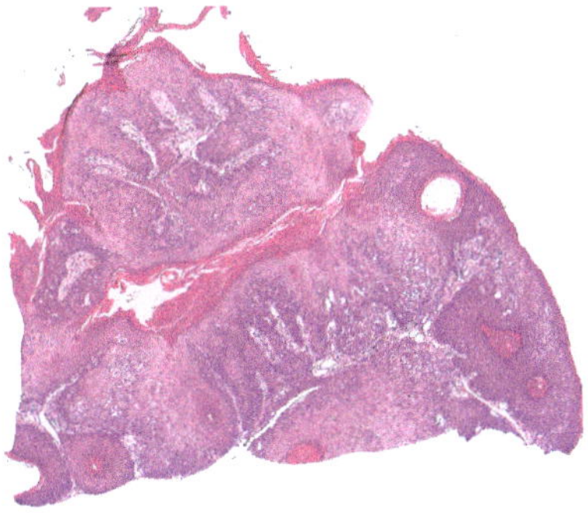

FIGURE 1: Inverted follicular keratosis: lesion shows proliferative downgrowths of mature squamous epithelium with infundibular keratinization (H&E ×40).

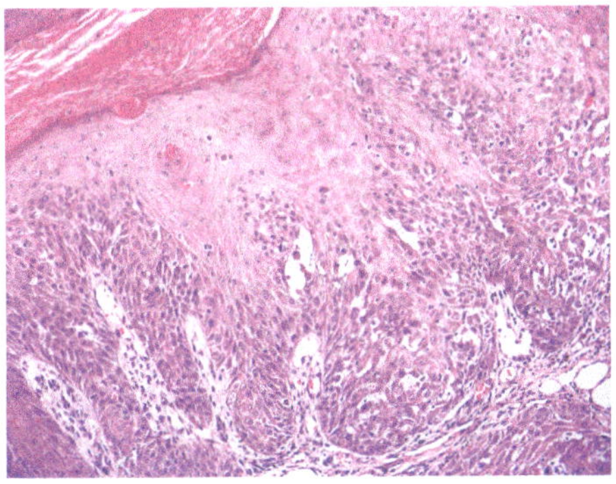

FIGURE 2: Inverted follicular keratosis: higher magnification showing squamous eddies (H&E ×200).

SCC, highlight diagnostic pitfalls, and suggest strategies for clinching the appropriate diagnosis.

2. Benign Squamoproliferative Lesions That Mimic SCC

2.1. Inverted Follicular Keratosis. Inverted follicular keratosis is a lesion that histopathologically shows downgrowths of follicular squamous epithelium and the adjacent epidermis [5]. It commonly occurs in middle-aged and elderly patients, presenting as a scaly papule, nodule, or plaque. It morphologically and conceptually overlaps with irritated seborrhoeic keratosis. In contrast to SCC, it has circumscribed borders, and significant cellular atypia is not seen (Figures 1 and 2).

A pitfall with regard to differential diagnosis of a supposedly benign squamous keratosis is when encountering a specimen of a superficial shave. Histologically, attention should be turned away from the hyperkeratotic superficial horn to the underlying lesional epithelium, which may be limited in amount in the specimen (Figure 3). The presence of significant atypia or abnormal maturation would raise the possibility of actinic keratosis or Bowen disease or even the superficial aspect of an invasive SCC.

2.2. Pseudoepitheliomatous Hyperplasia. Pseudoepitheliomatous hyperplasia (PEH) is a florid proliferation of the

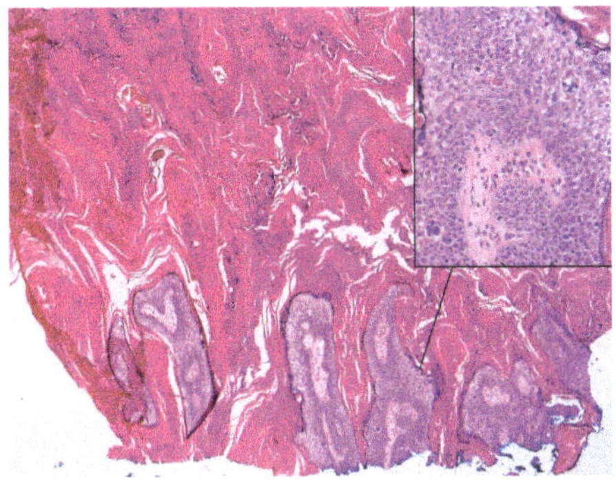

FIGURE 3: Bowen disease: Shave biopsy specimen showing mainly papillomatous epidermal lesion with hyperkeratotic horn. Inset: closer view of the underlying lesional epidermis shows cells with nuclear pleomorphism, prominent nucleoli, and frequent and abnormal mitotic figures. (H&E, ×20; Inset: ×400).

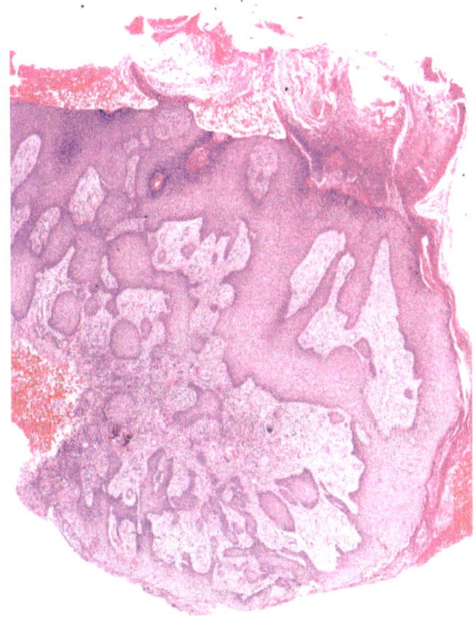

FIGURE 4: Pseudoepitheliomatous hyperplasia featuring acanthotic squamous epithelium showing irregular thick finger-like downgrowths into the underlying dermis. (H&E, ×20).

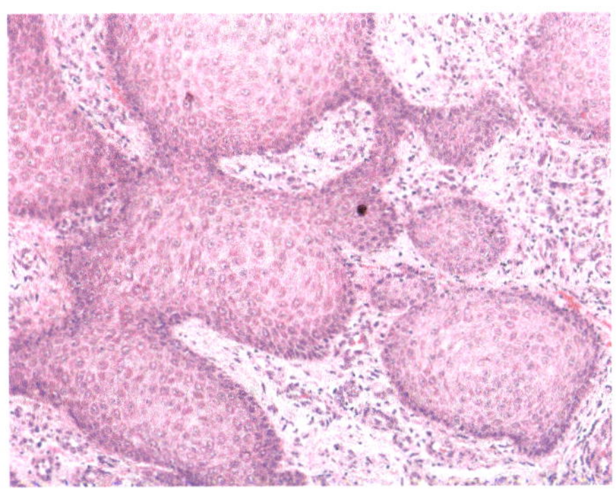

FIGURE 5: Pseudoepitheliomatous hyperplasia: higher magnification view showing reactive-appearing squamous downgrowths with no significant cytologic atypia. The dermis shows mild chronic inflammation and granulation tissue formation (H&E, ×200).

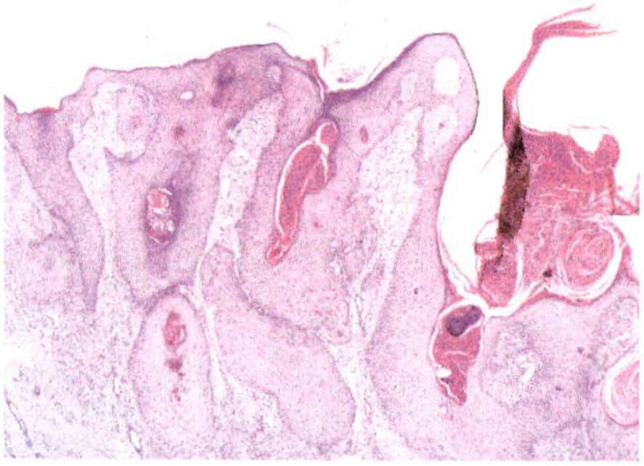

Figure 6: Infundibulocystic hyperplasia: skin lesion showing follicular proliferative process with bland squamous cells and formation of dilated canals containing keratotic material. (H&E, ×40).

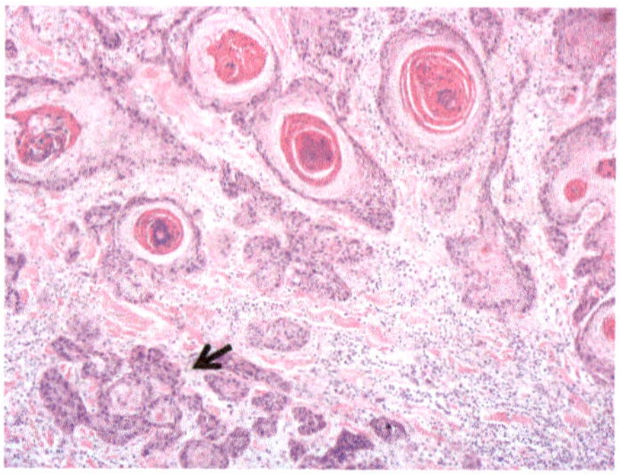

Figure 7: Infundibulocystic SCC: superficial areas showing infundibulocystic canals with deeper infiltrative squamous cell clusters featuring cellular atypia and mitoses (arrow). (H&E, ×100).

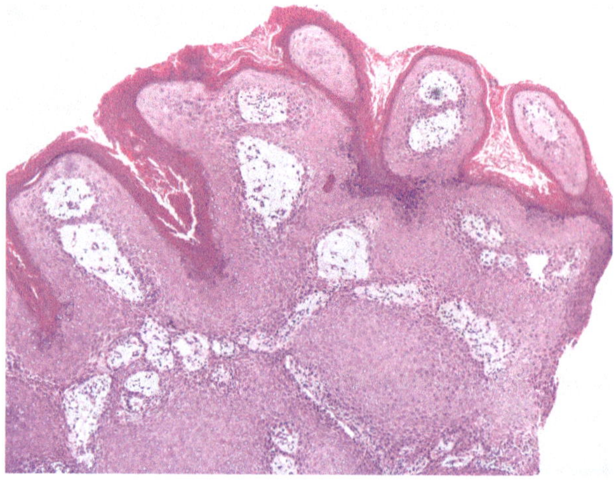

Figure 8: Verrucous hyperplasia: low power magnification view showing epidermal squamous proliferation with broad and superficial downgrowths of the epidermis. Overlying hyper-and parakeratosis is present. There is no atypia or koilocytes. (H&E, ×100).

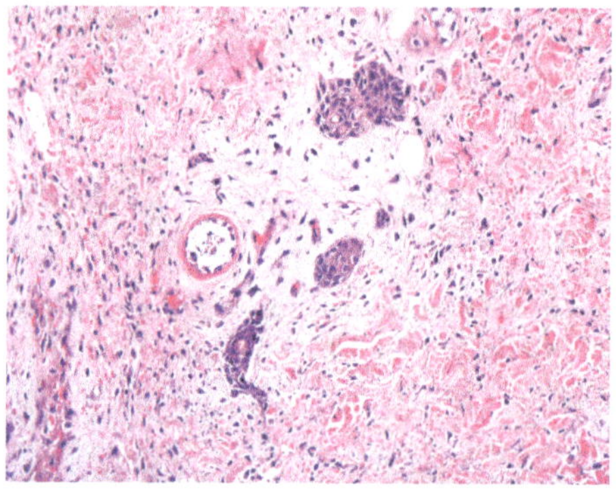

Figure 9: Eccrine squamous syringometaplasia: bland appearing squamous islands in the dermis centered around eccrine lumina. Scattered lymphocytes are present in the surrounding dermis. (H&E, ×200).

epidermis that may occur in the setting of chronic skin ulcers, abscesses, burns, and infections [6]. PEH with neutrophilic microabscesses is typically seen in halogenodermas, infections like chromomycosis and blastomycosis, granuloma inguinale, leishmaniasis, and pemphigus vegetans [7]. While the squamous epithelium of PEH can appear infiltrative, resembling well-differentiated SCC, careful attention should show that marked cellular atypia and abnormal mitotic activity are absent (Figures 4 and 5). A careful search for an inciting infective process should be carried out with examination of deeper levels and use of microbiological special stains. In challenging cases, close clinical correlation and followup are required; rare cases require repeat biopsy for evaluation.

2.3. Infundibulocystic Hyperplasia. Infundibulocystic hyperplasia is a distinctive follicular epithelial proliferative process with formation of dilated canals containing keratotic material [8]. Presenting clinically as a nodule or plaque, it features histologically bland lesional squamous cells and a relatively superficial noninfiltrative deep edge (Figure 6). When a short clinical evolution is noted and the lesion has a crateriform architecture, the features relate more to keratoacanthoma (*vide infra*). When marked cellular atypia or abnormal mitosis is noted, or if deeply infiltrative tongues are present, the lesion should be regarded as malignant, and an appropriate designation is infundibulocystic SCC (Figure 7) [8].

2.4. Verrucous Hyperplasia. Verrucous hyperplasia is another type of epidermal squamous proliferation typified by broad and superficial downgrowths of the epidermis (Figure 8). Overlying hyper- and parakeratosis are present. Atypia and koilocytes are absent. This condition usually occurs in the skin within and around the external genitalia and the oral cavity, in reaction to a variety of chronic irritative etiologies. It is distinguished from verrucous carcinoma, which has deeply pushing downgrowths. This feature can be difficult to assess in superficial or poorly oriented biopsies. Nevertheless, verrucous hyperplasia is well known to occur in close proximity, or to precede verrucous carcinoma [9]. Its presence in the context of a clinically worrying lesion should prompt close followup or a deeper and wider biopsy.

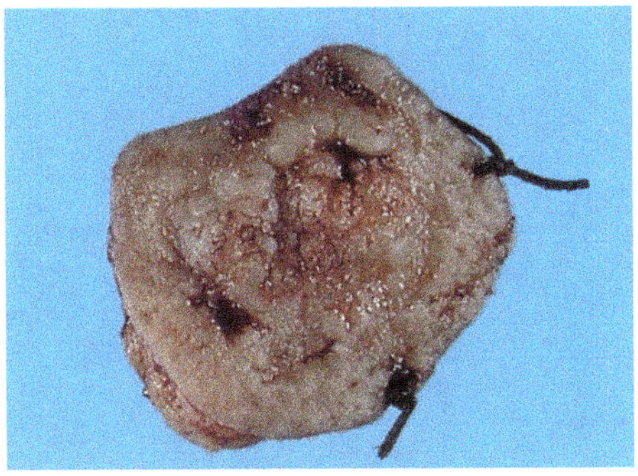

FIGURE 10: Desmoplastic trichoepithelioma: macroscopic picture showing an ulcerative nodular lesion with raised rolled edges features which mimic SCC or BCC.

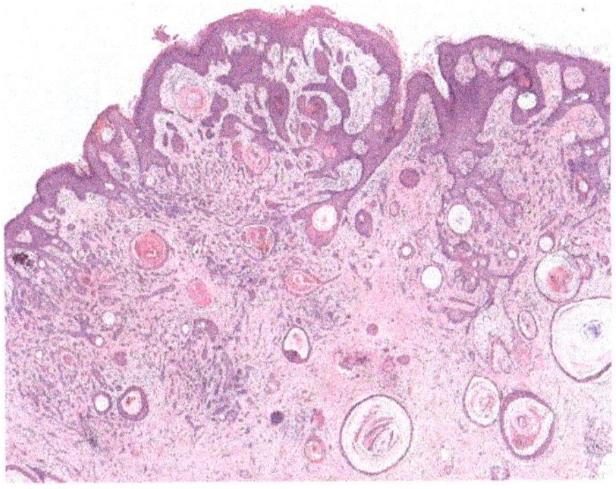

FIGURE 11: Desmoplastic trichoepithelioma: low power magnification showing hyperplastic downgrowths of epidermis with cords of basaloid tumor cells arranged in a pseudoinfiltrative pattern. (H&E, ×40).

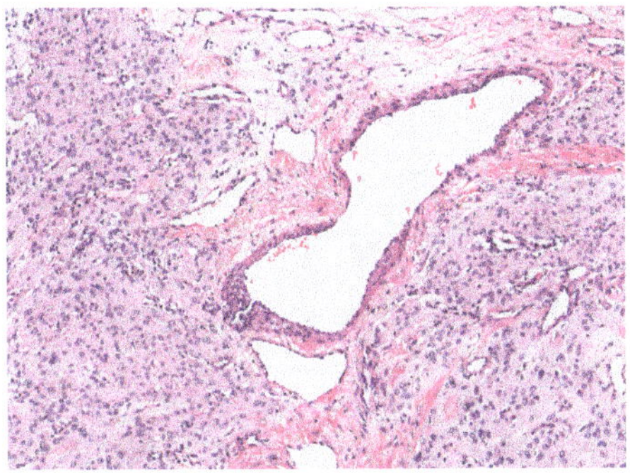

FIGURE 12: Meningioma: medium power magnification showing syncytial sheets and whorls of tumor cells with bland nuclear features. The presence of nuclear pseudoinclusions, psammoma bodies and the absence of atypia allow the distinction from SCC. (H&E, ×200).

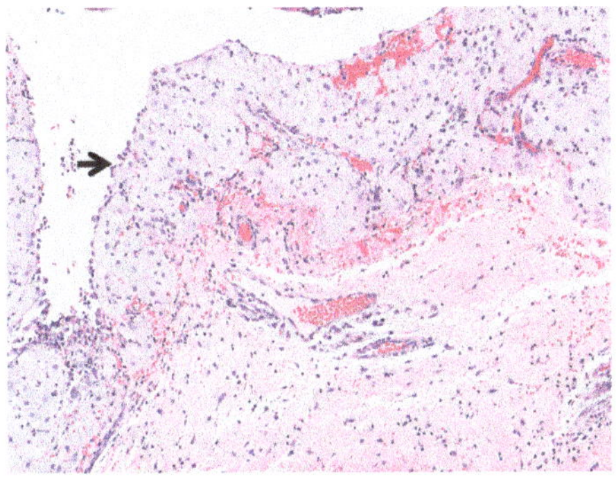

FIGURE 13: Endometriosis with decidualization: medium power magnification showing cystic space surrounded by large polygonal cells with basophilic cytoplasm and bland nuclei. The cyst wall is rimmed by a layer of endometrial cells (arrow). (H&E, ×200).

2.5. Eccrine Squamous Syringometaplasia. Eccrine squamous syringometaplasia (ESS) is a reactive process characterized by squamous metaplasia of eccrine ducts and glands [10, 11]. It commonly occurs in the axillary and groin regions and presents as nodules and plaques. EES is most well described as an adverse drug reaction, mostly to chemotherapeutic drugs [11]. It also occurs in the vicinity of burns, ulcers, and scars [10]. While it should not be confused with SCC clinically, it could cause some confusion histologically. The lesion features cytologically bland squamous islands in the dermis that are closely associated with eccrine lumina and conforming to a lobular configuration (Figure 9). An associated chronic inflammatory infiltrate is usually present.

2.6. Desmoplastic Adnexal Tumors. Some benign adnexal tumors may superficially resemble SCC. Desmoplastic trichoepithelioma presents clinically as an enlarging nodule and shows cords and nests of basaloid cells with horn cyst formation, embedded within a sclerotic dermal stroma (Figures 10 and 11) [12]. The overlying epidermis is often hyperplastic. On a superficial biopsy, the hyperplastic downgrowth of the epidermis and the cords of basaloid tumor cells give a pseudoinfiltrative appearance mimicking the features of SCC. The reassuring absence of significant atypia and the paucity of mitotic activity should be sought for.

Desmoplastic tricholemmoma is another adnexal tumor that can mimic SCC. The cohesive tumor cells growing as cellular sheets or cord-like manner streaming within a sclerotic dermis can appear concerning [13]. Squamous differentiation may also be present. Once again, the lesion should show cytological blandness. Areas of regular tricholemmoma disclosing epithelial cells with clear cytoplasm can usually be found.

3. Benign Nonsquamous Lesions That Mimic SCC

In unusual clinical contexts, benign lesions of varied nature may mimic SCC both clinically and histopathologically.

3.1. Extracranial Meningioma. Meningioma has been known to occasionally be located outside the intracranial location to involve the scalp [14]. Histopathologically, the syncytial sheets or whorled arrangement of tumor cells may impart a squamoid appearance (Figure 12). The presence of nuclear pseudoinclusions, psammoma bodies and the absence of significant atypia, in most cases, should allow distinction from SCC. Immunohistochemistry is of limited value in

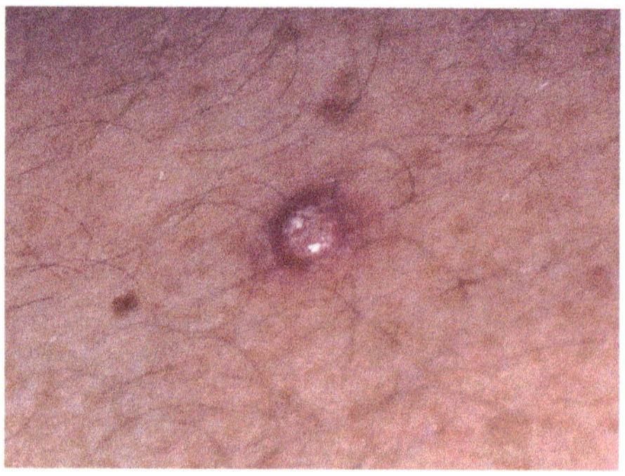

FIGURE 14: Keratoacanthoma: clinical photograph showing a well-circumscribed reddish nodule with erosion on the surface.

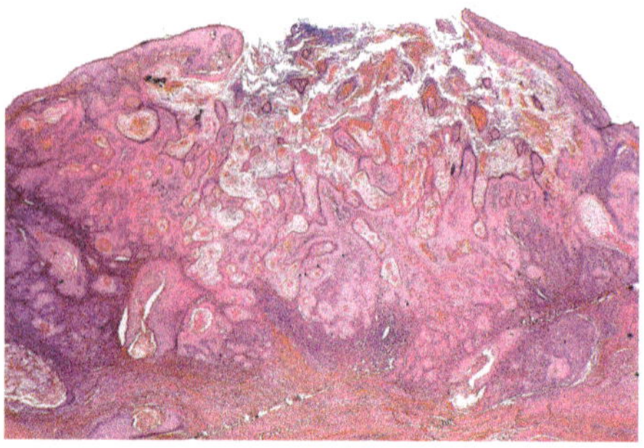

FIGURE 15: Keratoacanthoma: low power magnification showing a crateriform lesion which is filled with central keratinous plug and bounded by proliferative lesional squamous epithelium. (H&E, ×20).

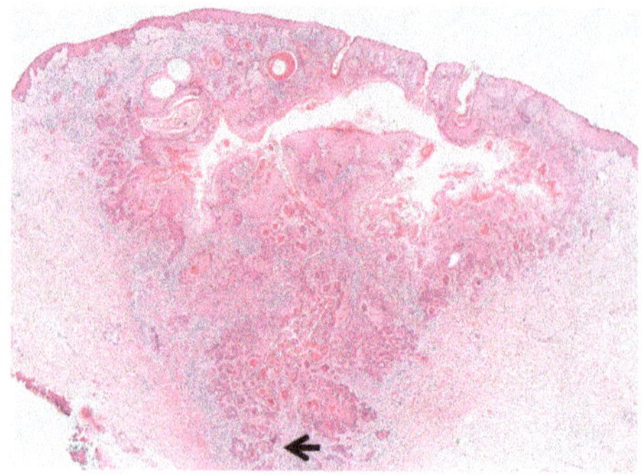

FIGURE 16: Keratoacanthoma-like SCC: low power magnification showing a crateriform lesion with infiltrative islands and clusters of squamous cells at the base (arrow). (H&E, ×20).

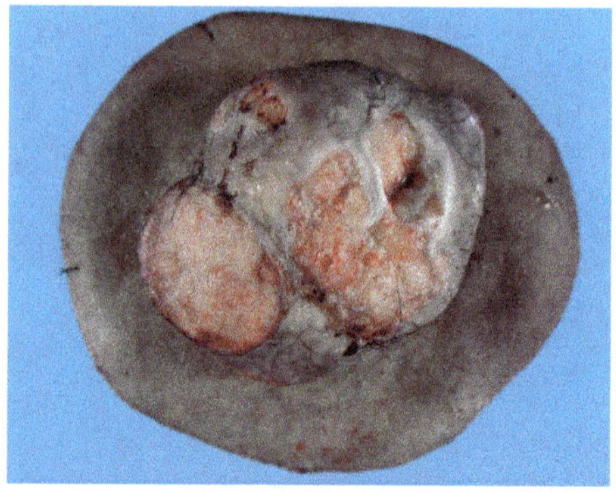

FIGURE 17: Proliferating tricholemmal tumor: macroscopic photograph showing a circumscribed cutaneous reddish-pink nodular tumor with surface erosions.

distinguishing the entities as both meningioma and SCC share expression of EMA, and the former is sometimes reactive for cytokeratins as well.

3.2. Decidualized Endometriosis. Another form of lesional tissue that may sometimes cause diagnostic confusion is decidualized endometrial tissue occurring outside the confines of the female genital tract [15]. The most common context of this is endometriotic deposits in the skin and soft tissue of the abdominal wall or perineum, where background therapy with progestational agents causes decidualization of the endometrial stromal component (Figure 13). Such decidualized cells are plump and form sheets, complete with well-defined intercellular borders, simulating SCC, if not for the notable absence of nuclear atypia.

4. Others Squamoproliferative Tumors That Mimic SCC

4.1. Keratoacanthoma. KA is a well-differentiated squamoproliferative tumor, with a fairly rapidly growing clinical course (Figure 14) [16]. Some authorities consider it a variant of SCC, while others regard it as a unique entity in view of its typically self-involuting course. Histopathologically, it features a cup-shaped or crateriform architecture, containing a central keratinous plug, bounded by lobules of lesional squamous epithelial cells (Figure 15). Features that favor a lesion as a KA rather than being an SCC include a limited pushing deep front, distinct tumour-stromal interface, and lesional squamous cells with abundant cytoplasm centrally. There is usually absence of stromal desmoplasia and of significant cellular atypia [17]. While there have been numerous studies investigating the differences between KA and SCC of the molecules involved in the regulation of cellular proliferation, apoptosis and the cell cycle, the histomorphology, as well as consideration of the clinical tempo of the lesion are still the most practical aspects in routine diagnosis.

An SCC can sometimes have a crateriform architecture mimicking a KA (KA-like SCC). In this regard, at least part of the tumor should have marked cytologic atypia, frequent or abnormal mitoses, or infiltrative margins (Figures 7 and 16). A shave biopsy that samples only the superficial part of a well-differentiated example of such a lesion could potentially lead to an underdiagnosis of an SCC (Figure 16). Where there is diagnostic doubt about a particular lesion, a complete excision should be recommended.

4.2. Proliferating Tricholemmal Tumor. Proliferating tricholemmal tumor (PTT), also known as proliferating pilar tumor or pilar tumor, is a well-circumscribed proliferation

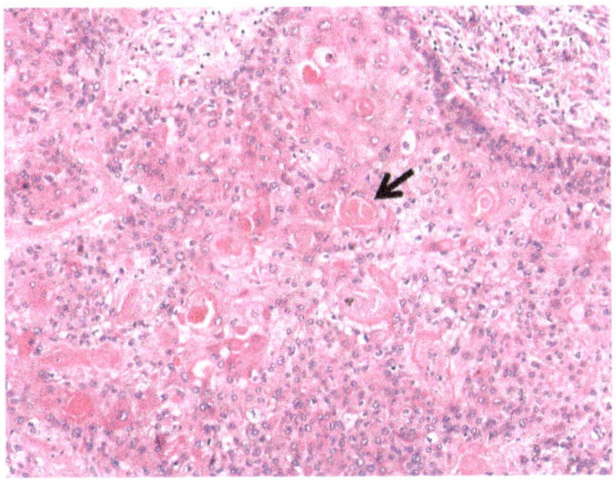

FIGURE 18: Proliferating tricholemmal tumor: the lesion shows proliferation of squamous cells with clear cytoplasm and abrupt pilar-type keratinization (arrow) (H&E, ×200).

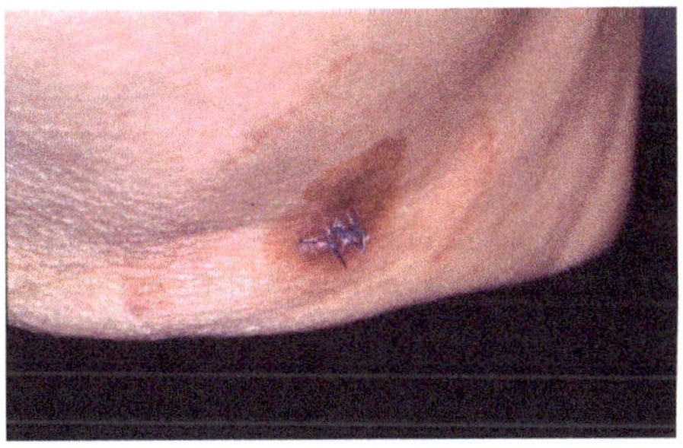

FIGURE 19: Clinical photograph showing a red, scaly plaque on the skin surface. The patient just had a biopsy performed with sutures still in place.

of squamous cells [18, 19]. It commonly occurs on the scalp or other parts of the head and neck as a gradually enlarging nodule or tumor (Figure 17). Histopathologically, apart from conventional squamous cells, the tumor shows cellular areas with characteristic clear cytoplasm and abrupt pilar-type keratinization (Figure 18). Calcification and an associated multinucleated cellular reaction are often present. There is a spectrum of appearances which may translate to different biologic behaviors. In a study by Ye et al., tumors that were well differentiated and well circumscribed behaved in a benign fashion [18]. Those with infiltrative borders but no significant atypia, increased mitoses, or necrosis had a local recurrence rate of 15%, while tumors which were infiltrative and which displayed cellular atypia, necrosis, and abnormal mitotic activity had a 50% chance of developing recurrence or metastasis to the regional lymph nodes. The latter category could be termed as a malignant PTT and viewed as equivalent to conventional SCC. Pathological examination of the entire lesion is necessary to assess the borders of the tumor as well as for the possible presence of necrosis and cytologic variation.

5. Bowen Disease (Squamous Cell Carcinoma *In Situ*)

Bowen disease clinically presents as a plaque in covered as well as uncovered skin areas (Figure 19). Histopathologically, it features full thickness dysplasia, incorporating loss of

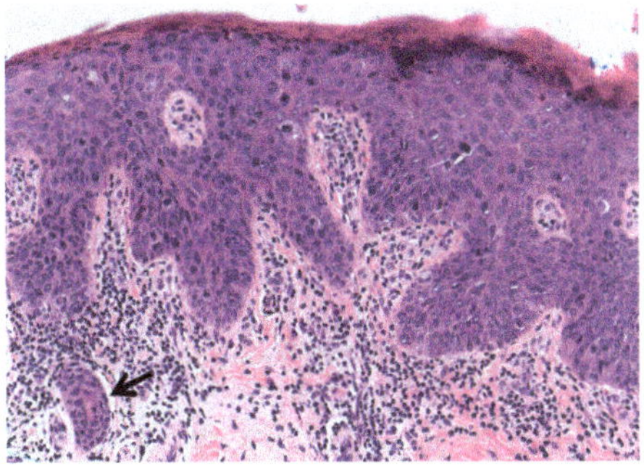

FIGURE 20: Bowen disease: medium-power magnification showing skin with full thickness epidermal dysplasia which is characterized by loss of the nuclear polarity, nuclear pleomorphism, and mitoses at all levels. The undulating deep epidermal contour and presence of eccrine ducts that have been colonized by the tumor cells (arrow) can potentially mimic invasion. (H&E, ×200).

polarity of the epidermis, nuclear pleomorphism, and mitosis at all levels (Figures 3 and 20). In usual cases, preinvasive malignancy is not in doubt in view of the previously described features. The differential diagnoses classically include extra-mammary Paget disease and melanoma *in situ* [20]. All three entities display single and groups of atypical cells within the epidermis. The tumor cells of Paget disease generally cluster above an intact basal layer of epidermis and may be demonstrated to contain mucin. Melanoma tumor cells often contain melanin although Paget cells have been known to show this feature as well. Immunohistochemistry helps to distinguish the entities: the tumor cells of Bowen disease are p63 positive, those of Paget's disease react for p-CEA, Ber-EP4, CK7, and CAM5.2, while melanoma cells are positive for S-100 and Melan-A [20].

Not uncommonly, Bowen disease shows a markedly undulating basal contour and can be associated with subjacent dermal fibroplasia, raising the possibility of whether early invasion has occurred. The neoplastic epithelium of Bowen disease can also colonize eccrine ducts, potentially exaggerating the incorrect impression of invasion (Figure 20). Examination of deeper levels or more blocks of tissue may reveal foci of convincing invasion, characterized by single or small jagged clusters of infiltrating tumor cells within unequivocally desmoplastic dermal stroma.

6. Other Malignant Tumors That Mimic Primary Cutaneous SCC

6.1. Basal Cell Carcinoma. Basal cell carcinoma (BCC) can sometimes mimic SCC. The typical BCC is characterized by basaloid cellular proliferation with peripheral palisading and tumor-stromal cleft formation. The infiltrating tumor cells may not uncommonly appear squamoid and raise the possibility of SCC. Immunohistochemistry can be helpful as BCC, and not SCC, is positive for Ber-EP4 and bcl-2 (Figure 21) [2].

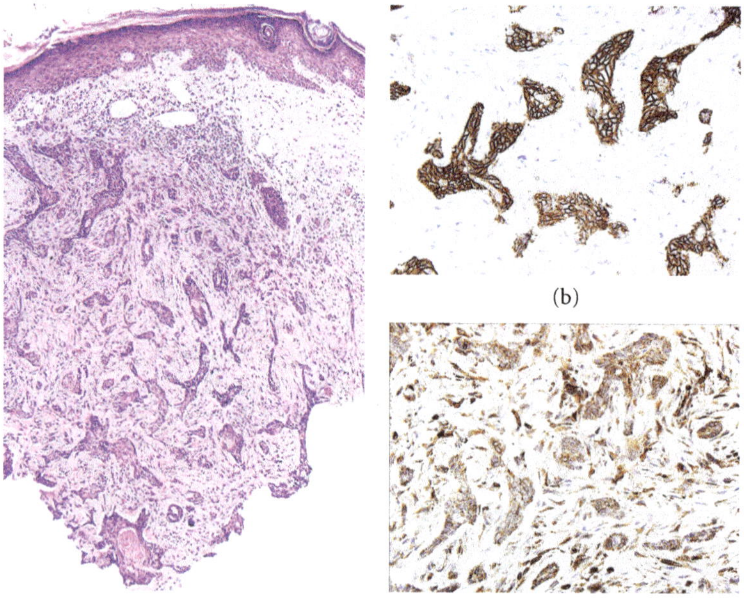

(a) (b) (c)

Figure 21: Basal cell carcinoma: (a) low power magnification showing infiltrative irregular islands of basaloid tumor cells which appear to have more ample eosinophilic cytoplasm mimicking the appearance of SCC (H&E, ×100). (b) Tumor cells are diffusely positive for Ber-EP4. (c) Tumor cells also show diffuse positivity for bcl-2.

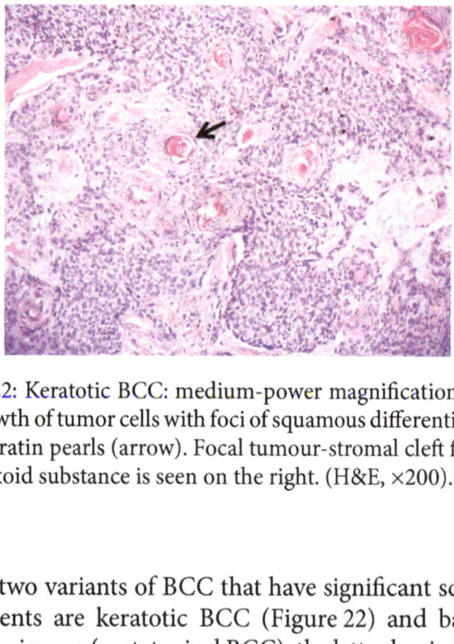

Figure 22: Keratotic BCC: medium-power magnification showing solid growth of tumor cells with foci of squamous differentiation featuring keratin pearls (arrow). Focal tumour-stromal cleft formation with myxoid substance is seen on the right. (H&E, ×200).

The two variants of BCC that have significant squamous components are keratotic BCC (Figure 22) and basosquamous carcinoma (metatypical BCC), the latter having a worse prognosis than BCC in general [21]. A careful assessment of the tumor would usually show areas of more typical BCC.

6.2. Sebaceous Carcinoma. The other skin cancer in the head and neck that occasionally mimics a poorly differentiated SCC is sebaceous carcinoma [22]. This tumor is disposed of in sheets and lobules of cells with bubbly cytoplasm that indent an atypical nucleus. Rarely, squamous differentiation may be present [23]. A basic immunochemistry panel can usually enable differentiation between SCC (EMA +ve, Ber-EP4 −ve), sebaceous carcinoma (EMA +ve, Ber-EP4 +ve), and BCC (EMA −ve, Ber-EP4 +ve) [22]. More recently, markers that have been found to be more specific for sebaceous carcinoma include adipophilin and androgen receptor, which in turn are usually negative in BCC and SCC [24].

6.3. Melanoma. Spindle cell melanoma is one of the classic differential diagnoses for pleomorphic spindle cell tumors of the skin [25]. While cytological features may not enable distinction from a spindle cell SCC and atypical fibroxanthoma (AFX), the presence of a junctional component helps delineate spindle cell melanoma (Figure 23). In contrast, careful examination of a spindle cell SCC may reveal overlying Bowen disease or actinic keratosis. By immunohistochemistry, expression of one or more of the cytokeratins helps distinguish the tumor from spindle cell melanoma which would instead express S-100. AFX is typically S-100 and cytokeratin negative and positive for CD10 and procollagen-1 [26].

6.4. Other Carcinomas with Squamous Differentiation. Other skin carcinomas that sometimes feature squamous differentiation include Merkel cell carcinoma (MCC), porocarcinoma, and sebaceous carcinoma [23, 27, 28]. This is likely a manifestation of divergent differentiation of the tumor or varied differentiation of tumor stem cells. Careful examination of MCC would usually show up the more typical malignant small round cells of MCC as well as dot-like expression of CK20 and positivity for the neuroendocrine markers synaptophysin, neurofilament protein, and CD56. As for porocarcinoma, the neoplastic poroid cells should be discernible with duct lumina formation decorated by EMA and p-CEA immunohistochemistry.

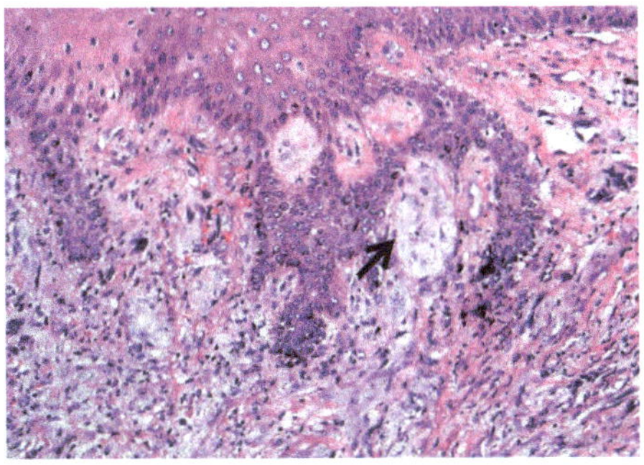

FIGURE 23: Spindle cell melanoma: medium-power magnification showing dermal pleomorphic spindle cell proliferation and focal junctional melanocytic nest (arrow). (H&E, ×100).

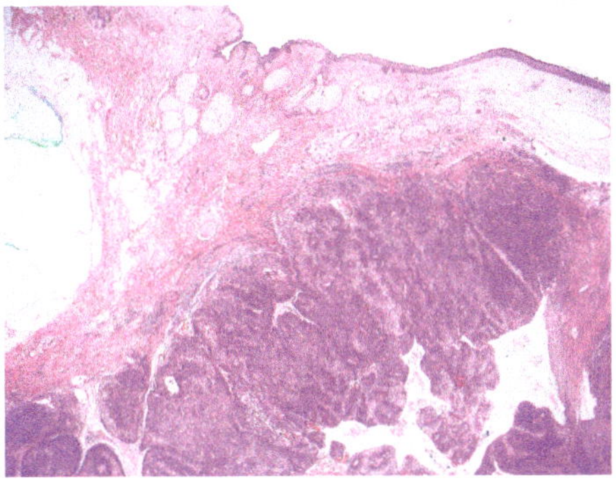

FIGURE 24: Metastatic SCC: low-power magnification showing solid growth of SCC which is predominantly located in the dermis and subcutaneous tissue. The overlying epidermis appears normal. This should raise suspicion of a metastatic deposit. (H&E, ×40).

6.5. Metastatic Squamous Cell Carcinoma to the Skin. An SCC present in the skin may occasionally represent direct invasion from an underlying malignancy or metastatic deposit. In such situations, the importance of clinical history and correlation cannot be overemphasized. The tumor tends to show a centre that is based in the dermis or subcutis (Figure 24). The overlying epidermis tends to show only reactive features or be ulcerated by the growth of the subjacent tumor.

6.6. Lymphoproliferative Disorders. Anaplastic large cell lymphoma and lymphomatoid papulosis are CD30-positive lymphoproliferative disorders that have reported cases being associated with epidermal hyperplasia [29]. While the epidermal hyperplasia is often mild in degree, it can be very florid with features of pseudoinfiltration which mimic SCC, raising the possibility of a collision between the carcinoma and lymphoproliferative process (Figure 25). Cellular atypia of the epidermal hyperplasia, while usually absent, has sometimes been reported. Mitoses of the squamous cells, if present, should be seen to be located at the basal layer of the squamous islands and not be abnormal in form.

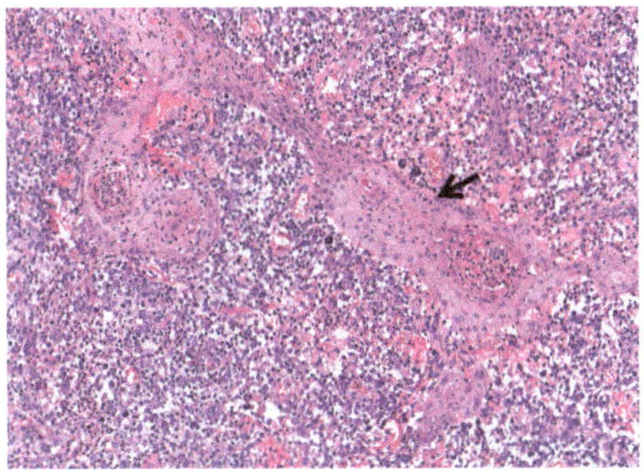

FIGURE 25: Cutaneous anaplastic large cell lymphoma: low-power magnification showing hyperplastic squamous islands (arrow) associated proliferation of large neoplastic lymphocytes. (H&E, ×100).

7. Collision Tumors

SCC can sometimes coexist with other malignant skin tumors within the same tumor mass, the most likely context being collision tumors. Combinations of SCC with melanoma or MCC are most well known [30, 31]. The practical importance is that on finding a prominent SCC component, the coexistence of a potentially more aggressive tumor, or a tumor that may require specific adjuvant therapy, should be sought for. Such a concurrence is not surprising as ultraviolet light exposure is a well known and common risk factor. Another plausible etiologic factor that has emerged more recently is that of human polyomaviruses. While the Merkel cell polyomavirus has been closely linked to MCC, its detection and role in SCC are less consistent and clear [31–33]. Interestingly, the virus has been detected in two cases of combined SCC and MCC [31]. The role of such human polyomaviruses in skin carcinogenesis deserves further investigation.

8. Conclusion

In summary, this review serves to highlight the spectrum of conditions that could mimic SCC: benign, preinvasive, and malignant. Being aware of the pertinent differential diagnoses provides the setting to minimize the pitfalls in the diagnosis of challenging cases which feature squamous proliferation. This, coupled with a systematic assessment for the criteria required for an SCC diagnosis, helps in the rendering of a correct diagnosis. Of the adjunctive studies, immunohistochemistry is the most widely used, helping to indicate the histogenesis of the lesional cells of nonsquamous mimics. In difficult cases, seeking a second opinion provides additional perspectives and insight.

Clinicopathological correlation is of paramount importance in the diagnosis of squamous epithelial lesions. A detailed and relevant history of cancers of the skin and other organs should be sought for. The clinical tempo of the lesion, knowledge of the site, size, and other characteristics are all critical pieces of information to the pathologist. If a lesion is clinically concerning, but the biopsy features are benign or nonspecific, further levels on the block often prove useful. Rarely, a summative assessment of inadequate material or of an atypical lesion that cannot exclude malignancy may have to be given with a recommendation for complete excisional biopsy. As always, this is balanced against the factors of cosmesis and practicability. On the one hand, the final reexcision specimen provides the opportunity for further evaluation of the residual lesion for definite diagnosis. On the other hand, the repeat excision often represents the definite surgical treatment for the lesion if it indeed turns out to be malignant. Such a pragmatic approach offers the rendering of a safe yet clinically useful diagnosis when diagnostically challenging cases are encountered.

References

[1] T. L. Diepgen and V. Mahler, "The epidemiology of skin cancer," *British Journal of Dermatology*, vol. 146, Supplement, no. 61, pp. 1–6, 2002.

[2] P. E. Swanson, M. M. Fitzpatrick, J. H. Ritter, E. J. Glusac, and M. R. Wick, "Immunohistologic differential diagnosis of basal cell carcinoma, squamous cell carcinoma, and trichoepithelioma in small cutaneous biopsy specimens," *Journal of Cutaneous Pathology*, vol. 25, no. 3, pp. 153–159, 1998.

[3] C. Garbe, K. Peris, A. Hauschild et al., "Diagnosis and treatment of melanoma. European consensus-based interdisciplinary guideline: update 2012," *European Journal of Cancer*, vol. 48, no. 15, pp. 2375–2390, 2012.

[4] D. Schrama, S. Ugurel, and J. C. Becker, "Merkel cell carcinoma: recent insights and new treatment options," *Current Opinion in Oncology*, vol. 24, no. 2, pp. 141–149, 2012.

[5] A. H. Mehregan, "Inverted follicular keratosis is a distinct follicular tumor," *The American Journal of Dermatopathology*, vol. 5, no. 5, pp. 467–470, 1983.

[6] M. Zayour and R. Lazova, "Pseudoepitheliomatous hyperplasia: a review," *The American Journal of Dermatopathology*, vol. 33, no. 2, pp. 112–126, 2011.

[7] D. M. Elston, T. Ferringer, C. J. Ko, S. Peckham, W. A. High, and D. J. Dicaudo, *Requisites in Dermatology: Dermatopathology*, Saunders, Philadelphia, Pa, USA, 2009.

[8] S. Kossard, K.-B. Tan, and C. Choy, "Keratoacanthoma and infundibulocystic squamous cell carcinoma," *The American Journal of Dermatopathology*, vol. 30, no. 2, pp. 127–134, 2008.

[9] J. I. Epstein and G. Mendelsohn, "Squamous carcinoma of the foot arising in association with long-standing verrucous hyperplasia in a patient with congenital lymphedema," *Cancer*, vol. 54, no. 5, pp. 943–947, 1984.

[10] T. Serrano, A. Saez, and A. Moreno, "Eccrine squamous syringometaplasia: a prospective clinicopathologic study," *Journal of Cutaneous Pathology*, vol. 20, no. 1, pp. 61–65, 1993.

[11] A. Martorell-Calatayud, O. Sanmartín, R. Botella-Estrada et al., "Chemotherapy-related bilateral dermatitis associated with eccrine squamous syringometaplasia: reappraisal of epidemiological, clinical, and pathological features," *Journal of the American Academy of Dermatology*, vol. 64, no. 6, pp. 1092–1103, 2011.

[12] J. Jedrych, D. Leffell, and J. M. McNiff, "Desmoplastic trichoepithelioma with perineural involvement: a series of seven cases," *Journal of Cutaneous Pathology*, vol. 39, no. 3, pp. 317–323, 2012.

[13] O. Tellechea, J. P. Reis, and A. P. Baptista, "Desmoplastic trichilemmoma," *The American Journal of Dermatopathology*, vol. 14, no. 2, pp. 107–114, 1992.

[14] S. K. Singh, B. K. Ojha, A. Chandra, M. Rastogi, M. Husain, and N. Husain, "Scalp meningioma," *Indian Journal of Dermatology*, vol. 53, pp. 196–198, 2008.

[15] S. E. Mills, "Decidua and squamous metaplasia in abdominopelvic lymph nodes," *International Journal of Gynecological Pathology*, vol. 2, no. 2, pp. 209–215, 1983.

[16] C. J. Ko, "Keratoacanthoma: facts and controversies," *Clinics in Dermatology*, vol. 28, no. 3, pp. 254–261, 2010.

[17] D. Weedon, *Weedon's Skin Pathology*, Churchill Livingstone, London, UK, 2010.

[18] J. Ye, O. Nappi, P. E. Swanson, J. W. Patterson, and M. R. Wick, "Proliferating pilar tumors: a clinicopathologic study of 76 cases with a proposal for definition of benign and malignant variants," *The American Journal of Clinical Pathology*, vol. 122, no. 4, pp. 566–574, 2004.

[19] A. A. Khoja, B. Yan, S. J. Lee, E. C. Cheong, and K. B. Tan, "Proliferating tricholemmal tumour: clinicopathological aspects of a case," *Singapore Medical Journal*, vol. 52, no. 12, pp. e255–e257, 2011.

[20] E. C. Wang, Y. C. Kwah, W. P. Tan, J. S. Lee, and S. H. Tan, "Extramammary Paget disease: immunohistochemistry is critical to distinguish potential mimickers," *Dermatology Online Journal*, vol. 18, no. 9, 4 pages, 2012.

[21] C. Garcia, E. Poletti, and A. N. Crowson, "Basosquamous carcinoma," *Journal of the American Academy of Dermatology*, vol. 60, no. 1, pp. 137–143, 2009.

[22] B. Sramek, A. Lisle, and T. Loy, "Immunohistochemistry in ocular carcinomas," *Journal of Cutaneous Pathology*, vol. 35, no. 7, pp. 641–646, 2008.

[23] M. Izumi, K. Mukai, T. Nagai et al., "Sebaceous carcinoma of the eyelids: thirty cases from Japan," *Pathology International*, vol. 58, no. 8, pp. 483–488, 2008.

[24] S.-I. Ansai, H. Takeichi, S. Arase, S. Kawana, and T. Kimura, "Sebaceous carcinoma: an immunohistochemical reappraisal," *The American Journal of Dermatopathology*, vol. 33, no. 6, pp. 579–587, 2011.

[25] M. B. Morgan, C. Purohit, and T. R. Anglin, "Immunohistochemical distinction of cutaneous spindle cell carcinoma," *The American Journal of Dermatopathology*, vol. 30, no. 3, pp. 228–232, 2008.

[26] K. Jensen, B. Wilkinson, N. Wines, and S. Kossard, "Procollagen 1 expression in atypical fibroxanthoma and other tumors," *Journal of Cutaneous Pathology*, vol. 31, no. 1, pp. 57–61, 2004.

[27] J. H. K. Hwang, K. Alanen, K. D. Dabbs, J. Danyluk, and S. Silverman, "Merkel cell carcinoma with squamous and sarcomatous differentiation," *Journal of Cutaneous Pathology*, vol. 35, no. 10, pp. 955–959, 2008.

[28] F. Mahomed, J. Blok, and W. Grayson, "The squamous variant of eccrine porocarcinoma: a clinicopathological study of 21 cases," *Journal of Clinical Pathology*, vol. 61, no. 3, pp. 361–365, 2008.

[29] J. J. Scarisbrick, E. Calonje, G. Orchard, F. J. Child, and R. Russell-Jones, "Pseudocarcinomatous change in lymphomatoid papulosis and primary cutaneous CD30 + lymphoma: a clinicopathologic and immunohistochemical study of 6 patients," *Journal of the American Academy of Dermatology*, vol. 44, no. 2, pp. 239–247, 2001.

[30] N. Mopuri, J. K. G. Laitung, and C. Cardozo, "Collision tumour of squamous cell carcinoma and invasive malignant melanoma of scalp: a case report," *Journal of Plastic, Reconstructive and Aesthetic Surgery*, vol. 62, no. 5, pp. e104–e105, 2009.

[31] C. Mitteldorf, K. D. Mertz, M. T. Fernández-Figueras, M. Schmid, M. Tronnier, and W. Kempf, "Detection of merkel cell polyomavirus and human papillomaviruses in merkel cell carcinoma combined with squamous cell carcinoma in immunocompetent European patients," *The American Journal of Dermatopathology*, vol. 34, no. 5, pp. 506–510, 2012.

[32] K. D. Mertz, A. Paasinen, A. Arnold et al., "Merkel cell polyomavirus large T antigen is detected in rare cases of nonmelanoma skin cancer," *Journal of Cutaneous Pathology*, vol. 40, no. 6, pp. 543–549, 2013.

[33] N. Scola, U. Wieland, S. Silling, P. Altmeyer, M. Stücker, and A. Kreuter, "Prevalence of human polyomaviruses in common and rare types of non-Merkel cell carcinoma skin cancer," *British Journal of Dermatology*, vol. 167, no. 6, pp. 1315–1320, 2012.

20

Safety and Efficacy of 188-Rhenium-Labeled Antibody to Melanin in Patients with Metastatic Melanoma

M. Klein,[1] M. Lotem,[1] T. Peretz,[1] S. T. Zwas,[2] S. Mizrachi,[1] Y. Liberman,[1] R. Chisin,[1] J. Schachter,[2] I. G. Ron,[3] G. Iosilevsky,[4] J. A. Kennedy,[4] E. Revskaya,[5] A. W. de Kater,[6] E. Banaga,[6] V. Klutzaritz,[6] N. Friedmann,[6] E. Galun,[1] G. L. DeNardo,[7] S. J. DeNardo,[7] A. Casadevall,[5] E. Dadachova,[5] and G. B. Thornton[6]

[1] *Hadassah Medical Center, Hebrew University, Kiryat Hadassah, 91120 Jerusalem, Israel*
[2] *Chaim Sheba Medical Center, Tel Hashomer, 52621 Ramat Gan, Israel*
[3] *Sackler Faculty of Medicine, Tel Aviv Medical Center, 69978 Tel Aviv, Israel*
[4] *Rambam Health Care Campus, 31096 Haifa, Israel*
[5] *Albert Einstein College of Medicine, 1300 Morris Park Avenue, Bronx, NY 10461, USA*
[6] *Pain Therapeutics, Inc., Austin, TX 78731, USA*
[7] *Davis Medical Center, University of California, Sacramento, CA 95817, USA*

Correspondence should be addressed to E. Dadachova; edadacho@aecom.yu.edu

Academic Editor: Silvia Moretti

There is a need for effective "broad spectrum" therapies for metastatic melanoma which would be suitable for all patients. The objectives of Phase Ia/Ib studies were to evaluate the safety, pharmacokinetics, dosimetry, and antitumor activity of ^{188}Re-6D2, a 188-Rhenium-labeled antibody to melanin. Stage IIIC/IV metastatic melanoma (MM) patients who failed standard therapies were enrolled in both studies. In Phase Ia, 10 mCi ^{188}Re-6D2 were given while unlabeled antibody preload was escalated. In Phase Ib, the dose of ^{188}Re-6D2 was escalated to 54 mCi. SPECT/CT revealed ^{188}Re-6D2 uptake in melanoma metastases. The mean effective half-life of ^{188}Re-6D2 was 12.4 h. Transient HAMA was observed in 9 patients. Six patients met the RECIST criteria for stable disease at 6 weeks. Two patients had durable disease stabilization for 14 weeks and one for 22 weeks. Median overall survival was 13 months with no dose-limiting toxicities. The data demonstrate that ^{188}Re-6D2 was well tolerated, localized in melanoma metastases, and had antitumor activity, thus warranting its further investigation in patients with metastatic melanoma.

1. Introduction

The incidence of melanoma is increasing worldwide, with a concomitant rise in mortality from metastatic disease. Patients who progress to stage IV metastatic melanoma (MM) have a median survival of less than 1 year [1]. In the United States, about 9,180 people will die from melanoma in 2012 (American Cancer Society, 2012). Until recently, treatment options for patients with stage IV disease were limited and offered marginal, if any, improvement in overall survival. This situation changed with the newly approved by FDA ipilimumab (anti-CTLA4 monoclonal antibody), an immunomodulator which in a phase III trial was shown to improve overall survival [2]. In addition, vemurafenib that inhibits mutated B-RAF protein offers hope for 40–60% melanoma patients carrying this mutation [3, 4]. However, the responses to the latter have been relatively short lasting followed by recurrences.

In our search for alternative therapeutic options for MM we turned to radioimmunotherapy (RIT). RIT takes advantage of the specificity of the antigen-antibody interaction to deliver cytotoxic radiation to tumors [5, 6]. The clinical success of FDA-approved drugs such as ibritumomab tiuxetan (anti-CD20 monoclonal antibody (mAb) labeled with ^{90}Yttrium) for treatment of primary, relapsed or refractory B-cell non-Hodgkin lymphoma demonstrates RIT potential as antineoplastic strategy. Unlike other therapies, RIT does not rely on specific genotypes, biochemical pathways, or the variability of an individual's immune response and thus can be offered to broad patient populations and is not a subject to multidrug resistance mechanisms which are already limiting the efficacy of vemurafenib.

Melanoma owes its name to melanin pigment with even "amelanotic" melanomas containing some melanin [7, 8]. Historically, melanin was not considered a target for RIT because of its intracellular location in melanosomes beyond the reach of melanin-specific mAbs. However, in rapidly growing melanoma tumors cell necrosis releases melanin into the extracellular space where it can be targeted for delivery of radiation by radiolabeled melanin-binding mAbs. Several mAbs to fungal melanin were generated in our laboratories [9]. We established the feasibility of targeting melanin in melanoma xenografts with melanin-binding mAb 6D2 IgM labeled with beta-emitting radionuclide ^{188}Re (E_{max} = 2.1 MeV, half-life 17.0 hrs) [10]. In spite of their fast clearance from the circulation which should result in favorable target to nontarget ratios, IgMs are often overlooked in radioimmunoimaging and RIT. Importantly, experiments with melanin-binding mAbs conducted in C57Bl6 black mice demonstrated that melanin in normal pigmented tissues such as retina of the eye, pigmented skin, or hair follicles is not accessible to the mAb by virtue of its intracellular location [10]. Preclinical development of ^{188}Re-6D2 resulted in developing cGMP-compatible radiolabeling methodology while computer-simulated tumor dosimetry demonstrated that ^{188}Re-6D2 could deliver tumoricidal doses to tumors within the wide range of melanin concentrations (up to 100 less melanin than in primary tumors) [11, 12]. Here we report the results of the recently completed consecutive Phase Ia and Ib trials of ^{188}Re-6D2 mAb in patients with MM.

2. Materials and Methods

2.1. Patients Eligibility and Screening. Patients were eligible for enrollment if they had histologically or clinically confirmed stage III (unresectable) or stage IV metastatic melanoma. The studies were conducted in accordance with International Conference on Harmonization guidelines and Good Clinical Practice guidelines. The studies were registered at clinicaltrials.gov and were numbered NCT00399113 and NCT00734188. The study protocols were approved by the Ethics Committees at Hadassah Medical Center, Jerusalem and Sheba Medical Center, Tel Hashomer, Israel where the study was conducted. All patients signed a written informed consent prior to participating in the study. Men and women (not pregnant or lactating, and following acceptable methods of birth control) were to be 18 years or older and have a life expectancy of at least 3 months. At least 4 weeks had to have elapsed since prior chemotherapy or radiation therapy and at least 1 week since IL-2 therapy. Patients had to have failed response to at least one previous therapy; adequate organ and marrow function and a negative human anti-mouse antibody (HAMA) result; no cerebral metastases by MRI or CT; no ocular diseases that may have led to an impaired blood-retinal brain barrier and no prior parenteral exposure to murine proteins.

2.2. Antibody, Radioisotope, and Radiolabeling. MAb 6D2, a murine IgM generated against fungal melanin, was previously described in references [8–12]. The clinical lot of 6D2 and all reagents used for manufacturing were produced in compliance with cGMPs by Goodwin Biotechnology Inc. (Plantation, FL). ^{188}Re was obtained from a ^{188}W/^{188}Re generator (Oak Ridge National Laboratory, Oak Ridge, TN, USA). The radiolabeling of 6D2 with ^{188}Re was performed as in [11]. The specific activity of ^{188}Re-6D2 in both Phase I studies was kept approximately at 1 mCi/mg to preserve 6D2 immunoreactivity towards melanin as was demonstrated in reference [11]. The highest level of activity achievable with ^{188}W/^{188}Re generators used in the study was 60 mCi/50 mg.

2.3. Phase I Study Objectives and Design. Both open-label Phase I studies had the following objectives: (1) characterization of pharmacokinetics and dosimetry to normal organs; (2) identification of the dose-limiting organs; (3) evaluation of the HAMA response; (4) determination of safety and tolerability; (5) evaluation of tumor localization and antitumor activity of ^{188}Re-6D2. The first Phase I study (phase Ia) had an additional objective of determining the effect of preload with "cold" (unlabeled) mAb on the biodistribution and pharmacokinetics of ^{188}Re-6D2 while the second phase I (phase Ib) study evaluated possible toxicities associated with increasing radioactive doses of ^{188}Re-6D2. Phase Ia enrolled 13 patients into 4 cohorts with each cohort receiving 10 mCi/10 mg ^{188}Re-6D2 preceded by either 0, 10, 20, or 50 mg of unlabeled 6D2 depending upon cohort. Seven patients in the Phase Ib were enrolled into 2 cohorts: 20–30 mCi and 40–60 mCi. Patients returned for posttreatment followup at 2 and 6 weeks after infusion (Phase Ia and Ib) and every 8 weeks thereafter until disease progression (Phase Ib).

2.4. Pharmacokinetics, Imaging, and Dosimetry for the Normal Organs. MAb pharmacokinetics was determined from blood samples taken at specified time intervals from predose to 48 h after ^{188}Re-6D2 administration. Biodistribution of ^{188}Re-6D2 was evaluated by whole body planar imaging. SPECT/CT scans were performed for the regions of interest after each planar imaging session as necessary. The percentages injected dose for the organs and whole body were calculated from regions of interest and fitted to an exponential kinetic model within the dosimetry code Organ Level Internal Dose Assessment (OLINDA) [13, 14].

2.5. Tumor Response Assessment. Tumor response (based upon evaluation of target, nontarget, and emergence of new lesions) was assessed utilizing RECIST version 1.0. Cutaneous melanoma lesions were measured and the longest diameter recorded in millimeters. Noncutaneous lesions were identified by radiologic assessment and measured. Tumors were recorded at baseline and tumor response was monitored at 2 and 6 weeks after infusion. In the Phase Ib, tumors

TABLE 1: Patients demographics.

	Phase Ia	Phase Ib
Age, mean (min, max)	64.2 (45, 83)	64.7 (54, 80)
Male	10 (76.9%)	5 (71.4%)
Caucasian	13 (100%)	7 (100%)
Stage IV	13 (100%)	6 (85.7%)
Prior therapies		
Chemotherapy	11 (84.6%)	3 (42.9%)
Immunotherapy	9 (69.2%)	6 (85.7%)
Radiotherapy	3 (23.1%)	4 (57.1%)
Surgery	13 (100%)	7 (100%)

continued to be monitored every 8 weeks until disease progression. In addition, whole body ^{18}FDG PET/CT scans were performed at baseline and approximately 2 and 6 weeks after infusion to observe the metabolic activity of the tumors.

2.6. Safety. Safety was evaluated by adverse event monitoring, vital signs, physical examinations, ECGs, and clinical laboratory tests which included HAMA and thyroid function. Safety assessments were part of patients followup.

2.7. Statistical Analysis. This study was not powered for conclusions regarding efficacy. Data were summarized descriptively. Data from patients receiving any amount of ^{188}Re-6D2 were included in safety summaries. A post hoc pooled analysis of overall survival was conducted among 17 subjects (12 from Phase Ia and 5 from Phase Ib). Overall survival, which was not a planned endpoint in either trial, was calculated as the time from ^{188}Re-6D2 administration until death. Subjects lost to followup or alive at the time of data cutoff were censored at the date of last contact. Median survival was estimated using Kaplan-Meier methods.

3. Results

3.1. Patient Demographics and Cohort Assignment. Hadassah Medical Center and Sheba Medical Center enrolled 20 MM patients who met the study eligibility criteria with 13 stage IV patients enrolled into Phase Ia and 7 stage IIIC/IV patients—into Phase Ib. Table 1 presents the patient demographic data. All patients had active metastatic disease at the time of accrual, and all had failed at least two previous treatments including Dacarbazine-containing regimens (13 patients) or ambulatory doses of IL-2 (4 patients).

In phase Ia all 13 patients received 10 mCi ^{188}Re-6D2 and an infusion of unlabeled 6D2 depending upon the cohort entered. Three patients entered cohort 1 and did not receive an infusion of unlabeled 6D2, 4 patients (cohort 2) received 10 mg 6D2, 3 patients (cohort 3) received 20 mg, and 3 patients (cohort 4)—50 mg. Two patients in cohort I received a second 10 mCi dose of ^{188}Re-6D2. In phase Ib, 4 patients (cohort 1) received 20–30 mCi ^{188}Re-6D2 and 3 patients (cohort 2)—41–54 mCi ^{188}Re-6D2.

3.2. Tumor Imaging and Absence of ^{188}Re-6D2 Localization in Normal Melanized Tissues. Whole body planar scintigraphy showed no uptake of ^{188}Re-6D2 in the normal melanized tissues like the retina of the eye, skin, and melanized neurons in brain (Figure 1(a)). Tumor targeting was visible on both whole-body planar scintigraphy and SPECT/CT. SPECT/CT of ^{188}Re-6D2 demonstrated targeting of various lesions: mediastinal and lung (Figure 1(b)), pelvic (Figure 1(c)), cutaneous, muscular, and nodal metastases. The highest uptake in the tumors was observed at 2 and 8 h after injection, with the tumor still visible 24 h after injection (Figure 1(b)).

3.3. Dynamics of ^{18}FDG Uptake after Treatment. ^{18}FDG PET/CT scans were performed prior to treatment and between 2 and 6 weeks after treatment for each patient. The maximum and the mean standardized uptake values (SUV_{max} and SUV_{mean}, resp.) were summed at baseline and at the last after treatment assessment to determine the percentage change from baseline. The results are shown in Figure 2. SUV_{max} was calculated for all 20 patients, whereas SUV_{mean} was only calculated for 12 patients. The results from these analyses are in concordance with the changes seen in target lesions after treatment per-RECIST. Based upon the SUV_{max} percent change from baseline, 15 patients experienced stable metabolic disease, 2 patients had progressive metabolic disease, and 3 patients experienced a partial metabolic response. Thirteen patients had stable metabolic disease. One patient from phase Ia and one from phase Ib experienced stable metabolic disease or partial metabolic responses in 100% of identified lesions. A complete metabolic response was observed in a single lesion in two additional patients, one from each study.

3.4. Pharmacokinetics of ^{188}Re-6D2. The effective half-life of ^{188}Re-6D2 was 12.2 h and the biological half-life 46.7 h (See Supplementary Table S1 available online at http://dx.doi.org/10.1155/2013/828329). The preload with 10–50 mg of unlabeled 6D2 had no effect on ^{188}Re-6D2 effective or biological half-lives compared to ^{188}Re-6D2 alone. Serum concentrations of 6D2 were quantifiable in all patients in both studies up to 48 hs after infusion of ^{188}Re-6D2.

3.5. Dosimetry to Normal Organs. The results from dosimetry calculations for ^{188}Re-6D2 are presented in Table 2. The radiation doses of ^{188}Re-6D2 (up to 54 mCi) administered in these two studies were determined to be safe when compared to the tolerance of normal tissue to therapeutic irradiation causing 50% complications in 5 years [15]. The kidneys and bone marrow had the highest radiation absorbed doses relative to MTDs for normal organs. At the highest doses administered in phase 1b, the kidneys absorbed 13.2 ± 1.9% of the maximum tolerated dose and the bone marrow absorbed 8.5 ± 0.9%. These are the potential dose limiting organs. Calculation of the total dose which could be delivered to

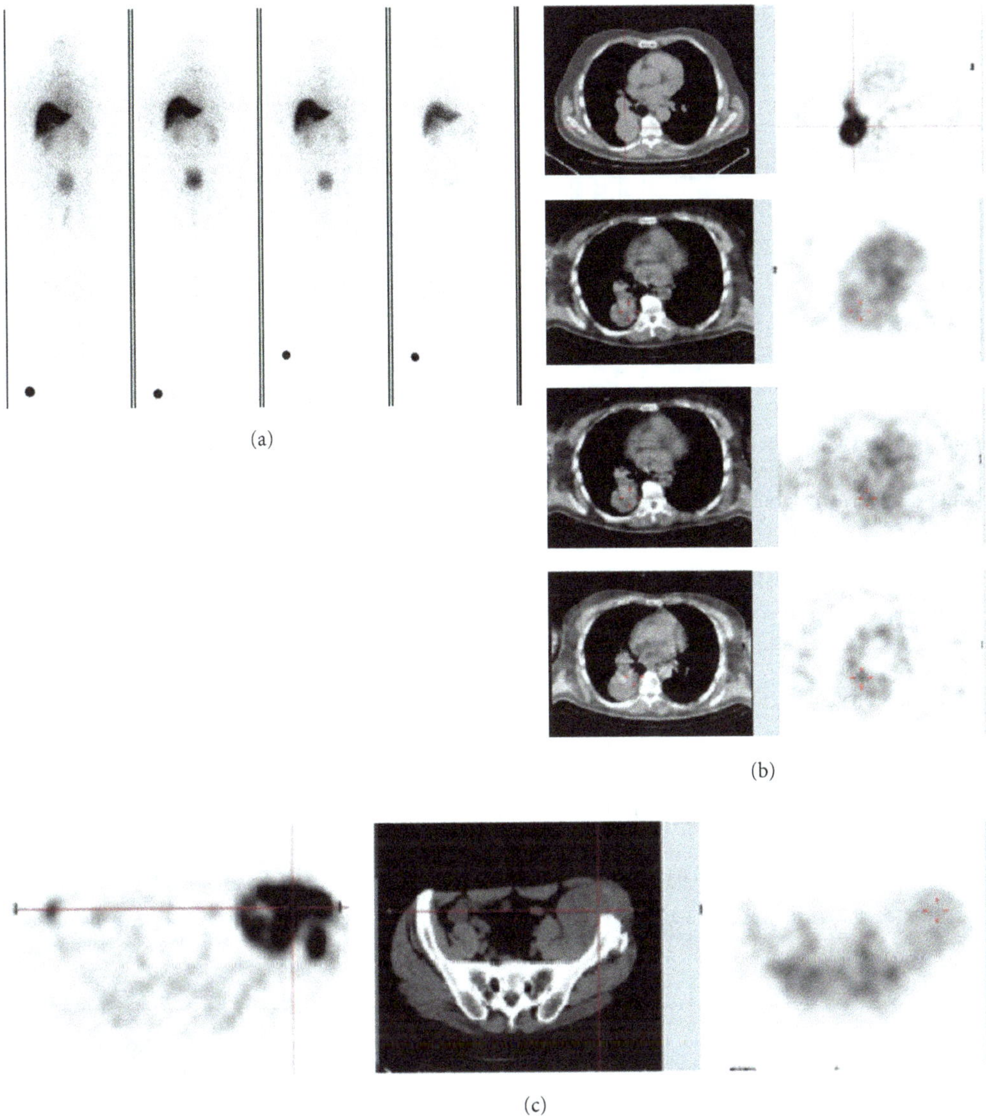

Figure 1: Imaging of patients with ^{188}Re-6D2 mAb. (a) Whole-body scintigraphic image of a patient from Phase Ia showing absence of ^{188}Re-6D2 uptake in normal melanized tissues: from left to right—0.4, 3, 5, and 20 hr images; (b) patient from Phase Ia study with mediastinal and lung metastases: top panel—^{18}FDG PET/CT 10 days before the study, lower panels—SPECT/CT of ^{188}Re-6D2 mAb at 2, 8, and 24 hrs after injection, respectively; (c) patient from Phase Ia study with large pelvic mass: from left to right—^{18}FDG PET/CT 10 days before the study, SPECT/CT of ^{188}Re-6D2 mAb 8 hrs after injection.

normal organs by 100 mCi ^{188}Re-6D2 demonstrated that doses to the critical organs would be 5 times below TD 50/5 and compare favorably to those from ibritumomab tiuxetan and tositumomab (Table 3).

3.6. Tumor Response to ^{188}Re-6D2 Administration and Survival. Although the efficacy was not the primary objective of these studies, antitumor activity of ^{188}Re-6D2 was evaluated within the confines of a phase I study (Supplementary Table S2). The 10 mCi ^{188}Re-6D2 in Phase Ia was not considered a therapeutic dose but was sufficient for imaging and pharmacokinetic analysis. After receiving 10 mCi, 9 patients demonstrated stable disease in target lesions at the conclusion of the 6-week followup period. At the conclusion of the 6-week followup period 3 patients met the RECIST criteria of stable disease and 8 patients had progressive disease. This is an encouraging observation as all patients had previously failed at least two standard therapies. During Phase Ib 4 patients met the criteria for stable disease through week 6. During continued followup one patient had an overall response of stable disease through followup week 22. Two patients continued to have an overall response of stable disease through week 14. Supplementary Figure S1 represents the data for the best percent change from baseline for the sum of the longest diameters (SLD) for the target lesions from each

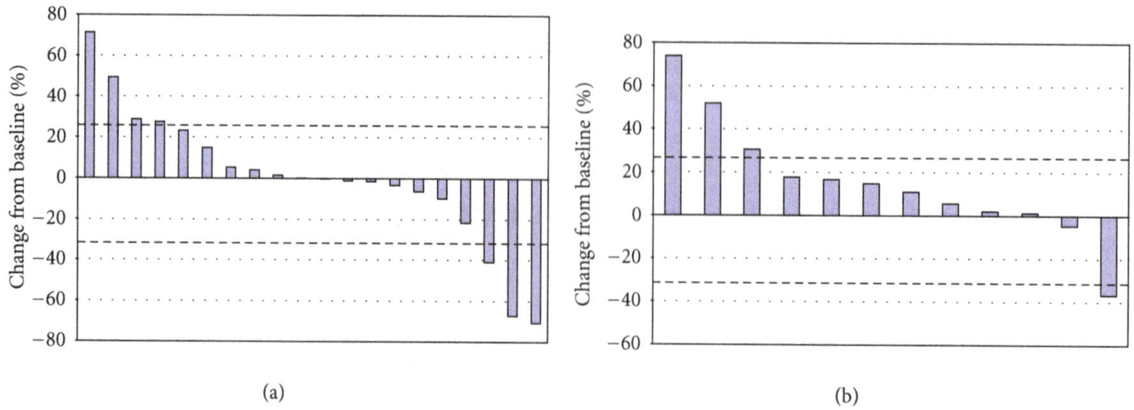

FIGURE 2: Waterfall plots of ^{18}FDG uptake in the tumors after treatment with ^{188}Re-6D2: (a) % change from baseline of SUV_{max}; (b) % change from baseline of SUV_{mean}. Every bar represents an individual patient. Dashed lines at 30% and −30% represent the separation from stable metabolic disease and progressive metabolic disease or partial metabolic response, respectively.

TABLE 2: Radiation-absorbed doses to organs from ^{188}Re-6D2 (mSv/MBq).

Cohort	Liver	Spleen	Kidneys	Bone marrow	Urine bladder wall	Whole body
Phase 1a						
Cohort 1	0.88 ± 0.13	0.86 ± 0.09	1.35 ± 0.05	0.09 ± 0.01	0.88 ± 0.23	0.16 ± 0.01
Cohort 2	0.89 ± 0.20	0.67 ± 0.05	1.11 ± 0.22	0.11 ± 0.02	1.01 ± 0.12	0.15 ± 0.03
Cohort 3	0.90 ± 0.08	0.73 ± 0.14	1.59 ± 0.01	0.11 ± 0.0	0.86 ± 0.14	0.13 ± 0.02
Cohort 4	1.04 ± 0.30	0.67 ± 0.30	1.29 ± 0.12	0.14 ± 0.03	1.02 ± 0.08	0.16 ± 0.04
Phase 1b						
Cohort 1	0.92 ± 0.20	0.93± 0.32	1.99 ± 0.17	0.11± 0.01	0.61 ± —*	0.14 ± 0.01
Cohort 2	0.77 ± 0.25	1.02 ± 0.35	1.75 ± 0.25	0.10 ± 0.01	0.95 ± 0.47	0.15 ± 0.03
Tositumomab	0.82	1.14	1.96	0.65	0.64	0.24
Ibritumomab tiuxetan	4.8	9.4	0.1	1.3	0.9	0.5

*Only one patient had sufficient data for calculation of urine bladder wall dose.

patient. The target lesions for 15 patients were considered stable disease by RECIST, 2 patients had partial responses in their target lesions, and 2 patients had progressive disease. The nontarget lesions in 8 patients showed progression and 9 patients developed new lesions (5 patients had both new lesions and nontarget progression).

Figure 3(a) shows ^{18}FDG PET/CT of a patient with massive lung and pleural involvement 10 days before the administration of ^{188}Re-6D2 mAb and 7 days after the 10 mCi dose. There was significantly decreased uptake in the tumor 7 days after ^{188}Re-6D2 mAb administration corresponding most likely to increased tumor necrosis seen on CT. The tumor necrosis could have been the result of radiation, considering the high uptake of the ^{188}Re-6D2 mAb in the lung mets, or a reflection of the natural history of the disease. Figure 3(b) shows the tumor in a patient who received 30 mCi/16 mg ^{188}Re-6D2 mAb and whose tumor was stable at 24 weeks after treatment. At the time of manuscript preparation, this patient was still alive with nonprogressive disease for 17 months. Figure 3(c) displays one tumor mass in the lung parenchyma of a patient with progressive disease who received 54 mCi/47 mg ^{188}Re-6D2 mAb.

A post hoc pooled analysis of overall survival (OS) performed in May 2011 established a median duration of OS at 13 months and mean OS—at 15.6 months. Ten out of 17 (59%) patients had an overall survival greater than 12 months, 3 patients (18%) greater than 24 months with one patient continued to be followed at month 42. Four patients still being followed as of May 2011 were at 22, 23, 25, and 42 weeks after ^{188}Re-6D2 mAb administration.

3.7. Toxicity, Adverse Effects, and HAMA. During the phase Ib no toxicities were observed for the administered doses including the maximum dose of 54 mCi ^{188}Re-6D2 manufactured during the study, suggesting that the doses of ^{188}Re-6D2 were well below MTD. All patients in both studies were negative for HAMA at baseline. Supplementary Table S3 displays the dynamics of the HAMA response in patients after receiving ^{188}Re-6D2 mAb in both studies. In the phase 1a study, 5 of 13 patients developed a positive HAMA response at 2 weeks after administration with this number decreasing to 3 patients at 6 weeks. Three patients who were HAMA positive at week 2 became negative by week 6. In the second trial, all 7 patients were negative for HAMA at 2 weeks after

TABLE 3: Radiation-absorbed doses of ^{188}Re-6D2 compared to tositumomab, ibritumomab tiuxetan, and normal organ tolerance TD 5/5 (cGy).

	Liver	Kidneys	Bone marrow	Urine bladder wall
Tositumomab 81 mCi	246	588	195	192
Ibritumomab tiuxetan 30 mCi	533	11	144	100
^{188}Re-6D2 40–60 mCi	130	305	17	158
^{188}Re-6D2 Estimated 100 mCi	344	650	42	350
Normal Organ Tolerance	3000	2300	200	6500

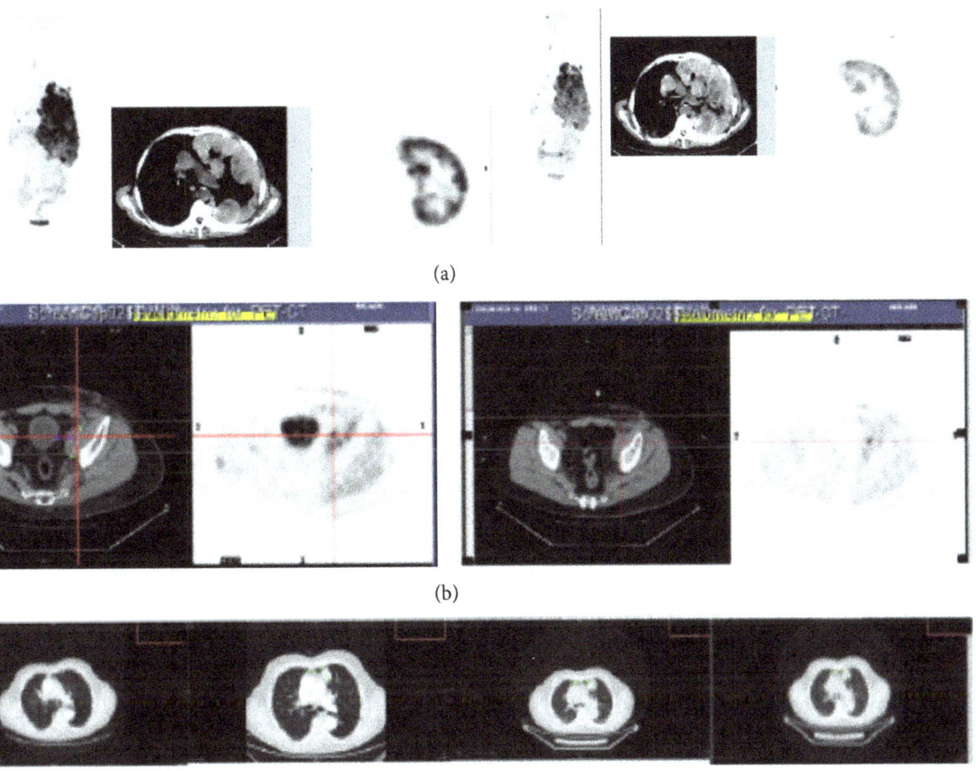

(a)

(b)

(c)

FIGURE 3: Tumor response to ^{188}Re-6D2 mAb in patients. (a) ^{18}FDG PET/CT of a patient from Phase Ia: left panel—10 days before the study showing coronal and transaxial views, right panel—7 days after the dose of ^{188}Re-6D2 mAb; (b) patient from Phase Ib with a stable disease who received 30 mCi/16 mg ^{188}Re-6D2 mAb: left panel—^{18}FDG PET/CT 10 days before the study; right panel—^{18}FDG PET/CT 24 weeks after the study; (c) patient from Phase Ib with progressive disease who received 54 mCi/47 mg ^{188}Re-6D2 mAb: panels from left to right—CT 6 months prior to study; 1 month prior to study; at the time of ^{188}Re-6D2 mAb administration; 1 month after administration.

infusion, with 2 patients developing a positive response at 6 weeks and another patient at 18 weeks. The 2 patients with a positive HAMA response at week 6 did not have any additional follow-up visits to determine if the response returned to negative. The one patient developing a positive HAMA response at week 18 returned to HAMA negative at week 26. There appeared to be no correlation between the ^{188}Re-6D2 dose and the prevalence of a HAMA response. Treatment with ^{188}Re-6D2 was safe and well tolerated in both studies (See Supplementary Table S4). No significant trends were noted in the types of adverse effects (AEs) at any dose level. In both studies serious AEs were considered to be unrelated to ^{188}Re-6D2.

4. Discussion

Even in the era of B-RAF inhibition, there continues to be an enormous need for effective "broad spectrum" therapies for MM which would be suitable for all patients diagnosed with the disease. In 1981 DeNardo et al. reported a curative therapy of murine melanoma with ^{131}I-labeled mAbs against P-51 murine melanoma [16]. RIT of melanoma moved into the clinical trial in 1985 when 50% tumor reduction was observed in a patient treated with ^{131}I-labeled Fab' fragments of a mAb against high molecular weight melanoma-associated antigen [17]. Despite early successes during the 80s, RIT of melanoma did not develop into a clinical modality for a variety of reasons that included disappointing results in clinical trials of different solid tumors during that time.

The availability of novel mAbs and radionuclides with optimal emission characteristics encouraged us to revisit the RIT for MM. We targeted melanin which is a novel antigen for radioimmunotherapy with an IgM mAb 6D2. IgMs are often overlooked in RIT despite fast blood clearance, ability to trigger ADCC and CDC immune responses, and early encouraging data in patients [18]. Though the doses of melanin-binding mAb ^{188}Re-6D2 were limited by the activity of the ^{188}W/^{188}Re generators at the time of the study, the combined survival data for the two studies demonstrated that the median survival of patients receiving ^{188}Re-6D2 was approximately 13 months which is longer than the 8.5 months for the MM patients receiving standard care. Although this result must be interpreted cautiously, the finding is encouraging. Importantly, no uptake in the healthy melanized tissues was observed which confirmed our prior observations in the melanoma animal models [10]. The treatment was not accompanied by the severe toxic effects. On the contrary, toxicity was very mild with no hematological AEs observed even in patients receiving the highest doses of ^{188}Re-6D2. Several factors contribute to the nontoxic nature of ^{188}Re-6D2: (1) fast clearance of ^{188}Re-6D2 from the blood which prevents harmful irradiation of bone marrow; (2) relatively short physical half-life of ^{188}Re (17.0 hrs) in comparison with 2.8 and 8 days for ^{90}Y and ^{131}I used in ibritumomab tiuxetan and tositumomab, respectively; (3) ^{188}Re nonresidualizing nature which results in its fast excretion through the kidneys; (4) the absence of 6D2 cross-reactivity with normal tissues leading to very low uptake of 6D2 in nontarget tissues. In this regard, the dosimetry calculations showed that up to 100 mCi ^{188}Re-6D2 could be safely administered to the patients which should further improve the therapeutic results.

HAMA in the majority of patients was transient and not dependent on the unlabeled mAb dose. In this regard it is important to emphasize that the mAb used in ibritumomab tiuxetan and tositumomab for treatment of NHL is also murine. One can suggest that the radiolabeled murine mAb to melanin can be administered safely to melanoma patients for up to two doses. The work on the conversion of the murine mAb into the human-mouse chimera which would allow for multiple administrations of the radiolabeled mAb to MM patients is currently ongoing in our laboratories.

Our study has some limitations with major ones being relatively small number of patients which precludes statistical analyses of the data and not achieving the maximum tolerated dose for the ^{188}Re-6D2 due to the technical restrictions of the ^{188}W/^{188}Re generators available to us at the time of the trial. The high activity/high specific activity ^{188}W/^{188}Re generators have become available commercially after the completion of this study which will ensure that higher doses could be administered to patients in the follow-up trials.

In conclusion, Phase I trials of ^{188}Re-6D2 mAb to melanin in patients with MM demonstrated tumor targeting and safety of the drug, as well as prolongation in survival. These results are encouraging and suggest the need for further investigation of this reagent by itself or in combination with other therapies.

Authors' Contribution

M. Klein and M. Lotem contributed equally to this paper.

Acknowledgment

The study was funded by Pain Therapeutics, Inc. At the time of the submission the technology is not licensed to any commercial company.

References

[1] E. Linos, S. M. Swetter, M. G. Cockburn, G. A. Colditz, and C. A. Clarke, "Increasing burden of melanoma in the United States," *Journal of Investigative Dermatology*, vol. 129, no. 7, pp. 1666–1674, 2009.

[2] F. S. Hodi, S. J. O'Day, D. F. McDermott et al., "Improved survival with ipilimumab in patients with metastatic melanoma," *The New England Journal of Medicine*, vol. 363, no. 8, pp. 711–723, 2010.

[3] A. Ribas, K. B. Kim, L. M. Schuchter et al., "BRIM-2: An open-label, multicenter phase II study of vemurafenib in previously treated patients with *BRAF* V600E mutation-positive metastatic melanoma," *Journal of Clinical Oncology*, vol. 29, supplement 1, abstract 8509, 2011.

[4] P. B. Chapman, A. Hauschild, C. Robert et al., "Phase III randomized, open-label, multicenter trial (BRIM3) comparing BRAF inhibitor vemurafenib with dacarbazine (DTIC) in patients with V600EBRAF-mutated melanoma," *Journal of Clinical Oncology*, vol. 29, supplement 1, abstract LBA4, 2011.

[5] D. E. Milenic, E. D. Brady, and M. W. Brechbiel, "Antibody-targeted radiation cancer therapy," *Nature Reviews Drug Discovery*, vol. 3, no. 6, pp. 488–498, 2004.

[6] R. M. Sharkey and D. M. Goldenberg, "Perspectives on cancer therapy with radiolabeled monoclonal antibodies," *Journal of Nuclear Medicine*, vol. 46, supplement 1, pp. 115S–121S, 2005.

[7] K. A. Cohen-Solal, S. M. Crespo-Carbone, J. Namkoong et al., "Progressive appearance of pigmentation in amelanotic melanoma lesions," *Pigment Cell Research*, vol. 15, no. 4, pp. 282–289, 2002.

[8] K. J. Busam, K. Hester, C. Charles et al., "Detection of clinically amelanotic malignant melanoma and assessment of its margins by in vivo confocal scanning laser microscopy," *Archives of Dermatology*, vol. 137, no. 7, pp. 923–929, 2001.

[9] A. L. Rosas, J. D. Nosanchuk, M. Feldmesser et al., "Synthesis of polymerized melanin by *Cryptococcus neoformans* in infected rodents," *Infection and Immunity*, vol. 68, no. 5, pp. 2845–2853, 2000.

[10] E. Dadachova, J. D. Nosanchuk, L. Shi et al., "Dead cells in melanoma tumors provide abundant antigen for targeted delivery of ionizing radiation by a mAb to melanin," *Proceedings of the National Academy of Sciences of the United States of America*, vol. 101, no. 41, pp. 14865–14870, 2004.

[11] E. Dadachova, E. Revskaya, M. A. Sesay et al., "Pre-clinical evaluation and efficacy studies of a melanin-binding IgM antibody labeled with ^{188}Re against experimental human metastatic melanoma in nude mice," *Cancer Biology and Therapy*, vol. 7, no. 7, pp. 1116–1127, 2008.

[12] A. D. Schweitzer, V. Rakesh, E. Revskaya, A. Datta, A. Casadevall, and E. Dadachova, "Computational model predicts effective delivery of 188-Re-labeled melanin-binding antibody to metastatic melanoma tumors with wide range of melanin concentrations," *Melanoma Research*, vol. 17, no. 5, pp. 291–303, 2007.

[13] M. G. Stabin, R. B. Sparks, and E. Crowe, "OLINDA/EXM: the second-generation personal computer software for internal dose assessment in nuclear medicine," *Journal of Nuclear Medicine*, vol. 46, no. 6, pp. 1023–1027, 2005.

[14] B. W. Wessels, W. E. Bolch, L. G. Bouchet et al., "Bone marrow dosimetry using blood-based models for radiolabeled antibody therapy: a multiinstitutional comparison," *Journal of Nuclear Medicine*, vol. 45, no. 10, pp. 1725–1733, 2004.

[15] B. Emami, J. Lyman, A. Brown et al., "Tolerance of normal tissue to therapeutic irradiation," *International Journal of Radiation Oncology *Biology* Physics*, vol. 21, pp. 109–122, 1991.

[16] S. J. DeNardo, K. L. Erickson, E. Benjamin et al., "Radioimmunotherapy for melanoma," *Clinical Research*, vol. 29, pp. 434–440, 1981.

[17] S. M. Larson, J. A. Carrasquillo, and R. W. McGuffin, "Use of I-131 labeled, murine Fab against a high molecular weight antigen of human melanoma: preliminary experience," *Radiology*, vol. 155, no. 2, pp. 487–492, 1985.

[18] W. C. Taddei-Peters, M. V. Haspel, P. Vente et al., "Quantitation of human tumor-reactive monoclonal antibody 16.88 in the circulation and localization of 16.88 in colorectal metastatic tumor tissue using murine antiidiotypic antibodies," *Cancer Research*, vol. 52, no. 9, pp. 2603–2609, 1992.

Prognostic Value of Melanoma Inhibitory Activity Protein in Localized Cutaneous Malignant Melanoma

Angela Sandru,[1] Eugenia Panaitescu,[2] Silviu Voinea,[1] Madalina Bolovan,[3] Adina Stanciu,[3] Sabin Cinca,[3] and Alexandru Blidaru[1]

[1] *Department of Surgical Oncology, "Carol Davila" University of Medicine and Pharmacy, "Alexandru Trestioreanu" Oncologic Institute, Fundeni Street, No. 252, Sector 2, 022328 Bucharest, Romania*
[2] *Department of Medical Informatics and Biostatistics, "Carol Davila" University of Medicine and Pharmacy, Bucharest, Romania*
[3] *Department of Carcinogenesis and Molecular Biology, "Alexandru Trestioreanu" Oncologic Institute, Bucharest, Romania*

Correspondence should be addressed to Angela Sandru; sandruangela@gmail.com

Academic Editor: Arash Kimyai-Asadi

Background. Cutaneous malignant melanoma (CMM) is a heterogeneous disease, acknowledged for its lack of predictability regarding clinical evolution. In order to appreciate a patient's individual prognosis, an attempt is made to find new tumor markers that parallel the disease progression. *Objective.* To identify if melanoma inhibitory activity (MIA) protein could represent a tool for selecting high risk early stages melanoma patients. *Method.* Between 2008 and 2013, 155 patients with CMM were treated in our clinic. 84 of them were classified into stages I and II, according to TNM 2009. MIA serum concentration was measured in all patients and 50 healthy donors. A cut-off value of 9.4 ng/ml was established using the ROC curve. *Results.* All patients were followed up by periodic investigations every 6 months. We have noticed that 66% of patients with MIA serum values at diagnosis greater than 9.4 ng/mL have relapsed, while only 5% of patients with MIA serum concentration below the estimated threshold, recurred during the follow-up period ($P = 0.000$). The death risk was 12 times higher in pathological MIA group of patients ($P = 0.0001$). *Conclusions.* Our data suggest that MIA is an independent prognostic factor for patients with localized CMM.

1. Introduction

Malignant melanoma represents the cutaneous neoplasia with the highest metastatic potential and a relatively unpredictable evolution, even in early stages. Fortunately, however, the detection of the disease in a localized phase allows it to be cured in most cases [1].

Statistics show that about 30% of people diagnosed with cutaneous malignant melanoma (CMM) develop metastases [2]. In these circumstances, finding new tools to identify those patients who although classified in stage I or II, so theoretically with a favorable outcome, still have a high risk of dissemination, represents a priority. A possibility in this regard might be the discovery of tumor markers whose expression in the blood stream would mirror the disease development.

Dozens of substances have been described which were deemed to have prognostic capacity in different stages of CMM. This presumed prognostic ability was suggested by the parallelism between serum concentration of these markers and body tumor burden that was noted in a significant percentage of cases. Nevertheless, only two of them are widely accepted: serum lactate dehydrogenase (LDH) and protein S100 [3, 4].

In recent years, researches in the field of autocrine growth-regulatory factors have led to the discovery of a new serum tumor marker, melanoma inhibitory activity (MIA), a protein synthesized by the malignant melanocytes and actively secreted in the extracellular compartment [5], from where a small amount reaches the bloodstream.

MIA has been isolated from the supernatant of malignant melanocytes cultures and initially it was thought to be a tumor suppressor factor, because, at this level, MIA was inhibiting the melanocytes proliferation by preventing their attachment to the culture plate [5, 6]. However, in vivo, MIA has a totally opposed action: its massive expression by

Table 1: Patient demographics ($N = 84$ patients).

Tumor characteristics	Stage I	Stage II
Number of patients	28 (33.3%)	56 (66.7%)
Mean age (years)	51.07 (±10.6)	53.40 (±13.5)
Sex		
Female (%)	17 (60.7%)	37 (66.1%)
Male (%)	11 (39.3%)	19 (33.9%)
Mean Breslow depth (mm)	1.42 (±1.1)	3.29 (±1.7)
Minimum/maximum	0.22 mm	12 mm
Localization		
Head/neck (%)	3 (10.7%)	4 (7.1%)
Trunk (%)	12 (42.9%)	35 (62.5%)
Extremity (%)	13 (46.4%)	17 (30.4%)

malignant melanic cells but not by the normal ones enables the malignant melanocytes to detach from the extracellular matrix components, thus increasing their mobility and implicitly their metastatic potential [5, 6].

MIA protein interacts with fibronectin, laminin, and tenascin and masks their binding sites with integrins situated on the melanocytes membrane [5, 6]. In this way, MIA induces a decrease by 30–50% of the attachments between malignant melanocytes and the adjacent conjunctive tissue [7]. Consequently, a high serum MIA concentration seems to indicate the presence of an aggressive tumor clone and the existence of a metastatic tumor phenotype.

Starting from these data, the present study intends to prospectively determine the clinical significance of MIA serum concentration in patients with localized CMM, in an attempt to answer the following questions.

(i) Is there a link between MIA serum concentration and survival of patients with early stage CMM?

(ii) Is a MIA value above the upper normal limit in a patient without evidence of disease a negative prognostic factor which should be taken into account in establishing the subsequent treatment and follow-up?

2. Material and Method

2.1. Group of Patients. Between June 2008 and May 2012, in Clinic II of Surgical Oncology of "Alexandru Trestioreanu" Oncologic Institute in Bucharest (IOB), 155 patients were diagnosed with CMM in various stages of disease and subsequently treated. Diagnosis of CMM was established, in most cases (153), by excisional biopsy of the primary tumor and patients were staged according to AJCC 2009. In order to characterize the status of the regional lymph nodes, lymphatic mapping and sentinel node biopsy were done for 61 patients with clinically and echographically normal regional lymphatic basins. The sentinel node was positive for malignant cells in only 10 cases.

For accurate staging, all patients were investigated by chest X-ray, abdominal and regional lymphatic basin ultrasound, and CT in suspected cases. After analyzing the obtained results, 84 of the subjects included in this study were classified in stages I and II. After surgery, they were submitted to periodic controls, every 6 months, which consisted in a complete physical exam, abdominal and regional lymphatic basin ultrasound, and, once a year, chest radiography.

2.2. MIA Samples. A number of 200 blood samples were obtained from 155 patients with CMM and 50 samples were obtained from healthy volunteers. Beforehand, patients were informed that they could participate in a clinical study and, in case of a positive response, a written approval was asked, in order to determine two blood tumor markers: MIA and S100 proteins (data referring to S100 are not presented in this paper).

After informed consent was obtained, 2 tubes of 5 mL blood were collected from each patient. For MIA samples, tubes with anticoagulant (EDTA) were used and the obtained plasma was kept at a temperature of −80°C for a variable period of maximum 12 months. Lipemic or strongly hemolyzed samples were eliminated from the work group. The samples processing was done in several batches within the IOB research laboratory. MIA serum value was measured with an ELISA type quantitative reaction of immunodetection by photometry, using a kit purchased from ROCHE Diagnostics, Roche Applied Science, Mannheim, Germany.

Regarding patients in stages I and II, MIA serum concentration was measured before surgery (excisional biopsy of the primary tumor or sentinel node biopsy). For some of the patients, multiple sampling was acquired during the postsurgical follow-up.

2.3. Statistical Analysis. For the statistical analysis the SPSS 15.0 system was used. For MIA values the receiver operating characteristics (ROC) and the area under the curve (AUC) were assessed. Survival time differences for the different MIA cut-offs were analyzed using the log rank test. Cox regression analyses were performed for the MIA cut-off value. As further multivariate method logistic regression was used, a P value of less than 0.05 was considered statistically significant.

3. Results

Of the 84 patients with localized disease, 54 were women and 30 men (Table 1). The mean age at diagnosis was 52.2 years. Primary tumor distribution varied with patients' sex: the most frequent localization on men was at the trunk level (46.7%) and on women at limbs level (64.8%). The recorded differences are very close to statistical significance ($P = 0.079$). The mean follow-up interval was 34.3 months, with a median of 32.8 months (the minimum surveillance period was 6.1 months).

Taking into account all MIA values (50 healthy donors and 155 patients with CMM), it was estimated, by using the ROC curve, that MIA cut-off value is 9.4 ng/mL. This cut-off point was calculated so that the sum of sensibility (76.7%) and specificity (94%) was maximum for patients with stage IV disease (Figure 1).

Table 2: Disease-free survival (DFS) rate of stages I and II melanoma patients according to MIA serum concentration.

MIA ng/mL	Number of patients	Number of relapses	1-year DFS	2-year DFS	3-year DFS	4-year DFS	Mean DFS (95% CI)	Median DFS (95% CI)
≥9.4	24	16	79.2%	58.3%	35.4%	30.3%	2.4 years [1.7–2.9]	2.2 years [0.9–3.5]
<9.4	60	3	98.3%	94.5%	94.5%	94.5%	4.4 years [4.1–4.6]	—

Table 3: Overall survival (OS) rate of stages I and II melanoma patients according to MIA serum concentration.

MIA ng/mL	Number of patients	Number of deaths	1-year OS	2-year OS	3-year OS	4-year OS	Mean OS (95% CI)	Median OS (95% CI)
≥9.4	24	14	87.5%	62.5%	43.8%	38.9%	2.9 years [2.3–3.6]	2.9 years [1.7–4.0]
<9.4	60	3	98.3%	96.2%	93.3%	93.3%	4.4 years [4.1–4.6]	—

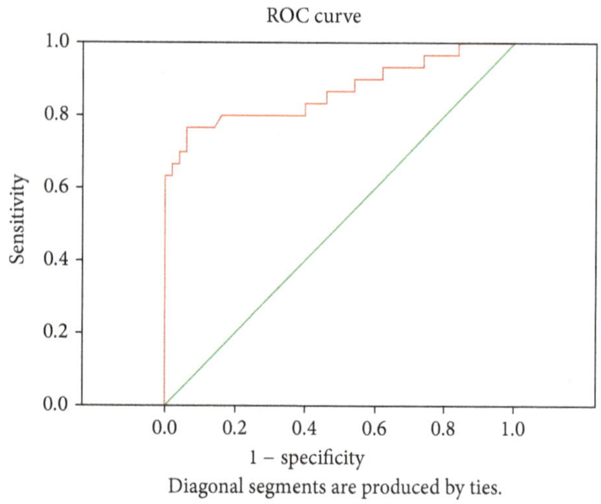

Figure 1: ROC curve for stage IV patients MIA values (AUC = 0.869).

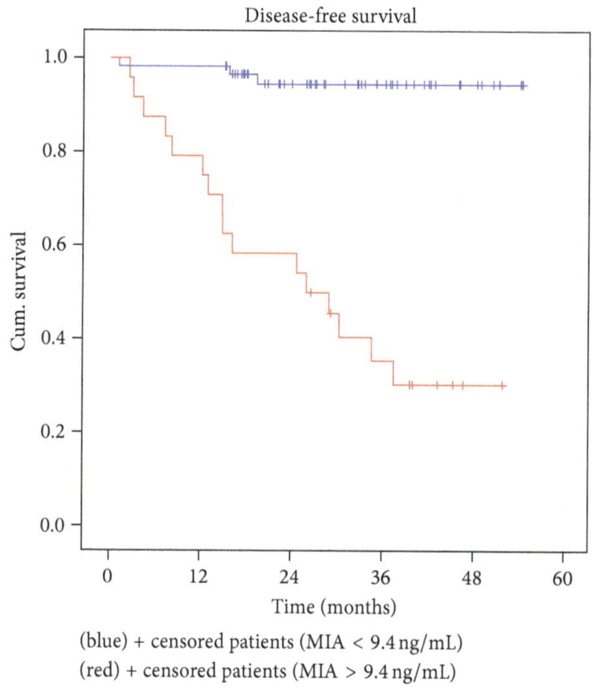

Figure 2: Kaplan-Meier disease-free survival for all stages I and II patients depending on MIA serum concentration. Red line: MIA serum concentration ≥ 9.4 ng/mL; blue line: MIA serum concentration < 9.4 ng/mL; $P = 0.000$.

In the group of stages I and II patients, 24 of them (~one-third) had a MIA serum concentration greater than 9.4 ng/mL preoperatively (Table 2). It is significant that 66.7% of these patients with elevated MIA values, that is, 16, developed regional or distance relapses, during the observation period. On the other hand, the disease evolved in only 5.0% of patients with MIA serum concentration within normal limits at diagnosis. Using univariate Cox analysis, we drew the conclusion that patients in stage I or II, with pathological MIA value before surgery, have a relapse rate 16 times higher than those with MIA within normal limits (hazard ratio = 16.11 with 95% CI = [4.68, 55.40]), which was translated in a significantly lower disease-free survival rate ($P = 0.000$) (Figure 2).

During the follow-up interval, 17 deaths were recorded in the group of patients enrolled in stages I and II; in other words, 20% of patients with localized disease died within 5 years of diagnosis (Table 3). The percentage is quite high compared with literature data and alarming at the same time. Trying to find an explanation for these unexpected and unpleasant results, we noted that, in 14 of the patients who died, the MIA serum concentration at diagnosis exceeded the threshold of 9.4 ng/mL, the highest measured value being 67.7 ng/mL. By analyzing the obtained data, we calculated that patients with localized CMM but with a MIA blood concentration greater than 9.4 ng/mL have 12 times higher death risk (hazard ratio = 12.30 with 95% CI = [3.53, 42.86]) compared to patients whose tumors do not overexpress MIA ($P = 0.0001$) (Figure 3).

Multivariate logistic regression was used to demonstrate that MIA serum concentration is an independent prognostic factor for survival, irrespective of TNM stage. For melanoma patients in the same stage of disease (stage I or II in this study), a MIA value greater than 9.4 ng/mL increases the death risk 33 times ($P = 0.0000$) (Table 4).

TABLE 4: Multivariate logistic regression of death risk for MIA cut-off value of 9.4 ng/mL and stages I and II patients.

Term	Odds ratio	95%	CI	Coefficient	S. E.	Z-statistic	P value
MIA ≥ 9.4 ng/mL	**33.1835**	7.2470	151.9457	3.5021	0.7763	4.5114	**0.0000**
TNM stage (I/II)	**7.4541**	1.2037	46.1601	2.0088	0.9303	2.1593	**0.0308**

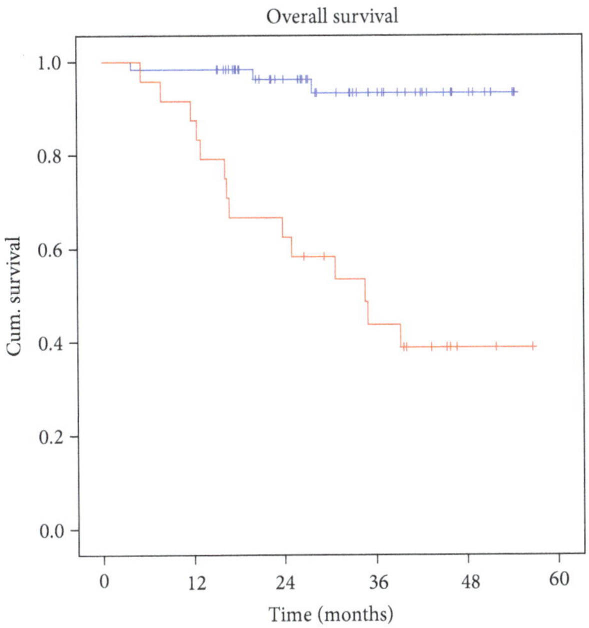

FIGURE 3: Kaplan-Meier overall survival for all stages I and II melanoma patients according to MIA serum concentration. Blue line: MIA serum concentration < 9.4 ng/mL; red line: MIA serum concentration ≥ 9.4 ng/mL; $P = 0.000$.

4. Discussions

The role of tumor markers in the initial stages of a neoplasia, regardless of its location, is still a subject of debate. As for CMM, both LDH and S100 have proven their utility in monitoring patients with metastasis [8] but have no role in the early stages of the disease. Actually, till now, no serum biomarker which might be able to suggest the evolution of patients with localized CMM has been identified [9].

In the complex network of autocrine and paracrine growth-regulatory factors involved in the progression of CMM, MIA seems to have a key role in the increase of malignant melanocytes motility and consequently in the initiation of the metastatic process. Therefore the hypothesis that an increased level of MIA protein in the blood of patients with localized CMM is associated with an increased risk of disease relapse seems plausible.

There is no unanimously accepted threshold for the upper limit of MIA serum concentration, as this varies between 6.5 ng/mL [10] and 18.7 ng/mL [11] in the literature. Within these limits each research team has set its own cut-off value depending on the number of investigated healthy volunteers, kits manufacturer's recommendations, and the calculation method applied. The most frequent upper limits used were 8.8 ng/mL [12], 10 ng/mL [13], 12 ng/mL [14], 14 ng/mL [15], and 15 ng/mL [12].

For the entire group studied by us, 155 patients with CMM and 50 healthy donors, we have established, using the ROC curve, a cut-off value of 9.4 ng/mL (data are not presented in this paper). Relating to this figure, we have assessed the recurrence and death risk for stages I and II patients from our group depending on diagnostic MIA serum concentration.

The data obtained suggests that there is a connection between the survival of patients with localized CMM and MIA serum concentration, a finding also presented in other papers [12, 13]. The 4-year disease-free survival was triple in the group of patients with MIA serum concentration in the normal range (Table 2, Figure 1), which is a further proof for MIA significant involvement in the processes of invasion and metastasis ($P = 0.000$).

Overall survival shows the same trend. Patients with CMM and MIA serum concentration at diagnosis lower than 9.4 ng/mL had a 4-year overall survival rate of 93.3% (Table 3, Figure 2), similar percentage to the literature data and significantly higher than that noted in patients with pathological MIA, 38.9% ($P = 0.0000$).

Multivariate analysis of the entire group of patients with CMM (155 patients in stages I–IV) revealed that MIA serum concentration represents an independent predictor for survival ($P = 0.0109$), together with the already acknowledged prognostic factors: clinical stage at diagnosis, sex of the patient, and lymphovascular invasion (data not shown in this paper).

5. Conclusions

A preoperative MIA serum concentration of 9.4 ng/mL or more in patients with localized CMM represents an alarm signal! In our study, elevated MIA values in patients with stages I and II CMM, properly staged, including sentinel node biopsy, have been associated with significantly lower DFS and OS. Therefore we consider that these patients should be monitored at shorter time intervals and thoroughly investigated in more detail in order to identify potential metastases.

Routine preoperative determination of MIA allows the selection of a group of patients with higher risk of relapse that might benefit from an adjuvant systemic treatment or participate in clinical trials. In our opinion MIA represents a useful tumor marker in both stratifying and adjusting the postoperative treatment and choosing the optimal follow-up for patients with localized CMM.

References

[1] S. Liu, P. Kirschmeier, J. Simon, C. Seidel-Dugan, and M. Puhlmann, "Prognostic and predictive molecular markers in cutaneous malignant melanoma: the first step toward personalized medicine," *Current Pharmacogenomics and Personalized Medicine*, vol. 6, no. 4, pp. 272–294, 2008.

[2] R. Essner, J. H. Lee, L. A. Wanek et al., "Contemporary surgical treatment of advanced-stage melanoma," *Archives of Surgery*, vol. 139, no. 9, pp. 961–967, 2004.

[3] C. M. Balch, J. E. Gershenwald, S. Soong et al., "Final version of 2009 AJCC melanoma staging and classification," *Journal of Clinical Oncology*, vol. 27, no. 36, pp. 6199–6206, 2009.

[4] S. Mocellin, G. Zavagno, and D. Nitti, "The prognostic value of serum S100B in patients with cutaneous melanoma: a meta-analysis," *International Journal of Cancer*, vol. 123, no. 10, pp. 2370–2376, 2008.

[5] A. Bosserhoff, "Melanoma inhibitory activity (MIA): an important molecule in melanoma development and progression," *Pigment Cell Research*, vol. 18, no. 6, pp. 411–416, 2005.

[6] A. K. Bosserhoff, "Mia1," *UCSD-Nature Molecule*, 2006.

[7] A.-K. Bosserhoff, R. Stoll, J. P. Sleeman, F. Bataille, R. Buettner, and T. A. Holak, "Active detachment involves inhibition of cell-matrix contacts of malignant melanoma cells by secretion of melanoma inhibitory activity," *Laboratory Investigation*, vol. 83, no. 11, pp. 1583–1594, 2003.

[8] S. Kruijff and H. J. Hoekstra, "The current status of S-100B as a biomarker in melanoma," *European Journal of Surgical Oncology*, vol. 38, no. 4, pp. 281–285, 2012.

[9] M. Al-Shaer, D. Gollapudi, and C. Papageorgio, "Melanoma biomarkers: vox clamantis in deserto (review)," *Oncology Letters*, vol. 1, no. 3, pp. 399–405, 2010.

[10] A.-K. Bosserhoff, M. Kaufmann, B. Kaluza et al., "Melanoma-inhibiting activity, a novel serum marker for progression of malignant melanoma," *Cancer Research*, vol. 57, no. 15, pp. 3149–3153, 1997.

[11] R. Meral, D. Duranyildiz, F. Tas et al., "Prognostic significance of melanoma inhibiting activity levels in malignant melanoma," *Melanoma Research*, vol. 11, no. 6, pp. 627–632, 2001.

[12] M. A. Hofmann, F. Gussmann, A. Fritsche et al., "Diagnostic value of melanoma inhibitory activity serum marker in the follow-up of patients with stage I or II cutaneous melanoma," *Melanoma Research*, vol. 19, no. 1, pp. 17–23, 2009.

[13] M. Essler, A. Link, B. Belloni et al., "Prognostic value of [18F]-fluoro-deoxy-glucose PET/CT, S100 or MIA for assessment of cancer-associated mortality in patients with high risk melanoma," *PLoS ONE*, vol. 6, no. 9, Article ID e24632, 2011.

[14] M. A. Hofmann, B. Schicke, A. Fritsch et al., "Impact of lymph node metastases on serum level of melanoma inhibitory activity in stage III melanoma patients," *Journal of Dermatology*, vol. 38, no. 9, pp. 880–886, 2011.

[15] J. M. Auge, R. Molina, X. Filella et al., "S-100β and MIA in advanced melanoma in relation to prognostic factors," *Anticancer Research*, vol. 25, no. 3, pp. 1779–1782, 2005.

22

Basal Cell Carcinoma of the Head and Neck Region: A Retrospective Analysis of Completely Excised 331 Cases

Duriye Deniz Demirseren,[1] Candemir Ceran,[2] Berrak Aksam,[2] Mustafa Erol Demirseren,[2] and Ahmet Metin[1]

[1] *Department of Dermatology, Ataturk Training and Research Hospital, Bilkent Way, 06800 Ankara, Turkey*
[2] *Department of Plastic Reconstructive and Aesthetic Surgery, Ataturk Training and Research Hospital, 06800 Ankara, Turkey*

Correspondence should be addressed to Duriye Deniz Demirseren; ddemirseren@yahoo.com

Academic Editor: Iris Zalaudek

The aim of the study is to analyze all completely excised BCCs in the head and neck region with regard to age, sex, personal and familial history, skin type, tumor localization and size, histopathological subtype of tumor, reconstruction method, and recurrence rates. Incompletely excised BCCs were not included in this study since incomplete excision is the most important preventable risk factor for recurrence. In 320 patients, 331 lesions were retrospectively evaluated by dividing into the following 8 subunits: scalp, frontotemporal, orbital, nose, cheek, auricula, perioral, and chin-neck area. Most of the patients were in 60–70 age group (34.7%). The nose (32.3%) was the most common site of presentation. Clinically, all lesions and, histopathologically, most of the lesions (42.2%) presented were of the nodular type. All cases of recurrence after complete excision ($n = 9$, 2.7%) were located in the median parts of the head and neck region and were mainly diagnosed histopathologically as sclerotic and micronodular. Even though completely excised, head and neck region BCCs, especially which are more prone to recurrence due to anatomical and histopathological properties, should be more closely monitored in order to decrease morbidity and health care costs.

1. Introduction

Basal cell carcinoma (BCC) is the most common type of skin cancer in the head and neck region. The incidence of BCC is on the rise, and it represents approximately 65% of all skin carcinomas [1–3]. BCC is not usually life threatening, unlike malignant melanoma, but it is locally invasive and may lead to considerable morbidity and complications [4]. BCC is the most frequent tumor type among the US population and also has a strongly rising incidence in Europe. Although, the incidence of BCC in Turkey is not accurately known, we think that there is a rise in the number of patients who are admitted to medical facilities [2]. With the increase in the incidence of BCC, even though mortality is relatively low, the morbidity and treatment-related costs represent a significant burden to health care systems. Treatment options include medical and surgical modalities. The first therapy of choice is generally surgical excision, with safe surgical margins. Recurrence is more common, especially with positive peripheral margins and certain types of BCC, like morpheaform forms. Recurrent BCC tends to be biologically more aggressive than primary lesions [1]. Positive surgical margins in primary BCC excisions in the head and neck region were reported to be 3–20% in the literature [5]. Recurrence rates in incompletely excised patients were also reported at 26–67% [6].

In our study, we present a case with a series of 320 patients with 331 BCCs, involving the head and neck region, and who were treated with complete surgical excision. The aim of this paper is to describe the clinical, histopathological, and epidemiological features of completely excised BCC and also to evaluate clinical features of the recurrent cases with previous histologically clear margins in the head and neck region.

2. Material and Methods

We performed a retrospective review of the database of our institution, Ataturk Training and Research Hospital, which has a wide acceptance of patients from the capital city Ankara and surrounding cities. All patients between January 2008 and January 2013 with head and neck BCCs were evaluated. Only completely excised primary cases with histopathologically confirmed BCCs were included in this study. Patients who were lost to follow-up before one year were not included.

All 331 lesions of 320 patients were categorized with regard to age, sex, personal and family history, skin type, tumor location, size, clinical and histopathological subtypes, reconstruction method, and recurrence rates. In order to achieve a systematic analysis of the collected data, the head and neck region were divided into the following 8 subunits: scalp, frontotemporal, orbital, nose, cheek, auricula, perioral, and chin-neck area. Lesions of each subunit were evaluated according to previously mentioned variables. The diagnosis of BCC was clinically undertaken first, but, in some cases when the clinical diagnose was not clear, the dermatologist performed a pretreatment biopsy. Most of the operations were performed under local anesthesia. Excision margins were planned, depending on the clinical features, size, and location of the lesion. With loupe (×5) magnification, the excision margin was marked in the dermatology department. While the 3 mm safe margin excision was used in small and well-defined lesions, where up to 10 mm safe margins were chosen for large tumors and unclear borders, deep margins were systematically located in the subcutaneous tissue or were more deeply situated, according to the tissue characteristics of the region. Incomplete excision was defined as a residual tumor at, or within, 1 mm of the lateral or deep incision margins. All incompletely excised lesions, whether or not they were reexcised, were excluded from the study. All excision materials underwent routine histopathological examination by the pathology department and were all confirmed as BCC. Methods of reconstruction were primary closure, skin grafts, and local and distant flaps. All patients were documented, and preoperative and postoperative photographs were taken. Routine outpatient controls were planned as postoperative one week, one month, three months, six months, and one year. Afterwards, the patients were called in for yearly controls. In some cases, extra control visits were added due to recurrence or a patient's need.

Statistical analysis was performed using SPSS 16.0 software (Chicago, IL, USA). Nonnormally distributed continuous variables were expressed as median, and categorical variables were expressed as numbers and percentages. Mann-Whitney U test was used in comparison with the continuous variables, while the chi-square test was used in comparison with the categorical variables. The level of statistical significance was considered as $P < 0.05$.

3. Results

A sample of 320 patients, presenting 331 histopathologically confirmed BCC of the head and neck, were identified in the retrospective review. There were 176 (55%) men and 144 (45%) women. In the whole head and neck region, there was no statistically significant difference between the male and female population. When the subunits were evaluated, scalp, frontotemporal, and auricular regions presented male predominance, while the perioral region presented female predominance ($P < 0.05$). The mean age of the patients was 67.3 ± 12.76. Tumors were rare below the age of 20, with only one case in the present study who revealed no history of an underlying disease such as nevoid BCC syndrome or xeroderma pigmentosum. Higher prevalence of patients (34.7%) was noted in the 60–70 age group which was found to be statistically significant ($P < 0.05$). There was no statistically meaningful difference noted among the subunits.

TABLE 1: Demographic analysis of patients.

	Total	Males	Females
Gender (%)	320	176 (55)	144 (45)
Age			
Mean	67.3	66.7	69.4
SD	12.76	12.11	13.32
Median	67	64	69
Range	18–95	28–90	18–95
Fitzpatrick skin type (%)			
1	9 (2.8)	3 (0.9)	6 (1.9)
2	129 (40.3)	69 (21.6)	60 (18.7)
3	165 (51.6)	93 (29.1)	72 (22.5)
4	17 (5.3)	11 (3.4)	6 (1.9)
Sun exposure history (%)	199 (62.2)	121 (37.8)	78 (24.4)
Systemic illness (%)	130 (40.6)	63 (19.7)	67 (20.9)
Family history (%)	22 (6.8)	8 (2.5)	14 (4.3)
Smoking history (%)	120 (37.5)	91 (28.4)	29 (9.1)

The personal history of chronic sun exposure which is defined by spending every working day in open areas due to occupational reasons was reported in 199 (62.2%) cases. One hundred and thirty (40.6%) patients had a coexisting systemic illness. None of the patients had a predisposing disease such as Gorlin's syndrome or xeroderma pigmentosum. Twenty-two (6.8%) patients had skin cancer in their family history. One hundred and twenty patients (37.5%) were smokers for more than ten years. The Fitzpatrick classifications of the patients were type 1 in 9 (2.8%) patients, type 2 in 129 (40.3%) patients, type 3 in 165 (51.6%) patients, and type 4 in 17 (5.3%) patients, respectively. There was no significant difference in the lesions that was related to a patient's skin type, in regard to subunits (Table 1).

Tumors most commonly occurred on the nose, with 107 (32.3%), followed by the orbital at 63 (19.1%), cheek 60 (18.1%), frontotemporal 42 (12.7%), auricular 23 (6.9%), scalp 21 (6.4%), perioral 9 (2.7%), and the chin-neck 6 (1.8%) regions. The size of the tumors was analyzed in 3 groups; 185 (55.9%) tumors were smaller than 10 mm in diameter, 143 (43.2%) were between 10 mm and 30 mm, and 3 (0.9%) were larger than 30 mm. In the nose and cheek regions the lesions were under 10 mm and in scalp region lesions between 10 and 30 mm were higher in number ($P < 0.05$).

Reports of clinical evaluation showed that all of the examined primary BCCs were of the nodular type and were either ulcerated or pigmented. With confirmation to histopathological analyses, 46 (13.8%) were of the mixed type (nodular + micronodular); 39 (11.7%) were of the micronodular type; 37 (11.2%) were of the superficial type; 31 (9.3%) were of the basosquamous type; 23 (6.9%) were of the adenoid type; 14 (4.2%) were of the sclerotic type of BCC. The rest of the lesions 141 (42.6%) were reported as being of the nodular type. Regarding the distribution of histopathologic patterns, no statistically significant difference was found in the entire head and neck region. In the scalp, frontotemporal, nose, and cheek regions, the nodular type tumor percentage was higher ($P < 0.05$). Two hundred and ninety-four excisions (88.9%) were undertaken under local anesthesia; 37 (11.1%) were done under general anesthesia.

The reconstruction method regarding the size of the defect was comprised of primary closure 84 (25.4%), full thickness skin grafting 54 (16.3%), and local flaps 192 (58%). One defect (0.3%) was reconstructed with the radial forearm free flap procedure (Table 2).

The mean follow-up time was at 33 ± 6.7 months. In nine lesions of the nine patients (2.7%) recurrence was observed. Recurrent lesions were in the scalp ($n = 3$), orbital ($n = 2$), and nose ($n = 4$) regions. The histopathological subtypes of these tumors were sclerotic ($n = 4$), micronodular ($n = 3$), mixed ($n = 1$), and nodular ($n = 1$). The recurrence time was between 6 months and 41 months (Table 3).

4. Discussion

BCC is the most common type of skin cancer in Caucasians, which predominantly occurs on the exposed parts of the body, with 75–85% of the lesions found in the head and neck regions [1, 2, 6–9]. According to our findings, more than half of the lesions are found in the nose (32.3%), orbital (19.1%), and cheek (18.1%) areas which are the most central and prominent parts of the entire head and neck region. These regions are also more prone to chronic sunlight exposure [2, 5, 10, 11].

Most of the BCC lesions are reported in the 40–79 age group, with the mean age of 62. In tropical regions and in patients with family history, BCC may occur in younger patients [2, 12]. We have had a statistically significant increase in the 60–70 age group (34.7%), in all the head and neck regions. But in other Mediterranean countries, the predominance is in the 70–80 age bracket [8, 13–15]. Regarding the patient's age and the location of the lesions, no significant difference was found. This can be explained with the siesta culture in these countries, which prevents their population from rush-hour sun exposure.

Men generally have up to 2 times higher rate of BCC [9, 10, 16]. In our study, when the whole head and neck region is encountered, there was no statistically significant difference between men (55%) and women (45%) that was consistent with other studies [10, 13, 17]. Most of our patients are from central Anatolia, where the population is generally comprised of men and women who both work during the daytime as farmers. When the subunits were evaluated, scalp, frontotemporal, and auricular lesions are more common in men, which can be explained by androgenic alopecia or short hair on men, when compared to the long hair or kerchief worn by women. Perioral lesions are found less in men, especially on the upper lip, which can be contributed to moustache on men. These findings are consistent with the report by Bastiaens et al. [18].

Phenotypic characteristics, such as fair skin type, red hair, and freckling are risk factors for BCC [9, 19]. Most of our patients were of type 2 (39.4%) and type 3 (51.6%), regarding the Fitzpatrick classification. This finding is similar to the literature [2, 10]. When the subunits were encountered, there was no significant difference in the lesions based on the patients' skin type.

Most of the lesions were found to be less than 10 mm in size (55.9%), when the whole head and neck region was evaluated. This finding is similar to other reports from Turkey [2]. This might be related to the recent increase in the public cognition of health issues and admission numbers at health facilities in Turkey. The ratio of tumors less than 10 mm was found to be higher in cosmetically more recognized regions, such as the nose and cheek (65.4% and 68.3%, resp.). This may be related to the social recognizability of the lesions.

Although a universally accepted classification scheme is lacking, commonly accepted clinical types are nodular, superficial, fibroepitelial, and morpheaform [9, 12]. Combinations of the latter three types with nodular BCC may occur. There are also histopathologic patterns, such as nodular, micronodular, adenoid, superficial, and sclerotic, which are referred to as subtypes of clinical type of nodular BCC [9, 20]. All of our patients were clinically evaluated as the nodular type BCC; histopathologically most of the lesions were nodular (42.2%). In the scalp, frontotemporal, nose, and cheek regions, a higher percentage of nodular type BCC was found.

The main goal of the BCC treatment is to eradicate the tumor with the safest and most cost-effective method available and to provide an aesthetically and functionally pleasant outcome. Even though different treatment modalities for BCC have been described, surgical excision is the most commonly preferred method for tumor removal [9].

In the literature, the 3 mm peripheral surgical margin is adequate for the clearance of 85% of small and well-defined BCCs, and the 4-5 mm margin will raise this to 95% [5]. It has been shown that loupe magnification can assist in reducing incomplete excision rates [20–22]. In our practice, with loupe magnification, the 3 to 10 mm excision margin was used, depending on the clinical features, size, and location of the lesion.

It has been shown that the recurrence rate for primary BCCs after surgical excision varies between 5% and 14% [1, 5]. Lesions in the head and neck region are at more risk for recurrence, when compared to lesions in trunk and extremities [1, 5, 7, 23]. Even though some factors, like anatomical localization, histopathological characteristics, and initial treatment strategy, have been proposed, there is lack of accepted understanding in the recurrence of the lesions [6]. Incomplete excision was reported as one of the risk factors for recurrence [6, 10, 20, 24]. The main difference of our study when compared with the previous studies is the

Table 2: Systematic analysis of patients' data with comparison to head and neck subunits.

Regions	Age					Sex		Size (mm)			Histopathological subtype							Anesthesia		Method of reconstruction			
(Patients/Tumors)	<50	50–60	60–70	70–80	80<	M	F	<10	10–30	<30	Nod	Mix	Mic	Sp	Bs	Ade	Sc	L	G	P	G	LF	DF
Scalp (21/21)	5	2	10	2	2	15	6	5	15	1	10	1	2	3	2	2	1	20	1	7	6	8	—
Frontotemporal (37/42)	5	4	17	12	4	31	11	20	21	1	14	3	6	7	3	4	5	34	8	15	10	16	1
Orbital (60/63)	6	11	21	19	6	30	33	32	31	—	25	7	9	5	10	5	2	51	12	16	13	34	—
Nose (104/107)	4	25	31	27	20	53	54	70	37	—	48	19	14	7	6	9	4	102	5	15	17	75	—
Cheek (60/60)	8	6	20	15	11	34	26	41	18	1	34	4	8	5	9	—	—	56	4	21	2	37	—
Auricula (23/23)	0	2	9	7	5	20	3	10	13	—	4	12		5	—	—	2	18	5	7	5	11	—
Perioral (9/9)	1	0	5	3	0	2	7	4	5	—	5	—		1	—	3	—	8	1	2	—	7	—
Chin-neck (6/6)	0	1	2	1	2	3	3	3	3	—	1	—		4	1	—	—	5	1	1	1	4	—
Total (320/331)	29	51	115	86	50	188	143	185	143	3	141	46	39	37	31	23	14	294	37	84	54	192	1

Nod indicates nodular; Mix: mixed; Mic: micronodular; Sp: superficial; Bs: basosquamous; Ade: adenoid; Sc: sclerotic; L: local; G: general; P: primary repair; G: full thickness skin graft; LF: local flap; and DF: distant flap.

TABLE 3: Clinical features of recurrent BCC.

	Regions	Specific localization	Age	Sex	Size (mm)	Histopathologic tumor type	Recurrence time	Treatment
1	Scalp	Left parietal	64	M	10–30	Nodular	36 months	Total excision
2	Scalp	Left parietal	66	F	<10	Sclerotic	25 months	Total excision
3	Scalp	Right parietal	62	M	10–30	Micronodular	41 months	Total excision
4	Orbital	Left medial cantus	63	M	10–30	Sclerotic	8 months	Total excision
5	Orbital	Right medial cantus	73	F	10–30	Sclerotic	6 months	Total excision
6	Nose	Dorsum	68	M	<10	Micronodular	18 months	Total excision
7	Nose	Right alar region	73	F	<10	Sclerotic	20 months	Total excision
8	Nose	Nose tip	71	F	<10	Mixed	22 months	Total excision
9	Nose	Left alar region	79	M	<10	Micronodular	9 months	Total excision

precise evaluation of the factors effective on recurrence in completely excised BCCs. In our series, the overall recurrence rate was 2.7%. Recurrent lesions were in the scalp ($n = 3$), orbital ($n = 2$), and nose ($n = 4$) regions. Interestingly, all recurrences were in the median parts of head and neck region; this may be attributed to high recurrence rates in embryonic fusion planes [9, 25–27]. Histopathological subtype of recurrent tumors was mainly micronodular and sclerotic, which is more difficult to eradicate and has high risk of recurrence [28].

Our study revealed that recurrence is related to the localization and histopathologic subtype, whereas they were not related to age, sex, and size of the lesion. The low recurrence rates in our series might be due to the relatively low rates of histopathologically aggressive subtypes, excision with appropriate margin, and no positive surgical margins after surgery.

5. Conclusion

In conclusion, this study presents a relatively large number of series of surgically treated BCCs in the head and neck region. We would like to emphasize the importance of the preoperative evaluation of the patient keeping the epidemiology in mind, defining the surgical margins in order to get lower recurrence rates, and by motivating the patient for follow-up visits, in order to evaluate outcomes and diagnose recurrences.

References

[1] L. Sartore, L. Lancerotto, M. Salmaso et al., "Facial basal cell carcinoma: analysis of recurrence and follow-up strategies," *Oncology Reports*, vol. 26, no. 6, pp. 1423–1429, 2011.

[2] Y. O. Tiftikcioğlu, O. Karaaslan, H. M. Aksoy, B. Aksoy, and U. Koçer, "Basal cell carcinoma in Turkey," *The Journal of Dermatology*, vol. 33, no. 2, pp. 91–95, 2006.

[3] A. W. Wilson, G. Howsam, V. Santhanam et al., "Surgical management of incompletely excised basal cell carcinomas of the head and neck," *British Journal of Oral and Maxillofacial Surgery*, vol. 42, no. 4, pp. 311–314, 2004.

[4] U. Leiter and C. Garbe, "Epidemiology of melanoma and non-melanoma skin cancer-the role of sunlight," *Advances in Experimental Medicine and Biology*, vol. 624, pp. 89–103, 2008.

[5] O. S. Janjua and S. M. Qureshi, "Basal cell carcinoma of the head and neck region: an analysis of 171 cases," *Journal of Skin Cancer*, vol. 2012, Article ID 943472, 4 pages, 2012.

[6] D. Farhi, N. Dupin, A. Palangié, A. Carlotti, and M.-F. Avril, "Incomplete excision of basal cell carcinoma: rate and associated factors among 362 consecutive cases," *Dermatologic Surgery*, vol. 33, no. 10, pp. 1207–1214, 2007.

[7] V. Smith and S. Walton, "Treatment of facial basal cell carcinoma: a review," *Journal of Skin Cancer*, vol. 2011, Article ID 380371, 7 pages, 2011.

[8] H. M. Gloster Jr. and K. Neal, "Skin cancer in skin of color," *Journal of the American Academy of Dermatology*, vol. 55, no. 5, pp. 741–760, 2006.

[9] H. P. Soyer, D. S. Rigel, and E. M. T. Wurm, "Actinic keratosis, basal cell carcinoma and squamous cell carcinoma," in *Dermatology*, J. L. Bolognia, J. L. Jorizzo, and J. V. Schaffer, Eds., pp. 1773–1793, Elsevier Saunders, Beijing, China, 2012.

[10] K. Seretis, V. Thomaidis, A. Karpouzis, D. Tamiolakis, and I. Tsamis, "Epidemiology of surgical treatment of nonmelanoma skin cancer of the head and neck in Greece," *Dermatologic Surgery*, vol. 36, no. 1, pp. 15–22, 2010.

[11] S. Cho, M.-H. Kim, K.-K. Whang, and J.-H. Hahm, "Clinical and histopathological characteristics of basal cell carcinoma in Korean patients," *Journal of Dermatology*, vol. 26, no. 8, pp. 494–501, 1999.

[12] J. J. Rippey, "Why classify basal cell carcinomas?" *Histopathology*, vol. 32, no. 5, pp. 393–398, 1998.

[13] R. Betti, E. Inselvini, M. Carducci, and C. Crosti, "Age and site prevalence of histologic subtypes of basal cell carcinomas," *International Journal of Dermatology*, vol. 34, no. 3, pp. 174–176, 1995.

[14] S. Boi, M. Cristofolini, R. Micciolo, E. Polla, and P. D. Palma, "Epidemiology of skin tumors: data from the cutaneous cancer registry in Trentino, Italy," *Journal of Cutaneous Medicine and Surgery*, vol. 7, no. 4, pp. 300–305, 2003.

[15] F. Revenga Arranz, J. F. Paricio Rubio, M. M. Vázquez Salvado, and V. del Villar Sordo, "Descriptive epidemiology of basal cell carcinoma and cutaneous squamous cell carcinoma in Soria (north-eastern Spain) 1998–2000: a hospital-based survey," *Journal of the European Academy of Dermatology and Venereology*, vol. 18, no. 2, pp. 137–141, 2004.

[16] Y. Scrivener, E. Grosshans, and B. Cribier, "Variations of basal cell carcinomas according to gender, age, location and histopathological subtype," *British Journal of Dermatology*, vol. 147, no. 1, pp. 41–47, 2002.

[17] D. Czarnecki, N. Collins, C. Meehan, T. O'Brien, S. Leahy, and C. Nash, "Basal-cell carcinoma in temperate and tropical Australia," *International Journal of Cancer*, vol. 50, no. 6, pp. 874–875, 1992.

[18] M. T. Bastiaens, J. J. Hoefnagel, J. A. Bruijn, R. G. J. Westendorp, B. J. Vermeer, and J. N. B. Bavinck, "Differences in age, site distribution, and sex between nodular and superficial basal cell carcinomas indicate different types of tumors," *Journal of Investigative Dermatology*, vol. 110, no. 6, pp. 880–884, 1998.

[19] M. Almahroos and A. K. Kurban, "Ultraviolet carcinogenesis in nonmelanoma skin cancer. Part I: incidence rates in relation to geographic locations and in migrant populations," *Skinmed*, vol. 3, no. 1, pp. 29–35, 2004.

[20] R. W. Griffiths, S. K. Suvarna, and J. Stone, "Basal cell carcinoma histological clearance margins: an analysis of 1539 conventionally excised tumours. Wider still and deeper?" *Journal of Plastic, Reconstructive and Aesthetic Surgery*, vol. 60, no. 1, pp. 41–47, 2007.

[21] D. J. Wolf and J. A. Zitelli, "Surgical margins for basal cell carcinoma," *Archives of Dermatology*, vol. 123, no. 3, pp. 340–344, 1987.

[22] N. Jallali, "Loupe magnification reduces the incidence of incomplete excision of basal cell carcinoma," *Plastic and Reconstructive Surgery*, vol. 113, no. 6, pp. 1887–1888, 2004.

[23] L. A. E. Sussman and D. F. Liggins, "Incompletely excised basal cell carcinoma: a management dilemma?" *Australian and New Zealand Journal of Surgery*, vol. 66, no. 5, pp. 276–278, 1996.

[24] R. W. Griffiths, S. K. Suvarna, and J. Stone, "Do basal cell carcinomas recur after complete conventional surgical excision?" *British Journal of Plastic Surgery*, vol. 58, no. 6, pp. 795–805, 2005.

[25] B. K. Goh, P. Ang, Y. J. Wu, and C. L. Goh, "Characteristics of basal cell carcinoma amongst Asians in Singapore and a comparison between completely and incompletely excised tumors," *International Journal of Dermatology*, vol. 45, no. 5, pp. 561–564, 2006.

[26] J. D. Richmond and R. M. Davie, "The significance of incomplete excision in patients with basal cell carcinoma," *British Journal of Plastic Surgery*, vol. 40, no. 1, pp. 63–67, 1987.

[27] D. P. Goldberg, "Assessment and surgical treatment of basal cell skin cancer," *Clinics in Plastic Surgery*, vol. 24, no. 4, pp. 673–686, 1997.

[28] R. Betti, S. Menni, G. Radaelli, C. Bombonato, and C. Crosti, "Micronodular basal cell carcinoma: a distinct subtype? Relationship with nodular and infiltrative basal cell carcinomas," *Journal of Dermatology*, vol. 37, no. 7, pp. 611–616, 2010.

23

Reducing Sun Exposure for Prevention of Skin Cancers: Factorial Invariance and Reliability of the Self-Efficacy Scale for Sun Protection

Steven F. Babbin,[1] Hui-Qing Yin,[2] Joseph S. Rossi,[2] Colleen A. Redding,[2] Andrea L. Paiva,[2] and Wayne F. Velicer[2]

[1] *Department of Psychiatry, Geisel School of Medicine at Dartmouth, Lebanon, NH 03766, USA*
[2] *Cancer Prevention Research Center and Department of Psychology, University of Rhode Island, Kingston, RI 02881, USA*

Correspondence should be addressed to Joseph S. Rossi; jsrossi@uri.edu

Academic Editor: Iris Zalaudek

The Self-Efficacy Scale for Sun Protection consists of two correlated factors with three items each for Sunscreen Use and Avoidance. This study evaluated two crucial psychometric assumptions, factorial invariance and scale reliability, with a sample of adults (N = 1356) participating in a computer-tailored, population-based intervention study. A measure has factorial invariance when the model is the same across subgroups. Three levels of invariance were tested, from least to most restrictive: (1) Configural Invariance (nonzero factor loadings unconstrained); (2) Pattern Identity Invariance (equal factor loadings); and (3) Strong Factorial Invariance (equal factor loadings and measurement errors). Strong Factorial Invariance was a good fit for the model across seven grouping variables: age, education, ethnicity, gender, race, skin tone, and Stage of Change for Sun Protection. Internal consistency coefficient Alpha and factor rho scale reliability, respectively, were .84 and .86 for Sunscreen Use, .68 and .70 for Avoidance, and .78 and .78 for the global (total) scale. The psychometric evidence demonstrates strong empirical support that the scale is consistent, has internal validity, and can be used to assess population-based adult samples.

1. Introduction

Skin cancer is a widespread, growing, and costly public health problem. Nonmelanoma skin cancers, which include squamous cell carcinoma and basal cell carcinoma, are the most common malignancies in the United States, with approximately 3.5 million new cases diagnosed each year [1]. Melanoma, although less common, is the deadliest form of skin cancer. Nearly 60,000 people are diagnosed and about 8,600 people die from melanoma each year [2]. Overall, skin cancer is the most common form of cancer in the United States, and incidence is increasing [1]. It results in significant potential years of life lost and billions of dollars in costs, including both medical costs and lost productivity costs [3, 4].

The burden of skin cancer can be reduced through prevention efforts. Exposure to ultraviolet radiation via the sun is the most important and avoidable cause of skin cancers. Unfortunately, the majority of adults in the United States do not protect themselves from the sun, and prevalence of at least one sunburn per year is over 50% [5, 6]. Sun protection behaviors, such as avoiding the sun, wearing protective clothing, and wearing sunscreen, can be emphasized in interventions designed to increase sun protection.

The Self-Efficacy Scale for Sun Protection was developed using the framework of the Transtheoretical Model of Behavior Change (TTM). The TTM is an integrative framework that consists of multiple dimensions that assess readiness to change [7, 8]. The core constructs of the TTM include stages of change, processes of change, decisional balance, and self-efficacy. Tailored, computerized interventions based on the TTM have been empirically validated and effective for a wide variety of behaviors [9–11], including sun protection behaviors [12–16].

The self-efficacy component of the TTM assesses an individual's perceived ability to perform healthy behaviors in difficult situations [17]. This component is based on self-efficacy as conceptualized by Bandura [18] and research on relapse prevention. The Self-Efficacy Scale for Sun Protection was designed to assess an individual's confidence to protect oneself from sun exposure [6, 19, 20]. Variations of this measure have been utilized in multiple population-based interventions that have demonstrated efficacy and effectiveness (e.g., [12–16]).

In a tailored intervention, different response patterns to the self-efficacy scale result in different, individualized feedback for participants. To confirm that the Self-Efficacy Scale for Sun Protection is useful and meaningful for intervention purposes across a wide range of potential target populations, the psychometric assumptions of factorial invariance and scale reliability were evaluated in the present study with a large, representative sample of adults ($N = 1356$) from across the United States involved in a tailored intervention study for exercise and sun protection. The psychometric assumptions of measurement invariance and scale reliability are crucial to the overall construct validity of the measure. A measurement model is called *factorially invariant* when the model is the same for different subgroups of a population. Three levels of factorial invariance, from the least restrictive to the most restrictive, were assessed. These levels have been used to test invariance of other TTM constructs [21–24]. Factorial invariance for the Decisional Balance for Sun Protection Inventory, a measure that was used in the same intervention study that provided data for the present study, was also tested with these three levels [25].

Each level adds more constraints to the model. The weakest level is *Configural Invariance*, which states that subgroups have zero loadings on the same constructs and unconstrained nonzero factor loadings [26]. Second is *Pattern Identity Invariance*, which requires the factor loadings to be equal across subgroups. Third, *Strong Factorial Invariance* requires factor loadings and error terms to be equivalent across subgroups. If a scale is factorially invariant across groups, the psychometric properties of the measure can be assumed equal across groups (e.g., factor correlations and internal consistency). Thus, comparisons between groups on the measure of interest can confidently be attributed to true differences in the construct and not simply to variance on the measure.

The present study was a secondary data analysis of a baseline sample of adults involved in a tailored intervention study. Factorial invariance was examined across age, education, ethnicity, gender, race, skin tone, and Stage of Change for Sun Protection. Internal consistency reliability of the scales was assessed with Cronbach's Coefficient Alpha. Scale reliability, based on results from confirmatory factor analysis (CFA), was assessed with the factor rho coefficient.

2. Methods

2.1. Participants. Baseline data from 1356 adults were used for this study. These participants were recruited from across the United States in 2010–2012 for a randomized, population-based, TTM-tailored intervention study [27]. The study evaluated a multimedia, computer-based intervention to increase exercise and sun protection. Recruitment was proactive, and participants were identified with screening calls. To be eligible for the study, participants had to be in preaction stages (precontemplation, contemplation, or preparation; [7, 8]) for both exercise and sun protection; eligible participants were not currently exercising and not currently protecting themselves from the sun. Additional inclusion criteria included age 18–75, willingness to provide basic demographic information, ability to participate in physical activity, and internet access. Participants that had a recent history of medical conditions (e.g., heart attack within the past six months, currently receiving chemotherapy or radiation, and pregnant women) or who had been advised by their doctor or health care provider to avoid exercise were excluded. All intervention materials and assessments were administered over the internet. Consent and other human subject protocols were approved by the University of Rhode Island Institutional Review Board, and research was conducted according to APA ethical guidelines. Demographic variables were utilized to create subgroups for invariance testing (see Table 1). Overall, the sample was 83% white and 63% female.

2.2. Self-Efficacy Scale for Sun Protection. The Self-Efficacy Scale for Sun Protection was designed to assess confidence in sun protection behaviors in adolescents and adults [6, 19, 20, 28] and was developed using the sequential method of scale development [29–31]. The scale can be modeled as a two-factor correlated model with six items: three items for Sunscreen Use and three items for Sun Avoidance (see Figure 1). For each item, participants rated how confident they were in their ability to protect themselves from sun exposure on a 5-point Likert scale, from 1, "not at all confident," to 5 "extremely confident." The scale can also be scored as a global measure of self-efficacy for sun protection by averaging (or summing) all six items into a single total score. In the computer-based assessments, participants could not skip scale items. Thus, there were no missing data from item nonresponse in this baseline sample.

2.3. Factorial Invariance. Three levels of invariance were tested in sequential order, with each level requiring more constraints: (1) Configural Invariance (unconstrained nonzero factor loadings); (2) Pattern Identity Invariance (equal factor loadings); and (3) Strong Factorial Invariance (equal factor loadings and measurement errors). Each invariance procedure was evaluated across specific subgroups.

Baseline variables were used to create subgroups (see Table 1). In general, when continuous variables were divided into categories (e.g., age and education), the goal was to avoid subgroup sizes of <100 to avoid convergence issues [32]. For other variables, subgroups that were too small for analysis were eliminated. Only complete cases were used for these subgroups. Thus, these subgroups vary in total sample size due to differences in missing data across subgroup variables. The sample was divided into five subgroups for age, three subgroups for education, two subgroups for ethnicity, two subgroups for gender, two subgroups for race, three subgroups for skin tone (untanned skin color, a proxy indicator of sun sensitivity [19]), and three subgroups for Stage of Change for Sun Protection (see Table 1). Despite

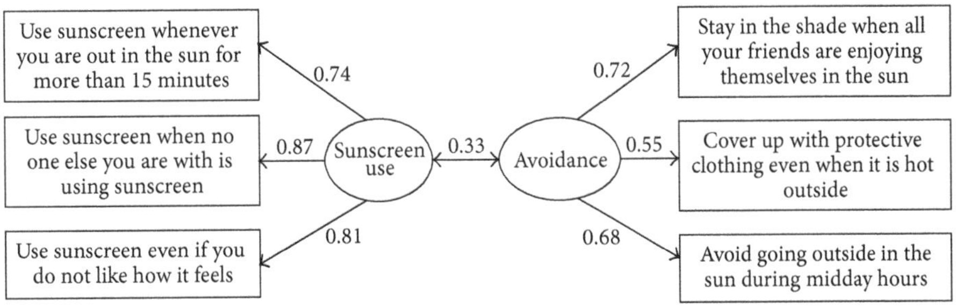

FIGURE 1: Model with standardized parameter estimates for the total sample ($N = 1356$).

TABLE 1: Sample sizes for subgroups included in invariance testing.

Variable Subgroup	n
Age (years)	
18–29	188
30–39	202
40–49	353
50–59	360
≥60	253
Total	*1356*
Education level (years)	
≤12	313
13–15	468
≥16	575
Total	*1356*
Ethnicity	
Hispanic	54
Non-Hispanic	1302
Total	*1356*
Gender	
Female	856
Male	500
Total	*1356*
Race	
White	1123
Black/African American	89
Total	*1212*
Skin tone (untanned skin color)	
Fair white	296
Medium white	598
Dark white (e.g., olive) and light brown	406
Total	*1300*
Stage of Change for Sun Protection	
Precontemplation	836
Contemplation	152
Preparation	367
Total	*1355*

the very small sample size of participants identified as Hispanic, the sample size was adequate for analysis. Demographic questions included more racial identities (American Indian or Alaskan Native, Asian, Native Hawaiian or other Pacific Islanders, and others), but no other subgroups had adequate sample sizes for analysis. Sample size for participants who identified skin tone as dark brown was not adequate for invariance testing ($n = 44$). Stage of Change for Sun Protection is a TTM construct that represents readiness to change sun protection behavior [6, 19]. The precontemplation stage included participants who were not consistently protecting themselves from the sun and were not intending to start within the next 12 months. The contemplation stage included participants who were not consistently protecting themselves but were seriously thinking about starting within the next 12 months. Preparation stage individuals were not currently protecting themselves but were planning to start within the next 30 days.

To test for factorial invariance, structural equation modeling (SEM) was employed using EQS 6.1 software [33]. Model fit was evaluated using the comparative fit index (CFI) and the root mean square error of approximation (RMSEA). For CFI, values closer to 1.0 indicate good fit and, for RMSEA, values closer to zero indicate good fit [34, 35]. The difference in CFI between a higher level model and a lower level of invariance (ΔCFI) was also calculated (e.g., Pattern Identity CFI-Configural CFI). A difference of .01 or smaller indicates that the null hypothesis of invariance should not be rejected and that the model demonstrates invariance [36]. The fit indices and invariance modeling procedures used in the present study are the same as included in recent psychometric assessments of self-efficacy measures for other behaviors [22, 23].

2.4. Scale Reliabilities. The internal consistency reliability of each subscale (Sunscreen Use and Sun Avoidance) and the total scale was assessed with Cronbach's Coefficient Alpha [37]. Confidence intervals for coefficient Alpha were also calculated [38]. The factor rho coefficient [34, 39–41] was calculated for each subscale and the total scale to assess scale reliability based on CFA results. Unstandardized model estimates were used to calculate rho. For both estimates of reliability, there are no strict cutoffs for acceptability [42], but values around .70 indicate adequate internal consistency, and values around .90 indicate excellent internal consistency [31, 34].

Table 2: Goodness-of-fit statistics for three invariance models.

	Model	χ^2	df	CFI	ΔCFI	RMSEA	[90% CI]
Age	Configural Invariance	112.424	40	.973	—	.082	[.064, .100]
	Pattern Identity Invariance	142.684	56	.968	−.005	.076	[.060, .091]
	Strong Factorial Invariance	173.593	80	.966	−.002	.066	[.052, .079]
Education	Configural Invariance	86.280	24	.977	—	.076	[.059, .093]
	Pattern Identity Invariance	99.994	32	.975	−.002	.069	[.054, .084]
	Strong Factorial Invariance	122.958	44	.971	−.004	.063	[.050, .076]
Ethnicity	Configural Invariance	81.672	16	.976	—	.078	[.061, .095]
	Pattern Identity Invariance	83.246	20	.976	.000	.068	[.053, .084]
	Strong Factorial Invariance	88.732	26	.977	.001	.060	[.046, .073]
Gender	Configural Invariance	91.839	16	.972	—	.084	[.067, .100]
	Pattern Identity Invariance	97.756	20	.971	−.001	.076	[.061, .091]
	Strong Factorial Invariance	112.064	26	.968	−.003	.070	[.057, .083]
Race	Configural Invariance	67.817	16	.978	—	.073	[.056, .091]
	Pattern Identity Invariance	69.539	20	.979	.001	.064	[.048, .080]
	Strong Factorial Invariance	89.886	26	.973	−.006	.064	[.049, .078]
Skin tone	Configural Invariance	124.397	24	.958	—	.098	[.081, .115]
	Pattern Identity Invariance	155.343	32	.948	−.010	.094	[.080, .109]
	Strong Factorial Invariance	201.558	44	.935	−.013	.091	[.078, .104]
Stage of Change	Configural Invariance	79.228	24	.974	—	.071	[.054, .089]
	Pattern Identity Invariance	88.925	32	.973	−.001	.063	[.047, .078]
	Strong Factorial Invariance	145.220	44	.953	−.020	.071	[.059, .084]

3. Results

3.1. Factorial Invariance. A total of 21 models were run, with three models (Configural Invariance, Pattern Identity Invariance, and Strong Factorial Invariance) for each of the seven subgroup variables. No constraints were dropped in any of the models to achieve a better fit. All sample sizes and results are summarized in Table 2.

3.1.1. Age. Sample size for invariance testing was adequate for the five subgroups: 18 to 29 years old, 30 to 39 years old, 40 to 49 years old, 50 to 59 years old, and 60 years old and over. The highest level of invariance, Strong Factorial Invariance, held across the subgroups with a good fit (CFI = .966; RMSEA = .066).

3.1.2. Education Level. Sample size was adequate for all three subgroups: 12 years of education or less, 13 to 15 years of education, and 16 years of education or more. Strong Factorial Invariance held across the subgroups with a good fit (CFI = .971; RMSEA = .063).

3.1.3. Ethnicity. Sample size was marginal for the Hispanic group, especially as compared to the non-Hispanic group, but there were no difficulties in fitting the models; thus, the sample size for Hispanics was considered acceptable. Strong Factorial Invariance fit well across the subgroups (CFI = .977; RMSEA = .060).

3.1.4. Gender. Sample size was adequate for both subgroups: female and male. Strong Factorial Invariance held across the subgroups (CFI = .968; RMSEA = .070).

3.1.5. Race. As with ethnicity, sample size was marginal but acceptable for the black/African American group and was large for the white subgroup. Strong Factorial Invariance fit well across the subgroups (CFI = .973; RMSEA = .064).

3.1.6. Skin Tone. Sample size was adequate for three subgroups: fair white, medium white, and dark white/light brown. Strong Factorial Invariance held across the three subgroups with a good fit (CFI = .935; RMSEA = .091).

3.1.7. Stage of Change for Sun Protection. Sample size was adequate for the three subgroups: precontemplation, contemplation, and preparation. Strong Factorial Invariance held across the subgroups (CFI = .953; RMSEA = .071).

3.2. Scale Reliabilities. Since Strong Factorial Invariance held for all of the subgroups, a CFA was performed on the total sample, and the final correlated model structure and parameter estimates are reported only for the total sample (see Figure 1). The total sample coefficient Alpha [95% confidence interval] was .84 [.82, .85] for Sunscreen Use, which indicates very good internal consistency reliability, and .68 [.65, .71] for Avoidance, which indicates adequate internal consistency reliability. Coefficient Alpha for the total six-item scale was good, $\alpha = .78$ [.76, .80]. The CFA-based factor rho coefficient was .86 for Sunscreen Use, which indicates very good scale reliability, .70 for Avoidance, which indicates adequate scale reliability, and .78 for the total six-item scale, which indicates good scale reliability. Considering the short length of the scale, the Alpha values, and the rho values, the Self-Efficacy Scale for Sun Protection demonstrates evidence of reliability.

4. Discussion

Assessments of factorial invariance and internal consistency suggest that the Self-Efficacy Scale for Sun Protection is a reliable and valid instrument and can be used across a full range of adult participants varying by age, educational level, skin tone, gender, ethnicity, race, and stage attributes. The scale demonstrates a high level of factorial invariance across subgroups. The highest level tested, Strong Factorial Invariance, required that factor loadings and error terms were equal across the subgroups. This demonstrated a good fit across age, education level, ethnicity, gender, race, skin tone, and Stage of Change for Sun Protection. Internal consistency reliability, as assessed by coefficient Alpha, was very good for the Sunscreen Use subscale, adequate for the Avoidance subscale, and good for the total six-item scale. Scale reliability, as assessed by the factor rho coefficient, was also very good for the Sunscreen Use subscale, adequate for the Avoidance subscale, and good for the total six-item scale. Overall, these results suggest that there is a consistent relationship between the two subscales (Sunscreen Use and Avoidance), as well as the six items that measure these factors.

The consistently good fit for Strong Factorial Invariance across seven subgrouping variables is very strong evidence that the scale is factorially invariant. The degree of fit does vary across the subgroups, however. For age, education level, ethnicity, gender, and race, CFI, ΔCFI, and RMSEA all indicated good fit for Strong Factorial Invariance. For skin tone and Stage of Change for Sun Protection, CFI and RMSEA suggested good fit, but the ΔCFI value was slightly more negative than –.01. This suggests that there may be some small differences in the factor model of the scale across levels of skin tone and Stage of Change for Sun Protection. But since most of the indices suggested good fit, Strong Factorial Invariance should not be rejected.

The high level of factorial invariance refers to the consistency in the factor structure. Such consistency in the measurement model is vital to valid research and intervention efforts. Since a population-based sample cannot be homogenous in every way, every sample will demonstrate some variation that is not related to the research question. Some subgroups may respond to the measurement instrument differently. Results from a factorially invariant model should not be biased by such differences. Strong Factorial Invariance suggests that the validity of the measurement should be the same regardless of the sample. However, since the focus is on the factor structure, the means were not assessed for equivalence across subgroups. Mean differences, in some cases, could be expected to be different. For example, one would anticipate that participants in the precontemplation stage for sun protection (not intending to start protecting themselves from the sun within the next 12 months) would have lower mean scores for confidence in Sunscreen Use and Avoidance than participants in the contemplation stage for sun protection (thinking about starting within the next 12 months). Testing such mean differences could be the focus of a future study.

The Self-Efficacy Scale for Sun Protection was developed to be consistent with self-efficacy theory [18]. The six items of the scale represent six different situations that represent obstacles and challenges to an individual's perceived ability to protect himself or herself from the sun. In general, self-efficacy scales developed for TTM studies involve a variety of situations related to one target behavior, such as smoking [17, 23] or alcohol use [22]. The Self-Efficacy Scale for Sun Protection, in contrast, involves multiple sun protection behaviors (wearing sunscreen, avoiding the sun, and wearing protective clothing). In the construction of the scale, including multiple behaviors was necessary due to the complex nature of sun protection; to be protected from the sun, an individual needs to perform multiple sun protection behaviors [6, 19, 20, 28]. Thus, this scale is more behaviorally defined and more operationalized in terms of behaviors than some other scales. Evidence from factorial invariance suggests that this larger emphasis on behavior does not impact the generalizability of the factor structure. Strong Factorial Invariance held across all subgroups, and this suggests that participants in different subgroups did not respond differently to items involving different behaviors. Regardless, the behaviorally defined nature of the scale may have some impacts on the measurement of self-efficacy that are beyond the scope of the present study but could be explored in future measurement studies. For example, some items related to specific behaviors may be more predictive of treatment outcome.

While reliability for the Confidence in Sunscreen Use subscale was good, reliability for the Avoidance subscale could be improved. Coefficient Alpha and coefficient rho were close to .70, which suggests that reliability was only adequate. The simplest solution to improving reliability would be to add items to the Avoidance subscale, as longer scales demonstrate greater reliability. However, the Self-Efficacy Scale for Sun Protection was intended to be brief, and an increase in reliability via more items would increase the time required to answer the scale and decrease the parsimony of the model. Past psychometric assessments of short TTM scales [21–25] have reported coefficient Alpha values ranging from .51 to .90, which suggests that an Alpha around .70 is consistent with similar measures. In addition to the two subscales, many applied researchers are likely to use the global (total) scale score as well, as an assessment of overall confidence in the ability to perform protective sun behaviors. The two measures of reliability, coefficient Alpha and coefficient rho, were good (nearly .80) for the total scale score. Both the total score and the subscale scores can be useful as intermediate level indicators of intervention effectiveness, prior to final intervention outcome assessments of behavior change [7, 8, 17].

The psychometric assessment of this scale was limited by some subgroup sample sizes. Most importantly, three subgroup variables could be improved with a larger, more diverse sample: ethnicity, race, and skin tone. The number of participants that identified their ethnicity as Hispanic was very small, and, therefore, the results of the invariance tests for ethnicity should be interpreted with caution. The number of participants identified as black or African American was also small. In addition to improving the sample size of this subgroup, a larger sample could cover a more comprehensive number of racial identities. Insufficient sample size also prevented participants who identified "dark brown" skin tones from being included in separate invariance analyses. A larger sample would improve the respective sample sizes for ethnicity, race, and skin tone and thus provide stronger evidence for validity.

The present study focused on invariance, internal consistency reliability, and scale reliability. These properties do not encompass all aspects of validity and reliability, and future investigations could test other psychometrics using assessment points beyond baseline. Test-retest reliability, or the stability of the measure over time, needs to be assessed. As the intervention was designed to promote sun protection, the factor means should change, but the overall factor structure should remain stable. Convergent validity could be assessed by comparing self-efficacy scores to self-reported sun protection behaviors at each assessment point. Predictive validity could be assessed by testing baseline self-efficacy scores as predictors of sun protection behaviors at future assessment points. Such efforts would further strengthen the evidence supporting the validity and reliability of this measure.

5. Conclusions

The Self-Efficacy Scale for Sun Protection demonstrates consistency and reliability. Ultimately, assessment of these psychometric properties provides strong empirical evidence for construct validity. This scale measures self-efficacy for sun protection as intended. It is short, psychometrically sound, and appropriate for research, providing a solid empirical foundation for the development of interventions to reduce the burden of skin cancer.

Disclosure

Preliminary results from this research were presented at the 34th Annual Meeting of the Society of Behavioral Medicine, San Francisco, USA, March 2013.

Disclaimer

NIH had no role in the study design, data collection, analysis, interpretation, paper writing, or the decision to submit the paper for publication.

Acknowledgments

This research was supported in part by NIH Grants R01CA119195 from the National Cancer Institute and G20RR030883 from the National Center for Research Resources. While revising this paper, Dr. Steven F. Babbin was supported by NIH Grant T32DA037202 (NIDA).

References

[1] H. W. Rogers, M. A. Weinstock, A. R. Harris et al., "Incidence estimate of nonmelanoma skin cancer in the United States, 2006," *Archives of Dermatology*, vol. 146, no. 3, pp. 283–287, 2010.

[2] U.S. Cancer Statistics Working Group, *United States Cancer Statistics: 1999–2008 Incidence and Mortality Web-Based Report*, Department of Health and Human Services, Centers for Disease Control and Prevention, and National Cancer Institute, Atlanta, Ga, USA, 2012, http://www.cdc.gov/uscs.

[3] D. R. Bickers, H. W. Lim, D. Margolis et al., "The burden of skin diseases: 2004," *Journal of the American Academy of Dermatology*, vol. 55, no. 3, pp. 490–500, 2006.

[4] G. P. Guy Jr. and D. U. Ekwueme, "Years of potential life lost and indirect costs of melanoma and non-melanoma skin cancer: a systematic review of the literature," *PharmacoEconomics*, vol. 29, no. 10, pp. 863–874, 2011.

[5] Centers for Disease Control and Prevention, "Sunburn and sun protective behaviors among adults aged 18–29 years—United States, 2000–2010," *Morbidity and Mortality Weekly Report*, vol. 61, no. 18, pp. 317–322, 2012.

[6] M. A. Weinstock, J. S. Rossi, C. A. Redding, J. E. Maddock, and S. D. Cottrill, "Sun protection behaviors and stages of change for the primary prevention of skin cancers among beachgoers in Southeastern New England," *Annals of Behavioral Medicine*, vol. 22, no. 4, pp. 286–293, 2000.

[7] J. O. Prochaska and W. F. Velicer, "The transtheoretical model of health behavior change," *The American Journal of Health Promotion*, vol. 12, no. 1, pp. 38–48, 1997.

[8] W. F. Velicer, J. O. Prochaska, J. L. Fava et al., "Using the transtheoretical model for population-based approaches to health promotion and disease prevention," *Homeostasis in Health and Disease*, vol. 40, no. 5, pp. 174–195, 2000.

[9] P. Krebs, J. O. Prochaska, and J. S. Rossi, "A meta-analysis of computer-tailored interventions for health behavior change," *Preventive Medicine*, vol. 51, no. 3-4, pp. 214–221, 2010.

[10] S. M. Noar, C. N. Benac, and M. S. Harris, "Does tailoring matter? Meta-analytic review of tailored print health behavior change interventions," *Psychological Bulletin*, vol. 133, no. 4, pp. 673–693, 2007.

[11] W. F. Velicer, J. O. Prochaska, and C. A. Redding, "Tailored communications for smoking cessation: past successes and future directions," *Drug and Alcohol Review*, vol. 25, no. 1, pp. 49–57, 2006.

[12] J. O. Prochaska, W. F. Velicer, J. S. Rossi et al., "Impact of simultaneous stage-matched expert system interventions for smoking, high fat diet and sun exposure in a population of parents," *Health Psychology*, vol. 23, no. 5, pp. 503–516, 2004.

[13] J. O. Prochaska, W. F. Velicer, C. Redding et al., "Stage-based expert systems to guide a population of primary care patients to quit smoking, eat healthier, prevent skin cancer, and receive regular mammograms," *Preventive Medicine*, vol. 41, no. 2, pp. 406–416, 2005.

[14] J. S. Rossi, M. A. Weinstock, C. A. Redding, S. D. Cottrill, and J. E. Maddock, "Effectiveness of stage-matched interventions for skin cancer prevention: a randomized clinical trial of high-risk beach bathers," *Annals of Behavioral Medicine*, vol. 19, supplement, p. s237, 1997.

[15] M. A. Weinstock, J. S. Rossi, C. A. Redding, and J. E. Maddock, "Randomized controlled community trial of the efficacy of a multicomponent stage-matched intervention to increase sun protection among beachgoers," *Preventive Medicine*, vol. 35, no. 6, pp. 584–592, 2002.

[16] G. J. Norman, M. A. Adams, K. J. Calfas et al., "A randomized trial of a multicomponent intervention for adolescent sun protection behaviors," *Archives of Pediatrics & Adolescent Medicine*, vol. 161, no. 2, pp. 146–152, 2007.

[17] W. F. Velicer, C. C. DiClemente, J. S. Rossi, and J. O. Prochaska, "Relapse situations and self-efficacy: an integrative model," *Addictive Behaviors*, vol. 15, no. 3, pp. 271–283, 1990.

[18] A. Bandura, "Self-efficacy: toward a unifying theory of behavioral change," *Psychological Review*, vol. 84, no. 2, pp. 191–215, 1977.

[19] J. S. Rossi, "Exploring behavioral approaches to UV risk reduction," in *Sunlight, Ultraviolet Radiation, and the Skin*, A. Moshell and L. W. Blankenbaker, Eds., pp. 91–93, National Institutes of Health, Bethesda, Md, USA, 1989.

[20] J. E. Maddock, C. A. Redding, J. S. Rossi, and M. A. Weinstock, "Development and validation of an appearance motivation attitudes scale for sun protection," *Psychology and Health*, vol. 20, no. 6, pp. 775–788, 2005.

[21] S. F. Babbin, M. Harrington, C. Burditt et al., "Prevention of alcohol use in middle school students: psychometric assessment of the decisional balance inventory," *Addictive Behaviors*, vol. 36, no. 5, pp. 543–546, 2011.

[22] M. Harrington, S. Babbin, C. Redding et al., "Psychometric assessment of the temptations to try alcohol scale," *Addictive Behaviors*, vol. 36, no. 4, pp. 431–433, 2011.

[23] H. A. McGee, S. F. Babbin, C. Redding et al., "Prevention of smoking in middle school students: psychometric assessment of the temptations to try smoking scale," *Addictive Behaviors*, vol. 37, no. 4, pp. 521–523, 2012.

[24] R. M. Ward, W. F. Velicer, J. S. Rossi, J. L. Fava, and J. O. Prochaska, "Factorial invariance and internal consistency for the decisional balance inventory—short form," *Addictive Behaviors*, vol. 29, no. 5, pp. 953–958, 2004.

[25] H.-Q. Yin, J. S. Rossi, C. A. Redding, A. L. Paiva, S. F. Babbin, and W. F. Velicer, "Validity and stability of the decisional balance for sun protection inventory," *Journal of Skin Cancer*, vol. 2014, Article ID 190541, 7 pages, 2014.

[26] W. Meredith, "Measurement invariance, factor analysis and factorial invariance," *Psychometrika*, vol. 58, no. 4, pp. 525–543, 1993.

[27] W. F. Velicer, C. A. Redding, B. Blissmer et al., "Using relational agents to increase engagement in computer-based interventions: preliminary outcomes," *International Journal of Behavioral Medicine*, vol. 21, supplement 1, p. S206, 2014.

[28] J. E. Maddock, J. S. Rossi, C. A. Redding, K. S. Meier, W. F. Velicer, and J. O. Prochaska, "Development of transtheoretical model constructs for sun protection behaviors among adolescents," *Annals of Behavioral Medicine*, vol. 20, p. S208, 1998.

[29] D. N. Jackson, "A sequential system for personality scale development," in *Current Topics in Clinical and Community Psychology*, C. D. Spielberger, Ed., vol. 2, pp. 61–96, Academic Press, New York, NY, USA, 1970.

[30] D. N. Jackson, "The dynamics of structured personality tests: 1971," *Psychological Review*, vol. 78, no. 3, pp. 229–248, 1971.

[31] C. A. Redding, J. E. Maddock, and J. S. Rossi, "The sequential approach to measurement of health behavior constructs: issues in selecting and developing measures," *Californian Journal of Health Promotion*, vol. 4, no. 1, pp. 83–101, 2006.

[32] W. F. Velicer and J. L. Fava, "Effects of variables and subject sampling on factor pattern recovery," *Psychological Methods*, vol. 3, no. 2, pp. 231–251, 1998.

[33] P. M. Bentler, *EQS 6.1 Structural Equations Program Manual*, Multivariate Software, Encino, Calif, USA, 2007.

[34] R. B. Kline, *Principles and Practice of Structural Equation Modeling*, Guilford Press, New York, NY, USA, 3rd edition, 2011.

[35] M. W. Browne and R. Cudeck, "Alternative ways of assessing model fit," in *Testing Structural Equation Models*, K. A. Bollen and J. S. Long, Eds., pp. 445–455, Sage, Newbury Park, Calif, USA, 1993.

[36] G. W. Cheung and R. B. Rensvold, "Evaluating goodness-of-fit indexes for testing measurement invariance," *Structural Equation Modeling*, vol. 9, no. 2, pp. 233–255, 2002.

[37] L. J. Cronbach, "Coefficient alpha and the internal structure of tests," *Psychometrika*, vol. 16, no. 3, pp. 297–334, 1951.

[38] L. S. Feldt, D. J. Woodruff, and F. A. Salih, "Statistical inference for coefficient alpha," *Applied Psychological Measurement*, vol. 11, no. 1, pp. 93–103, 1987.

[39] T. Raykov, "Scale reliability, Cronbach's Coefficient Alpha, and violations of essential tau-equivalence with fixed congeneric components," *Multivariate Behavioral Research*, vol. 32, no. 4, pp. 329–353, 1997.

[40] T. Raykov, "Behavioral scale reliability and measurement invariance evaluation using latent variable modeling," *Behavior Therapy*, vol. 35, no. 2, pp. 299–331, 2004.

[41] J. Wang and X. Wang, *Structural Equation Modeling: Applications Using Mplus*, John Wiley & Sons, 2012.

[42] M. M. Butts and L. C. Michels, "The sources of four commonly reported cutoff criteria: what did they really say?" *Organizational Research Methods*, vol. 9, no. 2, pp. 202–220, 2006.

24

Reporting Melanoma: A Nationwide Surveillance of State Cancer Registries

Kehinde O. Raji,[1] Lauren Payne,[2] and Suephy C. Chen[3,4]

[1]*Department of Internal Medicine, Scripps Clinic/Scripps Green Hospital, 10666 N. Torrey Pines Road, La Jolla, CA 92037, USA*
[2]*Department of Dermatology, Howard University, 2041 Georgia Avenue NW, Suite 2107, Washington, DC 20060, USA*
[3]*Division of Dermatology, Atlanta VAMC, 1670 Clairmont Road, Decatur, GA 30033, USA*
[4]*Department of Dermatology, Emory University, 1525 Clifton Road NE, 3rd Floor, Atlanta, GA 30322, USA*

Correspondence should be addressed to Suephy C. Chen; schen2@emory.edu

Academic Editor: Silvia Moretti

The goal of our study was to determine current melanoma reporting methods available to dermatologists and dermatopathologists and quantify changes in reporting methods from 2012 to 2014. A cross-sectional study design was utilized consisting of website perusal of reporting procedures, followed up by telephone and email inquiry of reporting methods from every state cancer registry. This study was conducted over a six-month period from February to August 2014. A previous similar survey was conducted in 2012 over the same time frame and results were compared. Kansas state cancer registry provided no data. As of August 2014, 96% of 49 state cancer registries had electronic methods available to all designated reporters. Seven (14%) states required an electronic-only method of reporting melanoma cases. Eighty-six percent allowed hard copy pathology report submission. Compared to the 2012 survey, 2 additional states were found to have initiated electronic reporting methods by 2014. In conclusion, a variety of methods exist for reporting diagnosed melanoma cases. Although most state cancer registries were equipped for electronic transmission of cases for mandated reporters, a number of states were ill-equipped for electronic submission from outpatient dermatologists. There was a general trend towards electronic versus nonelectronic reporting from 2012 to 2014.

1. Introduction

Over the last 10 years, incidence rates of melanoma have increased for both men and women in all age groups, and, according to the United States Cancer Statistics report, there will be an estimated 65,647 melanoma cases in 2014 [1, 2]. Previous studies attributed the increased rates to increased awareness and detection of thin (≤1 mm), perhaps less aggressive, lesions [3–5]. However, more recent studies have found a statistically significant increase in incidence for tumors of all varying histological subtypes and thickness, including tumors >4 mm, indicating that the incidence rates are a true increase [6, 7]. Melanoma, along with other cancers (not including basal or squamous cell carcinomas), is mandated by law to be reported by all physicians and treatment facilities to state cancer registries. However, reporting has been particularly challenging. The advent of new techniques such as Mohs micrographic surgery and the high percentage of melanomas found to be thin lesions, approximately 70% of invasive melanomas reported to the SEER in last decade, have led to decentralization of melanoma management from hospitals to outpatient settings [8, 9]. Also, given the relative ease of access to the skin, the cycle of care may not involve a hospital, as many dermatologists now utilize outpatient-based dermatopathologists and surgical options [10]. Most of the data compiled by state cancer registries are obtained from hospital cancer registries. Therefore, a lack of or delay in detection of many thin melanomas is likely to occur, resulting in underreporting of early stage melanoma [2, 8, 11]. Generating inaccurate trend estimates on melanoma incidence and burden will undermine efforts to effectively allocate resources and implement public health initiatives [8]. It is therefore crucial to focus resources on improving surveillance and reporting methods.

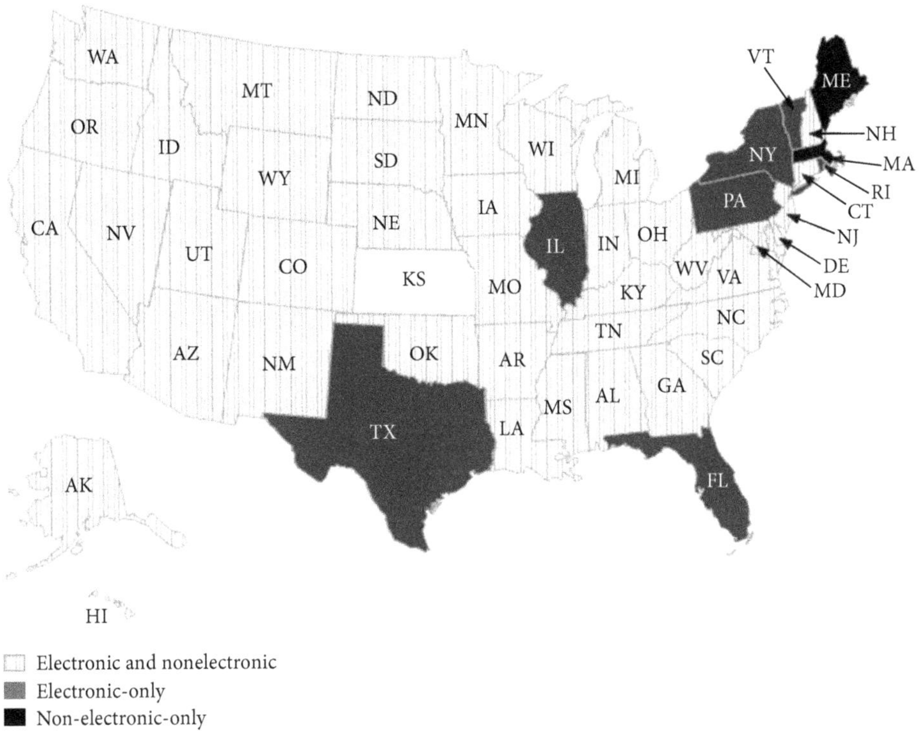

FIGURE 1: Distribution of reporting methods across state central cancer registries. Depiction of state cancer registries that allow reports of diagnosed melanoma cases in both an electronic or nonelectronic format, states that permit only electronic transmission, and states that are yet to have capabilities for electronic transmission.

Awareness of melanoma underreporting is emerging. A survey at a national conference found that 50% of dermatologists were unaware of mandated melanoma reporting and about 56% do not report newly diagnosed cases [12]. Tools to assist the practitioner awareness of methods to report to their state cancer registry may help narrow the knowledge and practice gaps. The purpose of this study is to generate a cross-sectional snapshot of the various reporting methods available to hospitals, outpatient dermatologists, and outpatient pathology labs for reporting diagnosed melanoma cases to their individual state cancer registries. Also, to investigate the dynamics of available reporting methods, we compared this snapshot to data that we obtained in 2012.

2. Methods

As this was publicly available information, IRB approval was not required. In order to accurately capture various reporting methods available to hospitals, independent pathology laboratories, and nonhospital affiliated physicians, we utilized a two-pronged approach. Initially, 50 state cancer registry websites were perused for reporting procedures. After this initial investigation, a brief query was made to every state cancer registry by either email or telephone inquiring about (1) available electronic reporting methods, (2) downloadable online reporting forms, and (3) submission of hard copy pathology reports. The contact information for each state cancer registry was obtained from their individual websites. "Hospital" here encompasses hospital-based pathology labs and hospital-affiliated physicians. "Pathology labs" and "physicians" refer to independent, non-hospital-affiliated entities. From the information gathered, a table of our data was generated depicting various reporting methods available to hospitals, independent pathology labs, and non-hospital-affiliated physicians. An identical survey that was conducted in 2012 was also perused to observe whether there had been a national shift towards electronic reporting methods for melanoma compared to our current survey.

3. Results

All US states were successfully contacted except Kansas despite multiple attempts. Forty-seven (96%) were equipped for electronic transmission of confirmed melanoma cases from hospitals, pathology laboratories, and physicians (Table 1). Maine and Massachusetts were the only 2 states that had yet to implement an electronic method of melanoma reporting (Table 1). Seven (14%) states accepted electronic-only transmittal methods while 40 states (82%) had options for both electronic and nonelectronic reporting methods such as submission of hardcopy pathology reports (Figure 1).

For states that allowed nonelectronic reporting, the alternative methods available to mandated reporters included submission of hard copy pathology reports, registries actively requesting pathology reports of diagnosed cases, and allowing reporters to request melanoma reporting forms. Forty-two (86%) state cancer registries permitted submission of hard copy pathology reports (Table 1). Twenty-seven (55%) state cancer registries actively requested pathology reports from dermatology practices by sending out periodic surveys

TABLE 1: Reporting methods available to mandated melanoma reporters across US state cancer registries.

States (all except Kansas)	Electronic reporting method available	Electronic-only	Non-electronic-only	Hardcopy path reports	Registry requests reports	Provider request reporting forms	Downloadable forms online
Alabama	‡			‡	*	‡	*
Alaska	‡			‡	*	*	‡
Arizona	‡			‡	‡	*	‡
Arkansas	‡			‡	‡	*	‡
California	‡			‡	‡	*	‡
Colorado	‡			‡	‡	‡	*
Connecticut	‡			‡	‡	*	*
Delaware	‡			‡	*	*	‡
Florida	‡	‡		*	*	*	*
Georgia	‡			‡	*	*	*
Hawaii	‡			‡	‡	*	*
Idaho	‡			‡	‡	*	‡
Illinois	‡	‡		*	*	*	*
Indiana	‡			‡	*	‡	‡
Iowa	‡			‡	‡	‡	*
Kentucky	‡			‡	‡	*	*
Louisiana	‡			‡	‡	*	*
Maine	*		‡	‡	*	*	‡
Maryland	‡			‡	‡	*	‡
Massachusetts	*		‡	‡	‡	‡	*
Michigan	‡			‡	*	*	‡
Minnesota	‡			‡	‡	*	*
Mississippi	‡			‡	‡	‡	*
Missouri	‡			‡	*	*	‡
Montana	‡			‡	‡	*	‡
Nebraska	‡			‡	‡	‡	*
Nevada	‡			‡	‡	‡	‡
New Hampshire	‡			‡	‡	*	‡
New Jersey	‡			‡	*	*	‡
New Mexico	‡			‡	‡	*	*
New York	‡	‡		*	*	*	*
North Carolina	‡			‡	‡	*	‡
North Dakota	‡			‡	‡	*	*
Ohio	‡			‡	*	*	‡
Oklahoma	‡			‡	*	*	*
Oregon	‡			‡	*	*	‡
Pennsylvania	‡	‡		*	*	*	*
Rhode Island	‡	‡		*	*	*	*
South Carolina	‡			‡	‡	‡	*
South Dakota	‡			‡	‡	*	*
Tennessee	‡			‡	‡	*	*
Texas	‡	‡		*	*	*	*
Utah	‡			‡	‡	*	‡
Vermont	‡	‡		*	*	*	*
Virginia	‡			‡	*	*	‡
Washington	‡			‡	‡	*	*
West Virginia	‡			‡	*	*	‡

Table 1: Continued.

States (all except Kansas)	Electronic reporting method available	Electronic-only	Non-electronic-only	Hardcopy path reports	Registry requests reports	Provider request reporting forms	Downloadable forms online
Wisconsin	‡			‡	*	*	‡
Wyoming	‡			‡	‡	*	*
Total N (%)	47 (96)	7 (14)	2 (0.04)	42 (86)	27 (55)	9 (18)	22 (45)

‡Available; *not available.

The "Electronic reporting method available" column elucidates the state cancer registries that have the capabilities for electronic reporting of diagnosed melanoma cases. The next two columns depict those states that allow an electronic-only transmission method and states that do not yet have capabilities for electronic transmission. The last four columns depict methods utilized by state cancer registries that allowed nonelectronic reporting. These include submission of hard copy path reports, periodic surveys to request pathology reports from practitioners, allowing providers to request melanoma reporting forms directly from their state cancer registries, and having melanoma reporting forms available for download on their websites.

(Table 1). Nine (18%) states allowed dermatologists to request melanoma reporting forms directly from them (Table 1), and 22 (45%) states had reporting forms available for download on their registry websites (Table 1).

Comparison data exploring shifts in allowable reporting methods showed an increase in electronic reporting methods. In 2012, 4 state cancer registries had non-electronic-only methods for reporting melanoma. In comparison, only 2 states were noted to have such restrictions during 2014. Also, since 2012, three additional state cancer registries have joined four others in requiring an electronic-only reporting method.

4. Discussion

The implementation of the National Program of Cancer Registries (NPCR) in 1992 signified a push to expand and augment state cancer registries and was a crucial step in developing a system that permitted up-to-date cancer surveillance. This, in turn, enhanced research efforts to shed light on cancer distribution, population heterogeneity, and environmental etiologies, all required for more efficient resource allocation for education and screening purposes [13–15]. To ensure that these registries obtain accurate and comprehensive data, it is crucial to recognize gaps in data reporting and generate tools targeted at minimizing this gap as much as possible. To address clinician knowledge and practice gaps, an easy-to-reference table depicting reporting method options may facilitate better data acquisition and thus more robust estimates of melanoma incidence. We propose that these data be made available on the American Academy of Dermatology (AAD) website.

Given the mandate of electronic health records, it is natural to expect that all state registries eventually adopt electronic methods for melanoma reporting. There was a variation in the actual methods each state registry utilized for data transmissions. Some state registries had developed their own software, while, more interestingly, some had implemented the ability for providers eligible for Meaningful Use stage 2 (MU-2) to report melanoma by transmitting their electronic health records directly to the registries. This latter method sounds the most feasible and efficient given the ever-increasing administrative burden on physician practices. However, such a streamlined process faces several challenges given that several facets have yet to be implemented including promotion of physician reporting, on-boarding new providers, and declaration of readiness from state cancer registries. The comparison data from 2012 and 2014 demonstrated an increased shift towards electronic reporting methods by more state registries; however this shift is mostly reflective of hospitals and independent pathology labs being able to report electronically. Outpatient dermatologists still do not have the means to report melanoma cases electronically in 11 states (data not shown) but we speculate a trend towards mandated electronic reporting from clinicians.

The main limitation of our study is the cross-sectional nature of data collection. While the purpose was to create a tool depicting state-specific reporting for dermatologists and independent pathology labs, to be most effective, there should be an ongoing, real-time update such that consumers (dermatologists and pathology labs) can reference current information. Until such a tool can be developed, depicting our data on the publicly accessible website of a national organization such as AAD will hopefully lead to ease of reporting. At the minimum, our results can be utilized in educational efforts of clinicians and dermatopathologists. These efforts will hopefully lead to increased melanoma reporting.

Abbreviations

CDC: Center for Disease Control
NCPR: National Program of Cancer Registries
NCI: National Cancer Institute
MU-2: Meaningful Use stage 2
SEER: Surveillance, Epidemiology, and End Results.

Acknowledgment

The authors are indebted to all the state central cancer registry personnel who responded to inquiries and were willing to share the information they sought.

References

[1] United States Cancer Statistics: 1999–2010 Incidence and Mortality Web-Based Report, US Cancer Statistics Working Group, 2013, http://www.cdc.gov/uscs.

[2] M. Watson, C. J. Johnson, V. W. Chen et al., "Melanoma surveillance in the United States: overview of methods," *Journal of the American Academy of Dermatology*, vol. 65, no. 5, supplement 1, pp. S6–S16, 2011.

[3] A. Jemal, M. Saraiya, P. Patel et al., "Recent trends in cutaneous melanoma incidence and death rates in the United States, 1992–2006," *Journal of the American Academy of Dermatology*, vol. 65, no. 5, supplement 1, pp. S17.e1–S17.e11, 2011.

[4] R. A. Swerlick and S. C. Chen, "The melanoma epidemic: more apparent than real?" *Mayo Clinic Proceedings*, vol. 72, no. 6, pp. 559–564, 1997.

[5] H. G. Welch, S. Woloshin, and L. M. Schwartz, "Skin biopsy rates and incidence of melanoma: population based ecological study," *The British Medical Journal*, vol. 331, no. 7515, article 481, 2005.

[6] E. Linos, S. M. Swetter, M. G. Cockburn, G. A. Colditz, and C. A. Clarke, "Increasing burden of melanoma in the United States," *Journal of Investigative Dermatology*, vol. 129, no. 7, pp. 1666–1674, 2009.

[7] US Department of Health and Human Services, *The Surgeon General's Call to Action to Prevent Skin Cancer*, US Department of Health and Human Services, Office of the Surgeon General, Washington, DC, USA, 2014.

[8] M. Cockburn, S. M. Swetter, D. Peng, T. H. M. Keegan, D. Deapen, and C. A. Clarke, "Melanoma underreporting: why does it happen, how big is the problem, and how do we fix it?" *Journal of the American Academy of Dermatology*, vol. 59, no. 6, pp. 1081–1085, 2008.

[9] P. A. Gimotty, D. Guerry, M. E. Ming et al., "Thin primary cutaneous malignant melanoma: a prognostic tree for 10-year metastasis is more accurate than American Joint Committee on cancer staging," *Journal of Clinical Oncology*, vol. 22, no. 18, pp. 3668–3676, 2004.

[10] L. A. Merlino, K. J. Sullivan, D. C. Whitaker, and C. F. Lynch, "The independent pathology laboratory as a reporting source for cutaneous melanoma incidence in Iowa, 1977–1994," *Journal of the American Academy of Dermatology*, vol. 37, no. 4, pp. 578–585, 1997.

[11] H. I. Hall, P. Jamison, J. P. Fulton, G. Clutter, S. Roffers, and P. Parrish, "Reporting cutaneous melanoma to cancer registries in the United States," *Journal of the American Academy of Dermatology*, vol. 49, no. 4, pp. 624–630, 2003.

[12] T. V. Cartee, S. P. Kini, and S. C. Chen, "Melanoma reporting to central cancer registries by US dermatologists: an analysis of the persistent knowledge and practice gap," *Journal of the American Academy of Dermatology*, vol. 65, supplement 1, no. 5, pp. S124–S132, 2011.

[13] J. N. Izquierdo and V. J. Schoenbach, "The potential and limitations of data from population-based state cancer registries," *American Journal of Public Health*, vol. 90, no. 5, pp. 695–698, 2000.

[14] B. K. Armstrong, "The role of the cancer registry in cancer control," *Cancer Causes & Control*, vol. 3, no. 6, pp. 569–579, 1992.

[15] P. A. Wingo, H. L. Howe, M. J. Thun et al., "A national framework for cancer surveillance in the United States," *Cancer Causes and Control*, vol. 16, no. 2, pp. 151–170, 2005.

25

Imaging in Patients with Merkel Cell Carcinoma

Elisabeth Enzenhofer, Philipp Ubl, Christian Czerny, and Boban M. Erovic

Department of Otolaryngology Head and Neck Surgery, Medical University of Vienna, Waehringer Guertel 18-20, 1090 Vienna, Austria

Correspondence should be addressed to Boban M. Erovic; boban.erovic@meduniwien.ac.at

Academic Editor: Justin Lee

Merkel cell carcinoma (MCC) is a rare, aggressive neuroendocrine tumor of the skin with a mortality rate of approximately 25% (Peloschek et al., 2010). Accurate assessment of nodal involvement in patients with MCC predicts significantly overall outcome (Smith et al., 2012 and Ortin-Perez et al., 2007). Due to the rarity of this highly aggressive disease, only a few imaging reports on MCC were published, and subsequently still to date no accepted imaging algorithm for MCC is available. For primary staging of MCC, general recommendations have included ultrasonography, chest X-ray CT, and MRI, but recent articles show that the use of sentinel node and FDG-PET/PET-CT is gaining more and more importance.

1. Introduction and Overview

Merkel cell carcinoma is a rare and highly aggressive neuroendocrine tumor of the skin. It develops predominantly on sun-exposed area of the head and neck [1, 2]. In 1972, Toker described an unknown, trabecular carcinoma of the skin in five caucasian patients [3]. In 1982, Tang and Toker proposed that the MCC derives from the Merkel cell, a mechanoreceptor of the hair follicle [3, 4].

MCC typically develops rapidly and manifests as firm, nontender, dome-shaped red, purple or violet nodule [5, 6]. The overlying skin is smooth and shiny, sometimes exhibiting ulcerative, acneiform, or telangiectatic features [5, 7].

MCC tends to metastasize to the regional nodes and in 50% of the patients it spreads hematogenously to other organs [8], that is, the liver, bone, brain, and lung [2]. In 1993, Haag and colleagues defined a commonly used staging system [2, 9]: stage I is defined by local disease without lymph node involvement or distant metastases, in stage II carcinoma has spread to lymph nodes but no systemic metastases are detectable, and in stage III distant metastases are detectable [9].

Diagnosis of MCC can be challenging because in many cases MCC lesions mimic benign skin lesions [10]. Unfortunately, in clinical practice, lesions highly suspicious for Merkel cell carcinoma are often biopsied or nonaccurately resected with close margins [2]. In fact, patients presenting with unclear new skin lesions should undergo clinical examination, and lesion still highly suspicious for Merkel cell carcinoma should be excised with clear and wide margins. Diagnosis and management of nodal metastasis in patients without a primary tumor can be challenging. In particular MCC metastasis can mimic metastasis from other small cell neoplasms, that is, for example lung carcinoma [3, 11]. In 2%–19% of the patients no primary tumor can be found—defined as MCC of unknown primary (MCCUP) [11]. Due to the rarity of this disease, the literature on MCCUP is very limited [12, 13].

Agelli performed multiple epidemiological studies showing that between 1986 and 2001 the age-adapted incidence of MCC has increased 3-fold with an annual increase of 8% [14]. This growing incidence rate has given a significant input for a growing interest in disease management of patients with Merkel cell carcinoma [15, 16].

Unfortunately, there is sparse literature on imaging algorithms in patients with Merkel cell carcinoma and no widely accepted guidelines for imaging of Merkel cell carcinoma are available [5, 8]. This paper reviews the literature on imaging of Merkel cell carcinoma discussing the role of the most recent imaging and diagnostic tools.

2. Ultrasonography

Ultrasonography is a highly accurate and cost-effective technique in tumor staging. In regard to Merkel cell carcinoma, work up and staging of the neck should be started with an ultrasonographic examination [2].

Primary skin lesions can appear as single or multicentric hypoechoic solid nodules arising from the dermis and extending in the subcutaneous fat, with variable degrees of posterior acoustic transmission [5, 8]. Ultrasonographic features of Merkel cell carcinoma appear similar to more common skin tumors such as melanoma or basal cell carcinoma [8]. It has been shown that in sonographically easy accessible regions, such as the neck, differentiation of malignant from benign lymph nodes can be achieved with an accuracy of 89%–94% [17, 18]. Furthermore, ultrasonography has a key role in real-time imaging during fine needle biopsy of nonpalpable lesions of Merkel cell carcinoma [8]. Except for a few published case reports, ultrasound guided and nonguided fine needle aspiration biopsy has been rarely described in MCC patients [19–23]. Definitive diagnosis of metastatic disease is challenging with fine needle aspiration cytology alone [20]. The cytomorphology resembles numerous other malignancies such as malignant lymphoma and malignant melanoma [23]. Nevertheless, FNA of MCC can provide an accurate and reliable diagnosis of primary or recurrent metastatic lesions [23]. In patients where positive nodes are proven, a full body imaging should be done to detect distant metastases [16].

3. Sentinel Node Biopsy (SLNB)

Sentinel lymph node biopsy provides the unique capacity to detect metastasis and micrometastasis and subsequently lymph metastasis node draining [5] in patients with melanoma [5], squamous cell carcinoma [24], and MCC [5] by using lymphoscintigraphy [25]. SLNB in patients with Merkel cell carcinoma appears to be a reliable staging technique, whereas the prognostic relevance of positive tumor status of the sentinel node still remains unclear [26].

In up to two-thirds of patients with stage I MCC disease, regional nodal spread has been diagnosed at initial presentation with SNLB, and in only 7%–31% nodes are clinically palpable in patients with stage II disease [5].

Lymphatic drainage pathways in the head and neck region are more variable than in any other location of the body and are challenging to be accurately predicted [27]. Occasionally, head and neck lymphoscintigrams fail to identify a definitive lymphatic drainage pattern [27]. In particular, unexpected nodal drainage is seen in 37%–84% of cases and is often missed without the use of lymphoscintigraphic guidance [5, 28]. Negative sentinel biopsy appears to be a relevant prognostic factor for disease-free survival [26]. Consequently, false-negative findings in lymphadenectomy are leading to inadequate staging of MCC and aggressive but unnecessary complete nodal dissection in patients with true stage I disease [5].

However, Stadelmann and colleagues showed that in 5%–6,8% of patients with melanoma or Merkel cell carcinoma of the head and neck region, no nodal disease could be detected [27]. In particular, in 5 out of 74 clinically node-negative patients who underwent preoperative lymphoscintigraphy, lymphoscintigram failed to identify positive nodes metastases [27]. In 2002, Nguyen and colleagues recommended lymphoscintigraphy in combination with perioperative lymphatic mapping.

4. Computed Tomography (CT)

Due to the usefulness of CT for imaging lymph nodes of the head and neck as well as for nodular metastases in subcutaneous fat and visceral metastases, several authors proposed that CT is a reliable imaging method for the initial staging of patients with Merkel cell carcinoma [2, 5, 8]. In particular, Colgan and colleagues proposed sensitivity and specificity rates of 47% and 97%, respectively, with positive and negative predictive values of 94% and 68%, respectively, for diagnosis of lymph node involvement by CT imaging [29]. However, Peloschek and coworkers claimed a specificity of 96.2% and a sensitivity of 89.1% for CT in diagnostic imaging of Merkel cell carcinoma including lymph node involvement as well as evaluation of distant metastasis [2].

Compared to the muscle, primary skin lesions appear as isodense to slightly hyperdense cutaneous rounded nodules extending below the skin [30]. Cutaneous fat stranding adjacent to the primary lesion suggests engorgement and edema from lymphatic invasion [8]. Furthermore, enhanced CT scan is able to demonstrate high-attenuation lymphadenopathy and soft CT scan is able to demonstrate high-attenuation tissue nodules, which are often clinically silent [5, 8, 30], suggesting focal metastases [30]. Lymphadenopathy mostly occurs in the neck, especially in the parotid region followed by the axilla, mediastinum, retroperitoneum, and groin. Distant metastases include local and retroperitoneal lymph nodes, liver, bone, brain, and lung [31]. Using CT-imaging, metastases of abdominal organs manifest as hypervascular lesions with ring-like enhancement [5]. Soft-tissue metastases may involve the chest wall or abdominal wall with musculoskeletal invasion. Gollub and colleagues conducted a study in 12 patients with MCC and showed the ability of CT scanning to detect visceral and nodal metastases. They suggest follow-up CT scans at 3, 6, 12, and 18 months after initial treatment to discover recurrent disease [30].

5. Magnetic Resonance Imaging (MRI)

There are only a few studies and case reports describing the usefulness of MRI in patients with MCC. In particular, case reports on large primary tumors of the sinonasal region [32], and abdominal wall [33] described MCC lesions as inhomogeneous in signal intensity on T1- and T2-weighted images [33, 34]. Focal central increased signal intensity on T2-weighted images within large lesions has been described as being associated with histologically proven central necrosis and hemorrhage [33, 34]. In MRI scans, lymphatic satellite lesions are reflected by reticular stranding and subcutaneous masses. The same appearance of satellite lesions can be observed by CT imaging. Large lymph node metastases appear as lesions with fine, compressed, retained fatty tissue [34].

Colgan showed in a study of 7 patients who underwent first MRI followed by sentinel lymph node biopsy or regional lymph node dissection a positive predictive value of 0% and a negative predictive value of 67% for the MRI [29]. However, Anderson and colleagues showed in 15 patients that MRI improves differentiation of distant metastases [34]. Furthermore, intramuscular masses and perifascial tumors were better defined on MRI than by CT imaging [34].

MRI in Merkel cell carcinomas is highly accurate for evaluating soft tissue metastases, as well as involvement of brain and bone marrow. Invasion of the central nervous system is rare; however, in case of neurologic symptoms, workup should be performed with MRI [5, 35].

6. Somatostatin Receptor Scintigraphy (SRS)

The rational for performing somatostatin receptor scintigraphy in MCC patients to detect locoregional and distant metastatic disease is based on the neuroendocrine characteristics of MCC. In 1992, Kweekeboom and colleagues presented data for the effectiveness of SRS in 4 patients with MCC. In all 4 patients, in whom the tumor was detected by CT and sonography, tumor sites were also detected in SRS. They showed that SRS had an equal or greater sensitivity than CT for imaging of MCC [36].

Nevertheless, more recent studies observed a limited sensitivity of SRS as well as a high rate of false positive and negative results [37–39]. Guiltera presented their 7-year experience with 20 patients with MCC. In particular, sensitivity of 78% and specificity of 96% for SRS of Merkel cell carcinoma could be observed [38].

A comparison between SRS, CT and MRI showed that tissue SRS is less affected by inflammation, edema, granulation tissue at surgically pretreated or irradiated sites [5]. However, there is a significantly limited value in organs showing a physiological uptake of radiolabelled octreotide such as liver, adrenal glands, pancreas, thyroid gland, and spleen [5, 37]. This causes a low tumor-to-background ratio, which hampers detection of metastasis near organs with a high physiological uptake of the tracer [37]. Further, other systemic diseases such as sarcoidosis, tuberculosis, Wegener's granulomatosis, non-Hodgkin lymphoma, or Hodgkin's disease have also led to false positive SRS results [37, 40].

Unfortunately, a limited use of SRS in diagnostic evaluation of Merkel cell carcinoma. Therefore many authors do not recommend SRS for routine imaging [37, 38].

7. Positron Emission Tomography (PET) and Positron Emission Computed Tomography (PET-CT)

Within the last years nuclear medicine, especially PET and PET-CT, has gained importance in diagnostic imaging of Merkel cell carcinoma. Since MCC is a rapid growing tumor, it is expected that tumor cells have an increased glycolysis [2].

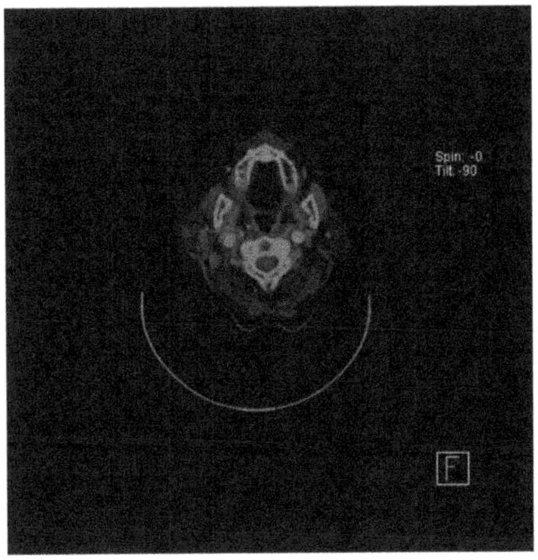

FIGURE 1: PET/CT: pathologic enhancement in the right parotideal region.

^{18}F-FDG is a glucose analog and a surrogate marker for glucose metabolism [41]. In particular, increased glycolysis in certain areas compared to healthy tissue is a distinctive feature of malignant transformation. Increased glycolysis can be captured using the FDG positron emission tomography (PET) technique allowing differentiation between normal and malignant tissue [5] as shown in Figure 1.

The main difficulty with PET alone is the lack of an anatomical reference frame. The hybrid of FDG-PET and the morphological data of CT have potential to improve specificity of PET [2].

Several studies in ^{18}FDG-PET and PET-CT supported the effectiveness in detecting locoregional nodal and distant metastatic disease and subsequently staging in patients with MCC [2, 42–47].

Unfortunately, only few data are available comparing ^{18}FDG-PET and PET-CT with the gold standard of histopathologic nodal evaluation and other imaging tools in MCC patients.

In a study comparing FDG-PET-CT, MRI, bone scan, and computerized tomography in 11 patients, the authors could show that FDG-PET has a sensitivity of 92% and specificity of 100%, and in 3 patients FDG-PET-CT allowed a more precise anatomic localization of lesions [42]. Furthermore, Concannon et al. found, in a retrospective study of 18 patients with MCC who underwent FDG-PET-CT imaging, that FDG-PET-CT resulted in altered staging in 33% of patients and in changes in disease management in 43% of the patients [36]. However, a retrospective study in 15 patients showed a significant advantage of FDG-PET-CT compared to clinical examination in 46% of patients, whereas sensitivity, specificity, and positive and negative predictive value were the same for PET-CT and CT, respectively [48].

In a retrospective study, Peloschek and colleagues described that FDG-PET has a sensitivity of 85,7% and a specificity of 96,2% compared to a sensitivity of 95,5% and specificity of 89,1% for conventional imaging methods [2]. In another study, Grewal et al. reported the sensitivity and specificity of FDG-PET in MCC as 79% to 92% [49].

The most significant drawback of this technique is the fact that in some cases metabolic trapping can be nonspecific and in addition to tumor cells it can also be found in sites of inflammation or infection [50]. In case of brain metastases FDG-PET scanning is significantly hampered due to the high metabolic rate. Subsequently high cerebral background impairs detection of metastatic lesions in the brain [51]. Furthermore, some authors describe a failure of FDG-PET-CT in detection of lymph nodes micrometastases and distant metastatic disease [29, 48].

7.1. Alternative Tracers. Biogenic amines are enhanced and accumulated in neuroendocrine tumors and are an alternative PET tracer for MCC to visualize malignant tissue [2]. A case report described that, due to the less intense uptake of ^{18}F-DOPA, it is more accurate in diagnosis of brain metastases ^{18}F-DOPA compared to FDG-PET and is as accurate in detection of more extracranial metastases [45]. However, Peloschek et al. showed in a study, superior value of FDG-PET in detection of malignant sites of MCC, showing two false negative regions in ^{18}F-DOPA-PET [2]. Furthermore, diffuse ^{18}F-DOPA uptake was ^{18}F-DOPA seen in a region pretreated with surgery and ^{18}F-DOPA irradiation, which was similar to that in FDG-PET that hampers the idea of a benefit of ^{18}F-DOPA. Thus, ^{18}F-DOPA-PET cannot be recommended for diagnostic imaging ^{18}F-DOPA in Merkel cell carcinoma [2].

7.2. Follow-Up Imaging. After treatment of primary lesions of MCC, a close monitoring is required.

For follow-up imaging, we would suggest a routine chest X-ray as well as a computed tomography of the head and neck region 3 months after therapy. Every year after therapy, a chest X-ray, CT and MRI of the head and neck region are recommended. 6, 9, 15, 18, 21, and 30 months after therapy a cervical ultrasonography and a chest X-ray should be performed. Because of the low cost of sonography, it has a high value in routine follow-up imaging of Merkel cell carcinoma [2]. Chest X-ray is a routine imaging technique to evaluate possible pulmonary involvement. Peloschek et al. recommend repetition of FDG-PET 3 months and 1 year after treatment [2].

8. Discussion

The key task of imaging in patients with Merkel cell carcinoma is staging at the initial presentation and post-therapeutical.

Early recommendations for imaging in MCC included ultrasonography CT, MRI, and octreotide scans [29]. Recently, ^{18}FDG-PET has become a valuable and useful imaging technique for staging in patients suffering from MCC. Its diagnostic value is comparable to conventional imaging methods that have a restricted field of view [2].

Peloschek et al. recommend that initial staging workup should be started with ultrasonography as it is cost-effective and an accurate imaging method in easy accessible lymph node regions such as the head and neck [2]. There is rarely literature available dealing with ultrasound-guided fine needle biopsy of Merkel cell carcinoma. Definitive diagnosis is difficult but possible and accurate with FNA [19, 20].

In oncologic patients with suspected distant metastases FDG-PET, CT or MRI imaging should be performed. Somatostatin receptor scintigraphy is no longer recommended for routine imaging of Merkel cell carcinoma, as studies showed a high rate of false-positive or false-negative results in detection of Merkel cell carcinomas and metastatic disease [37].

As Merkel cell carcinoma has a high rate of distant metastasis, PET scan has a particular value in imaging and staging workup.

MRI has a particular value in assessing soft-tissue involvement, whereas CT is used for imaging of thorax and abdomen. Three months and 1 year after treatment, FDG-PET should be repeated for follow-up imaging. Moreover, fusion of FDG-PET with CT or MRI would improve specificity of PET analysis [2].

Colgan et al. reported that the use of FDG-PET when compared with traditional computed tomography is significantly more sensitive and equally specific than FDG-PET alone in evaluation of regional lymph node basins in primary MCC [29].

The role of FDG-PET-CT in management of MCC remains to be a matter of debate. However, PET-CT has been shown to have a potential high impact of staging and management of MCC patients with stage I and II disease [43].

To date, there is still no imaging algorithm for Merkel cell carcinoma. Due to the rarity of Merkel cell carcinoma imaging, findings have been reported only in small trials and case reports. On the basis of the existing literature, we would recommend FDG-PET CT as first line imaging of Merkel cell carcinoma. It is a noninvasive imaging technique that has potential to detect occult lesions bigger than 5–8 mm in minimal diameter [48] that are not detectable by other imaging techniques. We suggest that further diagnostic imaging should be obtained depending on the results of lymph node involvement and distant metastases.

However, in case of negative lymph node involvement, we would recommend sentinel lymph node mapping with subsequently performing an ipsilateral neck dissection to confirm lymph node status histopathologically. In our opinion, due to the low morbidity of a neck dissection, it has a high diagnostic and preventive value.

In summary, Merkel cell carcinoma is a highly aggressive skin cancer with a high rate of metastasis and mortality. Since no imaging guidelines are available, more studies are required to define an evidence-based imaging algorithm.

References

[1] C. Suárez, J. P. Rodrigo, A. Ferlito, K. O. Devaney, and A. Rinaldo, "Merkel cell carcinoma of the head and neck," *Oral Oncology*, vol. 40, no. 8, pp. 773–779, 2004.

[2] P. Peloschek, C. Novotny, C. Mueller-Mang et al., "Diagnostic imaging in Merkel cell carcinoma: lessons to learn from 16 cases with correlation of sonography, CT, MRI and PET," *European Journal of Radiology*, vol. 73, no. 2, pp. 317–323, 2010.

[3] C. Toker, "Trabecular carcinoma of the skin," *Archives of Dermatology*, vol. 105, no. 1, pp. 107–110, 1972.

[4] C. K. Tang, C. Toker, A. Nedwich, and A. N. F. Zaman, "Unusual cutaneous carcinoma with features of small cell (oat cell-like) and squamous cell carcinomas. A variant of malignant merkel cell neoplasm," *American Journal of Dermatopathology*, vol. 4, no. 6, pp. 537–548, 1982.

[5] B. D. Nguyen and A. E. McCullough, "Imaging of merkel cell carcinoma," *Radiographics*, vol. 22, no. 2, pp. 367–376, 2002.

[6] C. L. Hitchcock, K. I. Bland, R. G. Laney, D. Franzini, B. Harris, and E. M. Copeland III, "Neuroendocrine (Merkel cell) carcinoma of the skin. Its natural history, diagnosis, and treatment," *Annals of Surgery*, vol. 207, no. 2, pp. 201–207, 1988.

[7] W. J. O'Connor and D. G. Brodland, "Merkel cell carcinoma," *Dermatologic Surgery*, vol. 22, pp. 262–267, 1996.

[8] F. Eftekhari, S. Wallace, E. G. Silva, and R. Lenzi, "Merkel cell carcinoma of the skin: imaging and clinical features in 93 cases," *British Journal of Radiology*, vol. 69, no. 819, pp. 226–233, 1996.

[9] M. L. Haag, L. F. Glass, and N. A. Fenske, "Merkel cell carcinoma: diagnosis and treatment," *Dermatologic Surgery*, vol. 21, no. 8, pp. 669–683, 1995.

[10] M. Heath, N. Jaimes, B. Lemos et al., "Clinical characteristics of Merkel cell carcinoma at diagnosis in 195 patients: the AEIOU features," *Journal of the American Academy of Dermatology*, vol. 58, no. 3, pp. 375–381, 2008.

[11] L. Jeremiah, J. L. Messina, S. S. Marzban et al., "Merkel cell carcinoma of unknown primary origin," *Annals of Surgical Oncology*, vol. 19, no. 7, pp. 2360–2366, 2012.

[12] E. J. Kim, H. S. Kim, H. O. Kim et al., "Merkel cell carcinoma of the inguinal lymph node with an unknown primary site," *Journal of Dermatology*, vol. 36, no. 3, pp. 170–173, 2009.

[13] I. S. Winer, F. Lonardo, S. C. Johnson, and G. Deppe, "Merkel cell carcinoma in a patient with noninvasive vulvular Paget's disease," *American Journal of Obstetrics & Gynecology*, vol. 207, no. 1, pp. e9–e11, 2012.

[14] M. Agelli, L. X. Clegg, J. C. Becker, and D. E. Rollison, "The etiology and epidemiology of merkel cell carcinoma," *Current Problems in Cancer*, vol. 34, no. 1, pp. 14–37, 2010.

[15] J. C. Becker, "Merkel cell carcinoma," *Annals of Oncology*, vol. 21, no. 7, pp. vii81–vii85, 2010.

[16] E. Ramahi, J. Choi, C. D. Fuller, and T. Y. Eng, "Merkel cell carcinoma," *American Journal of Clinical Oncology*, pp. 1–10, 2011.

[17] S. Jank, P. Robatscher, R. Emshoff, H. Strobl, G. Gojer, and B. Norer, "The diagnostic value of ultrasonography to detect occult lymph node involvement at different levels in patients with squamous cell carcinoma in the maxillofacial region," *International Journal of Oral and Maxillofacial Surgery*, vol. 32, no. 1, pp. 39–42, 2003.

[18] J. F. Griffith, A. C. W. Chan, A. T. Ahuja et al., "Neck ultrasound in staging squamous oesophageal carcinoma—a high yield technique," *Clinical Radiology*, vol. 55, no. 9, pp. 696–701, 2000.

[19] T. P. Jessup, W. Y. Wassef, R. K. Yantiss, and K. Bhattacharya, "Metastatic Merkel cell carcinoma diagnosed by EUS-guided FNA of a rapidly progressive peripancreatic mass," *Gastrointestinal Endoscopy*, vol. 63, no. 3, pp. 527–529, 2006.

[20] J. Bernstein, A. J. Adeniran, G. Cal et al., "Endoscopic ultrasound-guided fine needle aspiration diagnosis of merkel cell carcinoma metastatic to the pancreas," *Diagnostic Cytopathology*, 2012.

[21] S. Sanchez-Gàrcia, C. Manzanares-Campillo, P. Menéndez-Sànchez, V. Munoz- Atienza, and J. Martin-Fernández, "Merkel cell carcinoma and literature review," *Cirugia y Cirujanos*, vol. 80, no. 1, pp. 63–66, 2012.

[22] L. Stoll, S. Mudali, and S. Z. Ali, "Merkel cell carcinoma metastatic to the thyroid gland: aspiration findings and differential diagnosis," *Diagnostic Cytopathology*, vol. 38, no. 10, pp. 754–757, 2010.

[23] B. T. Collins, P. G. Elmberger, E. M. Tani, V. Bjornhagen, and R. R. Ramos, "Fine-needle aspiration of Merkel cell carcinoma of the skin with cytomorphology and immunocytochemical correlation," *Diagnostic Cytopathology*, vol. 18, no. 4, pp. 251–257, 1998.

[24] F. J. Civantos, S. J. Stoeckli, R. P. Takes et al., "What is the role of sentinel lymph node biopsy in the management of oral cancer in 2010?" *European Archives of Oto-Rhino-Laryngology*, vol. 267, no. 6, pp. 839–844, 2010.

[25] S. Brodsky, J. S. Zager, and C. G. Berman, "Imaging of merkel cell carcinoma," in *Merkel Cell Carcinoma: A Multidisciplinary Approach*, chapter 9, pp. 159–169, 2010.

[26] J. Ortin-Perez, M. C. van Rijk, R. A. Valdes-Olmos et al., "Lymphatic mapping and sentinel node biopsy in Merkel's cell carcinoma," *European Journal of Surgical Oncology*, vol. 33, no. 1, pp. 119–122, 2007.

[27] W. K. Stadelmann, L. Cobbins, E. J. Lentsch, and J. J. Disa, "Incidence of nonlocalization of sentinel lymph nodes using preoperative lymphoscintigraphy in 74 consecutive head and neck melanoma and Merkel cell carcinoma patients," *Annals of Plastic Surgery*, vol. 52, no. 6, pp. 546–550, 2004.

[28] S. P. L. Leong, T. A. Achtem, F. A. Habib et al., "Discordancy between clinical predictions vs lymphoscintigraphic and intraoperative mapping of sentinel lymph node drainage of primary melanoma," *Archives of Dermatology*, vol. 135, no. 12, pp. 1472–1476, 1999.

[29] M. B. Colgan, T. I. Tarantola, A. L. Weaver et al., "The predictive value of imaging studies in evaluating regional lymph node involvement in merkel cell carcinoma," *Journal of the American Academy of Dermatology*, vol. 67, no. 6, pp. 1250–1256, 2012.

[30] M. J. Gollub, D. R. Gruen, and D. David Dershaw, "Merkel cell carcinoma: CT findings in 12 patients," *American Journal of Roentgenology*, vol. 167, no. 3, pp. 617–620, 1996.

[31] L. I. Canales, A. Parker, and S. Kadakia, "Upper gastrointestinal bleeding from Merkel cell carcinoma," *American Journal of Gastroenterology*, vol. 87, no. 10, pp. 1464–1466, 1992.

[32] L. Azizi, K. Marsot-Dupuch, P. Bigel, S. Mzali, B. Meyer, and J. M. Tubiana, "Merkel cell carcinoma: a rare cause of hypervascular nasal tumor," *American Journal of Neuroradiology*, vol. 22, no. 7, pp. 1389–1393, 2001.

[33] P. Dunlop, H. Sapp, P. M. Logan, and N. M. G. Walsh, "Merkel cell carcinoma of the abdominal wall," *Skeletal Radiology*, vol. 27, no. 7, pp. 396–399, 1998.

[34] S. E. Anderson, K. T. Beer, A. Banic et al., "MRI of Merkel cell carcinoma: histologic correlation and review of the literature," *American Journal of Roentgenology*, vol. 185, no. 6, pp. 1441–1448, 2005.

[35] F. Ikawa, K. Kiya, T. Uozumi et al., "Brain metastasis of merkel cell carcinoma: case report and review of the literature," *Neurosurgical Review*, vol. 22, no. 1, pp. 54–57, 1999.

[36] D. J. Kwekkeboom, A. M. Hoff, S. W. J. Lamberts, H. Yoe Oei, and E. P. Krenning, "Somatostatin analogue scintigraphy: a simple and sensitive method for the In vivo visualization of Merkel

cell tumors and their metastases," *Archives of Dermatology*, vol. 128, no. 6, pp. 818–821, 1992.

[37] B. K. Durani, A. Klein, M. Henze, U. Haberkorn, and W. Hartschuh, "Somatostatin analogue scintigraphy in Merkel cell tumours," *British Journal of Dermatology*, vol. 148, no. 6, pp. 1135–1140, 2003.

[38] P. Guitera-Rovel, J. Lumbroso, M. S. Gautier-Gougis et al., "Indium-111 octreotide scintigraphy of Merkel cell carcinomas and their metastases," *Annals of Oncology*, vol. 12, no. 6, pp. 807–811, 2001.

[39] C. O. Wong, A. N. Pham, and H. J. Dworkin, "F-18 FDG accumulation in an octreotide negative merkel cell tumor," *Clinical Positron Imaging*, vol. 3, no. 2, pp. 71–73, 2000.

[40] E. G. Eising, D. Bier, E. J. Knust, and C. Reiners, "Somatostatin-receptor scintigraphy methods-indications-results," *Radiologe*, vol. 36, no. 1, pp. 81–88, 1996.

[41] V. A. Smith, E. Ramssay Camp, and E. J. Lentsch, "Merkel cell carcinoma: identification of prognostic factors unique to tumors located in the head and neck based on analysis of SEER Data," *Laryngoscope*, vol. 122, pp. 1283–1290, 2012.

[42] T. Belhocine, G. E. Pierard, J. Frühling et al., "Clinical added-value of 18FDG PET in neuroendocrine-merkel cell carcinoma," *Oncology Reports*, vol. 16, no. 2, pp. 347–352, 2006.

[43] R. Concannon, G. S. Larcos, and M. Veness, "The impact of 18F-FDG PET-CT scanning for staging and management of Merkel cell carcinoma: results from Westmead Hospital, Sydney, Australia," *Journal of the American Academy of Dermatology*, vol. 62, no. 1, pp. 76–84, 2010.

[44] A. Iagaru, A. Quon, I. R. McDougall, and S. S. Gambhir, "Merkel cell carcinoma: is there a role for 2-Deoxy-2-[F-18]fluoro-D-glucose-positron emission tomography/computed tomography?" *Molecular Imaging and Biology*, vol. 8, no. 4, pp. 212–217, 2006.

[45] J. N. Talbot, K. Kerrou, F. Missoum et al., "6-[F-18]fluoro-L-DOPA positron emission tomography in the imaging of Merkel cell carcinoma: preliminary report of three cases with 2-deoxy-2-[F-18]fluoro-D-glucose positron emission tomography or pentetreotide-(111In) SPECT data," *Molecular Imaging and Biology*, vol. 7, no. 4, pp. 257–261, 2005.

[46] S. G. Gupta, L. C. Wang, P. F. Peñas, M. Gellenthin, S. J. Lee, and P. Nghiem, "Sentinel lymph node biopsy for evaluation and treatment of patients with Merkel cell carcinoma: the Dana-Farber experience and meta-analysis of the literature," *Archives of Dermatology*, vol. 142, no. 6, pp. 685–690, 2006.

[47] J. L. Lampreave, F. Bénard, A. Alavi, J. Jimenez-Hoyuela, and D. Fraker, "PET evaluation of therapeutic limb perfusion in Merkel's cell carcinoma," *Journal of Nuclear Medicine*, vol. 39, no. 12, pp. 2087–2090, 1998.

[48] G. Maury, O. Dereure, A. Du-Thanh, D. Mariano-Goulart, and B. Guillot, "Interest of (18)F-FDG PET-CT scanning for staging and management of merkel cell carcinoma: a retrospective study of 15 patients," *Journal of the European Academy of Dermatology and Venereology*, vol. 25, no. 12, pp. 1420–1427, 2011.

[49] R. K. Grewal, N. Pandit-Taskar, M. Gonen, and S. M. Larson, "FDG-PET for evaluation of Merkel cell carcinoma," *Journal of Nuclear Medicine*, vol. 46, no. 2, abstract 137, 2005.

[50] O. Warburg, K. Posener, and E. Negelein, "The metabolism of cancer cells," *Biochemischen Zeitschrift*, vol. 152, pp. 129–169, 1924.

[51] G. Larcos and M. N. Maisey, "FDG-PET screening for cerebral metastases in patients with suspected malignancy," *Nuclear Medicine Communications*, vol. 17, no. 3, pp. 197–198, 1996.

26

Clinical and Demographic Features of Basal Cell Carcinoma in North Jordan

Firas Al-Qarqaz,[1] Maha Marji,[1] Khaldon Bodoor,[2] Rowida Almomani,[3] Wisam Al Gargaz,[4] Diala Alshiyab,[1] Jihan Muhaidat,[1] and Mohammad Alqudah[5]

[1]*Department of Dermatology, Jordan University of Science and Technology, P.O. Box 3030, Irbid, Jordan*
[2]*Department of Applied Biology, Jordan University of Science and Technology, P.O. Box 3030, Irbid, Jordan*
[3]*Department of Medical Laboratory Sciences, Jordan University of Science and Technology, P.O. Box 3030, Irbid, Jordan*
[4]*Department of Special Surgery, Jordan University of Science and Technology, P.O. Box 3030, Irbid, Jordan*
[5]*Department of Pathology, Jordan University of Science and Technology, P.O. Box 3030, Irbid, Jordan*

Correspondence should be addressed to Firas Al-Qarqaz; faalqarqaz@yahoo.com

Academic Editor: Arash Kimyai-Asadi

Basal cell carcinoma (BCC) is the most common cancer affecting humans. It almost has no tendency for metastasis; however it can be destructive to surrounding tissue. Patients with darker skin colors have lower risk of developing skin cancers and the clinical characteristics may differ from populations with lighter skin colors. *Methods*. This is a retrospective clinical study (2003–2017). Data on age, gender, and location of tumor were collected and analyzed. *Results*. 335 cases were identified. Males tend to get BCC at a younger age than females. Face was the most common site in both males and females. Cheeks and nose were the most likely areas of the face to be involved. Scalp was the most common extrafacial site to be involved in males; however in females scalp was much less likely to be involved. *Conclusion*. BCC is less common in populations with darker skin. Males were more affected and at an earlier age compared to females. Facial skin followed by scalp was the most common site affected. Skin phototype, cultural and religious dress type, and different sun exposure behavior may explain many of the clinical and demographic findings related to BCC in patients with darker skin tones.

1. Introduction and Background

Basal cell carcinoma (BCC) is the most common skin cancer especially in populations with fair skin color. The pathogenesis of BCC is linked to excessive sunlight exposure [1]. This explains the predominance of facial involvement by this cancer. Additional factors that increase the risk of BCC development include, among others, genetic alterations HPV infection and immune suppression [2, 3].

Despite being the most common skin cancer, BCC has almost no potential for metastasis and hence the mortality from this tumor is negligible. However, the morbidity from this slowly growing tumor can be significant due to local tissue damage [4, 5].

The incidence of BCC is on the rise worldwide; for example, in Netherlands the incidence increased by 3-fold between 1973 and 2008 from 40 to 148 per 100,000 in males and from 34 to 141 in females [6]. The true incidence is however even higher as these tumors are generally underreported.

The diagnosis of BCC is initially suspected based on the appearance of a slowly growing firm translucent nodule with surface telangiectasia and rolled margins; however there is some variation according to the type of BCC. Dermoscopic examination can provide additional important clues for diagnosis of BCC; however confirmation of diagnosis requires histopathologic examination. Comprehensive pathologic assessments, including histologic subtype, invasion behavior, among other features, are required as prognostic indicators to help predict recurrence and potential for invasion by the tumor cells [7, 8].

Several key genes have been implicated in BCC pathogenesis, especially protooncogenes and tumor suppressor genes.

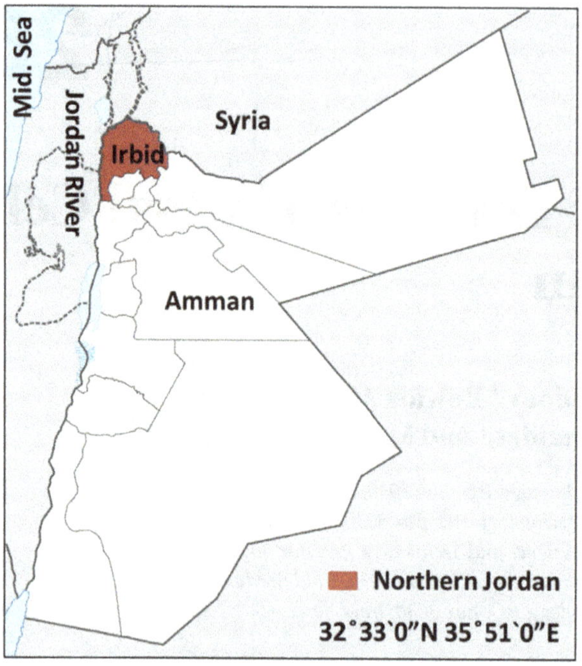

FIGURE 1: Map of Jordan showing the geography of the study area.

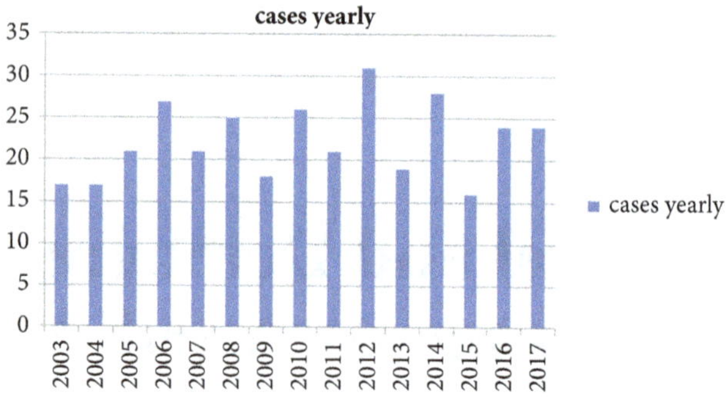

FIGURE 2: Number of BCC new cases over 15 years: 2003-2018.

These include, among others, PTCH1 and SMO genes which are key components of the Hedgehog (Hh) pathway, TP53 gene, and other RAS protooncogene family members [9, 10].

There is wealth of data on BCC in Caucasian skin with lighter skin colors but much less information exist on populations with dark skin [11–14]. It is clear that skin cancer is much less common of a problem in these populations which may explain why there are less interest and data populations with darker skins.

Northern Jordan is part of the Hawran plateau which covers northern Jordan and southwest Syria. The governorate is bordered by Syria (the Golan Heights) from the north, the Jordan River from the west, Mafraq Governorate from the east, and Jerash, Ajloun, and Balqa Governorates from the south (Figure 1). The geographic coordinates for Irbid are 32°33′0″N 35°51′0″E with altitude of around 620 meters. Northern Jordan has a hot-summer, Mediterranean climate with at least 4 months averaging above 30°C (June-September).

In this study we highlight the main demographic and clinical features of BCC in North Jordan population which predominantly has darker skin tones, mainly types 3 and 4.

2. Materials and Methods

This is a retrospective descriptive study. BCC cases were retrieved from the electronic records from the Department of Pathology at King Abdulah University Hospital in Irbid, north of Jordan, for the period 2004-2018. For the year 2003 BCC, cases were included for the calculation of the overall number but were not included in the age-adjusted incidence analysis because population data were missing from the national department of national statistics. The confirmed diagnosis of BCC at the final conclusion of pathology reports was used for the inclusion of these cases. The Pathology Department affiliated to Faculty of Medicine, Jordan University of Science and Technology, is the only pathology department for north of Jordan area with catchment area population of around 1,2 million. Clinicopathological and demographic parameters were statistically analyzed to identify significant correlations. *t*-test was used for calculation of p values using SPSS software package 17. P value was considered significant if it was less than or equal to 0.05. The study was approved by the Research Committee of the Faculty of Medicine and the IRB of the university.

3. Results

A total of 335 confirmed BCC cases were identified and included in the study. The cohort included 214 males and 121 female cases with male: female ratio of 1.76: 1. The mean age for females was 65.4 years (35-91 years), while the mean age for males was 61.9 years (27-96 years). The difference between means of age for males and females was statistically significant (P = 0.018). The average number of new cases of BCC is around 22.3 (16-31) cases per year (Figure 2). There was no significant variation in number of BCC cases over the 15 years (P value 0.31).

The incidence rates of BCC in northern Jordan ranged from 1.5 to 3 per 100,000 population for the years 2004 to 2017. However because BCC is usually increased with age, we also calculated the age-adjusted incidence rates for the study population. Based on the data from the Jordanian Department of Statistics [15], the age-adjusted incidence rates for BCC were calculated for the study population based on age categories: 0-19 years, 20-39 years, 40-64 years, and 65+ years. The age-adjusted incidence rates per 100,000 population results are shown in Table 1. For the age groups 0-39 years, the incidence rates were negligible (0-0.65 per 100,000 population). For the age group 40-65 years, the rates were between 2.4 and 7.7 per 100,000 population. However for the age group above 65 years the incidence rates were higher (9-31 per 100,000 population) as shown in Table 1.

In terms of tumor location, our data clearly shows that face was the most affected site in both males and females, accounting for 77% and 83% of all BCC cases, respectively

TABLE 1: Age adjusted incidence rates for BCC per 100,000 population (2004-2017)*.

	Age categories			
Year	0-19 (Y)	20-39 (Y)	40-64 (Y)	65+ (Y)
2004	0	0.00	4.60	20.86
2005	0	0.28	5.96	20.28
2006	0	0.27	7.71	24.62
2007	0	0.27	3.28	31.07
2008	0	0.26	5.00	30.15
2009	0	0.00	4.40	17.99
2010	0	0.24	5.55	26.15
2011	0	0.23	2.45	29.22
2012	0	0.66	6.93	19.65
2013	0	0.00	2.47	21.59
2014	0	0.00	5.52	18.24
2015	0	0.17	2.69	9.16
2016	0	0.50	3.50	13.41
2017	0	0.00	3.41	17.42

*Population Data for the year 2003 was absent from department of statistics and hence was not represented here.

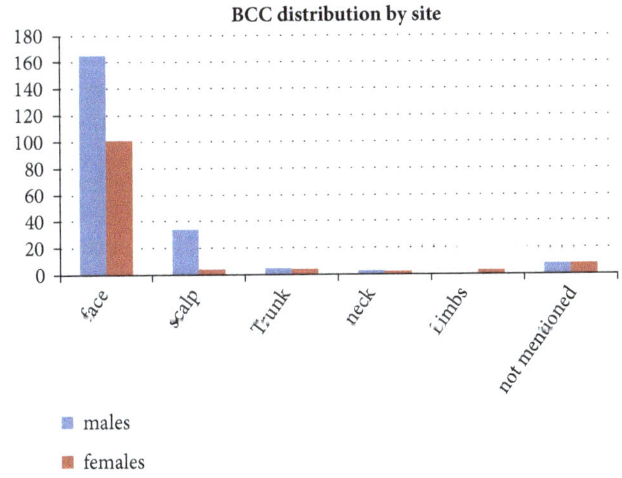

FIGURE 3: BCC distribution according to site.

(Figure 3). The most common nonfacial BCC was scalp in males accounting for 16% of cases, whereas, in females, nonfacial BCC did not show any strong predilection for specific sites with tumors scattered across various body sites (Figure 3).

Facial BCC mainly affected the centrofacial sites, namely, nose, cheeks, and eyelids skin (Figure 3). This distribution does however vary between males and females and this variation is statistically significant (p =0.01). The most important differences in distribution between males and females were related to forehead, ears, and temples being more affected in males but much less in females (18% versus 8% for these sites combined).

Of the 335 cases in this study, 12 cases (8 males and 4 females) had multiple BCCs while the remainder had only one BCC.

4. Discussion

The link between skin cancer and sunlight exposure is well established with increasing incidence of skin cancers in populations living near equator where there is stronger exposure to sunlight and this is especially manifested in populations with fair skin colors. However, in areas where the dominant skin color is dark, the risk for skin cancer is still generally low [16]. In a study from one center in Jordan a predominantly colored-skin population (types 3 and 4 mainly) there were 67 cases over 5 years (around 13 cases per year) [14].

In the current study, the cohort consisted mainly of skin phototypes 3 and 4 making around 82% of all cases. The annual number of new cases of BCC ranged from 16 to 31 with an average of around 22 cases. The difference over the years did not change significantly while in most countries with more fair skin color the incidence of BCC is increasing steadily [16–18].

In this population from north Jordan the overall incidence rate for BCC ranged from 1.5 to 3 per 100,000. In Saudi Arabia, a recent study has indicated incidence rates between 3.4 and 4.4 per 100,000 population [19]. Another study from Iran showed incidence rates for BCC between 10.05 and 15.57 per 100,000 population [20]. Additional studies from Jordan and neighboring countries with similar dark skin color are also in accordance with low incidence rates for BCC reported in this study [21–24]. It is worth noting that, in Caucasian skin populations, the incidence rates for BCC are much higher. For example, in Australia the incidence rate exceeds 1,000 per 100,000 population whereas in the United States the incidence rate is around 450 per 100.000 and in Europe the rate is around 100 per 100,000 [16].

The low incidence rates for BCC over the years in this population could be explained by the darker skin type, chronic rather than intermittent pattern of sun exposure, and generally clothes type covering most body parts except face and hands. Darker skin is more protected against damaging effects of ultraviolet radiation from solar light mostly due to protective effect by melanin [25, 26]. In this population, the general dress behavior pattern is more towards less exposed skin, i.e., long sleeves and long trousers, especially in the case of women who tend to cover almost all body and use head cover whenever they go out of their houses due to religious and social reasons. Additionally, the intermittent sun exposure "recreational" is not commonly seen on the contrary, and most people are chronically exposed to sunlight which implies more basal melanin production rates and hence more skin protection. Taken together, the aforementioned factors could be responsible for the low incidence of BCC in this population despite northern Jordan having sunny bright days during most of the year (average 310 sunny days/year).

In the current study, the average age at time of diagnosis was 61.9 years for males and 65.4 years for females. Males were more affected in this group than females; this is actually similar to what is reported from most countries [11, 27–29].

In terms of tumor location, face was the most common affected site in both males and females. This reflects again the importance of solar radiation as the main causative factor in the pathogenesis of this condition. Other sun-covered skin areas were much less commonly involved. As for extrafacial involvement, scalp was the next common site affected in males but not in females. Hair is an important photoprotector for the scalp and also many females in this population use head cover (scarf) whenever they are outdoors which could also explain the relative rarity of scalp involvement in women from this group.

Within the facial skin, the more sun-exposed regions were more likely to be affected with some variation between males and females. Nose, cheeks, and eyelids were the most sites affected in both sexes. In females, BCC in forehead, ears, and temples were less common than males (p= 0.01). This variation could also be explained by the head cover worn by many females in this population. Other studies have also demonstrated similar distribution of facial BCC with nose and cheeks being the more commonly involved sites [11, 30].

In this cohort, only 12 (3.6%) cases had multiple BCCs which is generally much less than reported by other studies [31, 32]. Multiple BCC is possibly linked to a number of risk factors including age, skin phototype (1 & 2), intermittent sun exposure and sunburns, history of radiotherapy, larger tumor size, truncal tumor, genetic factors, and geography of area especially high latitude [32, 33]. In this cohort, darker skin phototypes (3 & 4) are the most common, truncal BCCs were only seen in 9 patients (2.7%), the pattern of sunlight exposure is nonburning, non of these patients had prior radiotherapy treatment, and the geography of north Jordan is towards low altitude (620 meters). These factors could explain the low number of patients having multiple BCCs.

5. Conclusions

BCC in this population with darker skin color is much less common than in populations with fair skin color. The number of new cases did not change significantly over the past 15 years. Males are more affected and tend to be younger than females at time of diagnosis. Face is the most common site involved especially nose, cheeks, and eyelids. The darker skin color, type of clothing, and pattern of sunlight exposure are likely to explain the lower number of BCC cases and location distribution of BCC in this population.

References

[1] B. K. Armstrong and A. Kricker, "The epidemiology of UV induced skin cancer," *Journal of Photochemistry and Photobiology B: Biology*, vol. 63, no. 1–3, pp. 8–18, 2001.

[2] F. Rahnama, R. Toftgård, and P. G. Zaphiropoulos, "Distinct roles of PTCH2 splice variants in Hedgehog signalling," *Biochemical Journal*, vol. 378, no. 2, pp. 325–334, 2004.

[3] L. Parren and J. Frank, "Hereditary tumour syndromes featuring basal cell carcinomas," *British Journal of Dermatology*, vol. 165, no. 1, pp. 30–34, 2011.

[4] A. G. Marzuka and S. E. Book, "Basal cell carcinoma: pathogenesis, epidemiology, clinical features, diagnosis, histopathology, and management," *Yale Journal of Biology and Medicine*, vol. 88, no. 2, pp. 167–179, 2015.

[5] M. Mackiewicz-Wysocka, M. Bowszyc-Dmochowska, D. Strzelecka-Węklar, A. Dańczak-Pazdrowska, and Z. Adamski, "Reviews Basal cell carcinoma – diagnosis," *Współczesna Onkologia*, vol. 4, pp. 337–342, 2013.

[6] S. Flohil, E. Vries, H. Neumann, J. Coebergh, and T. Nijsten, "Incidence, Prevalence and Future Trends of Primary Basal Cell Carcinoma in the Netherlands," *Acta Dermato-Venereologica*, vol. 91, no. 1, pp. 24–30, 2011.

[7] C. Bichakjian, A. Armstrong, C. Baum et al., "Guidelines of care for the management of basal cell carcinoma," *Journal of the American Academy of Dermatology*, vol. 78, pp. 540–559, 2018.

[8] C. A. McKenzie, A. C. Chen, B. Choy, P. Fernández-Peñas, D. L. Damian, and R. A. Scolyer, "Classification of high risk basal cell carcinoma subtypes: experience of the ONTRAC study with proposed definitions and guidelines for pathological reporting," *Pathology*, vol. 48, no. 5, pp. 395–397, 2016.

[9] X. Bonilla, L. Parmentier, B. King et al., "Genomic analysis identifies new drivers and progression pathways in skin basal cell carcinoma," *Nature Genetics*, vol. 48, no. 4, pp. 398–406, 2016.

[10] E. H. Epstein, "Basal cell carcinomas: attack of the hedgehog," *Nature Reviews Cancer*, vol. 8, no. 10, pp. 743–754, 2008.

[11] C. Devine, B. Srinivasan, A. Sayan, and V. Ilankovan, "Epidemiology of basal cell carcinoma: a 10-year comparative study," *British Journal of Oral and Maxillofacial Surgery*, vol. 56, no. 2, pp. 101–106, 2018.

[12] V. Lai, W. Cranwell, and R. Sinclair, "Epidemiology of skin cancer in the mature patient," *Clinics in Dermatology*, vol. 36, no. 2, pp. 167–176, 2018.

[13] P. T. Bradford, "Skin Cancer in Skin of Color," *Dermatological Nursing*, vol. 21, no. 4, pp. 170–178, 2009.

[14] S. Weshah, R. Smadi, and M. Helalat, "Basal cell carcinoma: A retrospective analysis of 76 patients," *Pakistan Journal of Medical Sciences*, vol. 23, no. 4, pp. 556–560, 2007.

[15] Department of Statistics, 2018, http://dosweb.dos.gov.jo.

[16] Z. Apalla, A. Lallas, E. Sotiriou, E. Lazaridou, and D. Ioannides, "Epidemiological trends in skin cancer," *Dermatology Practical & Conceptual*, vol. 7, no. 2, pp. 1–6, 2017.

[17] U. Leiter, T. Eigentler, and C. Garbe, "Epidemiology of skin cancer," *Advances in Experimental Medicine and Biology*, vol. 810, pp. 120–140, 2014.

[18] D. Reinau, C. Surber, S. S. Jick, and C. R. Meier, "Epidemiology of basal cell carcinoma in the United Kingdom: incidence, lifestyle factors and comorbidities," *British Journal of Cancer*, vol. 111, no. 1, pp. 203–206, 2014.

[19] S. A. AlSalman, T. M. Alkaff, T. Alzaid, and Y. Binamer, "Nonmelanoma skin cancer in Saudi Arabia: single center experience," *Annals of Saudi Medicine*, vol. 38, no. 1, pp. 522–525, 2018.

[20] S. Razi, H. Rafiemanesh, M. Ghoncheh, Y. Khani, and H. Salehiniya, "Changing Trends of Types of Skin Cancer in Iran," *Asian Pacific Journal of Cancer Prevention*, vol. 16, no. 12, pp. 4955–4958, 2015.

[21] A. B. AlZou, M. A. Thabit, K. A. AlSakkaf, and H. O. Basaleem, "Skin Cancer: ClinicoPathological Study of 204 Patients in Southern Governorates of Yemen," *Asian Pacific Journal of Cancer Prevention*, vol. 17, no. 7, pp. 3195–3199, 2016.

[22] M. R. Hussein, "Skin cancer in Egypt: A word in your ear," *Cancer Biology & Therapy*, vol. 4, no. 5, pp. 593–595, 2005.

[23] M. S. Al-Zoubaidi, "Basal cell carcinoma and its subtypes in Iraqi population," *International Journal of Advanced Research*, vol. 4, no. 1, pp. 1002–1010, 2016.

[24] A. K. Omari, M. R. Khammash, and I. Matalka, "Skin cancer trends in northern Jordan," *International Journal of Dermatology*, vol. 45, no. 4, pp. 384–388, 2006.

[25] Y. Yamaguchi, J. Z. Beer, and V. J. Hearing, "Melanin mediated apoptosis of epidermal cells damaged by ultraviolet radiation: factors influencing the incidence of skin cancer," *Archives of Dermatological Research*, vol. 300, no. S1, pp. 43–50, 2008.

[26] Y. Yamaguchi, K. Takahashi, B. Z. Zmudzka et al., "Human skin responses to UV radiation: pigment in the upper epidermis protects against DNA damage in the lower epidermis and facilitates apoptosis," *The FASEB Journal*, vol. 20, no. 9, pp. 1486–1488, 2006.

[27] J. Callens, L. Van Eycken, K. Henau, and M. Garmyn, "Epidemiology of basal and squamous cell carcinoma in Belgium: the need for a uniform and compulsory registration," *Journal of the European Academy of Dermatology and Venereology*, 2016.

[28] H. W. Rogers, M. A. Weinstock, S. R. Feldman, and B. M. Coldiron, "Incidence estimate of nonmelanoma skin cancer (keratinocyte carcinomas) in the us population, 2012," *JAMA Dermatology*, vol. 151, no. 10, pp. 1081–1086, 2015.

[29] M. P. Staples, M. Elwood, R. C. Burton et al., "Nonmelanoma skin cancer in Australia: the 2002 national survey and trends since 1985," *The Medical Journal of Australia*, vol. 184, pp. 6–10, 2006.

[30] Y. Scrivener, E. Grosshans, and B. Cribier, "Variations of basal cell carcinomas according to gender, age, location and histopathological subtype," *British Journal of Dermatology*, vol. 147, no. 1, pp. 41–47, 2002.

[31] P. Wallberg, Taavi Kaaman, Magnus Lind, "Multiple basal cell carcinoma: a clinical evaluation of risk factors: Clinical reports," *Acta Dermato-Venereologica*, vol. 78, no. 2, pp. 127–129, 1998.

[32] Z Hallaji, H Rahimi, and M. Mirshams-Shahshahani, "Comparison of risk factors of single basal cell carcinoma with multiple basal cell carcinomas," *Indian Journal of Dermatology*, vol. 56, no. 4, p. 398, 2011.

[33] S. Ramachandran, A. A. Fryer, T. J. Lovatt et al., "Combined effects of gender, skin type and polymorphic genes on clinical phenotype: use of rate of increase in numbers of basal cell carcinomas as a model system," *Cancer Letters*, vol. 189, no. 2, pp. 175–181, 2003.

27

The use of BEREP4 Immunohistochemistry Staining for Detection of Basal Cell Carcinoma

Anthony Paulo Sunjaya, Angela Felicia Sunjaya, and Sukmawati Tansil Tan

Faculty of Medicine, Tarumanagara University, Jl. Letjen S. Parman No. 1, Jakarta 11440, Indonesia

Correspondence should be addressed to Anthony Paulo Sunjaya; anthonysjy@yahoo.com

Academic Editor: Mark Lebwohl

Basal Cell Carcinoma (BCC) is the most common type of malignant cancer found in the world today with a 3–10% increase in incidence each year. The American Cancer Society reported that 8 out of 10 patients with skin cancer are suffering from BCC with over 2 million new cases each year. BCC needs to be detected at the early stages to prevent local destruction causing disabilities to patients and increasing treatment costs. Furthermore, BCC patients who have undergone surgery are still at risk for recurrence, especially when the surgery performed fails to remove all the BCC cells, even when conventional histopathological testing after surgery has reported a surgically free margin. This review aims to evaluate studies on the use of BerEP4 immunohistochemistry staining on pathological sections of various types of BCC as well as its shortfalls. BerEP4 is a monoclonal antibody which detects specific epithelial-glycoprotein-adhesion-molecules (EpCAM) found on BCC cells. Various studies have shown that BerEP4 has a high sensitivity and specificity in detecting only BCC cells. The use of BerEP4 immunohistochemistry testing for the routine examination of cases of BCC is expected to be able to increase and improve early diagnosis as well as prevent recurrence after surgery.

1. Introduction

First discovered by Jacob et al. in 1827 and named *rodents ulcer*, basal cell carcinoma (BCC) is a type of nonmelanocytic malignant skin cancer. BCC arises from the basal cells of the epidermis and hair follicles. It is currently the most commonly found skin cancer in humans [1, 2].

The prevalence of BCC increases at a rate of 3–10% each year. The American Cancer Society (2012) reported that 8 out of 10 patients with skin cancer are suffering from BCC with more than 2 million new cases each year. BCC is also one of the main types of skin cancer found in Indonesia, constituting 36.67% of skin cancer patients, and more prevalent than any other types of skin cancers such as squamous cell carcinoma (11.4%) and melanoma (0.59%) [3–6].

The prevalence of BCC is also found to be twice more in men than in women, with increasing prevalence with older age. A higher incidence (more than 100-fold) of BCC was found in patients aged 55–70 years compared to those below 20 years old. BCC is rarely found in people under the age of 40 years, although, currently, the incidence in youth continues to rise due to increasing advances in the early diagnosis of BCC [3, 7].

BCCs are caused by frequent exposure to ultraviolet radiation, most commonly ultraviolet spectrum B (UV-B) with a wavelength of 290–320 nm, inducing mutations in tumor suppressor genes. Moreover, UV-B radiation damages the DNA and affects the immune system. In the long run, these genetic changes can cause neoplasms. Mutations in the p53 tumor suppressor gene have been found in approximately 50% of BCC cases. As a result, BCCs are mostly found in body parts frequently exposed to sunlight such as the face, scalp, and neck [1, 3].

2. Types of BCC

BCCs can be classified into several different types based on their morphologies as follows: nodular BCC, cystic BCC, infundibulocystic BCC, morpheaform/cicatricial BCC, infiltrative BCC, micronodular BCC, superficial BCC, pigmented

BCC, rodent's ulcer, fibroepithelioma of Pinkus, polypoid BCC, pore-like BCC, aberrant BCC, and solitary BCC. These various types of BCC exhibit different biologic behaviours with varying clinical, pathological profiles and prognoses [8].

The most aggressive BCCs are of the infiltrative and morpheaform type. Aberrant BCCs refer to those which are found in odd sites such as the scrotum, perineum, and axilla without direct or apparent exposure to carcinogenic factors such as radiation, arsenic, and chronic ulceration, whereas superficial BCCs are commonly found in immunocompromised hosts such as those with an underlying Human Immunodeficiency Virus (HIV) infection and patients with transplants [8].

3. Diagnosis

At present, histopathological examination using Hematoxylin and Eosin (H&E) is the gold standard to confirm the clinical and dermoscopic diagnosis of BCC. However, histopathological examination is not always able to accurately diagnose and distinguish some types of BCC morphologically similar to other types of carcinomas such as peripheral ameloblastoma or distinguish BCC with basosquamous carcinoma whose treatment should differ medically from BCC due to its higher metastasis capabilities [13–16].

4. Therapy and Prognosis

BCC has locally invasive properties as well as low metastatic ability and can easily be treated by surgical excision, provided it is diagnosed at an early stage. However, as they are often asymptomatic, patients often seek treatment in the later stages wherein the BCC has infiltrated the surrounding tissues. It has been found that the average duration from onset to diagnosis of BCC is 37.1 months. By this time the BCC would have been greater than 2 cm, increasing the risk of recurrence after therapy [2, 17].

Late diagnosis and management of BCCs can cause not only disability (scarring the appearance) but also functional impairments to vision, hearing, taste, and smell depending on the site of occurrence. Furthermore, later forms of BCCs pose greater difficulty in treatment. After therapy, these patients have a higher risk for recurrence especially when the results of histopathological examination on incision edges are positive for BCC cells. Even in those where histopathological examination of the edge of the incision has been declared free of BCC cells after surgery, the potential for recurrence remains. Recurrent BCCs area is associated with worse prognosis and a greater risk of metastasis [2].

Although improvements have been made in the prognoses of patients with BCC, recurrence still occurs due to the remnants of BCC cells that are not removed or detected by histopathological examination with H&E, the current gold standard. Research by Mosterd et al. (2011) showed that identification of primary BCC subtypes using conventional histopathological examination (H&E) has a diagnostic accuracy of 80.7%. Moreover, diagnosing recurrent BCC is even much more difficult due to its disjointed growth as a result of the formation of scar tissue [2, 18].

Therefore, as an adjunct to standard diagnostic techniques, an additional diagnostic test is needed that can detect BCC at its early stages as well as detect BCC cells that are not removed after surgical excision therapy. This test would need to be able to distinguish BCC from other carcinoma and skin disorders like squamous cell carcinoma, ameloblastoma, actinic keratosis, and so on. With increasing prevalence of BCC as a result of increased radiation due to global warming and an aging world, the issue of accurately diagnosing BCC is becoming more important than ever. This review aims to evaluate the potential of BerEP4 immunohistochemistry staining in detecting basal cell carcinoma at an early stage and preventing the recurrence of basal cell carcinoma after therapy.

5. Materials and Methods

The databases searched to obtain the articles included MEDLINE Full Text, Pubmed, Science Direct, Pro Quest, SAGE, Taylor and Francis Online, Google Scholar, High Wire, and Elsevier Clinical Key. The search strategies used included availability of full text written in English from 1 January 2000 till 31 December 2016.

Keywords used were "basal cell carcinoma" AND "BerEP4" AND "immunohistochemistry or synonyms." When multiple articles for a single study were found, the most recent publication was used. Relevance of studies was assessed by using an approach based on title, abstract, and full text. Studies were included if they were original studies of any design.

6. BerEP4 Immunohistochemistry

Immunohistochemistry is a technique that can be used to locate cell antigens, tissue, amino acids, proteins, and infectious agents found on specific cells. Presently, immunohistochemistry has become an important tool in medical research and serves as a companion in verifying differential diagnosis which cannot be determined by conventional analysis using H&E staining [19].

Morphologically BCC includes a group of intradermal tumors with cellular characteristics that resemble components of undifferentiated epidermal basal cells. BCCs are derived from stem cells or progenitor cells in the basal membrane enabling BCC to come in various forms and appearances. Some studies have shown that the majority of BCCs are monoclonal tumors and BCCs which differ anatomically may sometimes derive from the same cell origin [5].

All epithelial cells expressed cell adhesion molecules (CAMs) which can be subdivided into 4 families: cadherins, selectins, integrins, and immunoglobulins (Ig)-like-CAMs. Additionally, several CAMs can also be found that do not belong to these "classical" families of adhesion molecules, one of them known as EpCAM [20–22].

The study by Maetzel et al. (2009) showed that EpCAM has a role in cell signaling, proliferation, adhesion, migration, and differentiation. EpCAM was overexpressed in epithelial progenitor cells, carcinoma cells, and cancer triggering cells.

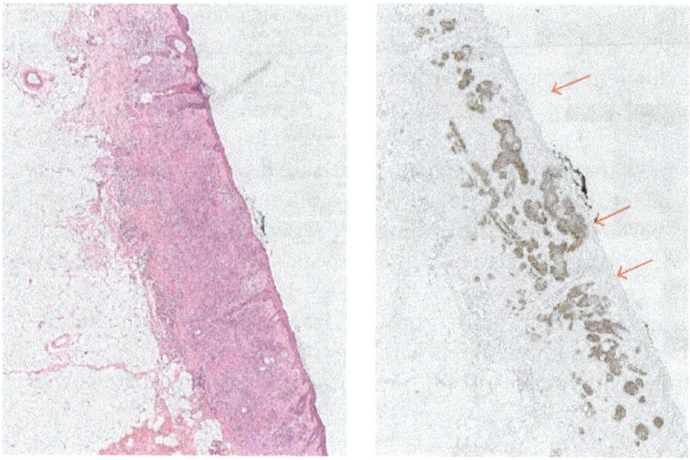

(a) (b)

Figure 1: Comparison H&E stain (a) with BerEP4 immunohistochemistry staining (b) on BCC pathological sections (10x magnification) [9].

Studies have found that EpCAM expression is high in proliferating cells and low in differentiated cells. It was also found to work as an oncogenic signaling molecule through the Wnt signaling pathway. The mechanism of EpCAM induced proliferation in cancer cells has been shown to involve regulated intracellular membrane proteolysis (RIP). EpCAM was found to be a cell surface glycoprotein highly expressed in nonsquamous epithelial cancers and at lower levels in normal simple epithelia [23, 24].

The above epithelial-specific antigen is also found in carcinomas of other organs such as ovarium, colon, prostate, stomach, and lung carcinoma. Currently, anti-EpCAM antibody has been available for use for histopathologic diagnosis and therapy in humans. BerEP4 is an anti-EpCAM antibody and has proven to be a sensitive marker towards BCC [25–27].

BerEP4 is a monoclonal antibody that can be used as a marker of BCC. It works by detecting the EpCAM antigen, a transmembrane epithelial glycoprotein cell adhesion molecule found in humans. BerEP4 is made from human mammary as well as mice carcinoma cell lining (MCF-7). This marker, which is a mouse IgG antibody, can detect glycopeptides with masses of 34 kD, 39 kD, and 40 kD [16, 24].

7. Study Results on BerEP4 Use in Detecting BCC

One of the first studies to evaluate the use of BerEP4 in detecting BCC cases was performed by Beer et al. (2000). It was reported that BerEP4 was able to detect all 39 BCC samples used in this study. The same result was obtained by Ishida et al. (2008) with studies being performed on 20 BCC samples. Krahl & Sellheyer (2007) also conducted tests with BerEP4 on 28 sclerosing and infiltrative BCCs. All 28 BCCs came with varying degrees of positive results, in which 27 have a degree of moderate to strong positives and one weak positive [29, 30, 37].

Another study conducted by Karahan et al. (2006) on 20 specimens of BCC also reported that BerEP4 was able to detect all the BCC specimens. Further research using BerEP4 immunohistochemistry consistently gave similar results; the study by Dasgeb et al. (2013) using BerEP4 to distinguish 24 BCC specimens with 88 common skin neoplasms, namely, trichoepithelioma, actinic keratosis, squamous cell carcinoma in situ, squamous cell carcinoma, seborrheic keratosis, lichen planus like keratosis, nevi, hemangioma, inverted follicular keratosis, sebaceous adenoma, and Merkel cell carcinoma (MCC) from dermatopathology files, also showed that it was able to diffusely stain all BCC sections. However, all trichoepitheliomas and MCCs were also diffusely stained while 1 squamous cell carcinoma and 1 sebaceous adenoma showed weak staining. The false positive rate was at 15% [16, 24].

Further immunohistochemistry tests were also conducted by Sellheyer, et al. (2013) to test the usefulness of BerEP4 in diagnosing morpheaform BCCs. The results showed that, among 17 specimens, 16 showed an immunological reaction of more than 75% while the other one showed an immunological reaction at over 25%. Ansai et al. (2012) in their study of 31 BCC cases, 18 cases of nodular type, 9 cases of superficial type, and 4 cases of morpheaform type, also reported a 97% sensitivity of BerEP4 in detecting BCC cells [34, 35].

Our previous study on BerEP4 use conducted by Tan & Sunjaya (2016) on 23 specimens with 394 microlesions also showed 100% positive results with 100% sensitivity and specificity. In the study, BerEP4 has been proven to detect and provide positive results in the early stages of BCC consisting of only several cells [9] (Figure 1).

7.1. Differentiating BCC from Squamous Cell Carcinoma (SCC). One of the main advantages of BerEP4 is the ability to distinguish BCC from squamous cell carcinoma (SCC) with high sensitivity and specificity. Both BCC and SCC arise from the epidermal layer with similar predilection on areas of the skin exposed to the sun; hence they both often show a similar clinical profile. Although SCCs which are

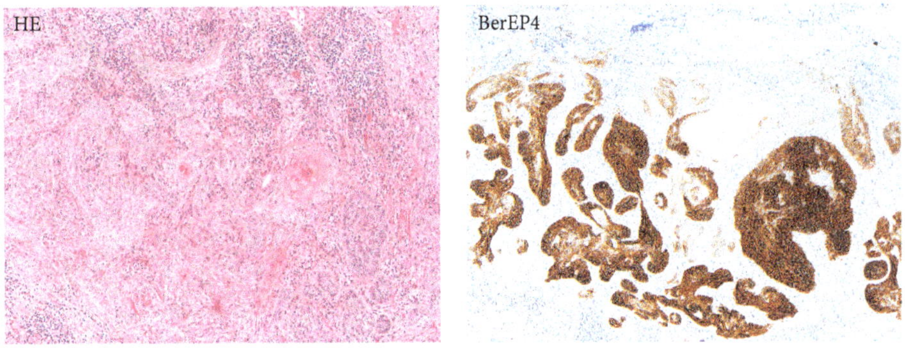

(a) (b)

FIGURE 2: Comparison H&E stain with BerEP4 immunohistochemistry staining on a pathological section having BCC with squamous cell metaplasia. Only BCC cells are stained with BerEP4. (100x magnification) [10].

similar in profile with BCCs rarely spread, they still do so more often than BCCs. As a result, these 2 disorders must be accurately differentiated to prevent misdiagnosis and incorrect treatment. Data from various studies compiled by Sellheyer et al. (2013) showed that all 75 cases of SCC stained with BerEP4 gave negative results. The same result was reported by Karahan et al. (2006) and Dasgeb et al. (2013). The above results are also supported by research performed by Ozawa et al. (2004) which showed that BerEP4 antigens are not found in normal keratinocytes and squamous cell carcinoma of the skin [16, 24, 34, 38].

Research by Mashhood et al. (2011) to find the sensitivity and specificity of BerEP4 in patients of Asian origin with SCC as control also reported that BerEP4 has a sensitivity and specificity of 100% [32]. These results do not differ much with the sensitivity and specificity calculated based on the summary of the studies on the usage of BerEP4 with SCC as control, showing the sensitivity of BerEP4 as 99.6% and specificity of BerEP4 as 99.2% with a positive predictive value of 99.6% and negative predictive value of 99.1% (Table 1).

7.2. Differentiating BCC from Basosquamous Carcinomas (BSC). In addition, BerEP4 also have important uses in diagnosing basosquamous carcinomas (BSC), which are currently difficult to identify and diagnose definitively. Definitive diagnosis of BCC and BSC is required and of great importance due to their differences in prognosis and treatment. A study by Karahan et al. (2006) showed that the identification of BSC can be facilitated by BerEP4 staining. This can be due to the fact that BSC is a tumor similar to BCC with squamous differentiation and therefore has an immunohistochemical profile that is similar to BCC. The difference between the results of staining BSC and BCC lies in the extent of staining of the specimen, in BSC, patchy stains were found which only cover part of the tumor studied [16].

7.3. Differentiating BCC from Collision Tumors. BerEP4 can also be used to distinguish collision tumors, a type of tumor that is a mixture of BCC and SCC. Areas of BCC will be strongly stained whereas areas of SCC will remain untainted by BerEP4 [16] (Figure 2).

TABLE 1: Sensitivity, specificity, positive predictive value, and negative predictive value of BerEP4 in detecting BCC with SCC as control.

Studies	BCC +	SCC + (control)
Karahan, et al. [16]	20/20	0/20
Fan, et al. [28]	51/51	-
Krahl & Sellheyer [29]	28/28	-
Ishida, et al. [30]	20/20	-
Filho, et al. [31]	20/20	-
Mashhood, et al. [32]	29/29	0/11
Tan & Sunjaya [9]	23/23	-
Kirzhner & Jakobiec [33]	13/13	-
Dasgeb, et al. [24]	24/24	1/11 (weak positive)
Patil, et al. [12]	9/9	-
Sellheyer, et al. [34]	17/17	0/75
Ansai, et al. [35]	30/31	-
BerEP4 positive	284	1
Ber EP4 negative	1	116
Total	**285**	**117**
Sensitivity	$284/285 \times 100 =$ **99.6%**	
Specificity	$116/117 \times 100 =$ **99.2%**	
Positive predictive value	$284/285 \times 100 =$ **99.6%**	
Negative predictive value	$116/117 \times 100 =$ **99.1%**	

7.4. Differentiating BCC from Basaloid Squamous Cell Carcinoma (bSCC). While previous studies have reported that BerEP4 can differentiate BCC from BSCs and collision tumors, Linskey et al. (2013) reported that BerEP4 alone was unable to differentiate bSCC and BSC as both were stained by BerEP4, although the mean percentage of cells stained was significantly higher in BSC group compared to bSCC. In detecting bSCC, BerEP4 was reported to have a sensitivity of 60%, specificity of 44%, positive predictive value (PPV) of 65%, negative predictive value (NPV) of 39%, and false positive rate of 25% [10].

7.5. Differentiating BCC from Sebaceoma. Research conducted by Fan et al. (2007) to compare the reaction of BerEP4

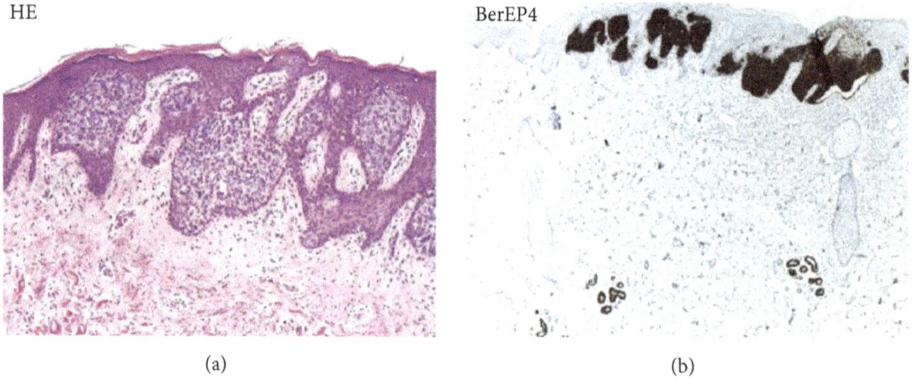

FIGURE 3: Comparison H&E stain (200x magnification) with BerEP4 immunohistochemistry staining (100x magnification) on superficial BCC pathological sections mimicking Bowen's Disease [11].

in BCC and sebaceoma showed that out of the 25 sebaceoma specimens tested, 24 were negative while one showed a weak positive result (<10% tumor cells stained) with a false positive rate of 4%. Meanwhile, all tested nodular BCC specimens (51 specimens) were moderately or strongly stained, with never less than 20% of the tumor stained by BerEP4 [28].

7.6. Differentiating BCC from Microcystic Adnexal Carcinoma (MAC). Other studies also showed that BerEP4 was able to distinguish BCC from microcystic adnexal carcinoma (MAC). Sellheyer et al. (2013) and Krahl et al. (2007) reported that BerEP4 was able to reliably differentiate MAC from BCC to the same extent as it distinguishes BCC from SCC. None of the MACs which were taken as control were stained in the study [29, 34].

7.7. Differentiating BCC from Bowen's Disease. Conflicting results have been reported with regard to BerEP4 use in distinguishing BCC from Bowen's Disease (BD). BerEP4 was found to be able to differentiate BCC from BD with a specificity and sensitivity of 100% in a study by Ansai et al. (2012), although a recent study by Kogut et al. (2016) reported that BerEP4 expression is not always helpful in distinguishing BD from BCC with around 26% of BD's reacting positively with BerEP4 (at least 5% staining) [39] (Figure 3).

7.8. Differentiating BCC from Other Epithelial Skin Disorders. Actinic keratosis [36], seborrheic keratosis [35], poroma [35], lichen planus like keratosis [24], nevi [24], hemangioma [24], inverted follicular keratosis [24], squamous intraepithelial neoplasia (SIN) [24], and sebaceous adenoma/hyperplasia [24] are a wide variety of epithelial skin disorders that have been proven to give negative results on BerEP4 testing (Table 2).

In addition to the studies above, various other studies and case reports also showed that BerEP4 can detect even rare forms of BCC such as perianal BCC, intraoral BCC, and axillary BCC with high sensitivity and specificity. In many cases, BerEP4 use has been of great help in preventing misdiagnosis of the skin disorders. The results of these studies are summarised below.

TABLE 2: Sensitivity and specificity of BerEP4 in differentiating BCC with the epithelial disorders below as control.

Epithelial skin disorder	Sensitivity (%)	Specificity (%)
Actinic keratosis	100 [36]	100 [36]
	100 [24]	100 [24]
Seborrheic keratosis	97 [35]	100 [35]
	100 [24]	100 [24]
Poroma [35]	97	100
Lichen planus like keratosis [24]	100	100
Nevi [24]	100	100
Hemangioma [24]	100	100
Inverted follicular keratosis [24]	100	100
Squamous intraepithelial neoplasia (SIN) [36]	100	100
Sebaceous adenoma/hyperplasia [24]	100	83.3

7.9. Perianal BCC. A study by Patil et al. (2013) used BerEP4 markers (Dako, Carpinteria, CA, USA) to identify BCC located in the anal region. These carcinomas are rarely found and hard to distinguish from basaloid squamous carcinoma without the use of biopsy techniques. In this study, specimens consisted of 9 BCC and 15 basaloid squamous carcinomas. The results show that BerEP4 staining was able to diffusely stain all BCCs. Interestingly, 40% of the basaloid specimens were also stained by BerEP4 in this study. A case report by Kreuter et al. (2012) also reported that immunohistochemical staining with BerEP4 on perianal tumors specimens showed strong positive results [12, 40] (Figure 4).

7.10. Intraoral BCC. Intraoral BCC case reports obtained also show that the use of BerEP4 can help distinguish intraoral BCC from peripheral ameloblastomas, both of which possess similar histological features. Of the four reported cases of intraoral BCC, all were initially misdiagnosed as peripheral

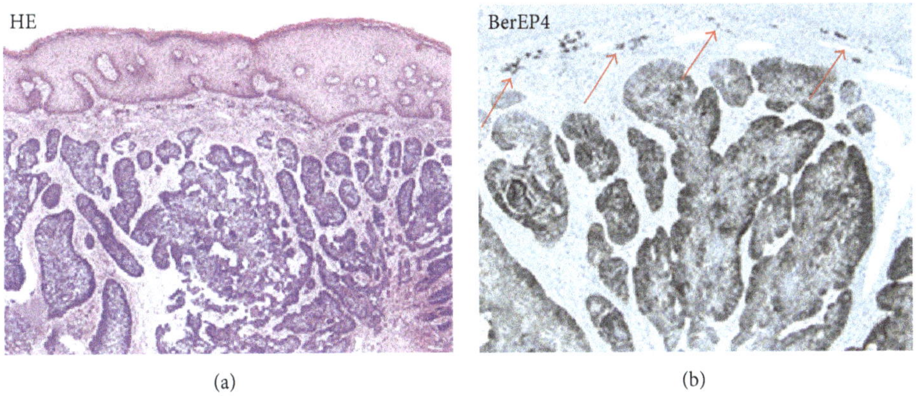

FIGURE 4: Comparison H&E stain with BerEP4 immunohistochemistry staining on perianal BCC pathological sections (20x magnification). Arrows show small groups of BCC cells difficult to differentiate with the H&E Stain [12].

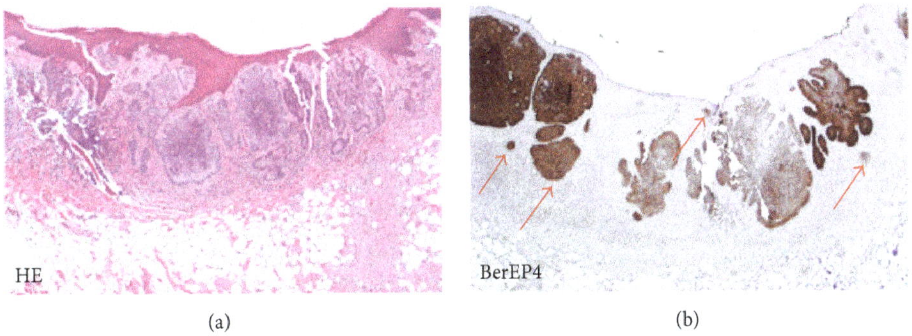

FIGURE 5: Comparison H&E stain with BerEP4 immunohistochemistry staining on intraoral BCC pathological sections (4x magnification). Arrows show small groups of basaloid cells difficult to differentiate with the H&E Stain [13].

ameloblastoma due to its similarity. The tumor can only be confirmed as intraoral BCC after immunohistochemical examination with BerEP4 marker yielded a positive result [13, 15].

Recent research conducted by Sook & Keun (2014) to compare protein expression between intraoral BCC and peripheral ameloblastoma detected with 50 different types of antisera also showed that intraoral BCC showed strong positive results against EpCAM [41] (Figure 5).

7.11. Axillary BCC. Due to the specificity and sensitivity of BerEP4 in detecting BCCs, some rare BCC cases can be ascertained and diagnosed as BCC only after BerEP4 immunohistochemical test results gave strong positive results. Axillary BCCs are rare as this region of the body is rarely exposed to the sun. Four cases of rare axillary, as well as one case of BCC who experienced postoperative recurrence and metastasis, have been diagnosed with the help of BerEP4 immunohistochemistry test [42, 43].

7.12. Metatypical and Granular BCC. Two metatypical BCC cases with a high rate of postoperative recurrence and metastasis risk [44, 45] as well as two cases of granular BCC found by Claassen et al. (2014) and Jedrych & Busam (2014) were also successfully diagnosed with the help of BerEP4 immunohistochemistry test [46, 47].

7.13. Eyelid BCC and in Epidermoid Cysts. Jakobiec et al. (2010) reported a case of BCC found in epidermoid cysts on the eyelids which was confirmed through BerEP4 immunohistochemistry test. Two years later, Kirzhner and Jakobiec (2012) retrospectively analysed 13 specimens of pigmented BCC specimens found in the eyelid. They reported that BerEP4 was found positive in all the lesions. BerEP4 was positive within the basaloid tumor cells but negative in metatypical and intratumoral melanocytes [33, 48].

8. BerEP4 Use after Surgery for Prevention of Recurrence

In accordance with the guidelines for handling BCC made by the British Association of Dermatologists, incision of small lesions (<20 mm) with clear boundaries with peripheral surgical margin of 3 mm will eliminate all BCC cells in 85% of cases, while a margin of 4-5 mm would eliminate all BCC cells in 95% of cases [49].

BCC patients are at risk for recurrence even after the incision edge has been declared free of BCC cells by H&E staining as several types of BCCs often have multiple microlesions which are spread out over the skin surface. These microlesions are difficult to detect and identify with normal staining as they are at times still a small group of cancer cells (Figure 6).

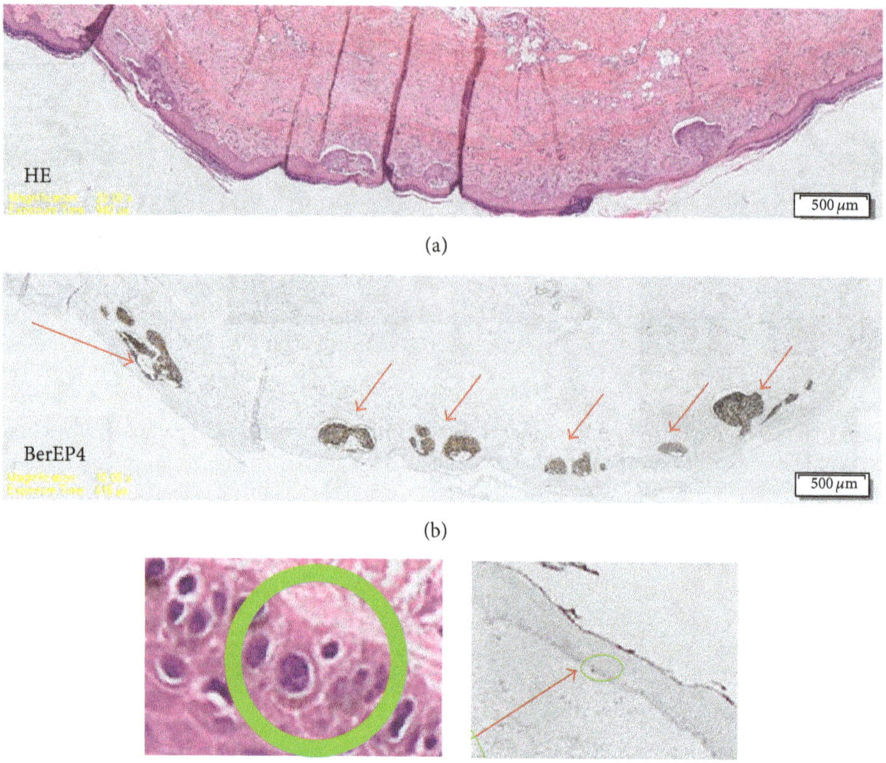

(a) (b) (c) (d)

Figure 6: Comparison H&E stain with BerEP4 immunohistochemistry staining on BCC pathological sections with Multiple microlesions [9]. ((a) 20x magnification, (b) 10x magnification, (c) 100x magnification, (d) 10x magnification).

In a study by Kist et al. (1997), 27 BCC specimens (15 nodular BCC, 11 Morpheaform BCC, and 1 Adenoid BCC) were examined for remaining BCC cells after Mohs Micrographic Surgery. Specimens were stained with BerEP4 and the results showed BCC cells remaining at 2 specimens that had previously been checked by H&E staining and provided negative results. In addition, BerEP4 also provides enhanced visualization of the 13 specimens previously reported positive with H&E staining, especially on the BCC specimens of the morpheaform type [50].

Filho et al. (2008) conducted a study using BerEP4 testing on 20 BCC specimens to ensure the edge of the incision has been free of BCC cells after curettage treatment and two cycles of electrofulguration. The test resulted in 5 BCC specimens (25%) being positive for remaining BCC cells [31].

Various studies have consistently reported that BerEP4 has a sensitivity of 100% and gives positive results in all BCC specimens examined. Besides being able to deliver positive results in frequent BCC locations such as the neck and face, BerEP4 also provide positive results in frequently found subtypes such as morpheaform BCC and nodular BCC, as well as positive results in rarely found BCC such as the axilla, intraoral, perianal, and granular BCC.

9. BerEP4 Limitations

However, BerEP4 was found to be unable to distinguish BCC from trichoepithelioma, trichoblastoma, Merkel cell carcinoma (MCC), and basaloid squamous cell carcinoma (bSCC). One of the reasons for this is that trichoepithelioma, trichoblastoma, and BCC are all epithelial neoplasms of follicular germinative cell differentiation. To distinguish trichoepithelioma and trichoblastoma with BCC requires the use of other immunohistochemistry test using pleckstrin homology-like domain (PHLDA1), whereas a panel of BerEP4, cytokeratin (CK) 14, and CK17 is needed to reliably differentiate BCC and BSCs from bSCCs [10, 24, 34, 35].

MCC is a malignant cutaneous neoplasm with epithelial and neuroendocrine differentiation. Therefore MCCs are positive for epithelial and neuroendocrine markers but are negative for lymphoid and melanoma markers. So far no single immunohistochemical examination method has been found which can accurately detect MCCs; the diagnosis can only be confirmed through the use of several immunohistochemical markers to exclude microscopically similar tumors such as melanoma, small cell metastatic lung carcinoma (SCLC), and BCCs. A combination of CK20 which is highly sensitive for MCCs, together with thyroid transcription factor-1 (TTF-1) and CK7 which are expressed in SCLCs but consistently absent in MCCs as well as HBM45, NKI/C3, and S-100 markers, which are positive in melanoma but negative in MCCs, can be used to identify MCCs [24, 51–53].

10. Practical Implications

From the various studies using BerEP4 immunohistochemistry explained above, differences remain to be found with regard to the sensitivity and specificity of results which can occur due to the use of different brands of BerEP4, differences in the original staining of the specimens, old specimens being analysed (especially when the specimens derive from dermatopathology archives), differences in staining techniques, the tools used, and the stage of the lesion being diagnosed.

The results of the studies found, however, suggest that immunohistochemistry testing using BerEP4 has a high sensitivity and specificity. BerEP4 use is therefore recommended especially in patients suspected of having BCC with multiple microlesions, infiltrative BCC, BCCs with mixed pathologies, and BCCs located in rare sites like the axilla, perianal region, and so on. In addition, BerEP4 can also be used to identify tumor excision margins especially in patients with recurring BCC lesions.

11. Conclusions

Currently, immunohistochemistry testing has become an important adjunct and tool for differential diagnosis especially for studying parameters that cannot be viewed, defined, or analysed with conventional staining. BerEP4 is a monoclonal antibody which can detect the presence of EpCAM antigen found on BCC cells. It has been proven to be able to reliably detect BCCs of all types and even those in rare locations including intraoral, axillary, metatypical, and granular BCC.

BerEP4 has been found to be able to differentiate BCC from other cutaneous pathologies such as squamous cell carcinoma, basosquamous cell carcinoma, collision tumors, sebaceoma, microcystic adnexal carcinoma, ameloblastoma, epidermoid cysts, actinic keratosis, seborrheic keratosis, poroma, lichen planus like keratosis, nevi, hemangioma, inverted follicular keratosis, squamous intraepithelial neoplasia, and sebaceous adenoma/hyperplasia. However, BerEP4 was found to be unable to distinguish BCC from trichoepithelioma, trichoblastoma, Merkel cell carcinoma, and basaloid carcinoma. Conflicting results have also been reported regarding BerEP4 use in differentiating BCC from Bowen's Disease. Despite its limitations, studies have shown that BerEP4 has the advantage of being able to detect small amounts of BCC cells making it suitable for early detection of BCC as well as in detecting BCC mixed with other cutaneous pathology. Moreover, it was able to accurately identify the presence of BCC cells after therapy and therefore is expected to reduce the incidence of recurrence after therapy.

References

[1] S. Kumar, B. B. Mahajan, S. Kaur, A. Yadav, N. Singh, and A. Singh, "A Study of Basal Cell Carcinoma in South Asians for Risk Factor and Clinicopathological Characterization: A Hospital Based Study," *Journal of Skin Cancer*, vol. 2014, Article ID 173582, 9 pages, 2014.

[2] V. P. Chinem and H. A. Miot, "Epidemiology of basal cell carcinoma," *Anais Brasileiros de Dermatologia*, vol. 86, no. 2, pp. 292–305, 2011.

[3] L. A. Goldsmith, S. I. Katz, B. A. Gilchrest, A. S. Paller, D. J. Leffel, and K. Wolff, Eds., *Fitzpatrick's Dermatology in General Medicine*, McGraw-Hill, 8th, 8th edition, 2012.

[4] S. C. Flohil, I. Seubring, M. M. van Rossum, J.-W. W. Coebergh, E. De Vries, and T. Nijsten, "Trends in basal cell carcinoma incidence rates: a 37-year dutch observational study," *Journal of Investigative Dermatology*, vol. 133, no. 4, pp. 913–918, 2013.

[5] M. Kasper, V. Jaks, D. Hohl, and R. Toftgård, "Basal cell carcinoma - Molecular biology and potential new therapies," *The Journal of Clinical Investigation*, vol. 122, no. 2, pp. 455–463, 2012.

[6] A. S. Suriadiredja, "Epidemiologi kanker kulit," *MDVI*, vol. 38, no. 2, article 61, 2011.

[7] R. S. Bader, L. Santacroce, L. Diomede, and A. S. Kennedy, *Basal Cell Carcinoma Medscape Emedicine*, 2014, http://emedicine.medscape.com/article/276624-overview.

[8] W. D. James, T. G. Berger, and D. M. Elston, *Andrew's Diseases of the Skin*, Saunders Elsevier, 11th edition, 2011.

[9] S. T. Tan and A. P. Sunjaya, "Pengunaan Uji Imunohistokimia (IHK) BerEP4 sebagai gold standard deteksi karsinoma sel basal (KSB)," *Indonesian Journal of Cancer*, vol. 10, no. 3, 2016.

[10] K. R. Linskey, D. C. Gimbel, L. R. Zukerberg, L. M. Duncan, P. M. Sadow, and R. M. Nazarian, "BerEp4, cytokeratin 14, and cytokeratin 17 immunohistochemical staining aid in differentiation of basaloid squamous cell carcinoma from basal cell carcinoma with squamous metaplasia," *Archives of Pathology & Laboratory Medicine*, vol. 137, no. 11, pp. 1591–1598, 2013.

[11] A. Alhumaidi, "Practical immunohistochemistry of epithelial skin tumor," *Indian Journal of Dermatology, Venereology and Leprology*, vol. 78, no. 6, pp. 698–708, 2012.

[12] D. T. Patil, J. R. Goldblum, and S. D. Billings, "Clinicopathological analysis of basal cell carcinoma of the anal region and its distinction from basaloid squamous cell carcinoma," *Modern Pathology*, vol. 26, no. 10, pp. 1382–1389, 2013.

[13] T. R. Woods, D. M. Cohen, M. N. Islam et al., "Intraoral Basal Cell Carcinoma, a Rare Neoplasm: Report of Three New Cases with Literature Review," *Head & Neck Pathology*, vol. 8, no. 3, pp. 339–348, 2014.

[14] G. Li, J. Tietze, and D. Kulichova, "High-Definition Optical Coherence Tomography in the Diagnosis of Basal Cell Carcinoma Evaluated by an Experienced Versus Inexperienced Investigator," *Journal of Clinical & Experimental Dermatology Research*, vol. 5, no. 4, 2014.

[15] I. G. Koutlas, C. A. Koch, R. A. Vickers, F. M. Brouwers, and A. O. Vortmeyer, "An unusual ostensible example of intraoral basal cell carcinoma," *Journal of Cutaneous Pathology*, vol. 36, no. 4, pp. 464–470, 2009.

[16] N. Karahan, S. Baspinar, M. Yildirim, and I. Barut, "The use of Ber-EP4 antigen in the differential diagnosis of basosquamous carcinoma from squamous and basal cell carcinoma," *Türk Patoloji Dergisi*, vol. 22, no. 2, pp. 87–91, 2006.

[17] K. Wolff and R. A. Johnson, *Fitzpatrick's Color Atlas & Synopsis of Clinical Dermatology*, McGraw-Hill, 7th edition, 2013.

[18] K. Mosterd, M. R. T. M. Thissen, A. M. W. van Marion et al., "Correlation between histologic findings on punch biopsy specimens and subsequent excision specimens in recurrent basal cell carcinoma," *Journal of the American Academy of Dermatology*, vol. 64, no. 2, pp. 323–337, 2011.

[19] L. L. de Matos, D. C. Trufelli, M. G. L. de Matos, and M. A. D. S. Pinhal, "Immunohistochemistry as an important tool in biomarkers detection and clinical practice," *Biomarker Insights*, vol. 2010, no. 5, pp. 9–20, 2010.

[20] U. Schnell, V. Cirulli, and B. N. G. Giepmans, "EpCAM: structure and function in health and disease," *Biochimica et Biophysica Acta*, vol. 1828, no. 8, pp. 1989–2001, 2013.

[21] P. A. Baeuerle and O. Gires, "EpCAM (CD326) finding its role in cancer," *British Journal of Cancer*, vol. 96, no. 3, pp. 417–423, 2007.

[22] M. Trzpis, P. M. J. McLaughlin, L. M. F. H. De Leij, and M. C. Harmsen, "Epithelial cell adhesion molecule: More than a carcinoma marker and adhesion molecule," *The American Journal of Pathology*, vol. 171, no. 2, pp. 386–395, 2007.

[23] D. Maetzel, S. Denzel, B. Mack et al., "Nuclear signalling by tumour-associated antigen EpCAM," *Nature Cell Biology*, vol. 11, no. 2, pp. 162–171, 2009.

[24] B. Dasgeb, T. M. Mohammadi, and D. R. Mehregan, "Use of Ber-EP4 and epithelial specific antigen to differentiate clinical simulators of basal cell carcinoma," *Biomarkers in Cancer*, vol. 5, pp. 7–11, 2013.

[25] G. Spizzo, P. Went, S. Dirnhofer et al., "Overexpression of epithelial cell adhesion molecule (Ep-CAM) is an independent prognostic marker for reduced survival of patients with epithelial ovarian cancer," *Gynecologic Oncology*, vol. 103, no. 2, pp. 483–488, 2006.

[26] P. Went, M. Vasei, L. Bubendorf et al., "Frequent high-level expression of the immunotherapeutic target Ep-CAM in colon, stomach, prostate and lung cancers," *British Journal of Cancer*, vol. 94, no. 1, pp. 128–135, 2006.

[27] S.-I. Ansai, H. Takeichi, S. Arase, S. Kawana, and T. Kimura, "Sebaceous carcinoma: an immunohistochemical reappraisal," *American Journal of Dermatopathology*, vol. 33, no. 6, pp. 579–587, 2011.

[28] Y. S. Fan, R. A. Carr, D. S. A. Sanders, A. P. Smith, A. J. F. Lazar, and E. Calonje, "Characteristic Ber-EP4 and EMA expression in sebaceoma is immunohistochemically distinct from basal cell carcinoma," *Histopathology*, vol. 51, no. 1, pp. 80–86, 2007.

[29] D. Krahl and K. Sellheyer, "Monoclonal antibody Ber-EP4 reliably discriminates between microcystic adnexal carcinoma and basal cell carcinoma," *Journal of Cutaneous Pathology*, vol. 34, no. 10, pp. 782–787, 2007.

[30] M. Ishida, R. Kushima, and H. Okabe, "Immunohistochemical demonstration of D2-40 in basal cell carcinomas of the skin," *Journal of Cutaneous Pathology*, vol. 35, no. 10, pp. 926–930, 2008.

[31] L. L. L. Filho, A. De Oliveira De Avelar Alchorne, G. C. Pereira, L. R. S. Lopes, and T. C. B. De Carvalho, "Histological and immunohistochemical evaluation of basal cell carcinoma following curettage and electrodessication," *International Journal of Dermatology*, vol. 47, no. 6, pp. 610–614, 2008.

[32] A. A. Mashhood, T. Sarfraz, M. Atique, and M. Asif, "Sensitivity and specificity of Ber-EP4 immunostaining in basal cell carcinoma cases in asian skin," *Pakistan Armed Forces Medical Journal*, vol. 3, 2011.

[33] M. Kirzhner and F. A. Jakobiec, "Clinicopathologic and immunohistochemical features of pigmented basal cell carcinomas of the eyelids," *American Journal of Ophthalmology*, vol. 153, no. 2, pp. 242–252, 2012.

[34] K. Sellheyer, P. Nelson, H. Kutzner, and R. M. Patel, "The immunohistochemical differential diagnosis of microcystic adnexal carcinoma, desmoplastic trichoepithelioma and morpheaform basal cell carcinoma using BerEP4 and stem cell markers," *Journal of Cutaneous Pathology*, vol. 40, no. 4, pp. 363–370, 2013.

[35] S.-I. Ansai, R. Takayama, T. Kimura, and S. Kawana, "Ber-EP4 is a useful marker for follicular germinative cell differentiation of cutaneous epithelial neoplasms," *The Journal of Dermatology*, vol. 39, no. 8, pp. 688–692, 2012.

[36] W. D. Tope, M. Nowfar-Rad, and D. A. Kist, "Ber-EP4-positive phenotype differentiates actinic keratosis from superficial basal cell carcinoma," *Dermatologic Surgery*, vol. 26, no. 5, pp. 415–418, 2000.

[37] T. W. Beer, P. Shepherd, and J. M. Theaker, "Ber EP4 and epithelial membrane antigen aid distinction of basal cell, squamous cell and basosquamous carcinomas of the skin," *Histopathology*, vol. 37, no. 3, pp. 218–223, 2000.

[38] M. Ozawa, S. Aiba, M. Kurosawa, and H. Tagami, "Ber-EP4 antigen is a marker for a cell population related to the secondary hair germ," *Experimental Dermatology*, vol. 13, no. 7, pp. 401–405, 2004.

[39] M. Kogut, F. Toberer, A. H. Enk, and J. C. Hassel, "Limitations of Ber-EP4 for distinction of Bowen disease from basal cell carcinoma," *Journal of Cutaneous Pathology*, vol. 43, no. 4, pp. 367–371, 2016.

[40] A. Kreuter, F. G. Bechara, M. Stücker, N. H. Brockmeyer, P. Altmeyer, and U. Wieland, "Perianal basal cell carcinoma - unusual localization of a frequent tumor," *JDDG: Journal der Deutschen Dermatologischen Gesellschaft*, vol. 10, no. 1, pp. 59–61, 2012.

[41] Y. S. Kim and S. K. Lee, "Different protein expressions between peripheral ameloblastoma and oral basal cell carcinoma occurred at the same mandibular molar area," *The Korean Journal of Pathology*, vol. 48, no. 2, pp. 151–158, 2014.

[42] M. Costescu, O. Andreia Coman, M. Tampa, I. Tudose, L. Coman, and S. Roxana Georgescu, "Axillary basal cell carcinoma - A rare form of a frequent kind of carcinoma," *Romanian Journal of Morphology and Embryology*, vol. 54, no. 3, pp. 851–856, 2013.

[43] R. N. Saladi, F. Singh, H. Wei, M. G. Lebwohl, and R. G. Phelps, "Use of Ber-EP4 protein in recurrent metastatic basal cell carcinoma: A case report and review of the literature," *International Journal of Dermatology*, vol. 43, no. 8, pp. 600–603, 2004.

[44] G. Tchernev, J. Ananiev, JC. Cardoso, and U. Wollina, "Metatypical basal cell carcinomas: a successful surgical approach to two cases with different tumor locations," *MAEDICA*, vol. 9, no. 1, pp. 79–82, 2014.

[45] M. Tarallo, E. Cigna, R. Frati et al., "Metatypical basal cell carcinoma: A clinical review," *Journal of Experimental & Clinical Cancer Research*, vol. 27, no. 1, article no. 65, 2008.

[46] S. L. Claassen, M. C. Royer, and W. L. Rush, "Granular cell basal cell carcinoma: Report of a case and review of the literature," *American Journal of Dermatopathology*, vol. 36, no. 7, pp. e121–e124, 2014.

[47] J. Jedrych and K. J. Busam, "Multiple lesions of granular cell basal cell carcinoma: A case report," *Journal of Cutaneous Pathology*, vol. 41, no. 1, pp. 45–50, 2014.

[48] F. A. Jakobiec, F. R. Zakka, and M. P. Hatton, "Eyelid basal cell carcinoma developing in an epidermoid cyst: A previously unreported event," *Ophthalmic Plastic & Reconstructive Surgery*, vol. 26, no. 6, pp. 491–494, 2010.

[49] N. R. Telfer, G. B. Colver, and C. A. Morton, "Guidelines for the management of basal cell carcinoma," *British Journal of Dermatology*, vol. 159, no. 1, pp. 35–48, 2008.

[50] A. K. El Tal, A. E. Abrou, M. A. Stiff, and D. A. Mehregan, "Immunostaining in Mohs micrographic surgery: A review," *Dermatologic Surgery*, vol. 36, no. 3, pp. 275–290, 2010.

[51] M. T. Bozinovic, D. Krasic, V. Katic et al., "Comparative analysis of clinicopathological and immunohistochemical characteristics of Merkel cell carcinoma," *Journal of B.U.ON.*, vol. 19, no. 2, pp. 530–534, 2014.

[52] L. A. Compton, G. F. Murphy, and C. G. Lian, "Diagnostic immunohistochemistry in cutaneous neoplasia: an update," *Dermatopathology*, vol. 2, no. 1, pp. 15–42, 2015.

[53] T. Jaeger, J. Ring, and C. Andres, "Histological, immunohistological, and clinical features of merkel cell carcinoma in correlation to merkel cell polyomavirus status," *Journal of Skin Cancer*, vol. 2012, Article ID 983421, 5 pages, 2012.

28

Assessing the Current Market of Sunscreen: A Cross-Sectional Study of Sunscreen Availability in Three Metropolitan Counties in the United States

Kyle T. Amber, Romi Bloom, Patrick Staropoli, Sonam Dhiman, and Shasa Hu

Department of Dermatology & Cutaneous Surgery, University of Miami Miller School of Medicine, 10660 SW 75th Avenue, Miami, FL 33156, USA

Correspondence should be addressed to Kyle T. Amber; kamber@med.miami.edu

Academic Editor: Günther Hofbauer

Sunscreen use is recommended for the prevention of sunburn and skin cancer. Little is known regarding sunscreen availability in high versus low income communities. We analyzed sunscreen availability in three large metropolitan counties to determine the relationship between availability and community demographics. We included sun care products in all pharmacies and supermarkets open as of July 2013 in representative high and low income zip codes in Cook County, Illinois, Miami-Dade County, Florida, and San Diego County, California. We recorded the percentage of tanning oil, sunscreens with a sun protection factor (SPF) < 15, SPF > 15, physical sunscreens, spray sunscreens, mean price per ounce (PPO), and mean SPF. Of the total products assessed, 11.0% were tanning oils, with physical sunscreens accounting for only 3.4% of the available sunscreens and 46.2% of sunscreens being spray-on. A comparison between higher and lower income zip codes demonstrated a significantly increased percentage of sunscreens with SPF < 15 in high income zip codes. Lower income zip codes had higher percentages of sunscreens with SPF > 15 and higher PPO, even when taking into account SPF. Further studies of sunscreen usage patterns in different populations must take into account sunscreen availability and price, as these significantly differ based on the community demographic.

1. Introduction

Both melanoma and nonmelanoma skin cancers (NMSC) are becoming increasingly prevalent [1, 2], with NMSC becoming the fifth most costly cancer in the United States [3]. Sunburn also accounts for a significant amount of lost work hours, resulting in an estimated economic impact for lost work and treatment in excess of $10 million [4]. Preventive measures against skin cancers and sunburn include sun avoidance during the peak hours, wearing protective clothing, and using sunscreen [5].

Broad spectrum sunscreen leads to a reduction in the formation of thymine dimers *in vivo* [6]. Routine use of sunscreen can prevent the development of NMSC [7, 8]. High sun protection factor (SPF) sunscreens have not been associated with increased sun exposure time in the general population [9]. Additionally, though controversial, regular sunscreen use may prevent the development of melanoma as well as nevi in fair-skinned children [10–12].

Sunscreen use habits can vary by region, education level, socioeconomic status (SES), racial/ethnic background, and age. Coups et al. found that young, Midwestern, non-Hispanic white (NHW), and less-educated males had the greatest number of skin cancer risk behaviors [13]. Buller et al., however, demonstrated that NHW, particularly males with higher incomes [14], experience higher rates of sunburn than Hispanic white (HW) [15]. Among Hispanics, acculturation appears to be positively associated with sunscreen use, with education level being a significant confounding variable [16].

Although the use of sunscreen for skin cancer prevention has been a topic heavily discussed in the media [17], there is little attention paid to the market availability of sunscreen and its possible effect on sunscreen usage. A study of female athletes demonstrated that the application of sunscreen significantly increased with improved access to sunscreen [18]. The cost of sunscreen, especially in the setting of daily use, can be expensive and unmanageable for certain patients who

TABLE 1: Demographics of selected zip codes.

	Cook County		San Diego County		Miami-Dade County	
Zip code	60611	60622	92127	92025	33156	33189
Median household income	$85,583	$64,037	$117,016	$45,998	$94,399	$51,677
Population	28,718	52,548	39,337	49,978	31,315	23,828
Median age	39.5	31.0	35.2	31.1	41.3	36.0
High school graduate or higher	99.5%	86.9%	96.6%	70.3%	93%	84%
Unemployed	6.7%	5.3%	5.4%	8.1%	5.4%	10.4%
Hispanic or Latino	4.9%	29.1%	9.5%	55.3%	47.9%	56.9%

require daily protection [19]. Sunscreen provided to study participants gratis correlated with increased usage with a decrease in sunburn, without an increase in sun exposure time [20]. Thus, the effect of cost on sunscreen usage could perhaps account for the finding that patients of lower SES, especially Hispanics, have a relatively larger proportion of nodular melanomas and relatively fewer superficial spreading melanomas [21].

Though the quality of available sunscreens has significantly improved over the course of the last 15 years, there is little data regarding the availability of quality sun protection in different communities. Wang et al. found marked improvements in sunscreen availability from 1997 to 2009 in the city of Cincinnati, with increases in SPF values and broad spectrum coverage, and a decrease in products with an SPF less than 15 [22]. As sunscreen availability likely varies by geographic location and local demographic characteristics, we sought to compare the availability of sunscreens in three large metropolitan counties in the USA and examine the relationship between sunscreen availability and community demographic characteristics.

2. Methods

2.1. Study Sites. We performed a cross-sectional study to evaluate sunscreens sold at pharmacies and supermarkets in Cook County in Illinois, San Diego County in California, and Miami-Dade County in Florida. Two zip codes, one with high income and the other with low income, were chosen from each county, based on the rank order provided by the U.S. Census [23]. To create a comparable match between the zip codes within each county, we chose zip codes of similar population size and geographic proximity such that the zip codes are not farther than 2 zip codes away from each other. Zip codes 92127 and 92025 (Cook County), 60611 and 60622 (San Diego County), and 33156 and 33189 (Miami-Dade County) were selected. The 2010 U.S. Census data, melanoma incidence [24], and geography of these zip codes are provided in Tables 1 and 2 and Figure 1, respectively.

We evaluated all pharmacies and supermarkets containing a sunscreen or sun care isle in the selected zip codes open as of July 2013. When more than one store of the same chain existed within the zip code, we randomly chose a single store location to include in the study. We evaluated products sold in the sunscreen or sun product isles only. Sunscreens were counted based on their visibility to a consumer. The depth of

TABLE 2: Melanoma incidence and demographic information of Miami-Dade, Cook, and San Diego Counties.

County	Melanoma incidence	Median household income[22]	High school degree or higher in 25+ year olds[22]	% White non-Hispanic[22]
	2006–2010	2007–2011	2007–2011	2012
Miami-Dade	8.7 per 100,000	$43,957	77.6%	16.3%
Cook	12.6 per 100,000	$54,598	83.7%	43.4%
San Diego	26.9 per 100,000	$63,857	85.3%	47.6%

the shelf was not recorded, but the width of the shelf was; for example, 3 identical sunscreens lined side-by-side would be counted as 3.

2.2. Measures. We quantified the market availability of sunscreen products by the percentage of tanning oil, sunscreens with an SPF less than 15 (SPF < 15), sunscreens with an SPF greater than 15 (SPF > 15), physical sunscreens, spray sunscreens, mean price per ounce, and mean SPF. As an SPF > 15 with proportional UV-A coverage has been recommended as a minimum requirement for sunscreens [25], our main outcome measures were the percentages of sunscreens with an SPF > 15, SPF < 15, and the price per ounce of each sunscreen between high and low income zip codes. Secondary measures included the percentage of tanning oils, physical blockers, spray sunscreens, and mean SPF between these high and low income zip codes. With the FDA proposing a cut-off at an SPF of 50+, we calculated a corrected SPF where original values greater than 50 were recorded as 50 [26]. Physical blockers were defined as those sunscreens containing zinc oxide and titanium dioxide. Sunscreens containing chemical UV absorbers or only the physical blocker titanium were considered to be chemical sunscreens, as these lack physical UV-A protection [27].

2.3. Statistical Analyses. We performed statistical analysis using the SPSS software version 21 (IBM Corporation, Chicago). To compare the percentage of sunscreens with SPF > 15, SPF < 15, tanning oils, physical blockers, and spray sunscreens between high and low income zip codes,

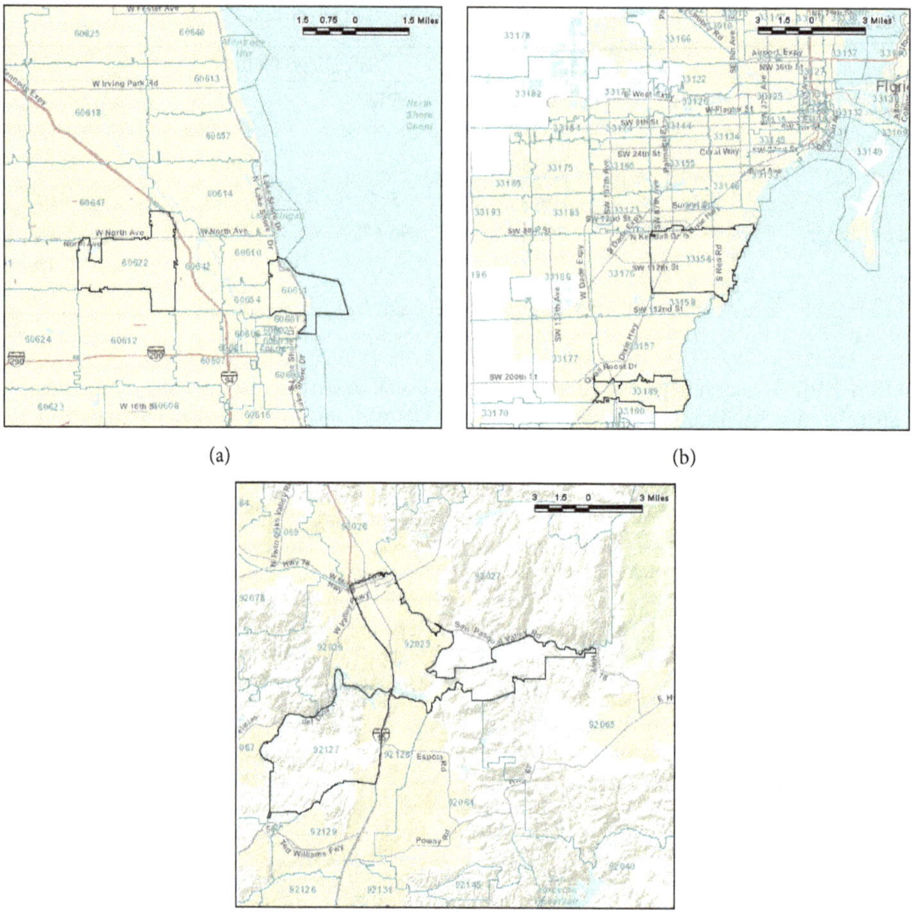

(a) (b) (c)

FIGURE 1: Selected zip codes in (a) Cook County, (b) Miami-Dade County, and (c) San Diego County.

we constructed a 2×2 contingency table and performed a χ^2 analysis. For tests failing to meet the χ^2 requirements, we used the Fischer-exact test. To compare price per ounce, price, and mean SPF we used an independent-samples t-test without the assumption of equal variances. All tests were two sided and significance was defined at the level of $P < 0.05$. A subgroup analysis was performed to evaluate for variations in each geographic location.

3. Results

A total of 1,660 sun products were assessed. Tanning oils accounted for 11.0% of total sun products. The percentages of products with SPF < 15 and SPF > 15 were 14.9% and 65.4%, respectively. Physical sunscreens accounted for 3.4% of available sunscreens and were significantly more expensive than chemical sunscreens. 46.2% of sunscreen were spray-on. Spray-on sunscreens were significantly cheaper than lotion sunscreens. The mean price per ounce of sunscreen was $2.10 with a mean SPF of 34.3. Chemical sunscreens and spray sunscreens were significantly cheaper than physical and lotion sunscreens, respectively (Table 3).

TABLE 3: Makeup of the sampled sunscreen isles with comparisons between the price per ounce, corrected for SPF, of physical versus chemical sunscreens and spray versus lotion sunscreens.

Sunscreens sampled $n = 1{,}660$	
% Tanning oils	11.0%
% SPF < 15	14.9%
% SPF > 15	65.4%
% Physical sunscreens	3.4%
Price per ounce · SPF physical = $0.10	
Price per ounce · SPF chemical = $0.07	
$P < 0.01$	
% Spray sunscreens	46.2%
Price per ounce · SPF lotion = $0.08	
Price per ounce · SPF spray = $0.03	
$P < 0.01$	
Mean price per Oz.	$2.10
Mean corrected SPF	34.3

A comparison between higher and lower income zip codes demonstrated a significantly increased percentage of

TABLE 4: Available sun products by zip code with comparisons between high and low income zip codes. "High income" zip codes represent the aggregates 92127, 33156, and 60611. "Low income" zip codes represent the aggregates 92025, 33189, and 60622.

	Zip code	Number of sunscreens sampled	Tanning oils %	SPF < 15%	SPF > 15%	Physical sunscreen %	Price per ounce	Spray %	Mean corrected SPF
Region	High income	552	16.3%	19.7%	59.6%	3.9%	1.97	40.3	30.8
	Lower income	1108	8.3%	12.2%	68.3%	3.1%	2.17	49.2	36.1
	P value		$P < 0.01$	$P < 0.01$	$P < 0.01$	$P = 0.40$	$P = 0.03$	$P < 0.01$	$P < 0.01$
San Diego County	92127	171	10.5%	20.5%	43.9%	4.6%	\$2.12	40.5%	33.4
	92025	475	3.6%	15.4%	55.4%	3.3%	\$2.25	48.7%	37.6
	P value		$P < 0.01$	$P = 0.15$	$P = 0.01$	$P = 0.62$	$P = 0.03$	$P = 0.10$	$P < 0.01$
Miami-Dade County	33156	259	23.9%	25.1%	59.5%	0.5%	\$1.87	39.6%	26.3
	33189	404	15.1%	11.9%	71.8%	0.6%	\$1.94	55.1%	32.6
	P value		$P < 0.01$	$P < 0.01$	$P < 0.01$	$P = 0.70^*$	$P = 0.01$	$P < 0.01$	$P < 0.01$
Cook County	60611	122	8.2%	7.4%	82.0%	8.9%	\$2.03	41.1%	36.6
	60622	229	6.1%	6.1%	89.1%	6.5%	\$2.19	40.9%	39.3
	P value		$P = 0.61$	$P = 0.82$	$P = 0.90$	$P = 0.53$	$P = 0.18$	$P = 0.92$	$P = 0.10$

*Fischer-exact test used in place of χ^2.

tanning oils and sunscreens with SPF < 15 in high income zip codes. Lower income zip codes had higher percentages of sunscreens with SPF > 15 and spray sunscreens, as well as a higher mean corrected SPF (Table 4). The price of sunscreen per ounce was significantly higher in the lower income zip codes than in the higher income zip codes. When price per ounce was adjusted with corrected SPF, the mean price per SPF ounce was still higher than in the lower income zip codes (0.094 versus 0.076, $P < 0.01$). There was no significant difference in the percentage of physical sunscreens among high and low income zip codes.

Subgroup analysis found similar stratification in sunscreen SPF and price only in Miami-Dade County. San Diego County demonstrated similar findings, except that there was no statistically significant difference in the percentage of sunscreens with an SPF > 15 or spray sunscreens. There was no statistically significant difference between the selected high and low income zip codes in Cook County.

3.1. Comment. We performed a cross-sectional study of sunscreens available in a representative high and low income zip codes in three major metropolitan counties in the United States. In the 3 counties surveyed, chemical sunscreens and spray sunscreens were more prevalent and inexpensive than physical sunscreens and sun lotions. Sunscreens sampled from San Diego County, the county with the highest incidence of melanoma amongst our sampled counties, had the lowest percentage of tanning oils (5.4%) yet the highest mean price per ounce (\$2.22). In contrast, Miami-Dade County, the county with the lowest incidence of melanoma amongst our sampled counties, had the highest percentage of tanning oil availability (18.5%), but the lowest price per ounce of sunscreen (\$1.91). From the three sampled counties, tanning oil availability appears to have a negative association with melanoma incidence while the price of sunscreen appears to have a positive association. Amongst all three counties sampled, lower income zip codes demonstrated an increased availability of sunscreens SPF > 15 with a smaller proportion of tanning oils. Prices were, however, higher for sunscreens in lower income zip codes than in higher income zip codes.

3.2. Physical versus Chemical Blocker. Sunscreens containing physical UV-A blockers were a lot less available compared to chemical sunscreens (3.4% versus 96.6%) in our study. Chemical sunscreens have certain limitations which makes the apparent lower market share of physical blockers concerning. Butyl methoxydibenzoylmethane (avobenzone) provides UV-A coverage in chemical sunscreens. However, it requires additional chemicals to increase its stability in sunlight [28, 29]. Without these photostabilizers or with the exhaustion of these stabilizers, UV-A protection can significantly decrease in as little as 60 minutes [30, 31]. This was confirmed in a study that demonstrated poor photostability of avobenzone in a majority of sunscreens in the market [32]. Additionally, chemical sunscreen is one of the most common causes of photoallergy [33, 34].

As opposed to chemical sunscreens that provide protection by mainly absorbing UV radiation, physical blockers absorb, reflect, and scatter UV radiation [35]. Physical blocks have superior photostability and are thus recommended for children and sunscreen allergic patients [36]. They are also recommended for use in patients with photoreactions towards visible light [37]. However, users may prefer chemical over physical blockers due to the thicker consistency of physical blocks [38]. This was similarly demonstrated in a study of facial sunscreen vehicles and usage patterns [39]. The significantly lower price per ounce of chemical blockers may additionally lead to increased availability.

3.3. Spray Sunscreens. Sunscreens dispensed by spray accounted for 46.2% of sampled sunscreen. The significantly lower price per ounce of spray-on sunscreen may account for its high availability. While spray-on sunscreens may account for a notable proportion of the sun care isle, little data is available regarding the actual amount of sunscreen successfully applied when using a spray sunscreen. Other delivery systems such as a lotion dispenser or stick have been shown to affect the amount of sunscreen users apply [40]. As sunscreen is already typically applied at far less than the thickness required to achieve the labeled SPF [41, 42], more data is needed on the efficacy of spray sunscreen. Additionally, there have been recent concerns regarding the risk of combustion and injury when using these sunscreens [43].

3.4. Differences in Sunscreens Offered by Zip Code. Though market availability of sunscreen is insufficient to conclude consumer habits and preventative behaviors, clear differences existed between sunscreen availability in high and low income zip codes overall as well as within Miami-Dade County and San Diego County. Tanning oil and sunscreens with SPF < 15 accounted for a greater proportion of sunscreens sold in the higher income, more educated zip codes, which notably had a higher mean age than their lower income and less educated counterparts. This is alarming given the higher sunburn prevalence in the higher income subset of non-Hispanic males [14, 44]. The relationship between sunburn prevalence and market availability of sunscreen SPF > 15 is not known and may be driven by consumer preference and sun protective behavior, but clearly the higher market share of SPF < 15 sunscreens in communities with higher levels of education and older communities needs to be addressed. As these higher income and more educated zip codes contain a larger percentage of non-Hispanics, it is possible that this is the determinate factor. Additionally, despite an increase of skin cancer risk factors in Midwesterners [13], our study notably demonstrated the lowest proportion of tanning oils and highest proportion of SPF > 15 sunscreens in Cook County provided the best coverage. Tanning oil availability does not appear from our limited sample, however, to be positively associated with melanoma incidence.

Perhaps the most concerning finding is the difference in pricing of sunscreen between high and low income zip codes. Even after correcting for the level of SPF in the sunscreen, lower income zip codes demonstrated a significantly elevated price of sunscreen per ounce. As price can often serve as a deterrent to sunscreen usage [19], this effect could be magnified in a low income community. Additionally, as price was the highest in the county with the greatest melanoma incidence and lowest in the county with the lowest melanoma incidence, further research is needed regarding the association between sunscreen prices and skin cancer.

3.5. Limitations. The use of a single high income and low income zip code could potentially bias our findings by not taking into account variability amongst all higher income zip codes and all lower income zip codes. The effect of this bias may be greatest when comparing findings between each county as a whole, as we only analyzed two zip codes from each county. To compare high and low income zip codes, however, we matched the zip codes by numerous demographic factors between each of the three counties to create an aggregate of high and low income zip codes. The exclusion of duplicate chain stores could have an effect on our results, potentially leading to a sample size from lower income zip codes that was twice that of high income zip codes. Nevertheless, the notable differences in sunscreens available by community demographics must raise further inquiry, as the supply of sunscreen could easily have an effect on consumer habits.

Though our study investigated 3 metropolitan counties, it can potentially extend beyond just large urban settings. In a study of sunscreen usage with planned exposure, rural residents were equally likely as urban residents to use sunscreen following the removal of confounding variables [45]. More research is needed to evaluate sales patterns within communities, and in areas outside of the large city setting to better understand the relationship between market availability and consumer habits and regional differences.

4. Conclusion

The market for sunscreens is constantly evolving, requiring further research to ensure the maintenance of adequate skin cancer and sunburn prevention. The study of changes in sunscreen patterns, however, requires an epidemiological approach, as community structure and regional differences noticeably alter the supply side of the sunscreen market. With this information, preventative education and initiatives can be tailored to individual community needs.

References

[1] A. Katsambas and E. Nicolaidou, "Cutaneous malignant melanoma and sun exposure. Recent developments in epidemiology," *Archives of Dermatology*, vol. 132, no. 4, pp. 444–450, 1996.

[2] T. Mudigonda, D. J. Pearce, B. A. Yentzer, P. Williford, and S. R. Feldman, "The economic impact of non-melanoma skin cancer: a review," *Journal of the National Comprehensive Cancer Network*, vol. 8, no. 8, pp. 888–896, 2010.

[3] B. O. Cakir, P. Adamson, and C. Cingi, "Epidemiology and economic burden of nonmelanoma skin cancer," *Facial Plastic Surgery Clinics of North America*, vol. 20, no. 4, pp. 419–422, 2012.

[4] M. M. Warthan, D. S. Sewell, R. A. Marlow, M. L. Warthan, and R. F. Wagner Jr., "The economic impact of acute sunburn," *Archives of Dermatology*, vol. 139, no. 8, pp. 1003–1006, 2003.

[5] S. Lautenschlager, H. C. Wulf, and M. R. Pittelkow, "Photoprotection," *The Lancet*, vol. 370, no. 9586, pp. 528–537, 2007.

[6] R. Bissonnette, S. Allas, D. Moyal, and N. Provost, "Comparison of UVA protection afforded by high sun protection factor sunscreens," *Journal of the American Academy of Dermatology*, vol. 43, no. 6, pp. 1036–1038, 2000.

[7] C. Ulrich, J. S. Jürgensen, A. Degen et al., "Prevention of non-melanoma skin cancer in organ transplant patients by regular use of a sunscreen: a 24 months, prospective, case-control study," *British Journal of Dermatology*, vol. 161, supplement 3, pp. 78–84, 2009.

[8] A. Green, G. Williams, R. Neale et al., "Daily sunscreen application and betacarotene supplementation in prevention of basal-cell and squamous-cell carcinomas of the skin: a randomised controlled trial," *The Lancet*, vol. 354, no. 9180, pp. 723–729, 1999.

[9] A. Dupuy, A. Dunant, and J.-J. Grob, "Randomized controlled trial testing the impact of high-protection sunscreens on sun-exposure behavior," *Archives of Dermatology*, vol. 141, no. 8, pp. 950–956, 2005.

[10] T. K. Lee, J. K. Rivers, and R. P. Gallagher, "Site-specific protective effect of broad-spectrum sunscreen on nevus development among white schoolchildren in a randomized trial," *Journal of the American Academy of Dermatology*, vol. 52, no. 5, pp. 786–792, 2005.

[11] J. S. Mulliken, J. E. Russak, and D. S. Rigel, "The effect of sunscreen on melanoma risk," *Dermatologic Clinics*, vol. 30, no. 3, pp. 369–376, 2012.

[12] J. K. Robinson and M. Bigby, "Prevention of melanoma with regular sunscreen use," *Journal of the American Medical Association*, vol. 306, no. 3, pp. 302–303, 2011.

[13] E. J. Coups, S. L. Manne, and C. J. Heckman, "Multiple skin cancer risk behaviors in the U.S. population," *The American Journal of Preventive Medicine*, vol. 34, no. 2, pp. 87–93, 2008.

[14] D. B. Buller, V. Cokkinides, H. I. Hall et al., "Prevalence of sunburn, sun protection, and indoor tanning behaviors among Americans: review from national surveys and case studies of 3 states," *Journal of the American Academy of Dermatology*, vol. 65, no. 5, supplement 1, pp. S114–S123, 2011.

[15] H. I. Hall, M. Saraiya, T. Thompson, A. Hartman, K. Glanz, and B. Rimer, "Correlates of Sunburn Experiences among U.S. Adults: results of the 2000 National Health Interview Survey," *Public Health Reports*, vol. 118, no. 6, pp. 540–549, 2003.

[16] V. A. Andreeva, M. G. Cockburn, A. L. Yaroch, J. B. Unger, R. Rueda, and K. D. Reynolds, "Preliminary evidence for mediation of the association between acculturation and sun-safe behaviors," *Archives of Dermatology*, vol. 147, no. 7, pp. 814–819, 2011.

[17] V. Cokkinides, D. Kirkland, K. Andrews, K. Sullivan, and J. L. Lichtenfeld, "A profile of skin cancer prevention media coverage in 2009," *Journal of the American Academy of Dermatology*, vol. 67, no. 4, pp. 570–575, 2012.

[18] L. E. Dubas and B. B. Adams, "Sunscreen use and availability among female collegiate athletes," *Journal of the American Academy of Dermatology*, vol. 67, no. 5, pp. 876.e1–876.e6, 2012.

[19] E. Mahe, A. Beauchet, M. F. de Maleissye, and P. Saiag, "Are sunscreens luxury products?" *Journal of the American Academy of Dermatology*, vol. 65, no. 3, pp. e73–e79, 2011.

[20] I. Nicol, C. Gaudy, J. Gouvernet, M. A. Richard, and J. J. Grob, "Skin protection by sunscreens is improved by explicit labeling and providing free sunscreen," *Journal of Investigative Dermatology*, vol. 127, no. 1, pp. 41–48, 2007.

[21] R. A. Pollitt, C. A. Clarke, S. M. Swetter, D. H. Peng, J. Zadnick, and M. Cockburn, "The expanding melanoma burden in California hispanics: importance of socioeconomic distribution, histologic subtype, and anatomic location," *Cancer*, vol. 117, no. 1, pp. 152–161, 2011.

[22] S. Q. Wang, P. R. Tanner, H. W. Lim, and J. F. Nash, "The evolution of sunscreen products in the United States—a 12-year cross sectional study," *Photochemical & Photobiological Sciences*, vol. 12, no. 1, pp. 197–202, 2013.

[23] Bureau USC, "Community Facts," Government Printing Office, Washington, DC, USA, 2010, http://factfinder2.census.gov.

[24] National Center for Health Statistics, "Incidence Rates Report," National Center for Health Statistics, 2013.

[25] H. W. Lim, M. Naylor, H. Hönigsmann et al., "American Academy of Dermatology consensus conference on UVA protection of sunscreens: summary and recommendations," *Journal of the American Academy of Dermatology*, vol. 44, no. 3, pp. 505–508, 2001.

[26] S. Q. Wang and H. W. Lim, "Current status of the sunscreen regulation in the United States: 2011 Food and Drug Administration's final rule on labeling and effectiveness testing," *Journal of the American Academy of Dermatology*, vol. 65, no. 4, pp. 863–869, 2011.

[27] P. Kullavanijaya and H. W. Lim, "Photoprotection," *Journal of the American Academy of Dermatology*, vol. 52, no. 6, pp. 937–958, 2005.

[28] E. Chatelain and B. Gabard, "Photostabilization of butyl methoxydibenzoylmethane (Avobenzone) and ethylhexyl methoxycinnamate by bis-ethylhexyloxyphenol methoxyphenyl triazine (Tinosorb S), a new UV broadband filter," *Photochemistry and Photobiology*, vol. 74, no. 3, pp. 401–406, 2001.

[29] L. R. Gaspar and P. M. B. G. Maia Campos, "Evaluation of the photostability of different UV filter combinations in a sunscreen," *International Journal of Pharmaceutics*, vol. 307, no. 2, pp. 123–128, 2006.

[30] H. Gonzalez, N. Tarras-Wahlberg, B. Strömdahl et al., "Photostability of commercial sunscreens upon sun exposure and irradiation by ultraviolet lamps," *BMC Dermatology*, vol. 7, article 1, 2007.

[31] A. Deflandre and G. Lang, "Photostability assessment of sunscreens. Benzylidene camphor and dibenzoylmethane derivatives," *International Journal of Cosmetic Science*, vol. 10, no. 2, pp. 53–62, 1988.

[32] H. Ou-Yang, J. W. Stanfield, C. Cole, and Y. Appa, "An evaluation of ultraviolet A protection and photo-stability of sunscreens marketed in Australia and New Zealand," *Photodermatology Photoimmunology and Photomedicine*, vol. 26, no. 6, pp. 336–337, 2010.

[33] E. Scheuer and E. Warshaw, "Sunscreen allergy: a review of epidemiology, clinical characteristics, and responsible allergens," *Dermatitis*, vol. 17, no. 1, pp. 3–11, 2006.

[34] D. Bilsland and J. Ferguson, "Contact allergy to sunscreen chemicals in photosensitivity dermatitis/actinic reticuloid syndrome (PD/AR) and polymorphic light eruption (PLE)," *Contact Dermatitis*, vol. 29, no. 2, pp. 70–73, 1993.

[35] K. Morabito, N. C. Shapley, K. G. Steeley, and A. Tripathi, "Review of sunscreen and the emergence of non-conventional absorbers and their applications in ultraviolet protection," *International Journal of Cosmetic Science*, vol. 33, no. 5, pp. 385–390, 2011.

[36] M. D. Palm and M. N. O'Donoghue, "Update on photoprotection," *Dermatology and Therapy*, vol. 20, no. 5, pp. 360–376, 2007.

[37] H. Moseley, H. Cameron, T. MacLeod, C. Clark, R. Dawe, and J. Ferguson, "New sunscreens confer improved protection for

photosensitive patients in the blue light region," *British Journal of Dermatology*, vol. 145, no. 5, pp. 789-794, 2001.

[38] B. L. Diffey and J. Grice, "The influence of sunscreen type on photoprotection," *British Journal of Dermatology*, vol. 137, no. 1, pp. 103–105, 1997.

[39] B. A. Solky, P. K. Phillips, L. J. Christenson, A. L. Weaver, R. K. Roenigk, and C. C. Otley, "Patient preferences for facial sunscreens: a split-face, randomized, blinded trial," *Journal of the American Academy of Dermatology*, vol. 57, no. 1, pp. 67–72, 2007.

[40] A. Diaz, R. E. Neale, M. G. Kimlin, L. Jones, and M. Janda, "The children and sunscreen study: a crossover trial investigating children's sunscreen application thickness and the influence of age and dispenser type," *Archives of Dermatology*, vol. 148, no. 5, pp. 606–612, 2012.

[41] R. Neale, G. Williams, and A. Green, "Application patterns among participants randomized to daily sunscreen use in a skin cancer prevention trial," *Archives of Dermatology*, vol. 138, no. 10, pp. 1319–1325, 2002.

[42] N. Bech-Thomsen and H. C. Wulf, "Sunbathers' application of sunscreen is probably inadequate to obtain the sun protection factor assigned to the preparation," *Photodermatology Photoimmunology and Photomedicine*, vol. 9, no. 6, pp. 242–244, 1992.

[43] FDA, *Use Sunscreen Spray? Avoid Open Flame*, Consumer Health Information, 2013.

[44] T. T. Brown, R. D. Quain, A. B. Troxel, and J. M. Gelfand, "The epidemiology of sunburn in the US population in 2003," *Journal of the American Academy of Dermatology*, vol. 55, no. 4, pp. 577–583, 2006.

[45] W. E. Zahnd, J. Goldfarb, S. L. Scaife, and M. L. Francis, "Rural-urban differences in behaviors to prevent skin cancer: an analysis of the Health Information National Trends Survey," *Journal of the American Academy of Dermatology*, vol. 62, no. 6, pp. 950–956, 2010.

29

Melanoma Disparities among US Hispanics: Use of the Social Ecological Model to Contextualize Reasons for Inequitable Outcomes and Frame a Research Agenda

Valerie M. Harvey,[1,2] Charlene W. Oldfield,[1] Jarvis T. Chen,[3] and Karl Eschbach[4,5]

[1] *Department of Dermatology, Eastern Virginia Medical School, Norfolk, VA, USA*
[2] *Hampton University Skin of Color Research Institute, Hampton, VA, USA*
[3] *Department of Social and Behavioral Science, Harvard School of Public Health, Boston, MA, USA*
[4] *University of Texas Medical Branch, Sealy Center on Aging, Galveston, TX, USA*
[5] *University of Texas Medical Branch, Center to Eliminate Health Disparities, Galveston, TX, USA*

Correspondence should be addressed to Valerie M. Harvey; harveyvm@evms.edu

Academic Editor: Mark Lebwohl

Cutaneous melanoma is a significant public health concern, accounting for thousands of deaths annually in the US. Early detection and diagnosis are critical given the poor prognosis and limited treatment options of advanced-stage disease. While non-Hispanic whites have higher incidence rates of melanoma, Hispanics are typically diagnosed at later disease stages and suffer higher morbidity and mortality. Currently, there is a paucity of literature investigating the root causes underlying these trends among Hispanics. Given that Hispanics are the most rapidly expanding demographic segment in the US, it is essential for cancer control efforts to elucidate the major determinants of their poor melanoma outcomes. Herein, we use the social ecological model as a framework to explore the multitude of influences on melanoma disparities among Hispanics and provide recommendations for planning future studies and interventions.

1. Introduction

Cutaneous melanoma (CM) is a significant public health concern, accounting for approximately 10,000 deaths annually in the United States (US) [1]. The poor prognosis and limited treatment options of advanced-stage disease make early detection and diagnosis critical. Although the incidence of melanoma is greatest in non-Hispanic whites (NHWs), numerous studies have shown that Hispanics diagnosed with melanoma are more likely to experience worse outcomes [2–7]. Surveillance, Epidemiology, and End Results data reveal that Hispanics diagnosed with melanoma are 2.4 times (age-adjusted odds ratio (OR), confidence interval (CI) 1.89–3.05) more likely to present with stage III disease [6] and 3.64 times more likely (CI 2.65–5.0) to have distant metastases than non-Hispanic whites (NHWs) [3, 4, 8–11]. Moreover, while the proportion of those with local-staged melanoma has increased significantly among NHWs, an opposing trend has been reported among Hispanic men living in California who were found to have thicker primary tumors at diagnosis [12]. Factors in the late presentation of CM in Hispanics may include lack of awareness and knowledge [6], lower rates of self-examinations and physician performed skin examinations [7], and differences in tumor biology [6]. For cancer control efforts to succeed, we must better understand the major causes of advanced presentation of melanoma in Hispanics (Hispanics and Latinos) who represent the most rapidly expanding demographic segment in the US.

The Hispanic category is multiethnic, encompassing populations with distinct national origins. Census Bureau data shows 55 million Hispanics living in the US, comprising of 35 million Mexican Americans, 8.7 million Puerto Ricans (including 3.4 million in Puerto Rico), 2 million Cubans, and 1.8 million Dominicans [13]. The recent immigration

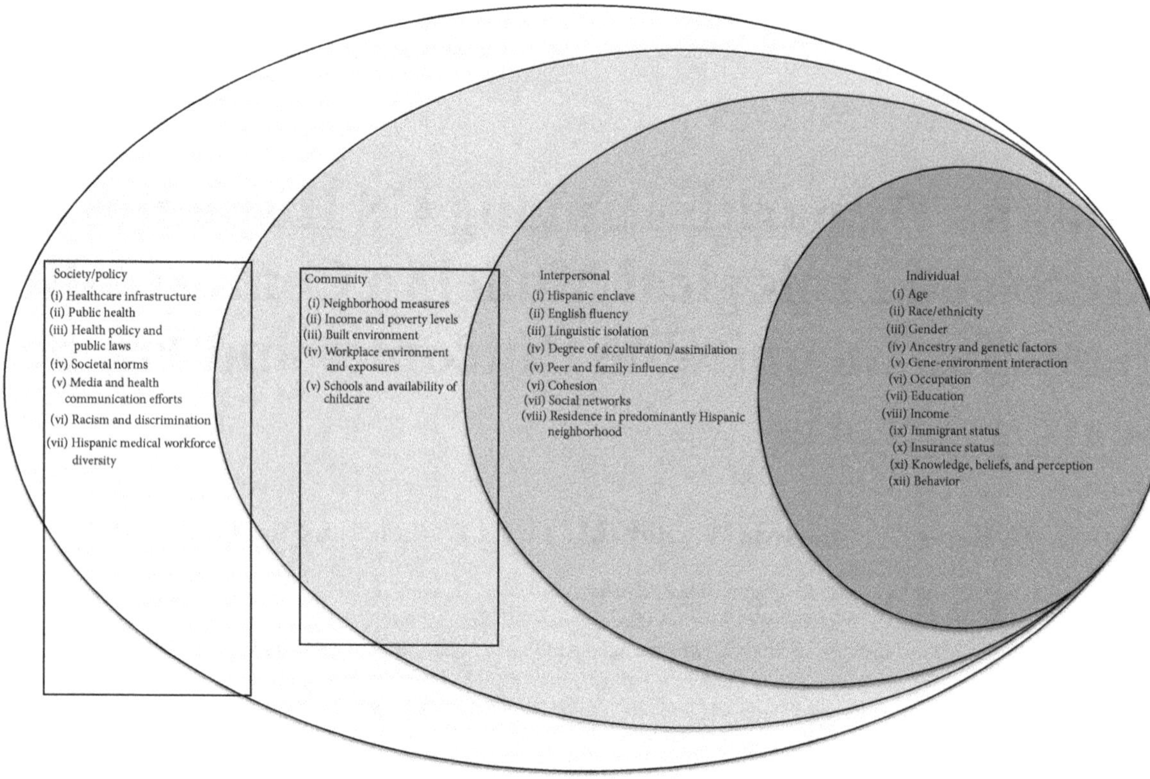

FIGURE 1: Social ecological model [88].

of over 8 million Hispanics from Central and South America has increased the diversity of the Hispanic population and even displaced Cubans as the third largest group [13]. These national origin groups are increasingly diverse, in nativity, primary language, acculturation, education, and occupation. Understanding the contributors to late-stage melanoma presentation in this heterogeneous group provides an opportunity to explore the effects of immigration and acculturation on determinants of cancer risk and outcomes. The objective of this article is to provide a framework for studying melanoma disparities in Hispanics and to provide recommendations for a research agenda to facilitate future research and interventions.

2. Conceptual Framework

The social ecological model (SEM) provides a dynamic and integrative framework for analyzing social and spatial variations in human health and disease [14, 15] (Figure 1). At the model's core lies the concept that health outcomes result from a unique combination of personal, interpersonal, and community attributes, thereby contextualizing the reciprocal interdependence of individuals and their environment. The individual level identifies biological and personal factors, including age, gender, genetics, knowledge, and behavior. The interpersonal level looks at how relationships with peers, partners, families, and social networks influence health. The community level examines settings such as the neighborhoods, schools, and workplaces within which disease occurs and seeks to identify the characteristics of these settings that promote or prevent disease. The policy/societal level investigates the broader structural determinants such as health system infrastructure, health care access, health care resources and utilization, health policies, workforce diversity, and societal norms. While numerous studies have documented connections between individual health outcomes and the influence of these social and spatial determinants [16–22], few have used this paradigm to understand the reasons for disparities in melanoma outcomes [23].

3. Individual Determinants

Individual attributes, including age, race/ethnicity, gender, beliefs/attitudes, behavior, and health insurance status are thought to impact cancer outcomes [24, 25]. While age-adjusted incidence rates of CM among Hispanics (4.8/100,000 for men and 4.5/100,000 for women) are lower than those for NHWs (33.6/100,000 and 20.2/100,000 for men and women, resp.) [26], Hispanics are more likely to be diagnosed at a more advanced stage and have thicker tumors than their non-Hispanic white counterparts [4, 6, 27]. Moreover, Hispanics have an increased mortality [4, 5]. The clinical presentation of CM also differs across race and ethnicity, with Hispanics having a higher incidence of lower extremity involvement (25% versus 9%; $P < 0.001$) [5], and a greater frequency of the acral lentiginous histological subtype than NHWs [5, 6]. The reasons for phenotypic variability are not entirely clear but may include genetic factors, gene-environment interaction, and/or inherent differences in the kinetics of tumor growth.

3.1. Health Insurance. Notably, Hispanics have the highest uninsured rate of any other racial/ethnic group in the US [28]. This is due in part to low-wage jobs without employer-based health benefits. Health insurance status has been shown to be a determinant of disparities in melanoma outcomes [29–31]. Intermittent and newly enrolled Medicaid CM patients were 2–13 times more likely, respectively, to have late-stage melanoma than those not on Medicaid. Medicare and Medicaid patients with CM were less likely than their privately insured counterparts to undergo sentinel lymph biopsies [29], indicating that publicly insured individuals may be understaged and possibly inadequately treated. Insurance may also attenuate disparities. For example, Hispanics enrolled in Medicare health maintenance organizations (HMOs) were diagnosed with CM at earlier stages and had decreased mortality than their age-matched controls in a Medicare fee-for-service program [32]. This observation may be in part due to the "HMO effect," meaning that those enrolled in an HMO will have more points of contact with their primary care provider and may therefore be more likely to undergo preventive services such as skin cancer screenings [32].

3.2. Knowledge and Awareness. Knowledge may be an important predictor of preventive behaviors and use of screening services for melanoma. Temoshok et al. found that low levels of CM knowledge and understanding were associated with greater tumor thickness at diagnosis [33]. Studies show that Hispanics have less melanoma knowledge and awareness than NHWs [34–38]. In general, Hispanics also have a low perception of personal cancer risk [34, 35, 39, 40]. Hispanics also believe they can do little to reduce their risk of skin cancer, primarily because the many recommendations make it hard for them to know which ones to follow [41]. Moreover, Hispanics are thought to ascribe to fatalism about skin cancer prevention [41, 42]. This passivity may explain why they are also less likely to seek medical care if they develop a suspicious skin lesion. Current evidence, however, is insufficient to determine how much these knowledge gaps contribute to CM inequities [43].

3.3. Behavior. Individuals who are knowledgeable and aware of the perils of melanoma are more likely to perform skin self-examinations [38, 44]. In general, compared to other racial and ethnic groups, Hispanics are less likely to comply with cancer screening guidelines [45] and have significantly lower rates of skin self-examination [27, 35, 46–49] and physician-assisted skin examination [49–51] than NHWs. Among Hispanics, factors associated with skin self-examinations and receipt of physician-assisted skin examinations include greater US acculturation, older age, an increased number of melanoma risk factors, physician recommendations [7, 40, 52], fewer skin self-examination barriers, [52] country of origin [7], tanning indoors, greater knowledge about skin cancer, greater perceived skin cancer severity, a low worry of skin cancer, and added physician-assisted skin examination benefits [52]. Hispanics cite lack of awareness of self-examination and lack of knowledge of how to conduct such an examination as primary reasons for not performing skin self-examinations [35, 40, 48]. The primary reasons for not receiving physician-assisted skin examinations were inadequate time with the physician and not knowing to ask or how to ask for an examination [40].

3.4. Occupation. A significant proportion of Hispanics work in outdoor occupations such as agriculture/landscaping, construction, maintenance, and transportation, all of which are associated with significant UV radiation and chemical exposure [53]. There is a paucity of data exploring occupational influences on skin cancer risk in this population. Day et al. found that a majority of outdoor Hispanic workers reported never wearing sunscreen, and 44% of study participants reported ever having a sunburn [54]. Similarly, 91% of migrant farmworkers in North Carolina reported never wearing sunscreen and had low levels of knowledge about melanoma [54, 55]. Melanoma risk has also been inconsistently linked to exposure to various chemicals, including arsenic and various pesticides [56]. Dennis et al. found significant associations between melanoma and several classes of pesticides in a large cohort from the Agricultural Health Survey [56]. Future longitudinal studies quantifying UV exposure as well as exposure to other environmental toxins in high risk occupations for skin cancer and melanoma development are warranted, although the low incidence of CM in this group may limit the feasibility of this type of prospective investigation [55].

3.5. Immigration Status. More than 19 million or 35% of the more than 55 million Hispanics in the US (excluding Puerto Rico) are foreign-born [57]. Of these, nearly 13 million or 23% are not US citizens [57]. The different Hispanic subgroups have very different settlement patterns and migration histories in the US. Virtually all Puerto Ricans, including the island-born, are native-born US citizens. More than two-thirds of Mexican Americans in the US were US-born. By contrast, all other major national origin groups are majority foreign-born. Each of the individual risks discussed above—insurance status, health related knowledge and behaviors, and occupational exposures—varies partially in relation to immigrant status. For example, in 2014, 14% of US-born Hispanics reported no current health insurance coverage, compared to 8% of all NHWs and 14.5% of all non-Hispanic Blacks. Among Hispanic immigrants who were citizens, 17% did not have health insurance coverage. However, more than half of noncitizen immigrants did not have health insurance, accounting for a majority of the uninsured Hispanics.

This heterogeneity provides opportunities for understanding and exploring how the genome, environment, and cultural factors contribute to CM development. It also creates important methodological challenges. The presence of a large undocumented population creates concerns about completeness of census counts supplying the denominators of incidence and mortality rates. Incidence counts may also be suppressed if a large undocumented and uninsured population has impaired access to screening and diagnosis. Mortality may be under ascertained in an immigrant population because of health selective return migration out of the US after a CM diagnosis. These issues have been recognized in the epidemiological literature, but empirical investigation of their net impact on the data has been limited [45].

4. Interpersonal Determinants

The SEM also considers how interpersonal determinants, or relationships with peers, family members, and the immediate social milieu influence health outcomes. Acculturation, the process by which immigrants and their families adopt the language, attitudes, behaviors, and norms of their host country, has been associated with behavioral changes in relation to skin cancer risk among Hispanics [55, 58–60]. US cultural norms favor sunscreen use and sun tanning more than Hispanic cultural norms [58]. Acculturation among Hispanics has been linked to higher perceived benefits of exposure to UV radiation [60], less worry about skin damage [60], higher rates of sunbathing [59], higher rates of indoor tanning [59], and an increased risk of sunburns [55]. One study found that more than half of acculturated Hispanics reported having sunburns in the past year, as compared to just 1 in 3 of less acculturated Hispanics [55]. Importantly, sun-protective behaviors vary by country of origin. Individuals from Central/South America, Puerto Rico, and Cuba reported lower rates of having a sunburn and decreased usage of sun-protective clothing than those from other Hispanic/Latino countries [55]. These examples highlight the importance of considering the diverseness of the Hispanic population when investigating health outcomes [55].

5. Community Determinants

Neighborhood measures of income, poverty, economic opportunity, and level of educational attainment are community factors shown to influence health and disease [5, 9, 10, 61, 62]. Little research exists on the community determinants of melanoma outcomes in Hispanics; what exists relies on composite measures from population-based cancer registry data. This approach makes it difficult to tease apart Hispanic subgroups and to decipher which determinants, either singly or in combination, result in melanoma inequities. Among NHWs, indicators of high socioeconomic status (SES) are associated with higher melanoma incidence rates; however, among Hispanics, 66% of the melanoma burden occurs within middle and low SES groups [5]. This opposing SES gradient in incidence suggests the existence of a unique set of exposure risks particular to Hispanics. Irrespective of race, ethnicity, or sex, patients from lower SES strata were more likely to present with thicker tumors (>2 mm) at diagnosis; however, the association of thicker tumors and low SES was most profound among Hispanic men (relative risk [RR] 2.18; confidence interval [CI] 1.73–2.74) and women (RR 1.98; 1.55–2.51), suggesting Hispanics may be disproportionately burdened by barriers to screening and care due to poverty [5]. In Florida, residence in an impoverished neighborhood was found to independently predict late-stage clustering of CM in Hispanics [63].

5.1. Education. Education helps individuals recognize the signs and symptoms that indicate the need for prompt medical attention and help them navigate through the health care system [64]. Cokkinides et al. examined age-adjusted mortality rate trends by level of educational attainment; they found that while melanoma mortality rates fell for highly educated individuals (greater than or equal to 13 years of education) over the 10-year study period, mortality for less-educated melanoma patients increased ($P = 0.17$) [65].

5.2. Access to Preventive Measures. Sunscreen availability differs across neighborhoods. To date, two studies have compared sunscreen accessibility within Hispanic and non-Hispanic communities. In Chicago, Hernandez et al. found that twice as many stores sold sunscreen in non-Hispanic neighborhoods with greater product diversity compared to Hispanic neighborhoods [66]. However, Sprague et al. were unable to replicate these results in Los Angeles, finding no significant difference in availability or diversity of sunscreen [67]. Further research is needed to elucidate the potential, if any, differences in sunscreen availability as well as the barriers to its usage and attainment that may influence CM outcomes.

6. Society and Policy Determinants

At the macro level, inequitable cancer health outcomes occur in the context of upstream societal and political factors. These elements include public/health policy and laws, health service infrastructure (financing, access, and quality), and societal norms (discrimination, racism, etc.).

6.1. Public Insurance Infrastructure. Hispanics face multiple barriers that impede access to quality healthcare. Although the rate of uninsured Hispanics among working age adults declined from 40% to 34% in 2014 with the implementation of the Patient Protection and Affordable Care Act (PPACA), Hispanics still have the highest uninsured rates of all major US racial or ethnic groups [68]. While half of uninsured Hispanics qualify for expanded Medicaid under PPACA, only 29 states and the District of Columbia enforce this provision [68]. Notably, Florida and Texas, two states which together account for a large proportion of the Hispanic populace, are among the states not participating in the Medicaid expansion. Among nonparticipating states, Hispanics continue to hold uninsured rates approaching 46% [68].

6.2. Immigration Status and Insurance. As discussed above, the low rate of health insurance coverage pertains primarily to noncitizen immigrants, of whom just less than half report

TABLE 1: Research questions and strategies by social ecological model levels of influence [89].

Research questions and strategies by SEM levels of influence		
Level of influence	Sublevel of influence	Future research questions and strategies
Society/policy	(i) Healthcare infrastructure (ii) Public health (iii) Health policy and public laws (iv) Societal norms (v) Media and health communication efforts (vi) Racism and discrimination (vii) Hispanic medical workforce diversity	(i) How does health system infrastructure impede access to dermatologic care among Hispanics? (ii) How can different media platforms be employed to increase knowledge and awareness among Hispanic subpopulations and influence CM societal norms? (iii) What are the most effective methods of dissemination of CM education? (iv) Can CM educational interventions designed for Hispanics influence outcomes? (v) How does racism/discrimination influence CM outcomes? (i) Training of physician extenders (and screen patients for skin cancer and melanoma. (ii) Implement policies that remove barriers to access of primary and specialty care. (iii) Diversification of the medical and dermatologic workforce to increase the representation of Hispanic care providers. (iv) Development of culturally and linguistically appropriate melanoma educational campaigns targeted to Hispanic subgroups. (v) Collaboration between Hispanic community stakeholders and professional medical organizations to facilitate dissemination of information/research findings to lay community.
Community	Neighborhood measures (i) Income/level of poverty (ii) Built environment (iii) Workplace environment and exposures (iv) Schools and availability of childcare	Are there unique environmental risk factors (aside from UV exposure) that increase CM risk among Hispanics? Develop longitudinal cohort studies quantifying workplace exposures and their impact on CM outcomes in Hispanics.
Interpersonal	(i) English language fluency (ii) Residence in predominantly Hispanic neighborhood (iii) Degree of assimilation (iv) Cohesion (v) Social networks (vi) Peer and family influence	What cultural factors contribute to CM risk/mortality? Do these factors vary by Hispanic country of origin? Are there components of Hispanic culture that influence participation in skin cancer screening or seeking medical care for skin conditions? How does melanoma risk vary by degree of acculturation? Develop more precise constructs to measure effects of acculturation. Development of community-based participatory research studies in which Hispanic stakeholders are included in early stages of study design.
Individual	(i) Age (ii) Race & ethnicity (iii) Gender (iv) Ancestry and genetic factors (v) Gene-environment interaction (vi) Immigration status (vii) Knowledge and behavior (viii) Insurance status (ix) Occupation (x) Health insurance status (xi) Income (xii) Education	What is the phenotypic profile of Hispanic patents with CM? Are kinetics of melanoma progression and metastasis different among Hispanics? How do CM risk and mortality vary by Hispanic subgroup? How does CM risk vary with immigration status and duration of time in US? How do fatalism and its impact on skin cancer perceptions vary between Hispanic subgroups? What role, if any, does fatalism play in CM inequities? How can melanoma knowledge and awareness be increased amongst Hispanic subgroups? Develop genetic studies (AIMS/GWAS) across Hispanic subgroups to understand the genetic basis for melanoma risk. Identification of biomarkers for melanoma disease progression within Hispanics. Case control studies of Hispanics with and without melanoma to help identify unique risk factors amongst this group. Efforts to increase recruitment of Hispanics melanoma patients into clinical trials. Transdisciplinary studies to understand the interlink between biological and social factors.

current health insurance coverage. Barriers are particularly high for the estimated 8 million undocumented immigrants from Latin America [69]. By law, undocumented immigrants are not qualified to attain health insurance through either the federal Marketplace [70] or Medicaid [71]. Medicaid also enforces a 5-year waiting period which may be waived for children, pregnant women, and certain "qualified noncitizens" (green card holders, lawful permanent resident, etc.) [70]. Overall, these policies impede primary care access. Over one-quarter of Hispanic adults lack a consistent primary care provider and are twice as likely as non-Hispanic blacks and three times as likely as NHWs to not have a regular healthcare provider [72]. Inconsistent primary care and dermatologic access have been linked to advanced melanoma at presentation [73] and decreased melanoma survival [74].

6.3. Hispanic Health Professional Shortage. Numerous studies have identified provider behaviors and bias as key contributing factors of health inequities, suggesting that cultural differences between patients and their providers impact healthcare outcomes [75–77]. Among Hispanics, race concordance is an important predictor of greater satisfaction with overall healthcare quality [78]. Hispanic physicians are more apt to provide medical care to minorities, low income, and non-English speaking patients and play a critical role in improving access to care among the underserved. Unfortunately, Hispanics are grossly underrepresented among the US physician workforce, comprising only 4.6% of US medical school graduates in 2014 [79].

6.4. Health Communication and Educational Campaigns. Health communication campaigns help shape health perceptions and risk behaviors, including those associated with melanoma. Studies demonstrate that mass media campaigns about health influence risky behaviors [80]. Previously, mass media campaigns have successfully increased screenings for cervical [81–83] and breast cancer [84]. Despite the plethora of public messaging on melanoma, most is geared towards middle aged whites [12, 85] with little being tailored towards the Hispanic population [12, 59, 85, 86]. While half of US adults report cancer-related internet searches on cancer [87], Hispanics may use it less than whites. Hay et al. found that nonwhite adults are more receptive to health information obtained via televised news [37]. Similarly, the Pew Hispanic Center and the Robert Wood Johnson Foundation found that 68% of Hispanic adults report obtaining their health information via television [72].

7. Conclusions and Recommendations

Hispanics diagnosed with melanoma typically present with advanced stages of disease and experience higher melanoma-specific mortality rates than NHWs. Yet, huge knowledge gaps exist regarding the contributors and solutions to melanoma disparities among this fast growing, understudied segment of the US population. In Table 1 we present research questions and strategies for promoting melanoma outcome equity, based on SEM level of influence. This approach highlights the need for a multidisciplinary approach spanning multiple levels of influence. Although the absolute frequency of melanoma is relatively low within the Hispanic population, melanoma studies in Hispanics (given their diverse genetic ancestry and migration) provide a unique opportunity for research to explicate melanoma etiology, benefiting Hispanics and non-Hispanics alike.

Competing Interests

The authors declare that they have no competing interests.

Acknowledgments

Funding for this project was provided by Grant no. U54MD008621 from the National Institutes of Health/ National Institute on Minority Health and Health Disparities.

References

[1] "What are the key statistics about melanoma skin cancer?" http://www.cancer.org/cancer/skincancer-melanoma/detailed-guide/melanoma-skin-cancer-key-statistics.

[2] C. M. Balch, J. E. Gershenwald, S.-J. Soong et al., "Final version of 2009 AJCC melanoma staging and classification," *Journal of Clinical Oncology*, vol. 27, no. 36, pp. 6199–6206, 2009.

[3] A. Katalinic, A. Waldmann, M. A. Weinstock et al., "Does skin cancer screening save lives? An observational study comparing trends in melanoma mortality in regions with and without screening," *Cancer*, vol. 118, no. 21, pp. 5395–5402, 2012.

[4] S. Hu, Y. Parmet, G. Allen et al., "Disparity in melanoma: a trend analysis of melanoma incidence and stage at diagnosis among whites, Hispanics, and blacks in Florida," *Archives of Dermatology*, vol. 145, no. 12, pp. 1369–1374, 2009.

[5] R. A. Pollitt, C. A. Clarke, S. M. Swetter, D. H. Peng, J. Zadnick, and M. Cockburn, "The expanding melanoma burden in California hispanics: importance of socioeconomic distribution, histologic subtype, and anatomic location," *Cancer*, vol. 117, no. 1, pp. 152–161, 2011.

[6] J. N. Cormier, Y. Xing, M. Ding et al., "Ethnic differences among patients with cutaneous melanoma," *Archives of Internal Medicine*, vol. 166, no. 17, pp. 1907–1914, 2006.

[7] E. J. Coups, J. L. Stapleton, S. V. Hudson, A. Medina-Forrester, J. S. Goydos, and A. Natale-Pereira, "Skin cancer screening among hispanic adults in the United States: results from the 2010 national health interview survey," *Archives of Dermatology*, vol. 148, no. 7, pp. 861–863, 2012.

[8] R. A. Pollitt, S. M. Swetter, T. M. Johnson, P. Patil, and A. C. Geller, "Examining the pathways linking lower socioeconomic status and advanced melanoma," *Cancer*, vol. 118, no. 16, pp. 4004–4013, 2012.

[9] C. A. Ortiz, J. S. Goodwin, and J. L. Freeman, "The effect of socioeconomic factors on incidence, stage at diagnosis and survival of cutaneous melanoma," *Medical Science Monitor*, vol. 11, no. 5, pp. RA163–RA172, 2005.

[10] S. D. Singh, U. A. Ajani, C. J. Johnson et al., "Association of cutaneous melanoma incidence with area-based socioeconomic indicators-United States, 2004–2006," *Journal of the American Academy of Dermatology*, vol. 65, no. 5, supplement 1, pp. S58–S68, 2011.

[11] R. A. Pollitt, C. A. Clarke, S. J. Shema, and S. M. Swetter, "California Medicaid enrollment and melanoma stage at diagnosis: a population-based study," *American Journal of Preventive Medicine*, vol. 35, no. 1, pp. 7–13, 2008.

[12] M. G. Cockburn, J. Zadnick, and D. Deapen, "Developing epidemic of melanoma in the hispanic population of California," *Cancer*, vol. 106, no. 5, pp. 1162–1168, 2006.

[13] Census Bureau, *HISPANIC OR LATINO ORIGIN BY SPECIFIC ORIGIN: 2014 American Community Survey 1 Year Estimates*, 2014.

[14] J. F. Sallis, N. Owen, and E. B. Fisher, "Ecological models of health behavior," in *Health Behavior and Health Education: Theory, Research and Practice*, K. Glanz, B. K. Rimer, and K.

Viswanath, Eds., Jossey-Bass, San Francisco, Calif, USA, 4th edition, 2008.

[15] D. Stokols, "Translating social ecological theory into guidelines for community health promotion," *American Journal of Health Promotion*, vol. 10, no. 4, pp. 282–298, 1996.

[16] M. A. Gerend and M. Pai, "Social determinants of black-white disparities in breast cancer mortality: a review," *Cancer Epidemiology Biomarkers and Prevention*, vol. 17, no. 11, pp. 2913–2923, 2008.

[17] P. Braveman, S. Egerter, and D. R. Williams, "The social determinants of health: coming of age," *Annual Review of Public Health*, vol. 32, pp. 381–398, 2011.

[18] H. K. Koh, S. C. Oppenheimer, S. B. Massln-Short et al., "Translating research evidence into practice to reduce health disparities: a social determinants approach," *American Journal of Public Health*, vol. 100, no. 1, pp. S72–S80, 2010.

[19] L. Márquez-Magaña, C. Samayoa, and C. Umanzor, "Debunking 'race' and asserting social determinants as primary causes of cancer health disparities: outcomes of a science education activity for teens," *Journal of Cancer Education*, vol. 28, no. 2, pp. 314–318, 2013.

[20] S. B. Wheeler, K. E. Reeder-Hayes, and L. A. Carey, "Disparities in breast cancer treatment and outcomes: biological, social, and health system determinants and opportunities for research," *Oncologist*, vol. 18, no. 9, pp. 986–993, 2013.

[21] D. R. Williams and M. Sternthal, "Understanding racial-ethnic disparities in health: sociological contributions," *Journal of Health and Social Behavior*, vol. 51, pp. S15–27, 2010.

[22] E. B. O'Keefe, J. P. Meltzer, and T. N. Bethea, "Health disparities and cancer: racial disparities in cancer mortality in the United States, 2000–2010," *Frontiers in Public Health*, vol. 3, article 51, 2015.

[23] J. A. Petersen, S. D. Quantz, F. D. Ashbury, and J. K. Sauvé, "The skin cancer prevention framework: a comprehensive tool for population-level efforts in skin cancer," *Canadian Journal of Public Health*, vol. 101, no. 4, pp. 128–132, 2010.

[24] R. L. Siegel, K. D. Miller, and A. Jemal, "Cancer statistics, 2015," *CA: Cancer Journal for Clinicians*, vol. 65, no. 1, pp. 5–29, 2015.

[25] X. Niu, K. S. Pawlish, and L. M. Roche, "Cancer survival disparities by race/ethnicity and socioeconomic status in New Jersey," *Journal of Health Care for the Poor and Underserved*, vol. 21, no. 1, pp. 144–160, 2010.

[26] "SEER Stat Fact Sheets: Melanoma of the Skin," http://seer.cancer.gov/statfacts/html/melan.html.

[27] M. Clairwood, J. Ricketts, J. Grant-Kels, and L. Gonsalves, "Melanoma in skin of color in Connecticut: an analysis of melanoma incidence and stage at diagnosis in non-Hispanic blacks, non-Hispanic whites, and Hispanics," *International Journal of Dermatology*, vol. 53, no. 4, pp. 425–433, 2014.

[28] Office of Minority Health, "Minority Population Profiles: Hispanic/Latino," 2015, http://minorityhealth.hhs.gov/omh/browse.aspx?lvl=3&lvlid=64.

[29] K. Y. Bilimoria, C. M. Balch, J. D. Wayne et al., "Health care system and socioeconomic factors associated with variance in use of sentinel lymph node biopsy for melanoma in the United States," *Journal of Clinical Oncology*, vol. 27, no. 11, pp. 1857–1863, 2009.

[30] M. McCarthy, "Surgery for melanoma is often delayed in Medicare patients, study finds," *The British Medical Journal*, vol. 350, Article ID h1886, 2015.

[31] A. Amini, C. G. Rusthoven, T. V. Waxweiler et al., "Association of health insurance with outcomes in adults ages 18 to 64 years with melanoma in the United States," *Journal of the American Academy of Dermatology*, vol. 74, no. 2, pp. 309–316, 2016.

[32] R. S. Kirsner, J. D. Wilkinson, F. Ma, H. Pacheco, and D. G. Federman, "The association of medicare health care delivery systems with stage at diagnosis and survival for patients with melanoma," *Archives of Dermatology*, vol. 141, no. 6, pp. 753–757, 2005.

[33] L. Temoshok, R. J. Diclemente, D. M. Sweet, M. S. Blois, and R. W. Sagebiel, "Factors related to patient delay in seeking medical attention for cutaneous malignant melanoma," *Cancer*, vol. 54, no. 12, pp. 3048–3053, 1984.

[34] F. Ma, F. Collado-Mesa, S. Hu, and R. S. Kirsner, "Skin cancer awareness and sun protection behaviors in white Hispanic and white non-Hispanic high school students in Miami, Florida," *Archives of Dermatology*, vol. 143, no. 8, pp. 983–988, 2007.

[35] M. Pipitone, J. K. Robinson, C. Camara, B. Chittineni, and S. G. Fisher, "Skin cancer awareness in suburban employees: a hispanic perspective," *Journal of the American Academy of Dermatology*, vol. 47, no. 1, pp. 118–123, 2002.

[36] C. E. Cheng, B. Irwin, D. Mauriello, L. Hemminger, A. Pappert, and A. B. Kimball, "Health disparities among different ethnic and racial middle and high school students in sun exposure beliefs and knowledge," *Journal of Adolescent Health*, vol. 47, no. 1, pp. 106–109, 2010.

[37] J. Hay, E. J. Coups, J. Ford, and M. DiBonaventura, "Exposure to mass media health information, skin cancer beliefs, and sun protection behaviors in a United States probability sample," *Journal of the American Academy of Dermatology*, vol. 61, no. 5, pp. 783–792, 2009.

[38] D. R. Miller, A. C. Geller, S. W. Wyatt et al., "Melanoma awareness and self-examination practices: results of a United States survey," *Journal of the American Academy of Dermatology*, vol. 34, no. 6, pp. 962–970, 1996.

[39] R. V. Kundu, M. Kamaria, S. Ortiz, D. P. West, A. W. Rademaker, and J. K. Robinson, "Effectiveness of a knowledge-based intervention for melanoma among those with ethnic skin," *Journal of the American Academy of Dermatology*, vol. 62, no. 5, pp. 777–784, 2010.

[40] C. Roman, A. Lugo-Somolinos, and N. Thomas, "Skin cancer knowledge and skin self-examinations in the hispanic population of North Carolina: the patient's perspective," *JAMA Dermatology*, vol. 149, no. 1, pp. 103–104, 2013.

[41] K. J. Buster, Z. You, M. Fouad, and C. Elmets, "Skin cancer risk perceptions: a comparison across ethnicity, age, education, gender, and income," *Journal of the American Academy of Dermatology*, vol. 66, no. 5, pp. 771–779, 2012.

[42] E. J. Coups, J. L. Stapleton, S. L. Manne et al., "Psychosocial correlates of sun protection behaviors among U.S. Hispanic adults," *Journal of Behavioral Medicine*, vol. 37, no. 6, pp. 1082–1090, 2014.

[43] V. M. Harvey, H. Patel, S. Sandhu, S. F. Wallington, and G. Hinds, "Social determinants of racial and ethnic disparities in cutaneous melanoma outcomes," *Cancer Control*, vol. 21, no. 4, pp. 343–349, 2014.

[44] M. Berwick, C. B. Begg, J. A. Fine, G. C. Roush, and R. L. Barnhill, "Screening for cutaneous melanoma by skin self-examination," *Journal of the National Cancer Institute*, vol. 88, no. 1, pp. 17–23, 1996.

[45] R. W. Haile, E. M. John, A. J. Levine et al., "A review of cancer in U.S. Hispanic populations," *Cancer Prevention Research*, vol. 5, no. 2, pp. 150–163, 2012.

[46] W. C. Black, R. T. Goldhahn Jr., and C. Wiggins, "Melanoma within a Southwestern Hispanic population," *Archives of Dermatology*, vol. 123, no. 10, pp. 1331–1334, 1987.

[47] P. Rouhani, P. S. Pinheiro, R. Sherman et al., "Increasing rates of melanoma among nonwhites in Florida compared with the United States," *Archives of Dermatology*, vol. 146, no. 7, pp. 741–746, 2010.

[48] M. R. Arnold and W. DeJong, "Skin self-examination practices in a convenience sample of US university students," *Preventive Medicine*, vol. 40, no. 3, pp. 268–273, 2005.

[49] J. Imahiyerobo-Ip, I. Ip, S. Jamal, U. Nadiminti, and M. Sanchez, "Skin cancer awareness in communities of color," *Journal of the American Academy of Dermatology*, vol. 64, no. 1, pp. 198–200, 2011.

[50] A. T. Pakilit, B. A. Kahn, L. Petersen, L. S. Abraham, G. A. Greendale, and P. A. Ganz, "Lifestyle high-risk behaviors and demographics may predict the level of participation in sun-protection behaviors and skin cancer primary prevention in the United States: results of the 1998 National Health Interview Survey," *Cancer*, vol. 92, no. 5, pp. 1315–1324, 2001.

[51] M. Saraiya, H. I. Hall, T. Thompson et al., "Skin cancer screening among U.S. adults from 1992, 1998, and 2000 National Health Interview Surveys," *Preventive Medicine*, vol. 39, no. 2, pp. 308–314, 2004.

[52] E. J. Coups, J. L. Stapleton, S. V. Hudson et al., "Skin cancer surveillance behaviors among US Hispanic adults," *Journal of the American Academy of Dermatology*, vol. 68, no. 4, pp. 576–584, 2013.

[53] United States Bureau of Labor Statistics, "Labor Force Characteristics by Race and Ethnicity," 2014, http://www.bls.gov/opub/reports/race-and-ethnicity/archive/labor-force-characteristics-by-race-and-ethnicity-2014.pdf.

[54] A. K. Day, J. L. Stapleton, A. M. Natale-Pereira, J. S. Goydos, and E. J. Coups, "Occupational sunscreen use among US Hispanic outdoor workers Cancer," *BMC Research Notes*, vol. 8, no. 1, article 578, 2015.

[55] E. J. Coups, J. L. Stapleton, S. V. Hudson, A. Medina-Forrester, A. Natale-Pereira, and J. S. Goydos, "Sun protection and exposure behaviors among Hispanic adults in the United States: differences according to acculturation and among Hispanic subgroups," *BMC Public Health*, vol. 12, article 985, 2012.

[56] L. K. Dennis, C. F. Lynch, D. P. Sandler, and M. C. R. Alavanja, "Pesticide use and cutaneous melanoma in pesticide applicators in the agricultural heath study," *Environmental Health Perspectives*, vol. 118, no. 6, pp. 812–817, 2010.

[57] United States Census Bureau, "Selected population profile in the United States 2014 American community survey 1-year estimates," http://factfinder.census.gov/faces/tableservices/jsf/pages/productview.xhtml?src=bkmk.

[58] V. A. Andreeva, J. B. Unger, A. L. Yaroch, M. G. Cockburn, L. Baezconde-Garbanati, and K. D. Reynolds, "Acculturation and sun-safe behaviors among US Latinos: findings from the 2005 Health Information National Trends Survey," *American Journal of Public Health*, vol. 99, no. 4, pp. 734–741, 2009.

[59] E. J. Coups, J. L. Stapleton, S. V. Hudson et al., "Linguistic acculturation and skin cancer-related behaviors among Hispanics in the southern and western United States," *JAMA Dermatology*, vol. 149, no. 6, pp. 679–686, 2013.

[60] C. J. Heckman and J. Choen-Filipic, "Brief report: ultraviolet radiation exposure, considering acculturation among hispanics (Project URECAH)," *Journal of Cancer Education*, vol. 27, no. 2, pp. 342–346, 2012.

[61] C. E. Ross and C.-L. Wu, "The links between education and health," *American Sociological Review*, vol. 60, no. 5, pp. 719–745, 1995.

[62] M. A. Winkleby, D. E. Jatulis, E. Frank, and S. P. Fortmann, "Socioeconomic status and health: how education, income, and occupation contribute to risk factors for cardiovascular disease," *American Journal of Public Health*, vol. 82, no. 6, pp. 816–820, 1992.

[63] S. Hu, R. Sherman, K. Arheart, and R. S. Kirsner, "Predictors of neighborhood risk for late-stage melanoma: addressing disparities through spatial analysis and area-based measures," *Journal of Investigative Dermatology*, vol. 134, no. 4, pp. 937–945, 2014.

[64] Office of Disea Prevention and Health Promotion, Healthy People 2020: Disparities, http://www.healthypeople.gov/2020/about/foundation-health-measures/Disparities.

[65] V. E. Cokkinides, A. C. Geller, and A. Jemal, "Trends in melanoma mortality among non-hispanic whites by educational attainment, 1993–2007," *Archives of Dermatology*, vol. 148, no. 5, pp. 587–591, 2012.

[66] C. Hernandez, D. Calero, G. Robinson, R. Mermelstein, and J. K. Robinson, "Comparison of sunscreen availability in Chicago Hispanic and non-Hispanic neighborhoods," *Photodermatology Photoimmunology and Photomedicine*, vol. 28, no. 5, pp. 244–249, 2012.

[67] J. Sprague, J. Obioha, and M. W. Chiu, "Availability of sunscreen in predominantly Hispanic neighborhoods vs. adjacent predominantly non-Hispanic neighborhoods in Los Angeles," *Photodermatology Photoimmunology and Photomedicine*, vol. 29, no. 5, pp. 279–282, 2013.

[68] B. M. M. Doty, S. Buetel, P. W. Rasmussen, and S. E. Collins, The Commonwealth Fund Blog: Latinos Have Made Coverage Gains but Millions Are Still Uninsured, http://www.commonwealthfund.org/publications/blog/2015/apr/latinos-have-made-coverage-gains.

[69] P. R. Center, "Pew Research Center Hispanic Trends: Unauthorized Immigrant Population Trends for States, Birth Countries and Regions," 2016, http://www.pewhispanic.org/2014/12/11/unauthorized-trends/.

[70] US Centers for Medicare & Medicaid Services, "Coverage for lawfully present immigrants," https://www.healthcare.gov/immigrants/lawfully-present-immigrants/.

[71] Centers for Medicuare & Medicare Services, "Eligibility for Non-Citizens in Medicaid and CHIP," http://www.medicaid.gov/medicaid-chip-program-information/by-topics/outreach-and-enrollment/downloads/overview-of-eligibility-for-non-citizens-in-medicaid-and-chip.pdf.

[72] G. Livingston, S. Minushkin, and D. Cohn, "Hispanics and Health Care in the United States: Access, Information and Knowledge," Pew Research Center Hispanic Trends, http://www.pewhispanic.org/2008/08/13/hispanics-and-health-care-in-the-united-states-access-information-and-knowledge/.

[73] M. L. Di Quinzio, R. A. Dewar, F. I. Burge, and P. J. Veugelers, "Family physician visits and early recognition of melanoma," *Canadian Journal of Public Health*, vol. 96, no. 2, pp. 136–139, 2005.

[74] M. L. Pennie, S. L. Soon, J. B. Risser, E. Veledar, S. D. Culler, and S. C. Chen, "Melanoma outcomes for medicare

patients: association of stage and survival with detection by a dermatologist vs a nondermatologist," *Archives of Dermatology*, vol. 143, no. 4, pp. 488–494, 2007.

[75] T. A. LaVeist and T. Carroll, "Race of physician and satisfaction with care among African-American patients," *Journal of the National Medical Association*, vol. 94, no. 11, pp. 937–943, 2002.

[76] T. A. LaVeist and A. Nuru-Jeter, "Is doctor-patient race concordance associated with greater satisfaction with care?" *Journal of Health and Social Behavior*, vol. 43, no. 3, pp. 296–306, 2002.

[77] T. A. LaVeist, A. Nuru-Jeter, and K. E. Jones, "The association of doctor-patient race concordance with health services utilization," *Journal of Public Health Policy*, vol. 24, no. 3-4, pp. 312–323, 2003.

[78] S. Saha, M. Komaromy, T. D. Koepsell, and A. B. Bindman, "Patient-physician racial concordance and the perceived quality and use of health care," *Archives of Internal Medicine*, vol. 159, no. 9, pp. 997–1004, 1999.

[79] Association of American Medical Colleges, *Table 30: Total Graduates by U.S. Medical School and Race and Ethnicity*, 2012, https://www.aamc.org/download/321538/data/factstableb6.pdf.

[80] M. A. Wakefield, B. Loken, and R. C. Hornik, "Use of mass media campaigns to change health behaviour," *The Lancet*, vol. 376, no. 9748, pp. 1261–1271, 2010.

[81] A. C. Marcus and L. A. Crane, "A review of cervical cancer screening intervention research: implications for public health programs and future research," *Preventive Medicine*, vol. 27, no. 1, pp. 13–31, 1998.

[82] M. E. Black, J. Yamada, and V. Mann, "A systematic literature review of the effectiveness of community-based strategies to increase cervical cancer screening," *Canadian Journal of Public Health*, vol. 93, no. 5, pp. 386–393, 2002.

[83] J. O. Anderson, R. M. Mullins, M. Siahpush, M. J. Spittal, and M. Wakefield, "Mass media campaign improves cervical screening across all socio-economic groups," *Health Education Research*, vol. 24, no. 5, pp. 867–875, 2009.

[84] R. J. Pasick, R. A. Hiatt, and E. D. Paskett, "Lessons learned from community-based cancer screening intervention research," *Cancer*, vol. 101, no. 5, pp. 1146–1164, 2004.

[85] S. Hu, R. M. Soza-Vento, D. F. Parker, and R. S. Kirsner, "Comparison of stage at diagnosis of melanoma among Hispanic, black, and white patients in Miami-Dade County, Florida," *Archives of Dermatology*, vol. 142, no. 6, pp. 704–708, 2006.

[86] R. Torrens and B. A. Swan, "Promoting prevention and early recognition of malignant melanoma," *Dermatology Nursing*, vol. 21, no. 3, pp. 115–123, 2009.

[87] L. J. F. Rutten, L. Squiers, and B. Hesse, "Cancer-related information seeking: hints from the 2003 Health Information National Trends Survey (HINTS)," *Journal of Health Communication*, vol. 11, supplement 001, pp. 147–156, 2006.

[88] Centers for Disease Control, "Colorectal Cancer Control Program (CRCCP): Social Ecological Model," 2015, http://www.cdc.gov/cancer/crccp/sem.htm.

[89] N. Krieger, "Defining and investigating social disparities in cancer: critical issues," *Cancer Causes and Control*, vol. 16, no. 1, pp. 5–14, 2005.

30

Basosquamous Carcinoma: A Single Centre Clinicopathological Evaluation and Proposal of an Evidence-Based Protocol

Jordan W. Oldbury,[1] Richard A. J. Wain,[1] Sameera Abas,[1] Christopher M. Dobson,[2] and Srinivasan S. Iyer[1]

[1]*Department of Plastic & Reconstructive Surgery, Royal Preston Hospital, Lancashire Teaching Hospitals NHS Foundation Trust, Sharoe Green Lane, Preston, Lancashire PR2 9HT, UK*
[2]*Department of Dermatology, Royal Preston Hospital, Lancashire Teaching Hospitals NHS Foundation Trust, Sharoe Green Lane, Preston, Lancashire PR2 9HT, UK*

Correspondence should be addressed to Jordan W. Oldbury; jordan.oldbury@doctors.org.uk

Academic Editor: Günther Hofbauer

Basosquamous carcinoma (BSC) is an uncommon skin malignancy with significant invasive and metastatic potential. There are currently no clear management guidelines. This study evaluates the management and outcomes of patients diagnosed with BSC over a 7-year period. We present an evidence-based unit protocol for the management of BSC. All patients treated for BSC between 2009 and 2015 were reviewed. Data collected included patient demographics, tumour-specific information, management strategy, presence of recurrence or metastasis, and details of follow-up. 74 patients were identified, making this one of the largest cohorts of BSC patients reported. Mean age at diagnosis was 75.4 years, with a male:female ratio of 1.6:1. The most common tumour site was the head and neck (n=43, 58.1%). All tumours were graded at pT1 (n=51) or pT2 (n=23). Inadequate excision occurred in 17 patients (23%). Mean excision margins were >4mm peripherally and deep. Inadequately excised BSCs were further treated with wide local excision (n=6) or radiotherapy (n=5), or both (n=1). There were no cases of local recurrence or metastatic disease. This study demonstrates a cohort of patients with BSCs that appear less aggressive than previously reported. Current management with surgical excision appears to produce adequate results. However, an evidence-based guideline is still lacking.

1. Introduction

Basosquamous carcinoma (BSC) is a rare form of skin cancer currently representing approximately 2% of all nonmelanoma skin malignancies [1–5]. The majority of cases are found in the head and neck region with preponderance for older Caucasian males [2, 6, 7]. Synonymously labelled metatypical basal cell carcinoma (BCC), BSCs are almost invariably clinically indistinguishable from BCCs but are said to be more aggressive and invasive than both BCCs and squamous cell carcinomas (SCCs) alone, with higher rates of recurrence (reported as up to 45%) and metastasis (approx. 5-10%) [2, 4, 5, 8].

Since its original description in 1910, there has been debate about the terminology, definition, and subsequent management of BSC [3, 9–11]. These tumours are of unpredictable behaviour and mixed morphology, demonstrating features of both BCC and SCC with, or without, a transition zone between the two cell types [8, 12]. Initially, it was suggested that BSCs represent "collision" tumours, whereby SCC and BCC tumours independently develop apposed to one another [5]. However, given the histological features of BSCs and their pluripotency, it has more recently led to the development of the squamatisation theory, which suggests that BSCs are actually basal cell carcinomas that undergo squamous differentiation [10]. This is supported by the definition provided by the World Health Organisation (WHO) [13], who have classified BSC as "basal cell carcinomas that are associated with squamous differentiation".

It is virtually impossible to clinically diagnose a BSC; however, the aid of dermoscopy alongside suspicious clinical behaviour might be beneficial. It has been shown that there are certain dermoscopic features which increase suspicion for BSC and enhance diagnostic accuracy [14], although histological confirmation by way of a punch or incision biopsy is essential prior to confirming diagnosis and initiating the correct treatment pathway. It should be noted, however, that easily excisable lesions or lesions with dermoscopic features suggestive of SCC should be excised as per the European Dermatology Forum (EDF) guidelines or the British Association of Dermatology (BAD) guidelines, dependent on country of practice (available from [15, 16]).

Whilst the ideal management strategy for BSC has not yet been established, the principal method apparent in the literature is surgical excision. Mohs micrographic surgery (MMS) has been shown to reduce recurrence rates when compared to standard excision and is the gold standard of treatment [1, 3, 8]; however, the inability to clinically distinguish BSC from BCC preoperatively, the minimal availability of MMS in the UK, and the current practice of excision biopsy of primary cutaneous lesions at presentation make patient selection challenging. Other techniques such as radiotherapy, laser ablation, cryotherapy, and chemotherapy have also been utilised in some cases, although mainly in stage 4 disease and without any significant evidence in literature [17].

It has been suggested that BSC requires a different approach with respect to treatment and follow-up than for BCC [18]. However, specific guidelines do not currently exist for management of BSC, and, given the inability to clinically distinguish BSC from BCC, histological confirmation is essential. We evaluated a cohort of patients with BSC over a 7-year period to determine the tumour characteristics, management strategies, follow-up regimens, recurrence rates, and incidence of metastasis. Data was compared to that available in the current literature, and an evidence-based unit protocol was devised.

2. Materials and Methods

This is a retrospective, monocentric study involving all patients treated for basosquamous carcinoma between 2009 and 2015 by our unit. Patients were identified using the institutional database in the Department of Pathology. Both clinical and histological characteristics reported at diagnosis were analysed. Exclusion criteria comprised those patients with an incomplete data set and patients lost to follow-up.

Clinical data was acquired from patient records and multidisciplinary team outcomes over several clinical sites. Variables including gender, age at diagnosis, primary tumour site, excision margins, need for wider excision or radiotherapy, follow-up regimen, and presence of recurrence and/or metastasis were recorded.

All histological specimens were excised as per BCC protocol and examined primarily by a dermatopathologist using haematoxylin and eosin (H+E) staining as a minimum. A small proportion of specimens were subsequently subjected to immunohistochemistry analysis using an anti-human epithelial antigen monoclonal antibody BerEP4, where the diagnosis was less clear. Diagnosis was made in accordance with the Royal College of Pathologists Standards for Histological Reporting of Primary Cutaneous BCC guidelines (available from [19]), and all diagnoses were reexamined by a specialist dermatopathologist through the specialist skin cancer multidisciplinary team to reconfirm diagnosis and establish a management plan. Excision margins, the presence of perineural or lymphovascular invasion, AJCC pT stage, and the status of reexcision specimens were also recorded when data was available.

Using a combination of the data collected, the results of this study, and current practices reported in recent literature, we have devised a new local protocol for the treatment and follow-up of this uncommon skin malignancy.

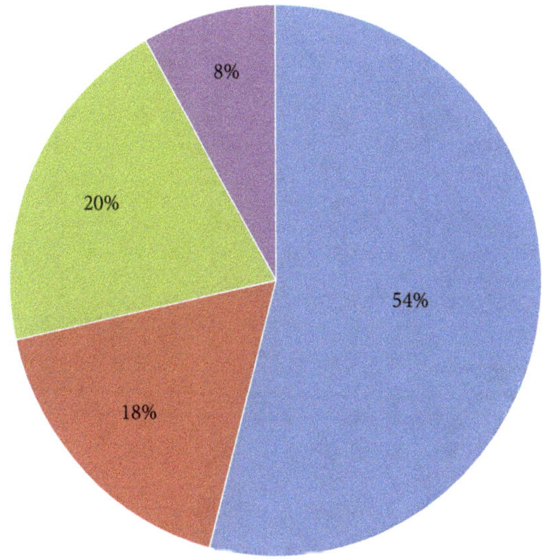

FIGURE 1: The most common area for BSC presentation was in the head and neck region (54% of cases), followed by the trunk.

3. Results

There were 74 patients included in the study with a male:female ratio of 1.6:1 and a mean age at diagnosis of 75.4 years (range 44-95 years). There were no re-referrals following discharge. There were no deaths during the follow-up period. The most common tumour site was the head and neck (58.1% (n=43)), followed by the trunk (20.3% (n=15)), lower limb (17.6% (n=13)), and upper limb (8.1% (n=6)). Figure 1 represents this data graphically. All lesions were pT1 (n=51) or pT2 (n=23), with 1 lesion displaying lymphovascular invasion and 4 lesions with (5.5%) perineural invasion. Mean excision margins were 4.5mm peripherally (range <1-13mm, SD 2.6mm) and 4.0 mm deep (range <1mm-16mm, SD 3.5mm). However, of the 73 patients for which we have data, the inadequate excision rate (defined as resection margins <1mm or involved margins) was relatively high (23%, n=17) with 59% (n=10) of these occurring at the deep margin, 29% (n=5) at both peripheral and deep margins, and 12% (n=2) at the peripheral margins alone.

Further treatment of inadequately excised BSCs (defined as margins ≤1mm) involved either wide local excision (WLE) (n=6), radiotherapy (n=5), or both WLE and radiotherapy (n=1). No further treatment was given to four patients due

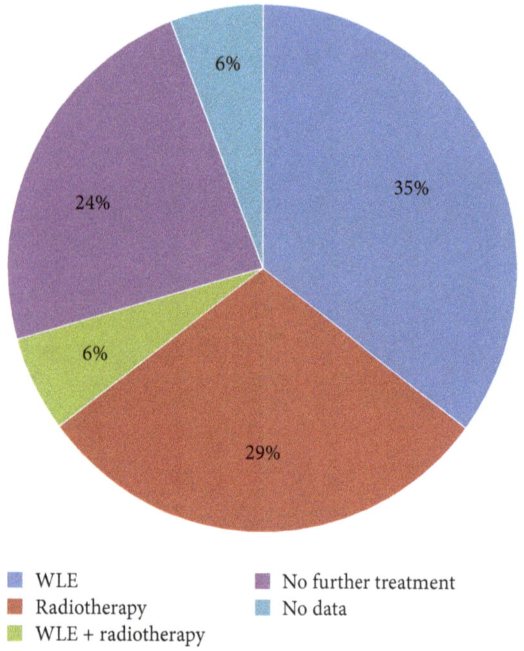

FIGURE 2: Follow-up and further treatment amongst patients with inadequately excised BCCs were heterogenous and varied.

to consultant decision to observe, and there was no data available for one patient (see Figure 2).

Only one of the WLE specimens showed evidence of residual malignancy. The duration of follow-up varied widely (5-60 months), with a mean length of follow-up of 20.2 months. Eight patients are still under review. Indeed, the interval between routine follow-up appointments following diagnosis also varied (3-6 months), with a mean of 4.4 months. There were no cases of local recurrence and no patients with metastatic disease at the time that the study was carried out.

4. Discussion

Basosquamous carcinoma is an uncommon, aggressive malignancy for which current literature has little consensus and is seen by some as a distinct pathology to both BCC and SCC [20]. However, there is long-standing discord over where BSC falls in the nonmelanoma skin cancer spectrum, and current consensus leans towards BSC representing a subtype of BCC. Early diagnosis and identification are key to optimal clinical outcome, given the reported aggressive nature of the disease and high risk of recurrence and metastasis. Due to experience and research with both BCCs and SCCs, surgical excision is currently the first-line treatment option, but a significant role has been demonstrated for radiotherapy and Mohs' micrographic surgery [5, 11, 21–24]. To date, there is no standardised treatment protocol for the management of basosquamous carcinoma [25].

The current study has demonstrated that primary excision of pT1 and pT2 BSC tumours can lead to good clinical outcome, with or without the need for further excision, with none of the 74 patients involved in this study developing metastasis or recurrence of disease. This is in line with Kececi *et al.*, who demonstrated no metastasis and a recurrence rate of only 4% in a series of 35 patients [7]; however, these figures are lower than other reported studies (see Table 1).

Previous reports demonstrate a strong male preponderance and an increased occurrence in the head and neck regions. Our study reflects these findings, albeit not as convincingly as the previous studies [4, 5, 7, 29]. These demographics are important to consider on clinical diagnosis of a skin malignancy given that a predisposition to development on the face leads to increased difficulty in resection and reconstruction, problems achieving adequate surgical margins, and issues in providing a good aesthetic outcome.

This is one of the largest reported studies involving only BSCs to date, and our findings are comparable with many previous studies. However, despite a large proportion of previous authors reporting high recurrence and metastasis rates, at the time that this study was carried out, we had not recorded a single patient within this cohort with recurrence or metastasis. We did not identify any patients with pT3 or pT4 tumours, which could account somewhat for this observation. Wermker *et al.* [2] reported a cohort of 89 patients, 18 patients of which were found to have pT3 or pT4 tumours. Of these patients, three patients (16.7%) developed lymph node metastases, whereas only 2/71 (2.8%) of those patients with pT1 or pT2 tumours developed lymph node metastases. Furthermore, the authors reported no change in progression-free survival at 18 months of follow-up in those diagnosed with pT1 and pT2 tumours. The findings of the current study, as well as those of Wermker *et al.*, go some way to explaining how we may have identified a cohort wherein recurrence and metastasis are unlikely to occur.

For the 71 patients for which we could collect data regarding subsequent treatment following the primary surgical excision, 17 patients had inadequately excised lesions, of whom nine (11.3%) patients had involved surgical margins. In this cohort, subsequent treatment varied widely. Previous reports have demonstrated positive margins in more than 30% of cases following primary excision, usually presumed due to the microscopic invasiveness of the disease, and this is well documented to be a significant risk factor for recurrence of disease [4, 7, 25, 30]. The most likely reason for this low incidence is the generally low clinical staging of disease, but this has yet to be tested and evaluated through further research.

Out of the 73 patients for which we had data in this cohort, four (5.5%) patients had histological evidence of perineural invasion, one of the significant risk factors for recurrence [1, 4]. Although the incidence in this cohort falls within previously reported incidence of perineural invasion (0-7.9%), it is likely that no recurrence has been seen in the current study due to the absolute number of BSCs demonstrating perineural invasion being small [1, 28]. It is possible that a larger cohort would demonstrate recurrence if the proportion of specimens demonstrating perineural invasion stayed the same.

4.1. Metastasis. Despite being relatively rare, the concerning aspect of BSC is its ability to metastasise. The treatment of

TABLE 1: A comparison of studies of the recurrence and metastatic rates of BSC following excision. NR = not recorded. * = only 25/35 patients available for follow-up, hence the higher percentage.

Study	No. of cases	Recurrence	LN/Distant Metastasis
Current study	74	0	0
Schuller *et al.*, 1979 [26]	33	4 (12%)	NR
Martin *et al.*, 2000 [4]	28	9 (32%)	5 (18%)
Bowman *et al.*, 2003 [5]	27	NR	2 (7.4%)
Leibovitch *et al.*, 2005 [1]	98	4 (4.1%)	0
Skaria, 2010 [27]	56	5 (8.9%)	NR
Mougel *et al.*, 2012 [28]	12	0	0
Betti *et al.*, 2013 [12]	35	2 (5.7%)	1 (2.9%)
Kececi *et al.*, 2014 [7]	35	1 (4%*)	0

metastatic BSC is complex with poor outcomes, with one study reporting an average life expectancy of 1.6 years at diagnosis [31]. This, however, appears to considerably underestimate the survival rate, with a further study reporting an overall survival rate in patients with significantly advanced diseased as 54% (95% CI, 19%-80%) [17].

The prevalence of metastasis in BSC is known to be higher than in BCC and SCC. In a case series of 1000 consecutive tumours treated with MMS, the authors report a significantly increased prevalence of metastasis in BSC (n=27; 2 (7.4%) with pulmonary metastasis) compared with SCC (n=228; 2 (0.87%) with pulmonary metastasis) [5]. This is supported by a case series of 28 patients, in which nine patients developed recurrent disease, five patients developed disease in the lymph nodes, and one developed pulmonary metastasis [4]. Wermker *et al.* [2] reported five lymph node metastases in a series of 89 patients, with progression-free survival time averaging 16.1 months (range: 8.1-24.1 months); of these, two patients had pT1/pT2 tumours, with the remaining three having pT3/pT4 disease. BCC is known to very rarely metastasise [20, 32].

There is no difference in the clinical characteristics between BSC and other types of BCC (with the exceptions of sclerosing BCC and pigmented BCC), but there is a significant difference in the histological phenotypes. This could suggest a difference in the genotypes of BSC compared with other subtypes of BCC, suggesting a possible explanation for the difference in rates of metastasis.

4.2. Recurrence. Previous studies have reported a wide range of local recurrence rates of between 4 and 47.1% (as reviewed by Kececi *et al.*, and Volkenstein *et al.*), and the risk of recurrence has been found to be increased by male gender, positive resection margins, and perineural and lymphatic invasion [5, 7, 11]. Clearly, a reduction in the rate of recurrence would lead to better clinical outcomes as well as reducing the rate of metastasis, and so care must be taken to ensure adequate surgical excision margins.

4.3. Mohs' Micrographic Surgery. Bowman *et al.* demonstrated that the number of stages of Mohs' micrographic surgery (MMS) required to achieve tumour-free margins in BSC was not significantly different to the number needed to treat SCC and BCC [5]. An initial randomised controlled trial studying the use of MMS for facial basal cell carcinoma in 408 patients with 30 months of follow-up demonstrated that the use of MMS slightly lowered the recurrence rates of BCCs, but this decrease did not reach statistical significance [33]. Subsequently, the same authors reanalysed the same population of patients and demonstrated a significantly lower rate of recurrence following MMS compared with surgical excision at 10 years of follow-up [24]. This robust study provided significant evidence for the use of MMS in nonmelanoma skin cancers; however, as the reported study did not look specifically at BSC, the results should be interpreted with caution in the context of the current study.

Whilst evidence suggests MMS may be the treatment of choice for these lesions with respect to recurrence rates and completeness of excision, the inability to clinically distinguish BSC from BCC preoperatively makes selection for MMS a technical and logistical challenge [1, 5]. Further considerations for the use of MMS for the treatment of BSC include identifying sources of funding and a much higher cost associated with MMS compared with surgical excision, the effect of a time-consuming surgery and its tolerability in an inherently elderly population, and the lack of national guidance in the treatment of BSC.

In this study, we demonstrated a perineural invasion rate of approximately 5.5%; this figure supports a potential role for MMS in the treatment of these skin lesions given that MMS ensures margin control in the excision of more aggressive tumours [34] and reduces recurrence rates in other cutaneous malignant lesions [24]. Currently, our service does not offer MMS for patients presenting with BCCs who are subsequently histologically diagnosed with BSCs, but this would be a valuable treatment option in the future when the service becomes available. The significant benefit of MMS is that the operating surgeon can more accurately secure disease-free margin, and the relatively high inadequate excision rate seen in this study would be significantly reduced.

4.4. Use of Radiotherapy. In our series, 6 (8.2%) patients were treated with adjuvant radiotherapy following primary surgical excision; however, there are currently no reports in the literature studying the use of radiotherapy in BSC. Cure rates of up to 91-93% have been seen with radiotherapy

At time of diagnostic surgery
(i) Punch or incision biopsy of suspicious lesion, or
(ii) If easily excisable measure and mark peripheral margins as per BCC guidance i.e. 4mm
(iii) Always ensure next clear anatomical plane is reached at the deep margin
(iv) If the lesion is suspicious of SCC, excise according to appropriate (EDF/BAD) SCC guidelines.
(v) In the case of confirmed BSC preoperatively, MMS should be offered where available
At first clinic review
(i) Explain difference between BSC and BCC i.e. whilst BSC has the potential for regional and distant metastasis, this is uncommon in pT1 & pT2 lesions, without deep invasion of the tumour
(ii) Full examination of excision site and regional nodes
Subsequent follow-up
(i) All patients to have full examination of excision site and regional nodes
(ii) Completely excised pT1 & pT2 BSC – follow up 3-4 monthly for 24 months, then discharge if well
(iii) Incompletely excised pT1 & pT2 BSC – offer wider excision or radiotherapy after Skin MDT discussion, follow up 3-4 monthly for 24 months, then discharge if well
(iv) All pT3 & pT4 BSCs, and those with invasion into deep structures e.g. fascia, muscle, cartilage or bone, require Skin MDT discussion, appropriate treatment and follow-up 3-4 monthly for 3 years, and then 6 monthly to total of 5 years follow up.

Box 1: Using the data presented in this study in conjunction with published reports, a proposed unit protocol has been designed to guide treatment and follow-up for patients diagnosed with BSC.

alone in treating BCC and that an approach utilising both surgery and radiotherapy together demonstrate cure rates of approximately 95% [35]. Given the close histological appearances between BCC and BSC, it would suggest that, in appropriate patient groups, treatment with radiotherapy either alone or in combination with surgery may be an appropriate option for the management of BSC if standard surgical excision or MMS is not possible [31].

4.5. Limitations. As demonstrated, our cohort of patients comprised only pT1 and pT2 cancers; therefore, reported rates of recurrence and metastasis would not accurately reflect the true recurrence/metastasis rate for the entire BSC population. We have also found that follow-up practices vary greatly, with variation between 5 and 60 months; this is a symptom of the lack of national guidance for the treatment of BSC. Additionally, the data used in this study is retrospective, heavily reliant on the availability of recorded data, and spread across multiple clinical sites. The findings of this study, therefore, must be interpreted with caution.

Given the methods by which the patients were identified in this study, it is possible, however unlikely, that the diagnosis of BSC has been missed in the full population of BCC patients in the time period identified. It should be noted that the number of BCCs excised in this time period is significant, and therefore subsequent reanalysis of all BCC specimens to identify any missed BSC diagnoses is not practical. All cases of BSC diagnosed in the time period were included. In cases where recurrence or metastasis was identified in patients originally diagnosed with BCC/SCC, the primary lesion was reexamined by an independent pathologist; no further cases of BSC were identified in this process. There were no cases of metastatic BCC at our centre in this time period.

It remains unclear whether BSC develops as a distinct clinical entity or whether BCC lesions undergo squamatisation. In this study, only those specimens in which the diagnosis was not clear on H+E staining were subjected to further analysis using BerEP4 immunohistochemistry staining. This anti-human epithelial antigen antibody labels the basaloid component of basal cell carcinoma, which in turn allows identification of a transition zone within the BSC itself [29]. When the transition zone is not present, the staining suggests the presence of collision tumours, as SCCs are typically negative for BerEP4 [11]; however, the lack of transition zone is not diagnostic [7]. Mougel *et al.* demonstrated in a 15 case series that 20% of those lesions initially labelled as basosquamous carcinoma were eventually diagnosed as SCC [28]. This was supported by a case series of 178 patients, wherein the initial diagnosis of BSC was only correctly given in 13.7% of cases [1]. Farmer *et al.* reanalysed cases of metastatic BCC and demonstrated that 80% of malignancies initially thought to be BCC had basosquamous differentiation on histology of metastases [31]. Given the retrospective nature of our evaluation of histological specimens, it is possible that some of the cases initially labelled as BSC were actually SCC and that some of the malignancies labelled as BCC and excluded were actually BSC. Future prospective studies should include immunohistological staining for BerEP4 as a standard to facilitate diagnosis of BSC [29].

4.6. Proposed Local Protocol. Whilst none of the available published studies have large numbers or prospective data collection [3], there are trends between the studies that can guide an approach to management and follow-up. In particular, the study by Wermker *et al.* [2] was conducted in a robust fashion and has shown a clear relationship between progression-free survival (PFS) and tumour stage, as well as between PFS and maximal vertical invasion of the tumour. Given the current lack of guidance available specifically for BSC, it would seem reasonable to base a unit BSC management protocol on the best available literature and the results of the current study. Our suggested unit protocol is demonstrated in Box 1.

5. Conclusion

In this patient group, BSCs appear less aggressive and less likely to recur or metastasise than those stated in the literature despite incomplete excision rates being comparable with other reported studies. Current management including surgical excision, with or without radiotherapy, appears to be the best method of management, with future consideration of inclusion of Mohs' micrographic surgery in the treatment protocol when the service becomes available. As Wermker *et al.* [2] noted, further prospective studies are needed, and practical, evidence-based protocols are pending the findings of these studies. Follow-up regimens locally are variable and require standardisation in the form of a guideline based on this study and the best available current literature. This is certainly necessary at a local level but perhaps could be used more widely. We propose a BSC management protocol for use in our unit in an attempt to standardise management and ensure improved quality care in this potentially challenging patient group.

Disclosure

Preliminary data from this study was presented at the British Association of Plastic, Reconstructive and Aesthetic Surgeons (BAPRAS) Winter Scientific Meeting, Victoria Park Plaza, London, November 2016.

Acknowledgments

The authors would like to thank the Department of Pathology at Lancashire Teaching Hospitals NHS Foundation Trust for their assistance in compiling the histological data for analysis.

References

[1] I. Leibovitch, S. C. Huilgol, D. Selva, S. Richards, and R. Paver, "Basosquamous carcinoma: Treatment with Mohs micrographic surgery," *Cancer*, vol. 104, no. 1, pp. 170–175, 2005.

[2] K. Wermker, N. Roknic, K. Goessling, M. Klein, H.-J. Schulze, and C. Hallermann, "Basosquamous Carcinoma of the Head and Neck: Clinical and Histologic Characteristics and Their Impact on Disease Progression," *Neoplasia*, vol. 17, no. 3, pp. 301–305, 2015.

[3] C. Z. Tan, K. E. Rieger, and K. Y. Sarin, "Basosquamous Carcinoma: Controversy, Advances, and Future Directions," *Dermatologic Surgery*, vol. 43, no. 1, pp. 23–31, 2017.

[4] R. C. G. Martin II, M. J. Edwards, T. G. Cawte, C. L. Sewell, and K. M. McMasters, "Basosquamous carcinoma: Analysis of prognostic factors influencing recurrence," *Cancer*, vol. 88, no. 6, pp. 1365–1369, 2000.

[5] P. H. Bowman, J. L. Ratz, T. G. Knoepp, C. J. Barnes, E. M. Finley, and J. Geisse, "Basosquamous carcinoma," *Dermatologic Surgery*, vol. 29, no. 8, pp. 830–833, 2003.

[6] A. De Stefano, F. Dispenza, A. G. Petrucci, L. Citraro, and A. Croce, "Features of biopsy in diagnosis of metatypical basal cell carcinoma (Basosquamous Carcinoma) of head and neck," *Otolaryngologia Polska*, vol. 66, no. 6, pp. 419–423, 2012.

[7] Y. Kececi, A. Argon, T. Kebat, E. Sir, M. Gungor, and E. Vardar, "Basosquamous carcinoma: Is it an aggressive tumor?" *Journal of Plastic Surgery and Hand Surgery*, vol. 49, no. 2, pp. 107–111, 2015.

[8] C. Garcia, E. Poletti, and A. N. Crowson, "Basosquamous carcinoma," *Journal of the American Academy of Dermatology*, vol. 60, no. 1, pp. 137–143, 2009.

[9] M. S. Jones, K. F. Helm, and M. E. Maloney, "The immunohistochemical characteristics of the basosquamous cell carcinoma," *Dermatologic Surgery*, vol. 23, no. 3, pp. 181–184, 1997.

[10] J. Burston and R. D. Clay, "The problems of histological diagnosis in baso-squamous cell carcinoma of the skin," *Journal of Clinical Pathology*, vol. 12, no. 1, pp. 73–79, 1959.

[11] S. Volkenstein, J. Wohlschlaeger, J. Liebau et al., "Basosquamous carcinoma-A rare but aggressive skin malignancy," *Journal of Plastic, Reconstructive & Aesthetic Surgery*, vol. 63, no. 3, pp. e304–e306, 2010.

[12] R. Betti, C. Crosti, S. Ghiozzi, A. Cerri, L. Moneghini, and S. Menni, "Basosquamous cell carcinoma: A survey of 76 patients and a comparative analysis of basal cell carcinomas and squamous cell carcinomas," *European Journal of Dermatology*, vol. 23, no. 1, pp. 83–86, 2013.

[13] P. E. LeBoit, International Agency for Research on Cancer, World Health Organization, International Academy of Pathology, European Organization for Research on Treatment of Cancer, and UniversitätsSpital Zürich, Eds., *Pathology And Genetics of Skin Tumours*, World Health Organization classification of tumours, IARC Press, Lyon, France.

[14] B. N. Akay, S. Saral, A. O. Heper, C. Erdem, and C. Rosendahl, "Basosquamous carcinoma: Dermoscopic clues to diagnosis," *The Journal of Dermatology*, vol. 44, no. 2, pp. 127–134, 2017.

[15] European Dermatology Forum, "Guidelines miscellaneous," 2018, http://www.euroderm.org/edf/index.php/edf-guidelines/category/5-guidelines-miscellaneous.

[16] British Association of Dermatologists, "Clinical Guidelines," 2018, http://www.bad.org.uk/healthcare-professionals/clinical-standards/clinical-guidelines.

[17] G. A. Zhu, C. Danial, A. Liu, S. Li, and A. L. Su Chang, "Overall and progression-free survival in metastatic basosquamous cancer: A case series," *Journal of the American Academy of Dermatology*, vol. 70, no. 6, pp. 1145-1146, 2014.

[18] M. Tarallo, E. Cigna, R. Frati et al., "Metatypical basal cell carcinoma: A clinical review," *Journal of Experimental & Clinical Cancer Research*, vol. 27, no. 1, article no. 65, 2008.

[19] "Dataset for the histological reporting of primary cutaneous basal cell carcinoma," 2018, https://www.rcpath.org/resourceLibrary/g123-data-set-basal-may-2014.html.

[20] D. Costantino, L. Lowe, and D. L. Brown, "Basosquamous carcinoma - An under-recognized, high-risk cutaneous neoplasm: Case study and review of the literature," *Journal of Plastic, Reconstructive & Aesthetic Surgery*, vol. 59, no. 4, pp. 424–428, 2006.

[21] I. Leibovitch, S. C. Huilgol, D. Selva, D. Hill, S. Richards, and R. Paver, "Cutaneous squamous cell carcinoma treated with Mohs micrographic surgery in Australia I. Experience over 10 years," *Journal of the American Academy of Dermatology*, vol. 53, no. 2, pp. 253–260, 2005.

[22] K. Mosterd, G. A. Krekels, F. H. Nieman et al., "Surgical excision versus Mohs' micrographic surgery for primary and recurrent basal-cell carcinoma of the face: a prospective randomised controlled trial with 5-years' follow-up," *The Lancet Oncology*, vol. 9, no. 12, pp. 1149–1156, 2008.

[23] I. Leibovitch, S. C. Huilgol, D. Selva, S. Richards, and R. Paver, "Basal cell carcinoma treated with Mohs surgery in Australia II. Outcome at 5-year follow-up," *Journal of the American Academy of Dermatology*, vol. 53, no. 3, pp. 452–457, 2005.

[24] E. Van Loo, K. Mosterd, G. A. M. Krekels et al., "Surgical excision versus Mohs' micrographic surgery for basal cell carcinoma of the face: A randomised clinical trial with 10 year follow-up," *European Journal of Cancer*, vol. 50, no. 17, pp. 3011–3020, 2014.

[25] R. L. Anand, D. Collins, and A. Chapman, "Basosquamous carcinoma: appearance and reality," *Oxford Medical Case Reports*, vol. 2017, no. 1, p. omw095, 2017.

[26] D. E. Schuller, J. W. Berg, G. Sherman, and C. J. Krause, "Cutaneous basosquamous carcinoma of the head and neck: a comparative analysis," *Otolaryngology—Head and Neck Surgery*, vol. 87, no. 4, pp. 420–427, 2016.

[27] A. M. Skaria, "Recurrence of basosquamous carcinoma after mohs micrographic surgery," *Dermatology*, vol. 221, no. 4, pp. 352–355, 2010.

[28] F. Mougel, J. Kanitakis, M. Faure, and S. Euvrard, "Basosquamous cell carcinoma in organ transplant patients: A clinicopathologic study," *Journal of the American Academy of Dermatology*, vol. 66, no. 5, pp. e151–e157, 2012.

[29] T. W. Beer, P. Shepherd, and J. M. Theaker, "Ber EP4 and epithelial membrane antigen aid distinction of basal cell, squamous cell and basosquamous carcinomas of the skin," *Histopathology*, vol. 37, no. 3, pp. 218–223, 2000.

[30] B. F. Johnson, P. J. Moore, J. R. Goepel, and D. N. Slater, "Basosquamous carcinoma, a wolf in sheep's clothing? Report of 3 cases.," *Postgraduate Medical Journal*, vol. 65, no. 768, pp. 750-751, 1989.

[31] E. R. Farmer and E. B. Helwig, "Metastatic basal cell carcinoma: A clinicopathologic study of seventeen cases," *Cancer*, vol. 46, no. 4, pp. 748–757, 1980.

[32] P. Piva de Freitas, C. G. Senna, M. Tabai, C. T. Chone, and A. Altemani, "Metastatic basal cell carcinoma: a rare manifestation of a common disease," *Case Reports in Medicine*, vol. 2017, Article ID 8929745, 4 pages, 2017.

[33] N. W. J. Smeets, G. A. M. Krekels, J. U. Ostertag et al., "Surgical excision vs Mohs' micrographic surgery for basal-cell carcinoma of the face: randomised controlled trial," *The Lancet*, vol. 364, no. 9447, pp. 1766–1772, 2004.

[34] I. Leibovitch, S. C. Huilgol, D. Selva, D. Hill, S. Richards, and R. Paver, "Cutaneous squamous cell carcinoma treated with Mohs micrographic surgery in Australia II. Perineural invasion," *Journal of the American Academy of Dermatology*, vol. 53, no. 2, pp. 261–266, 2005.

[35] M.-F. Avril, A. Auperin, A. Margulis et al., "Basal cell carcinoma of the face: surgery or radiotherapy? Results of a randomized study," *British Journal of Cancer*, vol. 76, no. 1, pp. 100–106, 1997.

31

Gender-Based Differences and Barriers in Skin Protection Behaviors in Melanoma Survivors

Jeffrey Chen,[1] Johnny Shih,[1] Andrew Tran,[1] Aaron Mullane,[1] Christina Thomas,[1] Nail Aydin,[2] and Subhasis Misra[2]

[1] *Texas Tech University Health Sciences Center, 1400 S. Coulter Street, Amarillo, TX 79106, USA*
[2] *Department of Surgery, Texas Tech University Health Sciences Center, 1400 S. Coulter Street, Amarillo, TX 79106, USA*

Correspondence should be addressed to Subhasis Misra; subhasis.misra@ttuhsc.edu

Academic Editor: Mark Lebwohl

Purpose. Skin protection behaviors and environmental exposure play a crucial role in the development and subsequent management of melanoma. This study investigates gender-based differences in skin protection behaviors after melanoma treatment. *Methods.* Patients diagnosed and surgically treated for cutaneous melanomas over the last six years in a geographically high risk area were surveyed over telephone using a standardized script. *Results.* Of 150 survey results obtained, there were 82 males and 68 females. Overall, 87% of participants reported skin self-examination for abnormal markings more often and 94% reported wearing skin protective clothing more often, with females being more than males. Females limited outdoor activity more often than males, 79% to 54%, $p < 0.05$. When outside, females sought shade more often than males, 75% to 56%, $p < 0.05$. However, males wore a wide brim hat more often than females, 52% to 28%, $p < 0.05$. Interestingly, 60% of participants reported wearing SPF 30 sunscreen less often, $p < 0.05$. *Conclusion.* Larger percentage of females adopted behavioral changes to prevent future melanoma. Those living in high risk areas and with outdoor occupations need particular attention to skin care. Population based screening should be adopted to deal with this rising public health crisis.

1. Introduction

Skin cancer is considered the most common cancer in the United States. Melanoma is a malignancy of melanocytes, pigment-producing cells that reside in the basal epidermal layer. Melanoma accounts for less than 2% of skin cancers but accounts for most skin cancer related deaths [1]. The incidence of melanoma has been increasing for the past 30 years [2]. In 2015 alone, there were approximately 74,000 newly diagnosed cases, 5% of which were from Texas [1, 3]. The Texas Panhandle has one of the highest incidence rates in the state with 21.5 per 100,000 persons compared to the state average of 14.1 per 100,000 [4]. The Texas Panhandle also claims melanoma death rates nearly twice the national average [5, 6]. The national incidence and mortality of melanoma vary by gender, accounting for the 5th and 7th most common cancers in men and women, respectively [7]. In 2015, 67% of melanoma deaths occurred in men [1].

Risk factors that increase the risk of developing melanoma include "blue or green eyes, light colored skin, dysplastic nevi, abnormal moles, blistering sunburns, excessive UV exposure, psoralen therapy with UVA light, immunosuppression, and habitation closer to the equator or at higher elevations" [8–12]. Studies have also isolated six high risk factors that independently increase the risk of getting melanoma. They are "actinic keratosis, blond or red hair, family history of melanoma, upper back freckles, three or more blistering sunburns prior to age 20, and three or more years of outdoor occupation as a teenager" [13–15]. Individuals with one or two of the risk factors have a tripled risk of developing melanoma compared to the rest of the population, and patients with previous melanoma have a ninefold increase in risk of developing subsequent melanoma compared to the rest of the population [9, 16]. Thus, skin protection behaviors and environmental exposure play a crucial role in the development and subsequent management of melanoma. Recommendations to reduce the risks of melanoma deaths and recurrence include routine self-examinations for suspicious lesions, sun avoidance, use of sunscreen, and protective clothing [17]. However, not much research is available on skin protection behaviors after melanoma treatment, especially between genders. This study aims to investigate gender differences in skin protection behaviors after melanoma treatment.

2. Methods

We looked at a representative sample of cutaneous melanoma cases diagnosed and surgically treated in the Texas Panhandle, a geographically high risk area. All patients were treated by surgical oncologists between 2008 and 2015. Inclusion was limited to living patients of 18 years or older with biopsy-proven and surgically treated melanoma. Telephone surveys lasting 8 to 10 minutes were conducted using a standardized script with three main categories consisting of health maintenance, skin protection, and sun avoidance as follows.

Telephone Survey Questions

Section I: Health Maintenance

(1) How often in the past year have you visited any physician for a skin examination?

(2) How often in the past year have you had a full body skin check by a healthcare provider?

(3) How often in the past year have you self-examined your skin for abnormal markings (changing color, getting bigger, new mole) for growths?

Section II: Skin Protection

(4) How often do you wear a hat with a wide brim all the way around?

(5) How often do you wear long sleeved shirts?

(6) How often do you wear sunscreen of at least SPF 30

(7) How often do you wear sunglasses?

(8) How often do you wear pants that reach your ankles?

Section III: Sun Avoidance Behavior

(9) How often do you limit your outdoor activity?

(10) When outside, how often do you seek shade?

(11) How often do you worry about developing another case of skin cancer?

(12) How often do you wear a hat, scarf, cap, or use an umbrella?

The Last 2 Questions Have Different Answer Choices

(13) Since being diagnosed with melanoma, how often do you take part in outdoor activities compared to before the diagnosis?

Significantly less, slightly less, the same, slightly more, significantly more

(14) Since being diagnosed with melanoma, how often do you worry about your melanoma compared to before the diagnosis?

I worry a lot less, I worry slightly less, I worry about the same amount, I worry slightly more, I worry a lot more

Table 1: Demographic characteristics.

	Number	%
Age		
Average	59.4	
Range	18–88	
Gender		
Male	82	55
Female	68	45
Stage		
Stage 0	38	25.3
Stage 1	91	60.7
Stage 2	7	4.7
Stage 3	4	2.7
Stage 4	0	0
Unstaged	10	6.7

Surveys were mailed in prepaid envelopes to those who did not respond to at least three of our phone calls. Data was evaluated and p values were calculated for each of the survey questions.

3. Results

Responses were collected from 150 of 500 contacted participants, a 30% return rate. The participants included 82 males and 68 females with ages ranging from 18 to 88 years (Table 1). Overall, 87% of participants reported skin self-examination for abnormal markings more often, with females self-examining more often than men (Table 2). Of all participants, 94% reported wearing skin protective clothing (sunglasses, pants that reach the ankles, and long sleeved shirts) more often, with females being more than males. Females limited their participation in outdoor activities after their diagnosis of melanoma to a greater degree than males, 79% to 54%, $p < 0.05$. When outside, females sought shade more often than males, 75% to 56%, $p < 0.05$. Of all participants, 81% worried more about their melanoma compared to before their diagnosis with females worrying more than males, 90% to 73%, $p < 0.05$. On the contrary, males wore wide brim hats more often than females, 52% to 28%, $p < 0.05$. Interestingly, 60% of participants reported wearing SPF 30 sunscreen less often, with 67% of males and 52% of females wearing sunscreen less often than prior to their melanoma diagnosis, $p < 0.05$. We also looked at age, separating the patients into two age groups, over 55 and under 55, but results were not statically significant.

TABLE 2: Results showed that a larger percentage of females compared to males adopted behavioral changes to prevent future cutaneous melanoma, with the exception of the wide brim hat. A majority of both females and males used sunscreen of at least SPF 30 less often than prior to diagnosis.

	Male (%)	Female (%)
More often		
Wear wide brim hat	52	28
Limit outdoor activity	54	79
Seek shade	56	75
Worry about recurrence	73	90
Less often		
Sunscreen SPF > 30	67	52

4. Discussion

In 2013, the American Association for Cancer Research reported that between 1990 and 2009, melanoma death rates increased by 10.5% in men, while in the same period, melanoma death rates decreased by 9.6% in women [1, 3]. Over the past decade, studies have reported a gender disparity in the biology of melanoma, with males having an increased risk of having thicker (>2 mm) tumors, higher risk of progression, and higher risk of metastasis [18, 19]. Our study looked into what seems to be lacking in the literature, to see whether or not there is a gender-based difference in behavior after the treatment of melanoma.

Results showed that a larger percentage of females compared to males adopted behavioral changes to prevent future cutaneous melanoma. Females were more likely to self-examine their skin for abnormal markings, and previous studies have shown a correlation between self- examinations and earlier melanoma diagnosis. Females were also more likely to wear protective clothing, limit their outdoor activity, and seek shade, which would ultimately lessen their exposure to UV radiation and decrease their risk of developing blistering sunburns, both of which are risk factors for melanoma. Women also worried more about their melanoma, which may be the underlying reason for their increased emphasis on preventative measures. One finding that seemed to deviate from the pattern was that men seem to wear a wide brim hat more often than females. This could possibly be due to behavioral change, but we hypothesize that it is more likely that males have careers involving agriculture or livestock in West Texas, so they are more likely to be outdoors for longer periods of time. Agriculture makes up the largest sector of the Texas Panhandle economy, and this predominately male workforce engaged in outdoor occupations including farming, ranching, and construction have a 6–8x higher UV exposure compared to workers in indoor occupations [20, 21].

Melanoma recurrence is higher than once thought, occurring in more than 6% of patients after 10 years, 6.8% of patients after 15 years, and 11.3% of patients after 25 years. Patients facing late recurrence were typically younger, with an average age of 41 to an average of 51 for early recurrence of melanoma [22, 23]. Studies have shown that sunscreen use decreases the incidence of sunburns. Sunburns, which can increase the likelihood of getting melanoma, are preventable, yet nearly 40% of the US population report getting sunburns each year [24, 25]. Thus, it is discouraging to find that more than half of the participants in both genders reported wearing sunscreen with greater than SPF30 less often than before their diagnosis of melanoma. We also looked at age to see if a certain age group was more or less likely to use sunscreen, but the data for two age groups, over 55 and under 55, was not statistically significant. The majority of respondents spent less time in outdoor activities after their diagnosis of melanoma. When asked about their sunscreen habits, the majority of those who spent less time outdoors believed that since they were outside for shorter periods of time, they no longer needed sunscreen. The second most popular response was that since sunscreen did not prevent melanoma in the first place, it probably was not going to prevent a recurrence.

Our results point to the need of stronger patient education on the possibility of melanoma recurrence and on proper sunscreen usage to dispel misconceptions surrounding application efficacy. Due to its preventable nature and its increasing incidence, melanoma has been labeled a public health crisis by the US Surgeon General because a person who dies from melanoma has lost on average 20 years of potential life [1, 26, 27]. While there are no national guidelines in the United States regarding skin cancer screening, developed countries around the world, such as Belgium, Germany, Australia, France, and Japan have adopted population based screening for skin cancer. Germany has seen a nearly 40% decrease in melanoma mortality as a result [28, 29]. Patient adherence to preventative measures such as sunscreen needs to be pursued more aggressively. With 67% of melanoma deaths occurring in men and with less male attention to health maintenance, skin protection, and sun avoidance after melanoma treatment, more needs to be done in terms of education and follow up, and mass population skin cancer screening should be adopted [1–3].

Disclosure

The work has been presented at the following meetings:

(i) Poster at Annual Meeting of the Society of Surgical Oncology on March 3, 2016, in Boston, Massachusetts.

(ii) Oral Presentation at Annual Meeting of the North Texas Chapter of the American College of Surgeons on Feb 19, 2016, in Dallas, Texas.

Competing Interests

The authors declare that there is no conflict of interest regarding the publication of this paper.

References

[1] Centers for Disease Control and Prevention, Skin Cancer Statistics, U.S. Cancer Statistics Working Group, http://www.cdc.gov/cancer/skin/statistics/.

[2] American Melanoma Foundation, *Facts About Melanoma*, http://www.melanomafoundation.org/facts/statistics.htm.

[3] American Cancer Society, *Cancer Facts & Figures 2015*, http://www.cancer.org/acs/groups/content/@editorial/documents/document/acspc-044552.pdf.

[4] Texas Cancer Registry, Age-Adjusted Invasive Cancer Incidence Rates by Council of Government in Texas, 2008–2012, http://cancer-rates.info/tx/.

[5] Texas Cancer Registry, *Age-Adjusted Cancer Mortality Rates by Metro Statistical Area in Texas, 2008–2012*, http://cancer-rates.info/tx/.

[6] E. Ramshaw, Health Care Sparse in Rural Texas. The Texas Tribune, http://www.texastribune.org/2010/01/04/health-care-sparse-in-rural-texas/.

[7] T. Thompson, M. Watson, G. Massetti et al., Vital Signs: Melanoma Incidence and Mortality Trends and Projections—United States, 1982–2030, http://www.cdc.gov/mmwr/pdf/wk/mm64e0602.pdf.

[8] D. S. Rigel, "Epidemiology of Melanoma," *Seminars in Cutaneous Medicine and Surgery*, vol. 29, no. 4, pp. 204–209, 2010.

[9] Z. Kutlubay, B. Engin, S. Serdaroğlu, and Y. Tüzün, "Current management of malignant melanoma: state of the art," in *Highlights in Skin Cancer*, P. Vereecken, Ed., chapter 4, InTech, Rijeka, Croatia, 2013.

[10] H. E. Kanavy and M. R. Gerstenblith, "Ultraviolet radiation and melanoma," *Seminars in Cutaneous Medicine and Surgery*, vol. 30, no. 4, pp. 222–228, 2011.

[11] S. C. Paek, A. J. Sober, H. Tsao et al., "Cutaneous melanoma," in *Fitzpatrick's Dermatology in General Medicine*, L. A. Goldsmith, S. I. Katz, B. Gilchrest, and A. S. Paller, Eds., pp. 1134–1157, McGraw Hill, New York, NY, USA, 7th edition, 2008.

[12] J. A. N. Bishop, "Lentigos, melanocytic naevi and melanoma," in *Rook's Textbook of Dermatology*, T. Burns, S. Breathnach, and N. Cox, Eds., pp. 54.32–54.56, Blackwell, London, UK, 8th edition, 2010.

[13] C. Garbe and U. Leiter, "Melanoma epidemiology and trends," *Clinics in Dermatology*, vol. 27, no. 1, pp. 3–9, 2009.

[14] C. Dahl and P. Guldberg, "The genome and epigenome of malignant melanoma," *APMIS*, vol. 115, no. 10, pp. 1161–1176, 2007.

[15] J. M. Bliss, D. Ford, A. J. Swerdlow et al., "Risk of cutaneous melanoma associated with pigmentation characteristics and freckling: systematic overview of 10 case-control studies," *International Journal of Cancer*, vol. 62, no. 4, pp. 367–376, 1995.

[16] H. W. Higgins, K. C. Lee, A. Galan, and D. J. Leffell, "Melanoma in situ: part I. Epidemiology, screening, and clinical features," *Journal of the American Academy of Dermatology*, vol. 73, no. 2, pp. 181–190, 2015.

[17] A. J. Sober, T.-Y. Chuang, M. Duvic et al., "Guidelines of care for primary cutaneous melanoma," *Journal of the American Academy of Dermatology*, vol. 45, no. 4, pp. 579–586, 2001.

[18] S. Swetter, C. Clarke, T. Keegan et al., "Why do men have worse melanoma survival than women? Is it behavior, biology, or both?" *The Melanoma Letter*, vol. 32, no. 2, 2014.

[19] A. Joosse, E. de Vries, R. Eckel et al., "Gender differences in melanoma survival: female patients have a decreased risk of metastasis," *Journal of Investigative Dermatology*, vol. 131, no. 3, pp. 719–726, 2011.

[20] D. E. Gaetano, B. Hodge, A. Clark, S. Ackerman, P. Burdick, and M. L. W. Cook, "Preventing skin cancer among a farming population: implementing evidence-based interventions," *AAOHN Journal*, vol. 57, no. 1, pp. 24–33, 2009.

[21] Texas State Historical Association, *Panhandle, Handbook of Texas Online*, http://www.tshaonline.org/handbook/online/articles/ryp01.

[22] S. Steen, X. Ye, and M. Sim, "Melanoma recurs after 10 years in more than 6 percent of patients," *Journal of the American College of Surgeons*, vol. 217, no. 1, pp. 27–34, 2013.

[23] B. Petersen and H. C. Wulf, "Application of sunscreen—theory and reality," *Photodermatology Photoimmunology & Photomedicine*, vol. 30, no. 2-3, pp. 96–101, 2014.

[24] M. Saraiya, K. Glanz, P. Briss, P. Nichols, C. White, and D. Das, "Preventing skin cancer: findings of the Task Force on Community Preventive Services on reducing exposure to ultraviolet light," *MMWR Recommendations and Reports*, vol. 52, no. 15, pp. 1–12, 2003.

[25] L. K. Dennis, M. J. Vanbeek, L. E. Beane Freeman, B. J. Smith, D. V. Dawson, and J. A. Coughlin, "Sunburns and risk of cutaneous melanoma: does age matter? A comprehensive meta-analysis," *Annals of Epidemiology*, vol. 18, no. 8, pp. 614–627, 2008.

[26] *The Surgeon General's Call to Action to Prevent Skin Cancer*, http://www.surgeongeneral.gov/library/calls/prevent-skin-cancer/exec-summary.html.

[27] D. U. Ekwueme, G. P. Guy Jr., C. Li, S. H. Rim, P. Parelkar, and S. C. Chen, "The health burden and economic costs of cutaneous melanoma mortality by race/ethnicity-United States, 2000 to 2006," *Journal of the American Academy of Dermatology*, vol. 65, no. 5, pp. S133–S143, 2011.

[28] A. Katalinic, A. Waldmann, M. A. Weinstock et al., "Does skin cancer screening save lives? An observational study comparing trends in melanoma mortality in regions with and without screening," *Cancer*, vol. 118, no. 21, pp. 5395–5402, 2012.

[29] E. W. Breitbart, A. Waldmann, S. Nolte et al., "Systematic skin cancer screening in Northern Germany," *Journal of the American Academy of Dermatology*, vol. 66, no. 2, pp. 201–211, 2012.

Permissions

All chapters in this book were first published in JSC, by Hindawi Publishing Corporation; hereby published with permission under the Creative Commons Attribution License or equivalent. Every chapter published in this book has been scrutinized by our experts. Their significance has been extensively debated. The topics covered herein carry significant findings which will fuel the growth of the discipline. They may even be implemented as practical applications or may be referred to as a beginning point for another development.

The contributors of this book come from diverse backgrounds, making this book a truly international effort. This book will bring forth new frontiers with its revolutionizing research information and detailed analysis of the nascent developments around the world.

We would like to thank all the contributing authors for lending their expertise to make the book truly unique. They have played a crucial role in the development of this book. Without their invaluable contributions this book wouldn't have been possible. They have made vital efforts to compile up to date information on the varied aspects of this subject to make this book a valuable addition to the collection of many professionals and students.

This book was conceptualized with the vision of imparting up-to-date information and advanced data in this field. To ensure the same, a matchless editorial board was set up. Every individual on the board went through rigorous rounds of assessment to prove their worth. After which they invested a large part of their time researching and compiling the most relevant data for our readers.

The editorial board has been involved in producing this book since its inception. They have spent rigorous hours researching and exploring the diverse topics which have resulted in the successful publishing of this book. They have passed on their knowledge of decades through this book. To expedite this challenging task, the publisher supported the team at every step. A small team of assistant editors was also appointed to further simplify the editing procedure and attain best results for the readers.

Apart from the editorial board, the designing team has also invested a significant amount of their time in understanding the subject and creating the most relevant covers. They scrutinized every image to scout for the most suitable representation of the subject and create an appropriate cover for the book.

The publishing team has been an ardent support to the editorial, designing and production team. Their endless efforts to recruit the best for this project, has resulted in the accomplishment of this book. They are a veteran in the field of academics and their pool of knowledge is as vast as their experience in printing. Their expertise and guidance has proved useful at every step. Their uncompromising quality standards have made this book an exceptional effort. Their encouragement from time to time has been an inspiration for everyone.

The publisher and the editorial board hope that this book will prove to be a valuable piece of knowledge for researchers, students, practitioners and scholars across the globe.

List of Contributors

Melinda B. Chu, Maulik M. Dhandha and Scott W. Fosko
Department of Dermatology, Saint Louis University, 1402 S. Grand Boulevard, 4th Floor, St. Louis, MO 63104, USA

Jordan B. Slutsky
Stony Brook School of Medicine, Department of Dermatology, 181 N. Belle Mead Road, Suite 5, East Setauket, NY 11733, USA

Brandon T. Beal
School of Medicine, Saint Louis University, 1402 S. Grand Boulevard, St. Louis, MO 63104, USA

Eric S. Armbrecht
Center for Outcomes Research, Saint LouisUniversity, 3545 Lafayette Avenue, 4th Floor, St. Louis, MO 63110, USA

Ronald J. Walker and Mark A. Varvares
Department of Otolaryngology-Head and Neck Surgery, Saint Louis University, 3635 Vista Avenue, St. Louis, MO 63110, USA

Matthew S. Ning and Thomas Andl
Division of Dermatology, Department of Medicine, Vanderbilt University Medical Center, Medical Center North, Room A2310A, 1161 21st Avenue South, Nashville, TN 37232-2600, USA

Annette S. Kim
Department of Pathology, Microbiology, and Immunology, Vanderbilt University Medical Center, Nashville, TN 37232-2600, USA

Nripesh Prasad
Department of Biological Sciences, University of Alabama in Huntsville, Huntsville, AL 35805, USA

Nripesh Prasad and Shawn E. Levy
HudsonAlpha Institute for Biotechnology, Huntsville, AL 35806, USA

Huiqiu Zhang
OrioR Lab, LLC, Rockville, MD 20852, USA

Farahnaz Fatemi Naeini and Bahareh Abtahi-Naeini
Skin Diseases and Leishmaniasis Research Center, Department of Dermatology, Isfahan University ofMedical Sciences, Isfahan, Iran

Bahareh Abtahi-Naeini and Hamidreza Sadeghiyan
Students' Research Committee, Isfahan University of Medical Sciences, Isfahan, Iran

Mohammad Ali Nilforoushzadeh
Skin and Stem Cell Research Center, Tehran University of Medical Sciences, Tehran, Iran

Jamshid Najafian
Cardiovascular Research Center, Cardiovascular Research Institute, Isfahan University of Medical Sciences, Isfahan, Iran

Mohsen Pourazizi
Students' Research Committee, Semnan University of Medical Sciences, Semnan, Iran

Jagdeep Rao
Department of Plastic Surgery, Sawai Man Singh Medical College, Jaipur, Rajasthan 300204, India

Harsh Deora
Department of General Surgery, Sawai Man Singh Medical College, Jaipur, Rajasthan 300204, India

G. Morand, D. Vital, T. Pézier, D. Holzmann and G. F. Huber
Division of Otolaryngology, Head and Neck Surgery, University Hospital Zurich, Frauenklinikstraße 24, 8091 Zurich, Switzerland

M. Roessle
Institute of Surgical Pathology, University Hospital Zurich, Frauenklinikstraße 24, 8091 Zurich, Switzerland

A. Cozzio
Division of Dermatology, University Hospital Zurich, Frauenklinikstraße 24, 8091 Zurich, Switzerland

Zhongyun Zhao, Song Wang and Beth L. Barber
Amgen Inc.,Thousand Oaks, CA 91320, USA

Karli Rosner, Evangelia Kirou, Jillian Frieder and Kelsey Lawrence
Laboratory for Molecular Dermatology, Barbara Ann Karmanos Cancer Institute, 110 East Warren Avenue, Detroit, MI 48201, USA

Karli Rosner, Darius R. Mehregan and Evangelia Kirou
Department of Dermatology, School of Medicine,Wayne State University, Detroit, MI 48201, USA

Karli Rosner
Center for Molecular Medicine and Genetics, School of Medicine,Wayne State University, Detroit, MI 48201, USA

Darius R. Mehregan
Pinkus Dermatopathology Laboratory, Monroe, MI 48162, USA

Judith Abrams and Seongho Kim
Biostatistics, Barbara Ann Karmanos Cancer Institute, Detroit, MI 48201, USA

Judith Abrams, Seongho Kim, Brittany Haynes andMalathy P. V. Shekhar
Department of Oncology, School of Medicine,Wayne State University, Detroit, MI 48201, USA

Malathy P. V. Shekhar
Department of Pathology, School of Medicine,Wayne State University, Detroit, MI 48201, USA Barbara Ann Karmanos Cancer Institute, Detroit, MI 48201, USA

Vanessa Shih, Renske M. ten Ham, Christine T. Bui, Dan N. Tran, Jie Ting and Leslie Wilson
Department of Clinical Pharmacy, University of California, San Francisco, 3333 California Street, Laurel Heights, San Francisco, CA 94143, USA

Inamaria Erovic
Medical University of Vienna, 1090 Vienna, Austria

Boban M. Erovic
Medical University of Vienna, Department of Otolaryngology, Head and Neck Surgery, 1090 Vienna, Austria

Richard L. Eckert, Gautam Adhikary, Christina A. Young, Ralph Jans and Wen Xu
Department of Biochemistry and Molecular Biology, University of Maryland, School of Medicine, 108 North Greene Street, Rm 103, Baltimore, MD 21201, USA

Richard L. Eckert
Department of Dermatology, University of Maryland, School of Medicine, Baltimore, MD 21201, USA
Department of Obstetrics and Genecology and Reproductive Sciences, University of Maryland, School of Medicine, Baltimore, MD 21201, USA

James F. Crish
Department of Cell Biology, Cleveland Clinic Foundation, Cleveland, OH 44106, USA

Ellen A. Rorke
Department of Microbiology and Immunology, University of Maryland, School of Medicine, Baltimore, MD 21201, USA

Ankit Sharma, Jitendra Singh Nigam, Shivani Rewri, Priyanka Bhatia Soni, Anita Omhare and Preethi Sekar
Department of Pathology, D.D.U. Hospital, Hari Nagar, New Delhi 110066, India

Deepak G. Paricharak and Ankit Sharma
Department of Pathology, Dr. D. Y. Patil Medical College, Kolhapur, Maharashtra 416006, India

LorenMasterson and Richard Keidan
Department of General Surgery, Beaumont Health System, Royal Oak, MI 48073, USA

Bryan J. Thibodeau, Laura E. Fortier, Timothy J. Geddes, Barbara L. Pruetz and George D.Wilson
Department of Beaumont BioBank, Beaumont Health System, 3811West 13 Mile Road 105-RI, Royal Oak, MI 48073, USA

Rajwant Malhotra
Department of Anatomic Pathology, Beaumont Health System, Royal Oak, MI 48073, USA

Alma C. Berlingeri-Ramos, Richard F. Wagner Jr. and Brent C. Kelly
Department of Dermatology, University of Texas Medical Branch, 301 University Drive, Galveston, TX 77555-5302, USA

Claire J. Detweiler
Department of Pathology, Duke University Medical Center, Durham, NC 27710, USA

Kathryn E. King, Linan Ha, Tura Camilli and Wendy C.Weinberg
Division of Monoclonal Antibodies, Office of Biotechnology Products, Center for Drug Evaluation and Research, US Food and Drug Administration, Bethesda, MD 20892, USA

Ievgenia Pastushenko, Tamara Gracia-Cazaña and Mariano Ara
Department of Dermatology, University Hospital "Clinico Lozano Blesa," Calle San Juan Bosco 15, 50009 Zaragoza, Spain

Sandra Vicente-Arregui and Steven J. Van Laere
Department of Pathology, University Hospital "Miguel Servet," Paseo Isabel la Católica 1-3, 50009 Zaragoza, Spain

Gert G. Van den Eynden and Peter B. Vermeulen
Translational Cancer Research Unit Antwerp, Oncology Centre, General Hospital Sint-Augustinus, Oosterveldlaan 24, 2610Wilrijk, Belgium

Francisco José Carapeto
Department of Medicine, Psychiatry and Dermatology, School of Medicine, University of Zaragoza, Calle Domingo Miral s/n, 50009 Zaragoza, Spain

Steven J. Van Laere
Department of Oncology, KU of Leuven, Herestraat 49, 3000 Leuven, Belgium

Everardo Macias, Dharanija Rao and John DiGiovanni
Division of Pharmacology and Toxicology, College of Pharmacy, The University of Texas at Austin, Austin, TX 78723, USA

John DiGiovanni
Department of Nutritional Sciences, College of Natural Sciences,The University of Texas at Austin, Austin, TX 78723, USA
Dell Pediatric Research Institute,The University of Texas at Austin, 1400 Barbara Jordan Boulevard, Austin, TX 78723, USA

Ryan K. Rader, Katie S. Payne and William V. Stoecker
Stoecker & Associates, LLC, 10101 Stoltz Drive, Rolla, MO 65401-7714, USA

Uday Guntupalli
Missouri University of Science & Technology, G20 Emerson Electric Co. Hall, Rolla, MO 65409-0040, USA

Harold S. Rabinovitz and Maggie C. Oliviero
Skin and Cancer Associates, 201 NW82nd Avenue, Bennett Medical Plaza, Suite 501, Plantation, FL 33324, USA

Rhett J. Drugge
Sheard & Drugge PC, 50 Glenbrook Road, Unit 1C, Stamford, CT 06902, USA

Joseph J. Malters
The Dermatology Center, LLC, 10101 Stoltz Drive, Rolla, MO 65401, USA

Farid Menaa
Department of Oncology, Stem Cells and Nanomedicine, Fluorotronics, Inc., 2453 CadesWay, Building C, San Diego, CA 92081, USA

Kong-Bing Tan, Sze-Hwa Tan and Yoke-Sun Lee
Department of Pathology, Yong Loo Lin School of Medicine, National University Health System, National University of Singapore, Lower Kent Ridge Road, Singapore 119074

Derrick Chen-Wee Aw and Huma Jaffar
University Medicine Cluster, National University Health System, Singapore 119074

Thiam-Chye Lim
University Surgical Cluster, National University Health System, Singapore 119074

Shu-Jin Lee
Departments of Otorhinolaryngology and Hand and Reconstructive Microsurgery, National University Health System, Singapore 119074

M. Klein, M. Lotem, T. Peretz, S. Mizrachi, Y. Liberman and R. Chisin
Hadassah Medical Center, Hebrew University, Kiryat Hadassah, 91120 Jerusalem, Israel

S. T. Zwas and J. Schachter
Chaim Sheba Medical Center, Tel Hashomer, 52621 Ramat Gan, Israel

I. G. Ron
Sackler Faculty of Medicine, Tel Aviv Medical Center, 69978 Tel Aviv, Israel

G. Iosilevsky and J. A. Kennedy
Rambam Health Care Campus, 31096 Haifa, Israel

E. Revskaya
Albert Einstein College of Medicine, 1300 Morris Park Avenue, Bronx, NY 10461, USA

A. W. de Kater, E. Banaga, V. Klutzaritz, N. Friedmann and G. B. Thornton
Pain Therapeutics, Inc., Austin, TX 78731, USA

G. L. DeNardo and S. J. DeNardo
Davis Medical Center, University of California, Sacramento, CA 95817, USA

Angela Sandru, Silviu Voinea and Alexandru Blidaru
Department of Surgical Oncology, "Carol Davila" University of Medicine and Pharmacy, Alexandru Trestioreanu"Oncologic Institute, Fundeni Street, No. 252, Sector 2, 022328 Bucharest, Romania

Eugenia Panaitescu
Department of Medical Informatics and Biostatistics, "Carol Davila" University of Medicine and Pharmacy, Bucharest, Romania

Madalina Bolovan, Adina Stanciu and Sabin Cinca
Department of Carcinogenesis and Molecular Biology, "Alexandru Trestioreanu" Oncologic Institute, Bucharest, Romania

Duriye Deniz Demirseren and Ahmet Metin
Department of Dermatology, Ataturk Training and Research Hospital, BilkentWay, 06800 Ankara, Turkey

Candemir Ceran, Berrak Aksam and Mustafa Erol Demirseren
Department of Plastic Reconstructive and Aesthetic Surgery, Ataturk Training and Research Hospital, 06800 Ankara, Turkey

Steven F. Babbin
Department of Psychiatry, Geisel School of Medicine at Dartmouth, Lebanon, NH 03766, USA

Hui-Qing Yin, Joseph S. Rossi, Colleen A. Redding, Andrea L. Paiva and Wayne F. Velicer
Cancer Prevention Research Center and Department of Psychology, University of Rhode Island, Kingston, RI 02881, USA

Kehinde O. Raji
Department of Internal Medicine, Scripps Clinic/ Scripps Green Hospital, 10666 N. Torrey Pines Road, La Jolla, CA 92037, USA

Lauren Payne
Department of Dermatology, Howard University, 2041 Georgia Avenue NW, Suite 2107,Washington, DC 20060, USA

Suephy C. Chen
Division of Dermatology, Atlanta VAMC, 1670 Clairmont Road, Decatur, GA 30033, USA
Department of Dermatology, Emory University, 1525 Clifton Road NE, 3rd Floor, Atlanta, GA 30322, USA

Elisabeth Enzenhofer, Philipp Ubl, Christian Czerny and Boban M. Erovic
Department of Otolaryngology Head and Neck Surgery,Medical University of vienna,Waehringer Guertel 18-20, 1090 Vienna, Austria

Firas Al-Qarqaz, Maha Marji, Diala Alshiyab and Jihan Muhaidat
Department of Dermatology, Jordan University of Science and Technology, Irbid, Jordan

Khaldon Bodoor
Department of Applied Biology, Jordan University of Science and Technology, Irbid, Jordan

Rowida Almomani
Department of Medical Laboratory Sciences, Jordan University of Science and Technology, Irbid, Jordan

Wisam Al Gargaz
Department of Special Surgery, Jordan University of Science and Technology, Irbid, Jordan

Mohammad Alqudah
Department of Pathology, Jordan University of Science and Technology, Irbid, Jordan

Anthony Paulo Sunjaya, Angela Felicia Sunjaya and Sukmawati Tansil Tan
Faculty of Medicine, Tarumanagara University, Jl. Letjen S. Parman No. 1, Jakarta 11440, Indonesia

Kyle T. Amber, Romi Bloom, Patrick Staropoli, Sonam Dhiman and Shasa Hu
Department of Dermatology & Cutaneous Surgery, University of Miami Miller School of Medicine, 10660 SW75th Avenue, Miami, FL 33156, USA

Valerie M. Harvey and Charlene W. Old field
Department of Dermatology, Eastern Virginia Medical School, Norfolk, VA, USA

Valerie M. Harvey
Hampton University Skin of Color Research Institute, Hampton, VA, USA

Jarvis T. Chen
Department of Social and Behavioral Science, Harvard School of Public Health, Boston, MA, USA

Karl Eschbach
University of Texas Medical Branch, Sealy Center on Aging, Galveston, TX, USA
University of Texas Medical Branch, Center to Eliminate Health Disparities, Galveston, TX, USA

Jordan W. Oldbury, Richard A. J. Wain, Sameera Abas and Srinivasan S. Iyer
Department of Plastic & Reconstructive Surgery, Royal Preston Hospital, Lancashire Teaching Hospitals NHS Foundation Trust, Sharoe Green Lane, Preston, Lancashire PR2 9HT, UK

Christopher M. Dobson
Department of Dermatology, Royal Preston Hospital, Lancashire Teaching Hospitals NHS Foundation Trust, Sharoe Green Lane, Preston, Lancashire PR2 9HT, UK

Jeffrey Chen, Johnny Shih, Andrew Tran, Aaron Mullane and Christina Thomas
Texas Tech University Health Sciences Center, 1400 S. Coulter Street, Amarillo, TX 79106, USA

Nail Aydin and Subhasis Misra
Department of Surgery, Texas Tech University Health Sciences Center, 1400 S. Coulter Street, Amarillo, TX 79106, USA

Index

www.ingramcontent.com/pod-product-compliance
Lightning Source LLC
LaVergne TN
LVHW060512210926
848485LV00005B/1070